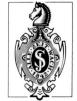

The Knee and the Cruciate Ligaments

Anatomy Biomechanics Clinical Aspects
Reconstruction Complications Rehabilitation

Edited by R. P. Jakob and H.-U. Stäubli
of the Orthopedic Study Group for the Knee

Translated by T. C. Telger

With 519 Figures in 1071 Separate Illustrations and 91 Tables

Springer-Verlag
Berlin Heidelberg New York London Paris
Tokyo Hong Kong Barcelona Budapest

Prof. Dr. R. P. Jakob
Department for Orthopedic Surgery, University of Bern
Inselspital, 3010 Bern, Switzerland

PD Dr. H.-U. Stäubli
Orthopedics/Traumatology, Tiefenau Hospital of the City of Bern
Tiefenaustrasse 112, 3004 Bern, Switzerland

Title of the original German edition: Kniegelenk und Kreuzbänder
© Springer-Verlag Berlin Heidelberg 1990

ISBN 3-540-53818-6 Springer-Verlag Berlin Heidelberg New York
ISBN 0-387-53818-6 Springer-Verlag New York Berlin Heidelberg

Library of Congress Cataloging-in-Publication Data
Kniegelenk und Kreuzbänder. English. The Knee and the cruciate ligaments: anatomy, biomechanics, clinical aspects, reconstruction, complications, rehabilitation / edited by R. P. Jakob and H.-U. Stäubli of the Orthopedic Study Group for the Knee; translated by R. C. Telger. p. cm. Includes bibliographical references and index.
ISBN 3-540-53818-6 (alk. paper). – ISBN 0-387-53818-6 (alk. paper)
1. Anterior cruciate ligament-Surgery. 2. Knee-Surgery. 3. Knee-Anatomy. I. Jakob, Roland. II. Stäubli, H.-U. III. Schweizerische Gesellschaft für Orthopädie. Orthopedic Study Group for the Knee. IV. Title. [DNML: 1. Knee Injuries-therapy. 2. Knee Joint-anatomy & histology. 3. Ligaments-physiopathology. 4. Ligaments-Surgery. WE 870 K685] RD561.K5913 1992 617.5'82059-dc20 DNLM/DLC 92-49767

Typesetting, printing, and binding: Appl, Wemding
24/3130-543210 – Printed on acid-free paper

To our families,
for their understanding, sacrifice,
and encouragement

"All in all you're just another brick in the wall."
Pink Floyd, *The Wall*

Foreword

This book summarizes the experience gained by the Orthopedic Study Group for the Knee (OAK) of the Swiss Orthopedic Society in dealing with knee problems relating to deficiencies of the cruciate ligaments. The editors, R.P. Jakob and H.-U. Stäubli, have collaborated with international authorities to produce this excellent work dealing with a great many aspects of knee surgery and especially the problems of the cruciate ligaments.

For clarity, the book begins with definitions and explanations of basic biomechanical terms. The chapters on Anatomy and Biomechanics present up-to-date scientific information based on anatomic and biomechanical principles as they are applied in modern knee surgery.

The second part of the book focuses on the OAK-sanctioned approach to knee documentation and evaluation, which is a valuable supplement to other knee evaluation schemes. The European Society for Knee Surgery (ESKA) and the American Orthopedic Society for Sports Medicine (AOSSM) are currently attempting to combine the advantages of the OAK system with an internationally valid evaluation scheme to create a standard evaluation and documentation system that will be acceptable to all physicians.

Next, Noesberger, Jakob, Stäubli and others take a comprehensive look at clinical diagnosis, pathomechanics, and pathomorphology. Arthroscopic and radiologic methods are described for documenting anterior subluxation of the tibia in patients with anterior cruciate ligament insufficiency. The authors use various methods to convey the techniques of knee stability testing in the position of near extension to medical students and younger clinical colleagues. Werner Müller describes in detail the various types of meniscus lesion that can develop in the anterior cruciate ligament-deficient knee. The natural history of untreated cruciate ligament insufficiency is reviewed by the editors and by Jean Yves Dupont, who gives us the perspective of the "French school." A long chapter is devoted to the treatment of acute anterior cruciate ligament insufficiency and associated injuries of the medial capsuloligamentous complex including meniscal tears. Various autologous, alloplastic, and synthetic ligament reconstructions are described in the chapter on Chronic Anterior Cruciate Ligament Insufficiency, which reflects state-of-the-art techniques practiced in Europe. Arthroscopically assisted techniques of cruciate ligament reconstruction – European modifications of American techniques and original innovations – are described in detail. A separate chapter is devoted to significant posterolateral injuries that can accompany lesions of the anterior and posterior cruciate ligaments, and another to synthetic cruciate ligament substitutes and their problems. Additionally, there are several chapters on late degenerative changes resulting from chronic cruciate ligament instability and on the complications that can follow specific reconstructive procedures.

This book is comprehensive enough to meet the needs and interests of a very wide readership. It is an excellent sourcebook on the status of reconstructive knee surgery as it is successfully practiced in Europe today.

Stockholm, Summer, 1992   Ejnar Eriksson

Introduction

In 1981 the Orthopedic Study Group for the Knee (OAK) held its first advanced training course on the anatomy and biomechanics of the knee. The course, in which anatomic specimens were used to demonstrate ligament reconstruction techniques, was quickly filled. It was repeated in 1982 and 1983, and in 1984 the OAK was officially established as a professional working group of the Swiss Orthopedic Society (SGO).

At the first congress of the European Society of Knee Surgery and Arthroscopy (ESKA) in 1984, the preliminary course on anatomy and biomechanics was again conducted chiefly by the OAK. This course, too, was highly successful.

More than 20 years ago, outstanding successes in the treatment of bone fractures and degenerative joint disease prompted a number of foreign scientists to visit Swiss orthopedic hospitals. While praising our methods of treating the spine, hip, knee and foot, these visitors also pointed out that newer methods had been devised for managing the soft tissues about the knee.

This led me, in April of 1971, to join several hundred colleagues from France, Belgium, Spain, and Italy in a visit to the Journes de Chirurgie du Genou in Lyon. To the credit of the great teacher Albert Trillat and his school, which is still active today, this was the first time that I truly appreciated the importance of the essential "third dimension" in knee surgery. Present-day exponents of the French school such as Henri Dejour, Pierre Chambat, Bernhard Myoen, Jean-Luc Lerat, and Jean-Yves Dupont, together with other OAK-affiliated European knee specialists such as Carl J. Wirth and Michael Wagner, are among the key contributors to this book.

Although the insights received at Lyon were important, the riddle of the knee was far from solved. Too many therapeutic outcomes appeared to be random in nature. There had to be hidden principles at work. Why, for example, was a pivot shift possible?

Biomechanics and kinematics, as elucidated by Alfred Menschik, provided the key that guided us to the explanation while deepening our knowledge of soft-tissue biodynamics and biomechanical dynamics.

The definitive step from the "bone age" to the "soft-tissue age" has already been taken in orthopedic surgery. One factor driving this development was sports medicine, which already had a significant head start in the USA.

The four-bar linkage of Menschik and the Weber brothers led us through coupling curves and envelope curves to the concept of isometry as a new quality in the healthy functioning of collagenous soft tissues like the ligaments. But isometry is too narrow and rigid a concept. We must adopt a broader functional view so that we can better grasp the new concepts of anatomometry and normometry.

W. Müller's book *The Knee – Form, Function, and Ligament Reconstruction*, published nearly a decade ago, offered the first comprehensive review of the problems of anatomy and function as they were understood at that time. Further basic research has confirmed older hypotheses and added new knowledge. Isometry, yes, but only in a limited sense and supported by tissue fibers that become tense when the laws of biomechanics demand a greater fiber potential to supply the necessary mechanical strength.

One lesson that can be drawn from these insights is that none of us can accomplish much by ourselves, and that only through cooperation in groups and across national boundaries can we achieve real progress in terms of improved patient care. Implicit in this awareness is the need to develop a common language for the complex nomenclature of the phenomena, and also for the documentation and qualitative evaluation of traumatic lesions and therapeutic outcomes.

In response to this need, the ESKA and the AOSSM (American Organization for Surgery in Sports Medicine) have founded the IKDC (International Knee Documentation Committee), in which 10 members each from the USA and Europe focus their professional efforts on solving the problems that are so familiar to us all.

Rik Huiskes from the team of Theo VanRens, the Cincinnati school of Frank Noyes and Ed Grood, and Russel Warren and Peter Torzilli and their colleagues at the Hospital for Special Surgery in New York have contributed much to the new discoveries in soft-tissue biomechanics. This research has laid vital foundations for the work of the IKDC. Fritz Hefti, Roland P. Jakob, Hans-Ulrich Stäubli, and Werner Müller of the OAK also have become members of the IKDC.

The knee continues to be of central importance in many respects:

- Anatomically, as the joint uniting the two longest lever arms of the musculo-skeletal system, the femur and tibia
- In sports traumatology, as the most commonly injured critical joint
- In an actuarial sense, as an object of contention in disability judgments
- In the treatment of degenerative joint disorders (e.g., after meniscectomy), ranking second only to the hip
- In individual cases where it is important to consider the possible effect of psychological factors on the knee joint and, conversely, the difficulty some patients may have in coping with a chronically painful "problem knee"

For the future, much remains to be improved, and basic research needs to be further refined. The evolutionary path will probably take us past the ligaments and menisci to the cartilage, to the functions of the synovial membrane including its eutrophic function in maintaining articular homeostasis and the destructive catabolic effects that occur in synovitis (e.g., due to abrasion of artificial ligaments), and finally to the still little-researched processes involved in proprioception.

With its comprehehsive, up-to-date summary of our knowledge of the knee and cruciate ligaments, this book will be a valuable aid in furthering our understanding and management of structures "about the knee."

Basel, Summer, 1992   Werner Müller

Preface

Members of the Orthopedic Research Group for the Knee (OAK) of the Swiss Orthopedic Society and experienced European knee specialists have pooled their authoritative knowledge to create *The Knee and the Cruciate Ligaments*, whose major emphasis is on diagnostic and therapeutic problems. Though a compilation, the work still manages to reflect the individual interpretive freedom of its contributors.

An introductory chapter on nomenclature is followed by numerous chapters, grouped by common themes, dealing with anatomy and biomechanics, diagnosis, pathomechanics, and pathomorphology of acute tears of the anterior cruciate ligament (ACL) and chronic knee instability.

Special attention has been given to the description of concomitant injuries of the collateral ligaments and menisci and to the various techniques of open and arthroscopically assisted ACL reconstruction. We have placed special emphasis on the treatment of posterolateral and posterior knee instability. Problems relating to the synthetic replacement of the ACL, chronic cruciate ligament insufficiency with osteoarthritis, and intra- and postoperative complications of reconstructions and their management are explored with the help of illustrative case materials. There is also a chapter on rehabilitation and evaluation in which therapeutic results, complications and their management are discussed on the basis of clinical series.

The editors of this volume – members of the International Knee Documentation Committee – have succeeded in incorporating the knowledge of that body into the documentation and evaluation of knee instabilities.

Our main purpose, and that of the book as a whole, is to help young surgeons and orthopedists to define indications while providing them with practical tools and precise details on operative and instrumental techniques.

Acknowledgments

We are sincerely grateful to all those who have contributed to the creation of this book: our secretaries Mrs. Charlotte Neuenschwander, Department of Orthopedic Surgery, Inselspital, and Mrs. Verena Oppliger, Orthopedics and Traumatology, Department of Surgery, Tiefenauspital, Bern; our illustrators Hans Holzherr, Christian Langenegger, and Willi Hess, Department of Instructional Media (AUM), University of Bern, Inselspital; and our photographers Mrs. Boa (Tiefenauspital), Mrs. Steiner (Inselspital), Mrs. Widmer (Inselspital), Mr. Huber (Inselspital), and Mr. Zimmermann (AUM).

Finally, we thank the staff at Springer-Verlag for their very high-quality production work.

Bern, Summer, 1992   R. P. Jakob H.-U. Stäubli

Table of Contents

Chronic Insufficiency of the Anterior Cruciate Ligament

Arthroscopic Techniques of Anterior Cruciate Ligament Reconstruction

Injuries of Posterolateral Structures and the Posterior Cruciate Ligament

Synthetic Materials for Ligament Reconstruction

Instability and Osteoarthritis

List of Contributors

Arnold-Schmiebusch, H., Dr.
Anatomisches Institut, Abt. Anatomie II, Albert-Ludwigs-Universität,
Albertstrasse 17, 7800 Freiburg i. Br., FRG

Bachelin, P., Dr.
Médecin-Chef Orthopédie, Hôpital de Zone, Saint-Loup Orbe, 1350 Orbe,
Switzerland

Ballmer, F.T., Dr.
Klinik und Poliklinik für Orthopädische Chirurgie der Universität Bern,
Inselspital, 3010 Bern, Switzerland

Ballmer, P.M., Dr.
Orthopädische Chirurgie, Grabenstr. 4, 3600 Thun, Switzerland

Baumgartner, R., Dr.
Orthopädie/Traumatologie, Kantonsspital, 4101 Bruderholz, Switzerland

Biedert, R., Dr.
Eidg. Turn- und Sportschule Magglingen, Hauptstrasse 243–245,
2532 Magglingen, Switzerland

Birrer, St., Dr.
Tiefenauspital der Stadt Bern, Tiefenaustrasse 112, 3004 Bern, Switzerland

Blankevoort, L., Dr.
Sectie Biomechanica, Institut voor Orthopaedie, KU-Nijmegen/St. Radboud
Ziekenhuis, P.B. 9101, 6500 Nijmegen, The Netherlands

Blatter, G., Dr.
Orthopädische Abteilung, Kantonsspital, 9007 St. Gallen, Switzerland

Bonnin, M., Dr.
Clinique de Chirurgie, Orthopédie et Traumatologie, Université Lyon 1,
Centre Hospitalier Lyon-Sud, 69310 Pierre-Bénite, France

Burch, H.B., Dr.
Ferpicloz, 1700 Fribourg, Switzerland

Burkart, P., Dr.
Orthopädische Chirurgie FMH, Obergrundstrasse 44, 6003 Luzern, Switzerland

Cartier, P., Dr.
Centre de Chirurgie du Genou, Clinique des Lilas, 41–49, Av. du Maréchal Juin,
9360 Les Lilas, France

Chambat, P., Dr.
Chirurgie Orthopédique, Traumatologie du Sport, Clinique Emilie de Vialar,
116, rue Antoine Charial, 69003 Lyon, France

Christen, S., Dr.
Turmstrasse 5, 3613 Steffisburg, Switzerland

Dejour, H., Prof. Dr.
Clinique de Chirurgie, Orthopédie et Traumatologie, Université Lyon 1,
Centre Hospitalier Lyon-Sud, Pavillon 3 A, 69310 Pierre-Bénite, France

Demottaz, J. D., Dr.
FMH für Orthopädische Chirurgie, 64, rue de Lyon, 1203 Geneva,
Switzerland

Drobny, T., Dr.
Orthopädische Klinik, Wilhelm-Schulthess-Klinik, Neumünsterallee 3,
8008 Zürich, Switzerland

Dupont, J. Y., Prof. Dr.
Clinique St. Michael & St. Anne, 51, rue de Kerjestin, B. P. 517,
29107 Quimper-Cédex, France

Fabbriciani, C., Prof. Dr.
Clinica Ortopedica della Università Cattolica, Largo A. Gemelli 8, 00168 Roma,
Italy

Fandrey, B.
Physiotherapie, Inselspital, 3010 Bern, Switzerland

Fasel, A., Dr.
Institut d'Anatomie de l'Université, 1700 Fribourg, Switzerland

Freudiger, S. N., Dipl. Ing. ETH
Protek AG, Stadtbachstrasse 64, 3012 Bern, Switzerland

Freuler, C., Dr.
Hôpital Cantonal Universitaire, Policlinique de Chirurgie, 24, rue Micheli-du-
Crest, 1211 Geneva 4, Switzerland

Friederich, N. F., Dr.
Orthopädische Abteilung, Kantonsspital Bruderholz, 4101 Bruderholz,
Switzerland

Fritschy, D., PD Dr.
Hôpital Cantonal Universitaire, Policlinique de Chirurgie, 24, rue Micheli-du-
Crest, 1211 Geneva 4, Switzerland

Gächter, A., Prof. Dr.
Orthopädische Abteilung, Kantonsspital Basel, 4000 Basel, Switzerland

Ganz, R., Prof. Dr.
Klinik und Poliklinik für Orthopädische Chirurgie der Universität Bern,
Inselspital, 3010 Bern, Switzerland

Gerber, C., Prof. Dr.
Orthopädische Klinik, Kantonsspital, 1700 Fribourg, Switzerland

Grünig, B.
Spiezbergstrasse 22, 3700 Spiez, Switzerland

Hackenbruch, W., Dr.
Orthopädie, Regionalspital, 4900 Langenthal, Switzerland

Hefti, F., PD Dr.
Kinderorthopädische Abteilung, Kinderspital, Römergasse 8, 4005 Basel,
Switzerland

Henche, H. R., PD Dr.
Kreiskrankenhaus Rheinfelden, Ortsteil Nollingen, 7888 Rheinfelden, FRG

Hey, W., Dr.
Kreiskrankenhaus Rheinfelden, Ortsteil Nollingen, 7888 Rheinfelden, FRG

Holzach, P., Dr.
Chirurgie, Spital, 7270 Davos, Switzerland

Huiskes, R., Prof. Dr.
Sectie Biomechanica, Instituut voor Orthopaedie, KU-Nijmegen/St. Radboud
Ziekenhuis, P. B. 9101, 6500 HB Nijmegen, The Netherlands

Hunziker, E. B., Prof. Dr.
M. E. Müller-Institut für Biomechanik, Universität Bern, Murtenstrasse 35,
3008 Bern, Switzerland

Jakob, R. P., Prof. Dr.
Klinik und Poliklinik für Orthopädische Chirurgie der Universität Bern,
Inselspital, 3010 Bern, Switzerland

Johner, R., Dr.
Chirurgien Orthopédique FMH, Av. Marc-Dufour 4, 1004 Lausanne, Switzerland

Kipfer, W. C., Dr.
Grafenriedstrasse 1, 3074 Muri, Switzerland

Lerat, J. L., Prof. Dr.
Hôpital Edouard Herriot, Pavillon I, Place d'Arsonval, 69374 Lyon Cédex 08,
France

Meystre, J.-L., Dr.
Orthopädische Klinik, Kantonsspital, 1000 Lausanne, Switzerland

Moyen, B., Prof. Dr.
Hôpital Edouard Herriot, Chirurgie Orthopédique, Médecine du Sport,
69374 Lyon Cédex 08, France

Müller, We., Prof. Dr.
Orthopädie/Traumatologie, Kantonsspital Bruderholz, 4101 Bruderholz,
Switzerland

Muller, H., Dr.
Hôpital Edouard Herriot, Chirurgie Orthopédique, 69374 Lyon Cédex 08, France

Munzinger, U., Dr.
Orthopädische Abteilung, Wilhelm-Schulthess-Klinik, Neumünsterallee 3,
8008 Zürich, Switzerland

Neyret, P., Dr.
Clinique de Chirurgie, Orthopédie et Traumatologie, Université Lyon 1,
Centre Hospitalier Lyon-Sud, 69310 Pierre-Bénite, France

Noesberger, B., Dr.
Orthopädie, Regionalspital Interlaken, 3800 Interlaken, Switzerland

O'Brien, W. R., Dr.
The Blazina Orthopaedic Clinic and Sherman Oaks Community Hospital,
Sherman Oaks, CA 91403, USA

Oransky, M., Dr.
Clinica Ortopedica della Università Cattolica, Largo A. Gemelli 8, 00168 Roma,
Italy

Oswald, M. H., Dr.
Chirurgische Klinik, Kantonsspital, 8200 Schaffhausen, Switzerland

Perren, S. M., Prof. Dr.
Schweizerisches Forschungsinstitut, Laboratorium für Experimentelle Chirurgie,
7270 Davos-Platz, Switzerland

Pradat, E., Dr.
Chirurgie Orthopédique, Traumatologie du Sport, Clinique Emilie de Vialar,
116, rue Antoine Charial, 69003 Lyon, France

Ramseier, E. W., Dr.
SUVA Direktion, Postfach, 6002 Luzern, Switzerland

Rodriguez, M., Dr.
Orthopädische Universitätsklinik Balgrist, Forchstrasse 340, 8008 Zürich,
Switzerland

Rogge, D., Dr. †
formerly: Unfallchirurgische Klinik, Medizinische Hochschule, Konstanty-
Gutschow-Strasse 8, 3000 Hannover 61, FRG

Scellier, C., Dr.
Clinique du Marais, 11bis, rue Barbette, 75003 Paris, France

Schabus, R., Dr.
Unfallchirurgische Universitätsklinik, Alser Strasse 4, 1097 Vienna, Austria

Schneider, B., Lic. phil. nat.
Seidenberggässchen 1, 3073 Gümligen, Switzerland

Spörri, S., Dr.
Tiefenauspital der Stadt und der Region Bern, Tiefenaustrasse 112, 3004 Bern,
Switzerland

Sprenger, F. B., Dr.
Orthopädische Chirurgie, Ärztehaus, Rorschacherstrasse 19, 9000 St. Gallen,
Switzerland

Stäubli, H.-U., PD Dr.
Orthopädie/Traumatologie, Tiefenauspital der Stadt und der Region Bern,
Tiefenaustrasse 112, 3004 Bern, Switzerland

Tscherne, H., Prof. Dr.
Unfallchirurgische Klinik, Medizinische Hochschule, Konstanty-Gutschow-
Strasse 8, 3000 Hannover 61, FRG

Wagner, M., Prof. Dr.
Landeskrankenhaus Salzburg, Unfallchirurgie, Müllner Hauptstrasse 48,
5020 Salzburg, Austria

Warner, J. P., Dr.
Center for Sports Medicine and Rehabilitation, Baum Boulevard at Craig,
Street, Pittsburgh, PA 15213, USA

Wirth, C. J., Prof. Dr.
Medizinische Hochschule, Heimchenstrasse 1–7, 3000 Hannover 61, FRG

Wirz, P., Dr.
Mühlenstrasse 30, 3076 Worb, Switzerland

Witschger, P., Dr.
M. E. Müller-Institut für Biomechanik, Universität Bern, Murtenstrasse 35,
3008 Bern, Switzerland

Zehnder, R., PD Dr. †
formerly: AO-Dokumentation, Murtenstrasse 35, 3008 Bern, Switzerland

Zuber, K., Dr.
Klinik und Poliklinik für Orthopädische Chirurgie der Universität Bern,
Inselspital, 3010 Bern, Switzerland

Terms, Definitions, and Glossaries

H.-U. Stäubli and R. P. Jakob

A review of the literature on the knee joint reveals significant discrepancies in the usage of many terms and definitions (American Academy of Orthopedic Surgeons 1984; American Academy of Orthopedic Surgeons 1985; American Medical Association 1966, Apley 1980, Feagin 1988; Hughston and Barrett 1983; Hughston et al. 1976a, b; Kennedy et al. 1978; W. Müller 1983; Noyes and Grood 1988; Wang and Walker 1974). These inconsistencies can cause confusion in attempts at communication. Precisely defined basic terms describing the dynamics and kinematics of the knee are essential for understanding the normal and abnormal motions and displacements of the knee joint (Noyes et al. 1989). The description and measurement of normal joint motion and of abnormal limits of motion with respect to a well-defined neutral position are essential for accurately characterizing the compartmental kinematics of the knee (Stäubli 1990).

The purpose of this introductory chapter is to present unambiguous definitions and descriptions of commonly used terms. For further clarity, glossary listings are presented which explain the origins and customary uses of the terms (Die anatomischen Namen 1965; Duden 1970; Duden 1963; Webster's 1988). The origins of the terms are explained both in a general biomechanical sense and specifically as they relate to the knee. Terms are presented under the following headings:

- Functional anatomy
- Biomechanics
- Basic positions
- Limb axes
- Kinematics
- Motion, displacement, and their measurement
- Dynamics: force, moments, and mass
- Stability/instability and laxity
- Properties of tendons and ligaments
- Functions of ligamentous elements
- Condition and functional competence of ligaments
- Preoperative diagnostic techniques
- Principles of reconstructive surgery

- Concepts in ligament healing
- Concepts in meniscal surgery
- Concepts in rehabilitation

Finally, the most common terms are summarized in a general glossary (p. 19 f.).

Essential basic terms were defined in collaboration with the International Knee Documentation Committee (IKDC) of the American Orthopedic Society of Sports Medicine (AOSSM) and the European Society of Knee Surgery and Arthroscopy (ESKA).

Terms defined according to the recommendations of F. Noyes, E. Grood, and P. Torzilli are marked with an asterisk in the glossary (Noyes et al. 1989).

Functional Anatomy

The anterior and posterior cruciate ligaments form the *central pivot* of the knee joint. The *anterior cruciate ligament* (ACL) controls the physiologic anterior motion of the joint. Loss of its restraining action permits anterior subluxation of the tibia with respect to the femur (Butler et al. 1980; Fukubayashi et al. 1982; Noyes and Grood 1988; Noyes et al. 1980; Torzilli et al. 1981). The *posterior cruciate ligament* (PCL), the meniscofemoral ligaments, and the popliteus tendon and its attachments control the physiologic posterior motion of the joint. Loss of the restraining action of the PCL and its reinforcing structures permits abnormal posterior tibial motion (Fukubayashi et al. 1982; Gollehon et al. 1987; Hughston and Jacobson 1985; Stäubli and Jakob 1990). Associated injuries of the arcuate ligament complex and of the popliteus tendon and its fascicles lead to a coupled posterolateral subluxation of the tibia with respect to the femur (Jakob et al. 1981; Stäubli and Birrer 1990).

The central pivot lies within the intercondylar notch of the distal femur. The intercondylar notch is bounded *superiorly* by the femoral roof of the notch, *anterosuperiorly* by the infrapatellar synovial plica and infrapatellar fat pad, *medially* by the intercondylar surface of the medial femoral condyle, and *laterally* by the intercondylar surface of the lateral femoral condyle. It is bounded *inferiorly* by the anterior and posterior intercondylar areas of the tibia and the intercondylar eminence. The central pivot, including the meniscofemoral ligaments, acts in concert with the menisci and the three-dimensional geometry of the articular surfaces to ensure a physiologic range of joint motion and keep it within normal limits.

Glossary: Functional Anatomy

Anterior intercondylar area: the anterior area between the tibial condyles (tibial insertion of the anterior cruciate ligament, attachments of the anterior horns of the medial and lateral menisci).

Posterior intercondylar area: the posterior area between the tibial condyles (tibial insertion of the posterior cruciate ligament, attachments of the posterior horns of the medial and lateral menisci).

Intercondylar eminence: prominence between the tibial condyles.

Intercondylar fossa: notch between the condyles of the femur.

Intercondylar surface of the lateral femoral condyle: femoral attachment of the anterior cruciate ligament.

Intercondylar surface of the medial femoral condyle: femoral attachment of the posterior cruciate ligament and the meniscofemoral ligaments

Cruciate ligaments

ACL: anterior cruciate ligament.

PCL: posterior cruciate ligament.

PCL + ACL: central pivot.

Pivot shift: displacement of the central pivot or center of rotation.

Popliteal: pertaining or belonging to the posterior fossa of the knee.

Popliteal sulcus: groove on the lateral surface of the lateral femoral condyle for the tendon of the popliteus muscle.

Sulcus statarius: indentation of the cartilage at the lateral margin of the lateral femoral condyle, caused by pressure from the popliteus tendon in extension ("orthostatic groove" of Fürst).

Biomechanics

The kinematics of the knee joint is described by 6 degrees of freedom with 12 limits of motion. The 6 degress of freedom in the knee consist of 3 translations and 3 rotations (Grood and Noyes 1987; Grood and Suntay 1983; Grood et la. 1988; Grood et al. 1979; Noyes et al. 1989) (Fig. 1).

The three translations are:

- Anterior-posterior
- Medial-lateral
- Proximal-distal

The three rotations are:

- Extension-flexion
- Adduction-abduction
- Internal-external rotation

Glossary: Biomechanics

Amplitude of motion: the excursion that occurs between two limits.

Limit of motion: extreme positions of motion that are possible in a given degree of freedom.

Motion segment: from L. *segmentum* (*secare* to cut) section, division. Excursion from the neutral position to the final or terminal position.

Pairs of terms relating to joint motion

Active motion: motion induced by intrinsic muscular forces and moments.

Passive motion: motion induced by extrinsic forces and moments.

Weight-bearing motion: motion occurring under an axial compressive load.

Non-weight-bearing motion: motion occurring without an axial load.

Coupled motion: motion in one degree of freedom is combined with motion in one or more other degrees of freedom.

Free motion: motion is possible in all degrees of freedom, without restriction.

Constrained motion: motion is restricted in one or more degrees of freedom.

Unconstrained motion: the degrees of freedom are not restricted.

Joint play: physiologic play between the limits of motion of the joint members in the three translational planes and about the three rotational axes.

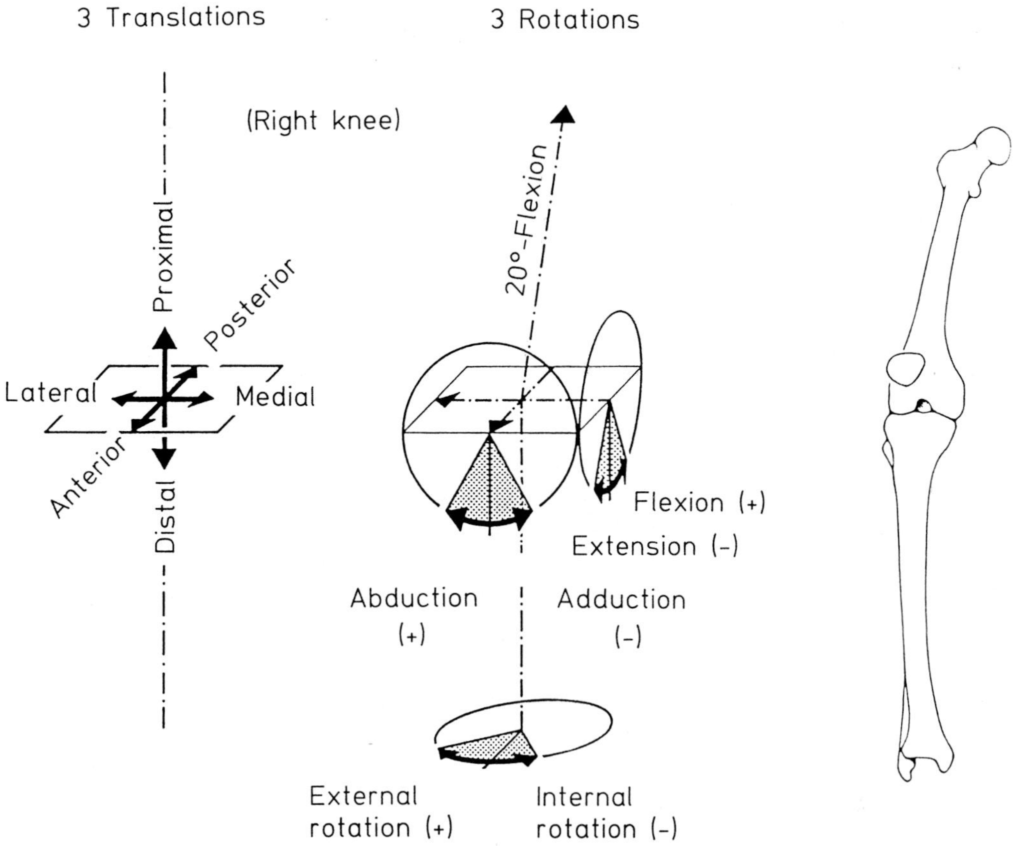

Fig. 1. The 6 degrees of freedom of knee motion: 3 translations, 3 rotations (right knee)

Abnormal motion: joint play that is excessive in one or more degrees of freedom, showing one or more abnormal limits of motion.

Central motion: relative displacement of a reference point at the center of the tibia with respect to a reference point at the center of the femur.

Compartmental motion: relative change in the position of reference points located in the medial and lateral femorotibial compartments. At least 2 reference points (2 on the femur, 2 on the tibia) must be defined for each moving body.

Biomechanics: the kinematics (motion geometry) and dynamics (study of masses and forces) of biologic systems.

Rotation: from L. *rotare* to turn. A type of motion or displacement in which all points on a body move about a fixed axis or center of motion. This axis is usually termed the axis of rotation. During a rotation, the various points on a body move in different directions and at different speeds. At each instant during the rotational motion, the points are moving in circles about the rotational axis. Knee rotation occurs about the cardinal axes of rotation.

Translation: from L. *trans* across, *latus* to carry.
Definition of translation (general): uniform displacement of a body in one direction along a defined plane.

Translation of the knee: equidistant, bicompartmental, unidirectional, uniplanar displacement of the tibia with respect to the femur (Stäubli 1990). At each instant during a translation, all points on the body are moving at the same speed and in the same direction. If the direction of motion is constant, the body moves in a straight path. If the direction changes with time, the body follows a curved path. Starting from the point of intersection of the translational planes, translation of the tibia with respect to the femur occurs along three mutually perpendicular planes.

Basic Positions

The *neutral position*, determined by the point at which the planes of translation and rotation intersect, refers to the compartmental alignment on the coronal, sagittal, and transverse planes when the knee joint is neutrally positioned on its three rotational axes. The gravitational force exerted on the knee varies with the position of the patient (supine, prone, right or left lateral decubitus). It is important to define the *starting position* (resting position) from which the active or passive testing of knee stability is performed.

When the patient is supine, the force of gravity produces a slight posterior sag of the tibia in relation to the femur. This posterior starting position (corresponding to the physiologic posterior limit of motion) must be distinguished from the posterior and anterior terminal positions. The *terminal position* (final position) is defined as the position in which the applied forces and moments are limited by capsuloligamentous restraint at the limit of the motion segment.

The clinical importance of the starting position (Stäubli and Jakob 1990) is as follows: When the PCL is deficient and the extensors are relaxed, gravity pulls the tibia into a posterior subluxated position when the distal femur is supported (Fig. 2a). Active quadriceps contraction moves the tibia from its sagging position through the neutral position into the physiologic anterior terminal position (assuming an intact ACL) (Fig. 2b). This posterior sag can be demonstrated with the knee slightly flexed (0°–20°) or at a large flexion angle (70°–90°) (Stäubli and Jakob 1990). The gravity-induced sag can be accentuated by passive anteroposterior pressure (Fig. 2c), while pressure in the opposite direction can reduce it through the neutral position to the physiologic anterior terminal position (Fig. 2d). The action of gravitational force (intrinsic limb weight) will change accordingly if the test is performed in a prone or lateral position.

Both the *position of the patient* and the *position of the knee joint* in relation to the applied force are significant factors in the analysis of physiologic joint play and abnormal motion patterns.

Another biomechanical concept involves defining the position of a body by the *location* of a point on the body and by the *orientation* of that body. The location of the tibia with respect to the femur can be defined by describing one or more points on the tibia. The location of the tibia is defined by three coordinates (anterior-posterior, medial-lateral, proximal-distal), which indicate where the tibia is located in relation to the femur. The *orientation* of the tibia with respect to

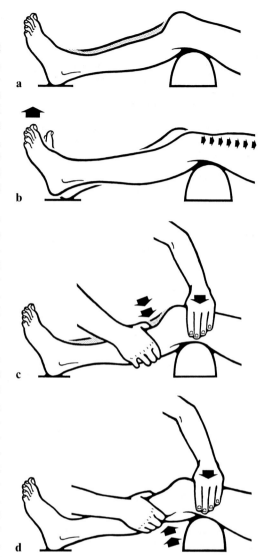

Fig. 2. a Starting position in a posterior cruciate-deficient knee: weight- or gravity-induced posterior subluxation of the tibia. **b** Active, quadriceps-induced *(arrows)* reduction from the subluxated position. **c** Passive posterior drawer test near extension. **d** Passive reduction of the posterior subluxation. (After Stäubli and Jakob 1990)

the femur is described by the three angles of flexion-extension, abduction-adduction, and internal-external rotation of the tibia. When the PCL is deficient, the tibia sags posteriorly under its own weight relative to the supported femur. The starting position of the tibia with respect to the femur changes, and this influences the measured direction of the displacement and the degree of displacement relative to the neutral position. The neutral position serves as the reference for defining the various motion segments.

Limb Axes on the Coronal, Sagittal, and Transverse Planes

In defining the limb axes, a distinction must be drawn between the *mechanical axis* and the *anatomic axis*. The *mechanical axis* of the limb is defined by a line connecting the center of the femoral head with the center of the ankle joint.

Morphotype or Limb Shape

Coronal plane: A *normal limb axis* is present when the mechanical axis passes through the center of the knee joint. *Genu varum* (bowleg) is present when the mechanical axis runs medial to the center of the knee, and *genu valgum* (knock knee) when the mechanical axis is lateral to the center of the knee.

Sagittal plane: The *normal limb axis* on the sagittal plane passes through the center of the knee joint. The normal posterior slope of the tibial plateau – the "physiologic retroversion" – generally equals 6°–9° (after the cessation of skeletal growth).

Genu recurvatum is present when the mechanical axis of the lower limb runs anterior to the center of the knee.
Genu recurvatum due to osseous deformity is characterized by a relative increase in the anterior tilt of both tibial plateaus (anteversion) relative to the physiologic posterior slope. In *genu antecurvatum*, the mechanical limb axis runs behind the center of the knee.
Genu antecurvatum due to osseous deformity is characterized by an excessive posterior slope (increased retroversion) of both tibial plateaus.

Transverse plane: The physiologic torsion of the femur on the transverse plane is distinguished from internal or external torsion of the femur. Analogously, normal tibial torsion is distinguished from excessive internal or external torsion of that bone.

Kinematics (Geometry of Moving Structures)

Normal Limits of Motion

In the knee with an *intact capsule and ligaments* and *normal joint play*, the *physiologic anterior compartmental motion limit* (starting from the neutral position) consists of a slight anterior displacement of the tibia ("anterior laxity") with respect to the femur. This displacement is coupled with a few degrees of internal rotation, depending on the angle of knee flexion (Fig.3).

As the anterior displacement proceeds, more and more structural elements are recruited to oppose the anterolateral motion. The *anterior limit of motion* is the point at which the sum of the applied forces and moments is neutralized by the sum of the active and passive restraining forces. This knee position represents the *anterior terminal position* or the *physiologic anterior limit of motion*. In clinical testing, the anterior terminal position is characterized by an increasingly palpable anterior terminal stiffness (assuming an intact end-point resilience of the ACL).

Starting from the neutral position, a *physiologic posterior compartmental motion limit* can be demonstrated. This normally consists of a slight posterolateral displacement. As the flexion angle increases, the posterior glide is coupled with an increasing external rotation of the tibia on the femur (see Fig.3). Starting from the neutral position, an anterior and a posterior motion segment, each with its associated anterior or posterior limit, are defined on the anteroposterior translational plane. The degree of the displacement, i.e. the path from the neutral position to the limit of motion, defines the motion segment. If the medial and lateral tibial plateaus move equal distances simultaneously in the same direction and plane, the motion is described as a pure anterior or posterior *translation*. In a *coupled motion*, the translation is combined with a simultaneous rotational component.

Displacement along the three translational planes and about the three rotational axes can be demonstrated during the testing of anteroposterior laxity, which is increased near extension with an altered end-point resilience in the opposite direction.

During the testing of anteroposterior laxity, the *neutral position* is distinguished from the *starting position* and from the *anterior* and *posterior terminal positions*. An anterior (forward) motion segment is distinguished from a posterior (backward) motion segment. Finally, the physiologic limit and the abnormal anterior or posterior limit of motion and the type of motion (in this case anterior translation) are distinguished from posterior translation (Fig.4). Translation is defined as an equidistant, bicompartmental, uniplanar displacement in the anterior or posterior direction until the corresponding limit of motion is reached.

Abnormal Limits of Motion

Concepts of coupled subluxations are detailed in Jakob et al. (1981), Losee et al. (1978), We. Müller et al. (1988), Noyes and Grood (1988), Noyes et al. (1989), and Stäubli (1990).

Anterolateral subluxation (Jakob et al. 1981; Kennedy et al. 1978; Losee et al. 1978): From the neutral position, both tibial plateaus undergo a combined anterior translation coupled with an internal rotation of the tibia through the anterior motion segment to the anterior terminal position. Anterolateral subluxation of the tibia, then, is defined as a motion couple consisting of anterior translation and internal rotation. The anterior displacement of the lateral tibial plateau is greater than that of the medial tibial plateau (Fig.5).

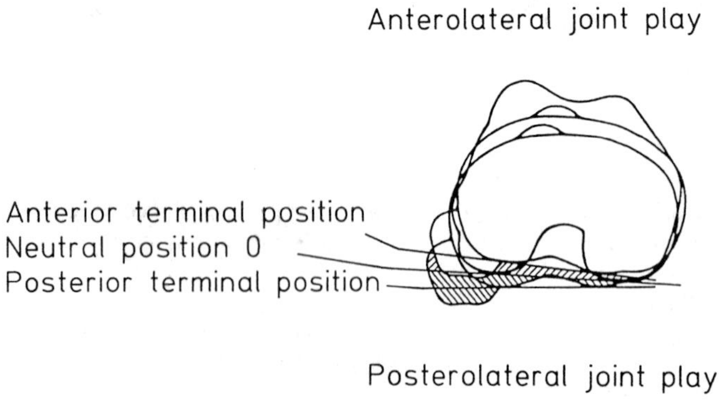

Anterolateral joint play

Anterior terminal position
Neutral position 0
Posterior terminal position

Posterolateral joint play

Fig.3. Physiologic anterolateral *(top)* and posterolateral *(bottom)* joint play

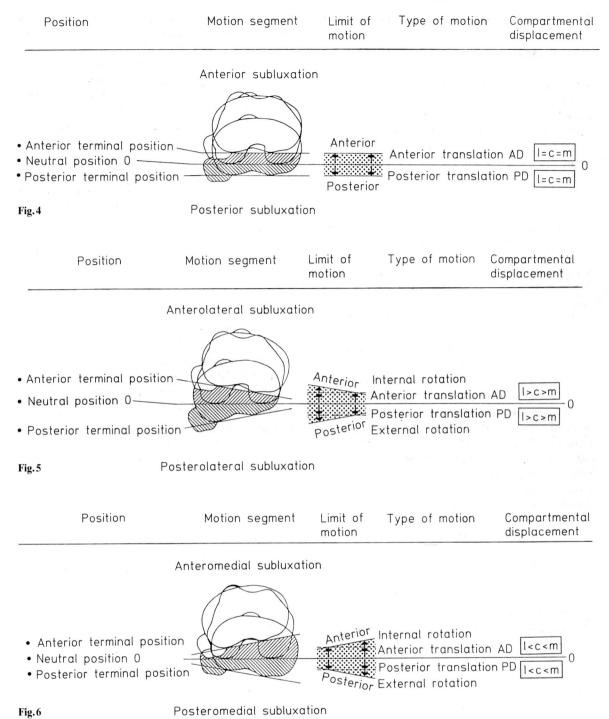

Fig. 4. Anterior subluxation, anterior translation, and bicompartmental equidistant anterior drawer near extension, here directed *upward*. Posterior subluxation is directed *downward* *AD*, Anterior drawer; *PD*, posterior drawer; *l*, lateral; *c*, central; *m*, medial

Fig. 5. Coupled anterolateral and posterolateral subluxations *AD*, Anterior drawer; *PD*, posterior drawer; *l*, lateral; *c*, central; *m*, medial

Fig. 6. Coupled anteromedial and posteromedial subluxations *AD*, Anterior drawer; *PD*, posterior drawer; *l*, lateral; *c*, central; *m*, medial

Posterolateral subluxation (Gollehon et al. 1978; Grood et al. 1988; Hughston and Jacobson 1985; Jakob et al. 1981): Posterolateral subluxation is present when increased posterior translation is coupled with external rotation of the tibia. It is defined as increased posterior motion of the lateral tibial plateau relative to the medial tibial plateau in comparison with the corresponding femoral condyles (see Fig. 5).

Anteromedial subluxation (Kennedy and Fowler 1971): From the neutral position, the anterior terminal position is reached by a combined anterior translation and external rotation of the tibia with respect to the femur. Anteromedial subluxation consists of an increased anterior displacement of the medial tibial plateau relative to the lateral tibial plateau in comparison with the corresponding femoral condyles (Fig. 6).

Posteromedial subluxation (Müller et al. 1988): Posteromedial subluxation is defined as the maximum position of subluxation at the limit of posterior motion when posterior translation of the tibia is coupled with internal rotation. This phenomenon occurs when the posterior displacement of the medial tibial plateau exceeds that of the lateral tibial plateau (see Fig. 6).

Displacement of the tibia from the neutral or starting position into the subluxated or terminal position (as determined by the limits of motion) is to be distinguished from the active or passive reduction of a subluxation to the neutral position or to the opposite physiologic terminal position. This is illustrated by the reduction of a gravity-induced posterior tibial subluxation in a PCL-deficient knee with an intact ACL. In this situation the tibia can be reduced actively (by quadriceps contraction) or passively (by the application of an anteriorly directed force) through the neutral position to the physiologic anterior terminal position (see Fig. 2a,d). Besides the concept of active vs. passively induced motion in stability testing, motion testing also may be characterized as free or coupled or as constrained or unconstrained depending on whether the examiner limits the amount of motion that occurs (Noyes et al. 1989).

Figure 1 illustrates the degrees of freedom in which the motions of translation (anterior-posterior, medial-lateral, proximal-distal) and rotation can be tested. Motion on the three rotational axes is tested about a mediolateral axis for flexion-extension, about an anteroposterior axis for abduction-adduction, and about a proximal-distal axis for internal-external rotation.

Glossary: Kinematics

Joint play: normal coupled motions of the tibia with respect to the femur, occurring within the physiologic limits of motion.

Compartment: from L. *compartimentum* (Fr. *compartire*). Separate division, part, or partition into which a closed space is subdivided. In the knee joint, a medial femorotibial compartment is distinguished from a lateral femorotibial compartment and an anterior femoropatellar compartment.

Compartmental displacement: relative motion between the medial and lateral femorotibial compartments.

Bicompartmental displacement: common displacement of the medial and lateral femorotibial compartments.

Unicompartmental: pertaining to one compartment.

Bicompartmental: pertaining to two compartments.

Tricompartmental: pertaining to three compartments. In degenerative joint diseases, unicompartmental disease, generally involving the medial femorotibial compartment, is distinguished from bicompartmental disease involving two of the joint compartments. Tricompartmental disease involves the medial and lateral femorotibial compartments in addition to the femoropatellar compartment.

Translation: equidistant, bicompartmental, unidirectional, uniplanar motion or displacement of two bodies.

Translation of the knee joint: the medial and lateral femorotibial compartments move the same distance (equidistant) on the same plane (uniplanar) in the same direction (unidirectional) with respect to the neutral position.

Coupled motion: motion in one degree of freedom is combined (coupled) with motion in one or more different degrees of freedom.

Couple: from L. *copula* bond, connecting band, cord, leash, Fr. *couple* connecting strap, pair.
Examples: The physiologic anterior joint play (starting from the neutral position) consists of a coupled anterior displacement and internal rotation of the tibia with respect to the femur. The physiologic posterior joint play consists of a coupled posterior displacement and external rotation of the tibia with respect to the femur (see Fig. 3).

Dynamics: Forces, Moments, and Masses

Active and passive forces and moments act upon the knee joint. In standard clinical tests of knee stability, forces and moments are applied to the tibia. The resulting displacement depends on the site of application of the force, its direction, magnitude, line of action, and cyclic initial loading. The unit of force measurement is the newton. A moment is defined by the location of the axis about which it occurs, the moment arm, the directional sense (clockwise or counterclockwise) of the moment, and its magnitude. The unit of the moment is the newton-meter. Depending on the position of the patient and the knee, gravitational forces can produce effects that must be taken into account during the testing of motion and stablity.

Glossary: Dynamics

Force: A force is defined by its action. The direction and magnitude of a force along a line of action defines the force. The SI unit of force is the newton (N).
One newton is defined as the force that imparts an acceleration of $1 \, ms^{-2}$ to a mass of 1 kg: $1 \, N = 1 \, m \, kg \, s^{-2}$.

Moment: A moment is defined by its action, which depends on the center of rotation, the moment arm, the magnitude of the moment, and the sense of the moment (clockwise or counterclockwise) about its line of action. The SI unit of moment is the newton-meter (Nm).

Mass M: SI unit is kg.

Gravitational force G: The gravitational force G is the effect of gravitational acceleration g along the gravitational line on the mass M:

$$G = m \times g \; [g = 9.812\,523 \, ms^{-2}]$$

Concepts in the Measurement of Motion and Displacement

Physiologic joint play (the motion segment from the neutral position to the physiologic limit of motion) is distinguished from an *abnormal range of motion* in which displacement progresses to an abnormal limit. A *normal range of motion* is distinguished from a *restricted range of motion.*

Examples of normal flexion-extension on the mediolateral rotational axis: A normal range of motion from 10° of hyperextension to 145° of flexion is denoted as follows (We. Müller et al. 1988):

	Extension	Neutral position		Flexion
• Normal range of motion	10°	0°		145°
• Extension deficit of 20°		0°	10°	145°
• Combined extension and flexion deficit		0°	10°	135°

Normal varus-valgus laxity of the joint (medial-lateral opening) is tested about the anteroposterior rotational axis. If an adducting moment is applied to the distal tibia with the knee flexed 20° while rotation is blocked (constrained test), a compressive force will act on the medial femorotibial compartment while a distracting force acts on the lateral femorotibial compartment. Known as the varus or adduction stress test, this maneuver angulates the tibia inward from the neutral position toward the center of the body. If an abducting moment is applied to the distal medial tibia, the lateral femorotibial compartment will be compressed while the medial compartment is distracted. This is known as the valgus or abduction stress test. Similarly, flexion-dependent internal-external rotation of the knee is tested with respect to the neutral position about a proximal-distal axis.

Concepts of Stability, Instability, and Laxity

The clinical examination of the injured knee includes comparison with the uninjured side. The constitutional laxity component is distinguished from the stability of the uninjured knee and the instability of the injured knee.

Glossary: Stability, Instability, Laxity

Stability: the quality of being stable.

Instability: the quality of being unstable.

Subluxation: partial loss of contact between members that normally articulate.

Dislocation: complete loss of contact between members that normally articulate.

Laxity: a constitutional quality of ligaments that depends on collagen composition, age, and gender.

Dynamic subluxation phenomena: transient clinical phenomena consisting of subluxation and reduction with respect to the neutral position. The direction of the reduction, the degree of the subluxation, and the type of coupled abnormal motion during the subluxation are defined. Examples: graded pivot shift (Jakob et al. 1987), flexion-rotation drawer (Noyes and Grood 1988); reversed pivot shift (Jakob et al. 1981).

Medial-lateral stability (medial-lateral opening, varus-valgus laxity): With the femur immobilized, forces and moments are applied to the medial or lateral aspect of the tibia to test for varus-valgus angulation; *opening (gapping) of the joint space* is tested on the *convex* side of the deforming forces, and *closure of the joint space* on the *concave* side.

When motion is tested on the planes of translation, the *total displacement* from the posterior to the anterior terminal position through the neutral position is subdivided into an *anterior* and a *posterior motion segment*. Each degree of freedom, i.e., each translation and each rotation, has two different limits of motion in opposite directions. As the translation proceeds, more and more fiber units are recruited against the displacement, i.e., the stiffness of the ligament structure or, conversely, its terminal compliance changes, the end point of the motion being characterized by the palpable end-point resilience.

Ligament laxity: an inherent increase in an individual's physiologic range of active and passive joint motion, where the limits of displacment and rotation are greater than normal in all planes and about all rotational axes. The term laxity should be distinguished from instability, which is the quality of being unstable (see below).

Instability: from L. *in* not, *stabilitas* firmness, steadiness. A joint condition characterized by abnormally increased limits of motion or displacement in one or more degrees of freedom due to insufficiency of one or more ligamentous structures.

In the literature, the term instability is used in two ways: (1) to describe an episode of giving way (subjective symptom), and (2) to describe a condition of excessive joint mobility (an objective physical sign). In the former case a symptom should be described either as a subjectively perceived functional instability with a sensation of unsteadiness or giving way, or as a partial or complete collapse of the knee joint. The symptom of giving way can also result from a patellar instability (subluxation), quadriceps weakness, or mechanical interference by loose osteochondral fragments or mobile meniscal tags within the joint.

The term instability should be reserved for the objective description of a state of abnormal stability with excessive limits of motion in the three translational planes and about the three rotational axes.

Instability can be described objectively as an increased or excessive displacement of the tibia with respect to the femur along the translational planes or about the rotational axes.

Laxity: from L. *laxare* to relax, slacken. In the medical literature, the term laxity refers to slackness or lack of tension in a ligament or to the looseness of a joint, which may be normal or abnormal. *Constitutional* laxity refers to an inherent quality of the ligaments relating to the constitution of the individual (i.e., age, gender, physique). A slight physiologic increase in ligament laxity may be observed in children and adolescents, in women, and under the influence of gestational hormones. An extreme form of increased abnormal constitutional laxity is seen in Ehlers-Danlos syndrome. Physiologic laxity is distinguished from abnormal laxity and from the decreased ligament laxity found in individuals with tight ligaments.

Dislocation: from L. *de* away from, *locare* to place. Dislocation (luxation) describes a state in which there is complete loss of contact between normally opposed articular surfaces. Dislocations of the knee are described in terms of the direction and degree of the dislocation and associated osteochondral, capsuloligamentous, and meniscal injuries. Congenital subluxations or dislocations can be distinguished from acquired (traumatic) forms. Usually a laxity component plays some etiologic role in both congenital and acquired traumatic dislocations.

Examples: patellar subluxation, patellar dislocation, subluxation or dislocation of the knee, fracture-dislocation of the knee.

Subluxation: from L. *sub* under, *luxare* to put out of joint. Subluxation denotes a state in which there is partial loss of contact between the normally opposed tricompartmental articular surfaces. A subluxation in the knee joint may involve the patellar facets and femoral trochlea in the femoropatellar compartment, or it may be bicompartmental, involving both the medial and lateral femorotibial compartments, due to rupture of the anterior or posterior cruciate ligament.

Properties of Tendons and Ligaments

Basic Concepts

The *stress* in a body is analogous to the pressure in a fluid (where pressure is defined as force per unit area). The difference is that the pressure in a fluid medium (liquid or gas) is hydrostatic, or independent of direction, and therefore always acts at right angles to the container walls, whereas the stress in a solid body is a highly directional phenomenon.

The stress in a body is defined as the force per unit cross-sectional area acting at a designated point in the body in the direction of its long axis (Fig. 7) (Gordon 1989). Expressed in physical symbols, the stress σ that is exerted by a force (F) upon an area (A) satisfies the equation

$$\sigma = F/A.$$

A tensile force gives rise to a positive stress, a compressive force a negative stress, and a shearing force a shear stress. In the International System of Measurements, stress, like pressure, is measured in pascals (Pa), where $1 \, Pa = 1 \, N/m^2$.

Strain is the effect that stress has upon a material. Defined as the ratio of length change to original length (Fig. 8), strain is a nondimensional quantity, a proportion. Strain is usually symbolized by the Greek letter ε. For a ligament of length L that is stretched by the amount l, the strain is given by the formula

$$\varepsilon = l/L.$$

Strain measures the relative elongation of a ligament under tensile stress. It is the ratio of the length change l to the original length L, expressed in percent (Gordon 1989).

Stiffness or elastic modulus (Butler et al. 1986; Gordon 1989; Markolf et al. 1976, 1981, 1984). Young's modulus (E) expresses the steepness of the stress-strain curve. It represents the ratio of stress (σ) to strain (ε) (Fig. 9).

$$\text{Young's modulus (E)} = \frac{\text{stress}(\sigma)}{\text{strain}(\varepsilon)}$$

Since strain is dimensionless, Young's modulus E has the dimension of stress and is measured in units such as pascals or MN/cm^2.

If a material has a low E modulus, it means that even a small load will generate a relatively high stress: The material is easily stretched or bent. Conversely, a high E modulus means that a large load is needed to

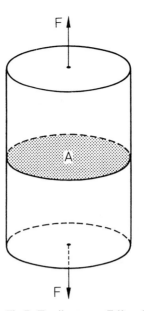

Fig. 7. Tensile stress = F (force) per unit area (A), shown schematically for a cylindrical ligamentous cross section. Simultaneous transverse contraction is disregarded

$$\text{Stress } \sigma = \frac{\text{force}}{\text{area}}$$

A = cross-sectional area
$1 \, kpm^{-2} = 9.80665 \, Pa$ (pascals)
1 MPA (megapascal) = $10.2 \, kg/m^{-2}$

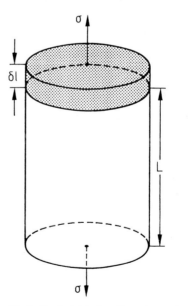

Fig. 8. Strain (ε) is the effect of stress in a material

$$\text{Strain } (\varepsilon) = \frac{\text{length change (l)}}{\text{original length(L)}}$$

Strain is defined as the ratio of a length change to the original length.

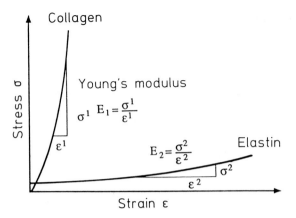

E_1 relatively large
E_2 relatively small

Fig.9. Young's modulus or elastic modulus. Comparison of the stress-strain behavior of collagen and elastin.

$$E_1 = \frac{\sigma_1}{\varepsilon_1} =$$

relatively small strain in response to a marked stress increase for collagen;

$$E_2 = \frac{\sigma_2}{\varepsilon_2} =$$

relatively large strain in response to a slight stress increase for elastin

achieve the same strain: The material is stiff and rigid.

Elasticity. A J-shaped stress-strain curve is characteristic of soft biologic tissues such as ligaments and tendons.

In the range of small stresses and strains, where the J curve is practically horizontal, the material has an extremely low shear modulus. The steep portion of the J curve, and thus the range of large stresses and strains, can be most clearly understood by picturing the material (a ligament) as a system of crosslinked fibers, fiber bundles, or molecular chains. When the initially recruited fiber units have come under strong tension, so that they are oriented approximately in the direction of the pull, a further increase in stress can produce only a small amount of additional elongation or strain (Gordon 1989). As the tensile stress increases, more and more fiber units are recruited to oppose the tensile stress (contribution of Friederich and O'Brien, p.78ff.). This mechanism underlies the function of the tendons and ligaments as "restraints" (Butler et al. 1980).

Biomechanical Properties of Ligaments and Tendons

Ligaments and tendons are *viscoelastic structures* with specific mechanical properties. Tendons are strong enough to withstand the tensile stresses exerted by the force of muscular contraction. At the same time, they are flexible enough to adjust their line of action to the changing position of the knee. The ligaments can deform and bend to allow for natural femorotibial joint play, yet they have the high structural strength and compliance needed to resist the forces and moments that act about the knee. When a ligamentous structure is tested to failure at a constant strain rate, a characteristic stress-strain curve can be derived. The four phases of the deformation curve are as follows (Fig. 10):

1. Phase of physiologic compliance: With a low E modulus and small tensile forces, the ligament undergoes a relatively large degree of strain.
2. Linear phase: Fiber strain is associated with a progressive increase in ligament stiffness and a progressive recruitment of more and more fiber bundle units.
3. Phase of permanent plastic deformation and initial microtearing.
4. When the maximum rupture strength is exceeded, the continuity of the ligament is disrupted: complete ligament rupture with loss of restraining action.

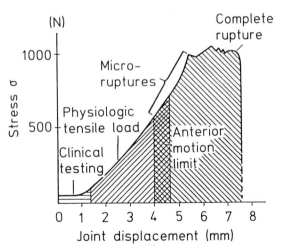

Fig.10. Tensile stress-displacement curve and structural integrity of ligamentous structures. In clinical stability testing, the examiner applies relatively low tensile stresses that elicit little displacement (physiologic joint play with intact ligaments). As tensile stress is increased, more and more ligamentous elements are recruited (linear portion of curve). If the physiologic strain limit is exceeded, partial and ultimately complete ruptures ensues. (Modified from Noyes et al. 1980)

Condition and Functional Competence of the Ligaments

A ligament is *intact* when its structural integrity and physiologic restraining action are preserved. A ligament is said to be *insufficient* (deficient, incompetent) when it can no longer function as a restraint due to partial or complete loss of its structural integrity. Normally a ligamentous structure can be stretched elastically by 13%–15% of its original length (Butler et al. 1986). If stretched beyond its elastic reserve, the ligament will undergo permanent plastic deformation with partial loss of its efficacy as a restraint and partial structural damage. We call this lesion a *partial rupture*. If the degree of plastic deformation exceeds the normal compliance and stiffness of the ligament, a *complete rupture* occurs, and the ligament is functionally incompetent; the restraining action intrinsic to the ligament is completely lost. Besides a partial or complete rupture leading to partial or complete loss of ligamentous restraint, other types of ligament injury are *overstretching* ("mild sprain") and *avulsion*, where the ligament is torn from its bony attachment. A bony avulsion may occasionally coexist with overstretching.

Function and Properties of Ligamentous Structures

The role of the cruciate ligaments as the primary restraints to knee motion depends on the anatomic configuration of their attachments, i.e., their three-dimensional geometry. The mechanical properties of the cruciate ligaments are based on the biochemical crosslinking of the various collagenous structures. The unidirectional, uniplanar restraining forces that act in one direction or on one plane (Butler et al. 1980) are based on the mechanical properties of the primary restraint and its ability to delimit joint motion in various degrees of freedom.

Besides the interaction between gravity, patient position, knee position, and the applied active and passive forces and moments, the viscoelastic properties of the primary and secondary restraints play an essential role. The intact restraining function of the capsule and ligaments is important in its interaction with the three-dimensional geometry of the joint surfaces and their capacity for elastic deformation under loading. *Ligament strain* (elongation relative to initial length), *stiffness* (increasing restraining force with displacement), *compliance* (distensibility), and *terminal stiffness* are important functional properties of ligaments along with their capacity for elastic and plastic deformation. Viewing the mechanical functions of ligaments as a three-dimensional phenomenon leads to the concept of *recruitment*, or the tightening of more and more ligament fibers as displacement proceeds.

The behavior of the ACL as the knee is extended and then hyperextended from a position of 30° flexion illustrates the process of recruitment, or the progressive tightening of ligamentous structural elements. As the knee approaches terminal extension, increasing numbers of ACL fiber bundle units are recruited, i.e., more and more fiber bundle units act mechanically to oppose the forces of extension. Hyperextensibility is ultimately limited by the configuration of the intercondylar roof, the ACL and the three-dimensional geometry of its attachments, and by the spatial orientation of the PCL and popliteus system. If the imposed physical forces outstrip the restraining forces (despite maximal recruitment of all capsuloligamentous elements), the structures will become stretched beyond their viscoelastic capacity, and a partial or complete rupture will occur. If the primary ligament restraint cannot neutralize the energy acting on the joint, the damage will extend to involve secondary restraints according to the position of the joint and the mechanism of injury.

Understanding the basic terms that describe functional anatomy (Kennedy et al. 1974) and kinematics is an essential prerequisite for understanding both the physiologic and nonphysiologic motions of the knee.

Preoperative Diagnostic Techniques

Imaging Procedures

Conventional X-ray studies are supplemented by *functional radiographic techniques. Stressradiography* under anesthesia documents the direction, degree, and nature of an altered compartmental position. *Sonography* (diagnostic ultrasound), computed tomography (CT), *magnetic resonance imaging* (MR, MRI), and *nuclear medicine studies* such as radionuclide bone scanning can provide useful adjuncts to the clinical examination.

Arthroscopy

Arthroscopy of the knee is important for the functional probing of the articular cartilage surfaces, menisci, cruciate ligaments, and popliteus tendon in designated joint positions.

Principles of Reconstructive Surgery

Techniques of ACL reconstruction may be described as *intraarticular* or *extraarticular.* In *intraarticular* techniques the ACL is reconstructed in its natural course between the tibial and femoral sites of insertion. *In extraarticular* reconstructions, portions of the iliotibial tract, fascia lata, biceps tendon (Marshall et al. 1972), or portions of the extensor apparatus are rerouted outside the joint to stabilize it against anterolateral or combined anteromedial, posteromedial and posterolateral subluxation. A distinction may be drawn between an *anatomic reconstruction* and an *anatomic-like reconstruction.* The "over-the-top" method is a nonanatomic, nonisometric technique of ACL reconstruction in which the graft is routed over the posterosuperior border of the lateral femoral condyle.

Surgical Options

Open surgical procedures in which the knee joint is opened by a formal "conventional" arthrotomy are distinguished from *arthroscopically assisted* procedures. Reconstructions that combine video arthroscopic control with open approaches are becoming increasingly important. The following surgical options are available for the treatment of ACL insufficiency:

- *Primary repair:* An ACL that has been avulsed from the femur, preferably with a flake of bone and periosteum, and is not overstretched can be repaired by transfemoral reattachment.
- *Osseous reattachment:* A bony avulsion of the ACL from the anterior intercondylar area of the tibia ("eminence avulsion" in children or adolescents) can be reattached transosseously by an open or arthroscopically assisted procedure.
- *Reattachment with recession:* If a bony avulsion coexists with elongation of the ACL, the tibial attachment can be transposed to a lower site following curettage of the bony bed. The recession technique is also used in the repair of peripheral structures.
- *Augmentation:* Reinforcement of the primary repair with biologic or synthetic tissue.

Reconstruction of the ACL refers to the use of biologic tissue (autologous, homologous, heterologous) to reconstitute an ACL that has been completely torn through its substance or partly or completely resorbed. *Substitution* denotes replacement of the ACL using an intra- or extraarticular technique.

Graft selection. Autologous (autogenous) grafts are distinguished from *homologous* (allogenous) and *heterologous* (xenogenous) grafts. *Synthetic materials* can be used as a ligament substitute or to reinforce a repair.

Graft length and tension. The concept of isometry, or the maintenance of a constant ligament length as the knee moves through flexion and extension, must be distinguished from the concept of the *"most isometric"* attachment (Hefzy et al. 1989) and the *functional isometry* of Friederich and O'Brien (see contribution p. 78 ff.).

Isotony, or a state of constant ligament tension as the knee moves through flexion and extension, is distinct from the concept of *"most isotonic"* ligament tension and a state of *functional tension.*

Graft fixation. A graft may be fixed with sutures or wire loops secured to anchoring screws or an osseous bridge, or with interference screws inserted between a bone block and the wall of the bone tunnel.

One-tunnel, two-tunnel and blind-hole technique. Drilling the bone over an axial Kirschner guide wire or through a drill guide in one direction with the knee in a specified position is called the *one-tunnel technique*, in which the femoral and tibial tunnels are aligned. In the *two-tunnel technique*, the tibial and femoral tunnels are drilled separately from each other. In the *blind-hole technique* a partial-depth femoral channel is drilled from the intercondylar notch.

In the "trough technique" the tunnel is open at the side to form a groove for an over-the-top (femur) or over-the-bottom (tibia) reconstruction.

An ideal method of cruciate ligament reconstruction is based upon the following concepts:

- Functional anatomy (see contribution of Friederich and O'Brien, p. 78 ff.)
- Concept of isometric and "most isometric" sites of attachment (Hefzy et al. 1989)
- "Most physiologic" ligament tension
- Widening and reconfiguring of the intercondylar notch (notch plasty)
- Biologic ligament remodeling and *neoenthesis* (formation of new attachment between the ligament and bone)
- Primary stable graft fixation allowing for early functional rehabilitation

---

Glossary: Principles of Ligament Reconstruction

Augmentation: from L. *augmentum* reinforcement.

Ligament augmentation: reinforcement of a ligament using biologic or synthetic tissue.

Recession: from L. *recedere* to recede.

Ligament recession: posterior or distal transposition of a ligament attachment.

Reconstruction: from L. *re* again, *construere* build; restoration, reconstitution, reapproximation.

Ligament reconstruction: restoration of ligament integrity.

Refixation: from Fr. *refixer* (fr. L. *fixus* firm) reattachment.

Substitution: from L. *substituire* to replace, exchange. Ligament substitution: complete replacement of the original ligament.

Concepts in Rehabilitation

The various terms and concepts pertaining to rehabilitation are summarized in the glossary.

Glossary: Concepts in Rehabilitation

Agonists and antagonists: from Gr. *ágein* to act, *anti*
against. The muscle group acting in one direction of motion or plane and the muscle units acting in opposition to
that group lead to an interplay of active forces and
counterforces.

Concepts in therapeutic mobilization

CPM: Continuous passive motion – the continuous,
passive, postoperative mobilization of the knee on a motion splint for the purpose of improving cartilage nutrition
and preventing the formation of adhesions (Salter et al.
1980).

IPM: Intermittent passive motion – periods of passive
knee mobilization separated by rest periods with the joint
in ligament tension-adapted positions.

Coactivation: simultaneous isometric contraction of the
hamstring and quadriceps muscles. Coactivation of the
quadriceps and adductor group: The simultaneous contraction and innervation of these muscle groups, which
develop from similar myotomes, can potentiate the toni-
cizing effect of the vastus medialis and vastus medialis obliquus to promote the restoration of full active extension.

Concept of early functional rehabilitation: early postoperative, limited therapeutic exercise at an amplitude that
does not place exorbitant stresses on reconstructed elements.

Continuous postoperative epidural analgesia: concept of
Arvidsson and Eriksson (1988) to avoid pain-induced
muscle inhibition after surgery.

Contraction: from L. *contrahere* to draw together; active
muscular tension.

Contracture: fixed condition of being shortened or drawn
together.

Cryotherapy: therapeutic application of cold.

Hydrotherapy: Therapy in water. Hydrotherapy using
cruciate ligament-sparing knee positions and full under-
water weight bearing (buoyancy principle) can be safely
initiated soon after surgery to prevent postoperative adhesions and stimulate physiologic ligament forces.

Joint immobilization: The principle of continuous or intermittent mobilization must be distinguished from the
principle of temporary joint immobilization. The joint
may be immobilized by an external plaster cast or by temporary external skeletal fixation that bridges the joint
(e.g., a one-bar external fixation device mounted on the
anterior side).

Neutral quadriceps angle: knee flexion angle of 70°. When
the quadriceps apparatus is actively innervated with the
knee flexed 70° (and the cruciate ligaments are intact),
there will be no actively induced anterior or posterior
drawer motion of the tibia with respect to the femur. This
concept of the "neutral Q angle" is useful in early rehabilitation as a means of protecting the anterior cruciate ligament substitute (duck standing, duck walking, and duck
running).

PNF: proprioceptive neuromuscular facilitation.

Postisometric relaxation: Elongation of the musculotendinous unit following isometric muscle contraction.

Prophylaxis: prevention.

Prophylactic braces: uniaxial, biaxial, or multiaxial knee
braces, recommended by some to avoid injury (controversial).

Concepts in Ligament Healing

The *spontaneous healing* of a ligament is distinguished from the healing that follows reapproximation of the torn ends. *Remodeling* describes the functionally adapted structural changes that accompany
natural healing processes; *regeneration,* the restoration of a ligament's structural properties. *Ligamentization* and *neoligamentization* refer to the remodeling, alignment, and maturation of collagenous
structures under functional loading. *Ligament resorption* refers to dissolution of the ligament stumps following a complete rupture.

Concepts in Meniscal Surgery

Anatomy

The medial (C-shaped) and lateral (O-shaped) menisci consist of two incomplete annular segments. Their
principal sites of attachment are in the anterior intercondylar area (anterior horn) and posterior intercondylar area (posterior horn). Additional attachments
to the anterior horns of the medial and lateral menisci
(transverse ligament of the knee), the meniscofemoral and meniscotibial capsuloligamentous attachments, the various fascicles that attach to the menisci,
and the meniscofemoral ligaments (of Humphry and
Wrisberg) ensure the transmission of the physiologic
hoop tension to these wedgelike fibrocartilaginous
structures.

The surfaces of the menisci are concave superiorly
and flat inferiorly. Compressive stresses predominate

at the center of the menisci, while a combination of compressive and radially directed tensile stresses act at the periphery. The large area of tibiomeniscofemoral stress transfer is made possible by the intact hoop tension, by the congruence-enhancing shape of the menisci, and by their viscoelastic properties.

Functions of the Menisci

The mobility of the menisci in the three translational and three rotational degrees of freedom is a factor in determining the physiologic limits of joint motion. While important as secondary restraints, the menisci also perform a chondroprotective, biomechanical, and chondronutritive function (wetting or "lubrication" of the articular surfaces). Joint displacement exceeding the normal limits of motion gives rise to shearing forces and combined compressive and distractive forces at the periphery or center of the meniscal substance that can lead, acutely or through recurrent microtrauma, to various types of meniscal tear. These lesions may be complete or incomplete and may involve the peripheral, vascularized portion of the meniscus or the central avascular portion.

Meniscal tears are also classified by their direction, length, and extent. Incomplete or complete stable tears are distinguished from complete unstable tears. The loss of annular tension due to pouting of the inner border of the meniscus and unstable, subluxating, spontaneously reducing meniscal segments are distinguished from temporarily subluxated tears and tags that become incarcerated in the intercondylar notch (e.g., a displaced peripheral, wide-based bucket handle tear of the medial meniscus). An incarcerated bucket handle fragment may later rupture through its center to form anteriorly and posteriorly based flaps.

Meniscus Surgery

The two broad categories of surgical procedures on the menisci are (1) partial or total meniscectomy (meniscal resection) and (2) meniscus-conserving procedures such as meniscal repair, reconstruction, and replacement.

Stimulation of Reparative Mechanisms

Various procedures have been recommended for the stimulation of reparative processes in damaged menisci: supra- and submeniscal abrasion of the highly

vascular perimeniscal synovium (synovial abrasion), freshening the surfaces of the meniscal substance adjacent to the tear (meniscal rasping), the application of an exogenous fibrin clot, and the use of biologic adhesives (fibrin glue). A stable meniscus repair that anatomically coapts the torn surfaces helps to ensure a favorable rate of healing.

Meniscus-conserving procedures may be open, arthroscopic, or combined using a retractor to protect neurovascular tissues. The principle of compartmental distraction (manual or with an external distraction device) helps to protect the articular cartilage during meniscal rasping, the reduction of displaced bucket handle fragments, and the placement of meniscal sutures. The principle of compartmental compression (manual or with an external fixation device used in the compression mode) is useful for coapting the articular surfaces or approximating torn meniscal surfaces and facilitates the extraarticular tying of absorbable or nonabsorbable sutures. Recent trends in meniscus-conserving knee surgery include the creation of pedicled synovial or fat flaps for the revascularization of tears in the avascular meniscal substance, the conversion of unstable meniscal segments to stable ones, interconnecting annular segments with autologous tissue (fascia lata, gastrocnemius tendon), the placement of collagen templates to direct the ingrowth of fibroblast-inducing scar tissue, and the replacement of menisci by homologous meniscal tissue.

Glossary: Meniscus Surgery

Meniscal segments

Lateral meniscus: consists of the anterior horn and its attachment, the middle third with the inferior popliteomeniscal fascicle (inlet of popliteal hiatus), the posterior horn with its superior popliteomeniscal fascicle, the posterior meniscofemoral ligament (of Wrisberg), the anterior meniscofemoral ligament (of Humphry), and the attachment of the posterior horn.

Medial meniscus: consists of the anterior horn and its attachment, the middle third, and the posterior horn and its attachment along with the fascicles that project into that area.

Meniscal configuration (meniscal shape): The medial meniscus is crescent or C-shaped on the transverse plane, while the lateral meniscus is approximately O-shaped. Both represent incomplete annular segments. On the coronal plane the menisci are wedge-shaped or wedge-like with a concave superior surface and flat inferior surface.

Meniscal functions: The functions of the menisci include the transmission of forces between the tibia and femur, increasing the congruity of the femorotibial joint surfaces, secondary restraint, and protection and nutrition of the articular cartilage. The menisci also appear to have an important function in the wetting or "lubrication" of the joint surfaces.

Terms in meniscal surgery

Meniscectomy: from Gr. *ek* out, *tomein* to cut. Surgical or microsurgical removal of meniscal tissue.

Meniscus-conserving procedures: surgical procedures that preserve functionally important meniscal segments by repair, reattachment, reconstruction or augmentation, or replace those segments with meniscus-like tissue.

Meniscal resection: from L. *resecare* to cut off, cut away. Synonym for meniscectomy.

Extent of meniscectomy

Partial meniscectomy: removal of irreparable meniscal segments, generally avascular, that interfere with joint mechanics.

Subtotal meniscectomy: almost complete removal of the meniscus.

Total meniscectomy: complete removal of the meniscal substance. The immediate effect of complete meniscectomy is a loss of stability, followed years later by postmeniscectomy osteoarthritis chiefly affecting the ipsilateral compartment.

Types of meniscus-conserving procedure

Meniscal allograft: replacement of the meniscus with an allograft from a suitable organ donor.

Meniscal augmentation: reinforcement of a meniscal repair by the use of autologous material (e. g., fascia lata, portions of the lateral gastrocnemius tendon).

Meniscal reattachment: Reattachment of a peripheral meniscal tear or horn detachment.

Meniscal reconstruction: restoration of the meniscal structure and function.

Meniscal repair: generally refers to the suture repair of peripheral meniscal tears.

Meniscal substitution: replacement of the meniscus with a collagen template.

Types of meniscal lesion

Avascular zone: portion of the meniscal substance that lacks a microvascular blood supply.

Basal: synonymous with "peripheral" when applied to menisci.

Bucket handle tear: generally a vertical or oblique tear through the *peripheral* vascular zone with displacement of the meniscal segment beneath the femoral condyle to-

ward the intercondylar notch. A subluxating bucket handle tear that has lost partial contact with the articular surfaces is distinguished from a dislocated tear that has completely lost its normal meniscotibial and meniscofemoral relationship. A *central* bucket handle tear occurs through the avascular part of the meniscus.

Central meniscal lesion: lesion involving the substance of the meniscus, generally the avascular zone.

Discoid meniscus: disk-shaped lateral meniscus.

Dissected bucket handle fragment: Combination of a bucket handle tear with a radial tear in which the center of the bucket handle fragment ruptures transversely, creating a pair of anteriorly and posteriorly based flaps or tags.

Flap tear: flap- or tag-shaped tear of the meniscus.

Fresh lesion: meniscal lesion that is diagnosed or treated within 7 days of the injury.

Horizontal tear: a cleavage tear, usually degenerative, running parallel to the superior or inferior surface of the meniscus and generally involving its avascular substance.

Meniscal substance: three-dimensional body of the meniscus, whose shape is determined by the configuration of the collagen fiber bundles.

Meniscocapsular: pertaining to the area of attachment of the meniscal substance to the capsule, the meniscofemoral and meniscotibial ligament (coronary ligament).

Mesial: toward the free inner border of the meniscus.

Oblique tear: generally a tear running obliquely from the center of the meniscal undersurface toward the periphery of the superior surface and occurring at the junction of the vascular and avascular zones.

Old lesion: meniscal lesion that is diagnosed or treated more than 1 week postinjury.

Peripheral meniscal lesion: from Gr. *peripherein* to carry around. Describes a lesion located at the periphery or outer circumference of the meniscus, near the junction of the meniscal substance with the meniscocapsular fibers.

Radial tear: tear that divides the meniscus into an anterior and posterior segment.
Radial tear of the lateral meniscus: generally occurs opposite to the popliteal hiatus (see also annular tension, meniscal fascicle).

Vascular zone: from L. *vas* vessel, *zona* band. The microvascular blood supply of the meniscus dwindles from the inner border of the meniscus toward the periphery, except in early childhood when the entire meniscus has a microvascular supply. With aging, the portion of the meniscus that has a blood supply recedes toward the periphery. The **vascular zone** refers to the outer circumferential third or fourth of the meniscal substance that has a microvascular blood supply. The sites of attachment of the anterior and posterior horns are vascularized better than the middle third. An avascular zone is located opposite to the popliteal hiatus.

Vertical tear: generally a longitudinal tear through the peripheral vascular zone of the meniscus.

White rim: zone from the microvascular arcades, visible

on the meniscal surface by arthroscopy, to the location of a vertical or oblique tear in the meniscal substance.

Complete and incomplete tears

Complete tear: tear extending completely through the periphery or substance of a meniscus.

Incomplete tear: tear involving the superior or inferior meniscal surface but not extending completely through the meniscus.

Meniscal stability

Displaced meniscus: meniscal segment showing complete loss of normal femorotibial contact.

Dissected meniscal tear: from L. *dissecare* to cut apart, separate. Radial tear of a subluxatable or subluxated bucket handle fragment, forming anteriorly and posteriorly based flaps.

Stable meniscus: meniscus that shows normal mobility of its segments upon probing.

Subluxatable meniscus: meniscal segment that is abnormally mobile on probing, with partial loss of normal contact with the femoral and tibial surfaces.

Tear size: The length of a meniscal tear (in millimeters), together with the location of the tear in relation to the vascular or avascular zone and meniscal stability (stable, subluxatable, or displaced), determines whether a meniscus can be repaired or whether a partial, subtotal, or total meniscectomy is required.

Techniques of meniscal repair

"Inside out": transarthroscopic technique in which the suture-armed meniscal repair needle is passed from inside to outside.

"Outside in": technique in which the needle is passed from outside to inside (special repair technique used on the anterior and posterior horns).

Meniscal healing: documented full meniscal healing is achieved when arthrography (meniscography) or arthroscopy with probing confirms that the repair is healed over its entire length and on its superior and inferior surfaces.

No healing: arthrography or arthroscopy shows no discernible healing of the meniscal tear.

Partial healing: arthrography or arthroscopy demonstrates *incomplete healing* of the former tear.

Retearing: recurrence of tearing at the site of an old lesion in response to an adequate or nonadequate second trauma.

Factors stimulating meniscal healing

Abrasion: from L. *abradere* to scrape off. Abrasive removal of excess meniscal scar tissue using a meniscal or synovial shaver.

Meniscal debridement: from Fr. *débridement* removal of a rein or bridle. Removal and smoothing of small meniscal tags or irregularities that have little effect on stability.

Submeniscal: located below the meniscus or pertaining to its inferior surface.

Suprameniscal: located above the meniscus or pertaining to its superior surface.

General Glossary

This chapter concludes with a general glossary covering terms that are frequently encountered in the evaluation and treatment of knee disorders.

Anatomy: from Gr. *ana* up and *tomein* to cut, cut up. The art of dissection.

Arthrography: from Gr. *árthron* joint, *gráphein* to write. Radiographic visualization of a joint after the intraarticular injection of contrast medium.

Arthrometry: from Gr. *árthron* joint, *metron* measure. The measurement of joint displacement. Generally one sensor is placed on the anterior patellar surface and another on the tibial tuberosity. Physically defined forces are applied in designated joint positions, and the resulting patellotibial displacement in millimeters is read from an indicator dial (Daniel et al. 1985).

Arthroscopy: from Gr. *árthron* joint, *skopeín* to look. In knee arthroscopy the interior of the knee joint is examined through an optical instrument, and a probe is inserted through a separate portal to palpate the joint surfaces, test the stability of the menisci, and test the functional integrity (restraining force) of the cruciate ligaments and popliteus tendon.
Diagnostic arthroscopy: arthroscopy for diagnostic purposes.
Interventional arthroscopy: arthroscopy performed for an operative procedure.

Arthrotomography: from Gr. *tomeín* to cut. Sectional radiographs of a joint.

Electrogoniometer: measuring instrument for the continuous, computer-compatible monitoring of the six degrees of freedom of knee motion during specific subluxation and reduction maneuvers.

Examination under anesthesia: elimination of active muscular forces and muscle tonus by the induction of general endotracheal intubation anesthesia or regional (spinal or peridural) anesthesia. Knee stability can be objectively tested and measured with little or no pain and no muscular resistance.

Hemarthrosis: from Gr. *haíma* blood, blood in the joint.

Hemarthrosis with fat globules: presence of fat droplets in the intraarticular blood due to an intraarticular fracture, a ligament avulsion that has opened the cancellous trabeculae, or a bony ligament avulsion.

Knee joint effusion: intraarticular fluid collection.

Lesion: from L. *laesio* (fr. *laesus, laedere* to hurt). A trauma- or disease-related abnormality in an organ or any of its parts.

Meniscus: from Gr. *meniskos* crescent. One of two (lateral and medial) crescent-shaped disks of fibrocartilage attached to the superior articular surface of the tibia.

Pivot: a person, thing, or factor having a major or central role; a center of rotation; to turn as if on a pivot.

Pivot shift: a shift in the position of the center of rotation of the knee joint.

Pivot shift grading: grading the pivot shift tested in internal, neutral, and external rotation.

Reversed pivot shift: A reversal of the pivot shift phenomenon, signifying posterolateral subluxation or reduction.

Serosanguinous effusion: from L. *sanguis* blood. Serous effusion containing blood.

Serous knee effusion: from L. *serum* milk, whey. Serum is the watery constituent of blood. Increased production of synovial fluid in the knee joint.

Stressradiography: functional radiographic technique for assessing coupled translation and rotation in the knee by the measurement of compartmental femorotibial displacement (Stäubli 1990).

Syndesmoplasty: from Gr. *plásein* to form. Construction of a ligament substitute.
Aplasia: complete failure of development of a part.
Hypoplasia: incomplete development of a part.
Hyperplasia: excessive or overdevelopment of a part.

Synthetic knee effusion: type of effusion caused by particulate abrasion (after implantation of prosthetic ligaments).

X-ray stereophotogrammetry: procedure, introduced by Selvik in 1974, for studying the kinematics of the skeletal system.

References

American Academy of Orthopaedic Surgeons (1984) Athletic training and sports medicine. The American Academy of Orthopaedic Surgeons, Chicago

American Academy of Orthopaedic Surgeons (1985) Glossary of spinal terminology. The American Academy of Orthopaedic Surgeons, Chicago

American Medical Association (1966) Standard nomenclature of athletic injuries. American Medical Association, Chicago

Apley AG (1980) Instability of the knee resulting from ligamentous injury. A plea for plain words. J Bone Joint Surg [Br] 62: 515-516

Arvidsson I, Eriksson E (1988) Counteracting muscle atrophy after ACL injury: Scientific bases of a rehabilitation program. In: Feagin JA (ed). The crucial ligaments. Churchill Livingstone, New York Edinburgh London Melbourne, pp 451-464

Butler DL, Noyes FR, Grood ES (1980) Ligamentous restraints to anterior-posterior drawer in the human knee. A biomechanical study. J Bone Joint Surg [Am] 62: 259-270

Butler DL, Kay MD, Stouffer DC (1986) Comparison of material properties in fascicle-bone units from human patellar tendon and knee ligaments. J Biomech 19: 425-492

Daniel DM, Malcom LL, Losse G, Stone ML, Sachs R, Burks R (1985) Instrumented measurements of anterior laxity of the knee. J Bone Joint Surg [Am] 67: 720-726

Die anatomischen Namen (1965). Ihre Ableitung und Aussprache (Hrsg H Triepel). 27. Aufl. von R Herrlinger. Bergmann, München 1965

Duden (1970) Band 2: Das Stilwörterbuch, 6. Aufl. Bibliographisches Institut, Mannheim

Duden (1963) Band 7: Das Herkunftswörterbuch: Eine Etymologie der deutschen Sprache. Bibliographisches Institut, Mannheim

Feagin JA jr (1988) The crucial ligaments. Diagnosis and treatment of ligamentous injuries about the knee. Churchill Livingstone, New York Edinburgh London Melbourne

Fukubayashi T, Torzilli PA, Sherman MF, Warren RF (1982) An in vitro biomechanical evaluation of anterior-posterior motion of the knee. J Bone Joint Surg [Am] 64: 258-264

Gollehon DL, Torzilli PA, Warren RF (1987) The role of the posterolateral and cruciate ligaments in the stability of the human knee. A biomechanical study. J Bone Joint Surg [Am] 69: 233-242

Gordon JE (1989) Strukturen unter Streß: mechanische Belastbarkeit in Natur und Technik. Spektrum der Wissenschaft, Heidelberg

Grood ES, Noyes FR (1987) Diagnosis of knee ligament injuries. Biomechanical precepts. In: Feagin JA jr (ed). The crucial ligaments. Churchill Livingstone, New York, pp 245-260

Grood ES, Suntay WJ (1983) A joint coordinate system for the clinical description of three dimensional motions: Application to the knee. J Biomech Eng 105: 136-144

Grood ES, Suntay WJ, Noyes FR, Butler DL, Miller EH, Malek M (1979) Total motion measurement during knee laxity. Orthop Trans 3: 179-180

Grood ES, Stowers SF, Noyes FR (1988) Limits of movement in the human knee. Effect of sectioning the posterior cruciate ligament and posterolateral structures. J Bone Joint Surg [Am] 70: 88-97

Hefzy MS, Grood ES, Noyes FR (1989) Factors affecting the most isometric femoral attachments. Part III: The anterior cruciate ligament. Am J Sports Med 17: 208-216

Hughston JC, Barrett GR (1983) Acute anteromedial rotatory instability. Long-term results of surgical repair. J Bone Joint Surg [Am] 65: 145-153

Hughston JC, Jacobson KE (1985) Chronic posterolateral rotatory instability of the knee. J Bone Joint Surg [Am] 67: 351-359

Hughston JC, Andrews JR, Cross MJ, Moschi A (1976a) Classification of knee ligament instabilities. Part I. The medial compartment and cruciate ligaments. J Bone Joint Surg [Am] 58: 159-172

Hughston JC, Andrews JR, Cross MJ, Moschi A (1976b) Classification of knee ligament instabilities. Part II. The lateral compartment. J Bone Joint Surg [Am] 58: 173-179

Jakob RP, Hassler H, Stäubli H-U (1981) Observations on rotatory instability of the lateral compartment of the knee. Acta Orthop Scand 52 [Suppl 191]: 1-32

Jakob RP, Stäubli H-U, Deland JT (1987) Grading the pivot shift. Objective tests with implications for treatment. J Bone Joint Surg [Br] 69: 294-299

Kennedy JC, Fowler PJ (1971) Medial and anterior instability of the knee. An anatomical and clinical study using stress machines. J Bone Joint Surg [Am] 53: 1257-1270

Kennedy JC, Weinberg HW, Wilson AS (1974) The anatomy and function of the anterior cruciate ligament. As determined by clinical and morphological studies. J Bone Joint Surg [Am] 56: 223-235

Kennedy JC, Stewart R, Walker D (1978) Anterolateral rotatory instability of the knee joint. An early analysis of the Ellison procedure. J Bone Joint Surg [Am] 60: 1031-1039

Losee RE, Johnson TR, Southwick WO (1978) Anterior subluxation of the lateral tibial plateau. A diagnostic test and operative repair. J Bone Joint Surg [Am] 60: 1015-1030

Markolf KL, Mensch JS, Amstutz HC (1976) Stiffness and laxity of the knee − The contributions of the supporting structures. A quantitative in vitro study. J Bone Joint Surg [Am] 58: 583-594

Markolf KL, Graff-Radford A, Amstutz HC (1978) In vivo knee stability. A quantitative assessment using an instrumented clinical testing apparatus. J Bone Joint Surg [Am] 60: 664-674

Markolf KL, Bargar WL, Shoemaker SC, Amstutz HC (1981) The role of joint load in knee stability. J Bone Joint Surg [Am] 63: 570-585

Markolf KL, Kochan A, Amstutz H (1984) Measurement of knee stiffness and laxity in patients with documented absence of the anterior cruciate ligament. J Bone Joint Surg [Am] 66: 242-253

Marshall JL, Girgis FG, Zelko RR (1972) The biceps femoris tendon and its functional significance. J Bone Joint Surg [Am] 54: 1444-1450

Müller We (1983) The knee. Form, function and ligament reconstruction. Springer, Berlin Heidelberg New York

Müller We, Biedert R, Hefti F, Jakob RP, Munzinger U, Stäubli H-U (1988) OAK Knee Evaluation. A new way to assess knee ligament injuries. Clin Orthop 232: 37-50

Nomina anatomica (1977) Fourth Edition. Excerpta Medica, Amsterdam Oxford 1977

Noyes FR, Grood ES (1988) Diagnosis of knee ligament injuries: Clinical concepts. In: Feagin JA jr (ed) The crucial ligaments. Churchill Livingstone, New York Edinburgh London Melbourne, pp 261-285

Noyes FR, Grood ES, Butler DL, Paulos LE (1980) Clinical biomechanics of the knee − Ligament restraints and functional stability. In: Funk FJ (ed) The American Academy of Orthopaedic Surgeons: Symposium on the Athlete's Knee. Surgical repair and reconstruction. Mosby, St. Louis, pp 1-35

Noyes FR, Grood ES, Torzilli P (1989) Current concepts review: The definitions of terms for motion and position of the knee and injuries of the ligaments. J Bone Joint Surg [Am] 71: 465-472

Salter RB, Simmonds DF, Malcolm BW et al. (1980) The biological effects of continuous passive motion on the healing of full thickness defects in articular cartilage. J Bone Joint Surg [Am] 62: 1232-1251

Segond P (1897) Recherches cliniques et expérimentales sur les épanchements sanguins du genou par entorse. Progres Med Paris 7: 379-381

Shoemaker SC, Markolf KL (1985) Effects of joint load on the stiffness and laxity of ligament-deficient knees. An in vitro study of the anterior cruciate and medial collateral ligaments. J Bone Joint Surg [Am] 67: 136-146

Stäubli H-U (1990) The limits of compartmental knee motion. Acta Orthop Scand [Suppl]: in press

Stäubli H-U, Birrer S (1990) The popliteus tendon and its fascicles at the popliteal hiatus. Gross anatomy and functional arthroscopic evaluation with and without anterior cruciate ligament deficiency. J Arthroscop Rel Surg Vol 6 Nr 3 209-220

Stäubli H-U, Jakob RP (1990) Posterior instability of the knee near extension. J Bone Joint Surg [Br] 72: 225-230

Torzilli PA (1986) Biomechanical analysis of knee stability. The lower extremity and spine in sports medicine, Vol. 1. Mosby, St. Louis

Torzilli PA, Greenberg RL, Insall J (1981) An in vivo biomechanical evaluation of anterior-posterior motion of the knee. Roentgenographic measurement technique, stress machine and stable population. J Bone Joint Surg [Am] 63: 960-968

Walker PS, Erkman MJ (1975) The role of the menisci in force transmission across the knee. Clin Orthop 109: 184-192

Wang CJ, Walker PA (1974) Rotatory laxity of the human knee joint. J Bone Joint Surg [Am] 56: 161-170

Webster's (1988) Ninth new collegiate dictionary. Merriam-Webster, Springfield MA

Wissenschaftliche Tabellen Geigy (1977) Einheiten im Meßwesen, Körperflüssigkeiten, Organe, Energiehaushalt, Ernährung, 8. Aufl. Basel, Ciba-Geigy

Historical and Current Perspectives in the Treatment of Anterior Cruciate Ligament Insufficiency

R. P. Jakob and J. P. Warner

Historical Perspectives

The treatment of anterior cruciate ligament (ACL) insufficiency continues to be a significant problem in orthopedic practice. Although the current problems are well known and have been identified, many questions remain unanswered. Major procedural differences and the contradictory results of many workers attest to the fact that there is still no general consensus regarding the natural history, management, and biomechanics of the knee with anterior instability. To appreciate the complexity of these problems, we must first understand the historical foundations laid by our predecessors. Otherwise we risk repeating previous mistakes or making "new" discoveries that actually are rediscoveries of previously known facts. A grasp of history is essential if we are to explore new areas in ACL surgery. A chronologic summary of historical milestones relating to the ACL and its injuries is presented in Table 1. Galen of Pergamum and Rome is credited with first describing the anatomy and nature of the ACL. Before Galen it was thought that the cruciate ligaments were part of the nervous system and had contractile properties. Galen developed the concept of these ligaments as static stabilizing structures that limit abnormal motion in diarthrotic joints. During the next 1600 years, scant attention was given to the knee ligaments except in descriptions of dislocations and severe sprains.

Stark, in 1850, was the first to describe a rupture of the ACL. He treated the injury by immobilizing the knee in plaster and subsequently found only slight residual disability. Battle (1900) published the first report of a repair of an acutely torn ACL. In 1903 Mayo Robson published an 8-year follow-up of a combined repair of the anterior and posterior cruciate ligaments. The patient, a miner, was able to return to work without significant disability. In 1913 Goetjes performed the first studies in cadaveric knees and investigated the mechanism of ACL rupture in 37 cases. He recommended examination under anesthesia when the diagnosis was in doubt, and he advocated the early surgical repair of acute ruptures. In

1917 Hey Groves published a case report describing an intraarticular reconstruction of the ACL using a strip of fascia lata. The strip was left attached to a distal pedicle and routed through a tibial tunnel. In 1919 he presented 14 additional cases in which the procedure was modified by detaching the fascia lata graft distally rather than proximally. This technique is thought to be the precursor of all modern intraarticular reconstructions.

In 1918 Alwyn Smith published an up-to-date review of the anatomy, biomechanics, mechanism, diagnosis, and treatment of ACL injuries. He modified the Hey Groves operation by pulling the graft medially through the medial femoral condyle to reinforce the medial collateral ligament, and by advancing the insertion of the sartorius muscle for extraarticular reinforcement. Unlike Hey Groves, Smith advocated reconstruction for chronic ruptures of the ACL. He also was the first to attempt reconstruction of the ligament using a silk band. Though it failed, this was the first attempt at prosthetic replacement. Jones and Smith, with their description of the "rocking knee" in 1913, provided early insight into the pathomechanics and diagnosis of ACL injuries. As quoted by Arnold et al. (1979), these authors also published the first description of the "pivot shift" phenomenon:

"... placing the hands on the joints, the femur seemed to be suddenly displaced inward, just before extension was completed, constituting the slipping of which the patient complained."

In 1920 Hey Groves published another description of the "giving way" phenomenon in the symptomatic ACL-deficient knee. Today this description is counted among the classic works of orthopedic literature.

Between 1919 and 1930, the procedures of arthroscopy and arthrography were introduced and technically refined. These procedures were to revolutionize the diagnosis and treatment of ACL pathology. The pioneers of these new methods were Eugen Bircher of Switzerland and Kenji Takagi of Japan. Takagi was the first to examine the interior of the knee with a cystoscope in 1918. However, the 7.3-mm caliber of

Table 1. Significant historical events relating to the anterior cruciate ligament

2nd century A.D.	Galen	First description of the anatomy and function of the anterior cruciate ligament (ACL)	1936, 1939	Campbell	First report on ACL reconstruction using the patellar tendon, and description of concomitant MCL injuries
1850	Stark	First description of ACL rupture	1934	Felsenreich	First German-language description of the pivot shift
1900	Battle	First report of ACL repair			
1903	Mayo Robson	8-year follow-up of repair	1936	Bosworth and Bosworth	Description of the first extra-articular reconstruction
1905	Werndorff and Robinson	First gas arthrogram of the knee	1937	Sommer	Use of the 3.1-mm arthroscope for examination and the 4.7-mm arthroscope for photography
1913	Goetjes	Cadaveric study of mechanism of ACL rupture			
1913	Jones and Smith	First description of the pivot shift phenomenon	1937	Cubbins, Callahan and Scuderi	Recommendation for immediate repair of the ruptured ACL
1917	Hey Groves	Case study of the first intra-articular ACL reconstruction	1938	Palmer	Publication of the dissertation *On the Injuries to Ligaments of the Knee Joint*
1918	Takagi	First examination of a cadaveric knee with a cystoscope			
1918	Alwyn Smith	General review of the anatomy, biomechanics, mechanisms, diagnosis and treatment of ACL injuries	1939	Wilke	Review of current arthroscopic technique (in German and English)
			1941	Brantigan and Voshell	Publication of "The mechanics of the ligaments of the knee joint"
1920	Hey Groves	Description of the clinical importance of the pivot shift	1950	O'Donoghue	Essay on the treatment of severe ligamentous knee injuries
1920	Bircher	Arthroscopy of the knee in vivo	1952	Augustine	Concept of "dynamic reconstruction" using the semitendinosus tendon
1921	Bircher	First publication on arthroscopy			
1922	Bircher	Essay on the pathology and treatment of meniscal injuries (20 knees)	1955	Watanabe	First arthroscopic knee operation (removal of a benign tumor)
1925	Kreuscher	First English-language work on knee arthroscopy	1962	Watanabe	First partial medial meniscectomy performed by arthroscopy
1930	Bircher and Oberholzer	Description of double-contrast artrography of the knee	1969	Watanabe, Takeda and Ikeuchi	Atlas of arthroscopic surgery
1931	Takagi, Watanabe, Takeda and Ikeuchi	First description of triangulation in arthroscopy	1967	Lemaire	First French-language description of the pivot shift phenomenon
1931	Burman, Finkelstein and Mayor	English-language work on arthroscopic technique	1972	Galway, Beaupr and MacIntosh	Classic description of the pivot shift phenomenon

the instrument made it too large for practical clinical use. In 1919 Bircher, working independently of Takagi, first experimented on cadaveric knees using the Jacobeus laparoscope, and this was soon followed by endoscopic examinations in patients. In his classic publication, the first on knee arthroscopy in general, Bircher described 13 correct diagnoses in 18 arthroscopically examined knees. The 13 diagnoses were later confirmed by open arthrotomy. In 1922 he praised the value of this technique:

"Arthroscopy permits us to visualize the interior of the joint and evaluate pathologic changes, and thus to establish a diagnosis by visual observation. In this respect it is superior to all other methods of examination and, like endoscopy of the bladder, can be used to define certain indications for surgery. Also like cystoscopy, it will meet with resistance but undoubtedly will

gain in popularity and develop until it becomes as indispensable as cystoscopy itself" (quoted in Henche and Holder 1988, p. 3).

Bircher's prophetic forecast was followed in 1925 by the first English-language description of arthroscopy by P.H. Kreuscher, and in 1930 by Bircher and Oberholzer's description of double-contrast arthrography. The triangulation technique of arthroscopic surgery was popularized by the Japanese surgeons Takagi, Watanabe, Takeda, and Ikeuchi.

Numerous case reports were published in the 1930s detailing various operative procedures for the treatment of ACL insufficiency. The first use of the patellar tendon to reconstruct the acutely ruptured ACL was described by Campbell in 1936 and in 1939. He also noted the relative frequency of associated tears of the medial collateral ligament and medial meniscus. In 1936 Bosworth and Bosworth described the first extraarticular reconstruction of the ACL using strips of fascia lata placed on the medial and lateral sides of the joint. Cubbins et al. concluded in 1937 that early surgical repair of the acutely torn ACL and reconstruction of a chronically deficient ligament would yield the best results. They also emphasized the need for at least one year's postoperative rehabilitation following such a procedure.

Before Ivar Palmer published his classic work *On the Injuries to the Ligaments of the Knee Joint*, studies in this area were limited to case reports and descriptions of new surgical techniques. Palmer's 282-page work, published in 1938, was a landmark in terms of deepening our understanding of ligamentous knee injuries. The nine chapters of the book set forth detailed clinical and experimental studies on the anatomy, biomechanics, diagnosis, and treatment of ACL injuries. Palmer designed a drill guide that was reproduced in many other countries.

Palmer's book also laid the groundwork for the classic paper "The mechanics of the ligaments and menisci of the knee joint," published by Brantigan and Voshell in 1941. This work dealt with the instabilities that developed following the systematic sectioning of various knee ligaments. The 1950s and 1960s marked the start of the modern era of cruciate ligament surgery. O'Donoghue's classic work (1950) was the first of a long series of scientific publications. O'Donoghue took a very optimistic stance toward the surgical treatment of cruciate ligament injuries. He presented the results of 22 knee injuries in athletes treated by ligament repair, and he stressed the advantages of early diagnosis and treatment. During this same period Watanabe perfected the use of the arthroscope for the surgical treatment of internal disruptions of the knee. In 1967 Lemaire published the first French-language description of the pivot shift, and in 1972 Galway et al. published a description of the phenomenon that is still considered valid today.

Current Perspectives

As Dye has pointed out, the human knee joint is the result of 400 million years of tetrapod evolution. The brief period of human investigation of this unique structure has been unable to provide definitive answers to questions relating to the form and function of the normal and disordered knee. Basic controversies persist regarding the pathologic anatomy, mechanics, natural history, diagnosis, and surgical treatment of the ACL-deficient knee.

The evolution of our "modern" understanding of ACL insufficiency began during the 38 years from Palmer's publication to the classification of knee instabilities published by Hughston in 1976. Hughston's study consisted of a correlation of clinical and intraoperative findings. In the early 1960s, O'Donoghue and Rockwood presented guidelines for the surgical treatment of acute cruciate ligament injuries and offered criteria for patient selection. This marked the start of a period of aggressive treatment for these injuries. The advent of arthroscopy led to the principle of the "aggressive diagnostic approach" to acute knee injuries. The concept of the "isolated tear of the ACL," first popularized by Feagin, was qualified by the frequent observation of concomitant intraarticular lesions by many examiners. This fact also promoted both the use of diagnostic arthroscopy and the treatment of ligamentous injuries.

The past few decades also have been marked by close cooperation between natural scientists and clinicians. By adopting precise terminology and technical terms from the engineering field, we have been able to define knee joint mobility more objectively and identify patterns of knee instability with greater precision. Even so, there are still many scientific publications in which terms such as "deceleration," "twist," "wrench," and "jump" are applied to knee injuries. Purely descriptive terms such as these make it difficult to compare clinical results for epidemiologic and pathomechanical analysis. Despite numerous clinical observations and extensive documentation on the pathomechanics of ACL insufficiency by various authors, questions and confusion remain.

Feagin's observation that it has been impossible in the past to identify athletes with an increased risk of ACL rupture remains true today. Without knowing the exact frequency with which ACL injuries occur, it is virtually impossible to define the "natural history" of untreated ACL insufficiency. Nevertheless, countless studies have attempted to present data on the course of this condition. Almost all of these studies were deficient in their methodology and design, however, especially in terms of divergent patient populations, variations in patient activity levels and compliance, and poorly comparable investigative and interpretive criteria. Feagin and Curl (1976) found in a retrospective study that rupture of the ACL can lead to a progressive deterioration of joint function. On the other hand, Chick and Jackson (1979) noted that 83% of their patients with minimal instability were able to resume full participation in sports after an average interval of 2.6 years. It should be emphasized, however, that their study focused on the activity level of each individual patient, and that their observation period was relatively short. Fetto and Marshall (1980) showed that the chronic course of recurrent giving-way episodes and periarticular changes was associated with progressive functional disability. Noyes et al. (1983a, b) showed in a prospective and retrospective study that ACL insufficiency has a high association with meniscal lesions and osteochondral defects. Departing from these somewhat pessimistic studies, McDaniel and Dameron (1980) reported good 10-year outcomes in 50 patients with untreated ruptures of the ACL. Seventy-two percent of these patients resumed strenuous athletic activity, and 47% could participate in sports with no limitations. But despite these optimistic findings, mild complaints persisted in 73% of cases, effusion was present in 58%, giving way in 43%, and radiographic signs of osteoarthritis in 73%. This underscores the fact that the resumption of athletic activity at the preinjury level is not a very good indicator of the patient's true functional status.

Published reports continue to differ with regard to indications for surgical treatment and the definition of functional disability in the deficient knee. Viewing the situation from a historical perspective, however, we can observe a marked change of attitude regarding the operative treatment of ACL insufficiency.

The initially strong trend toward immediate surgical repair of the ACL gave way to a somewhat nihilistic attitude as it was discovered that the operative treatment of tears was not always successful. The change to a more conservative approach was also motivated by confusion about the natural history of ACL insufficiency.

The poor correlation between the clinical features and functional stability of the operated and nonoperated knees added further to the confusion. Experimental and clinical data gave no indication that the "one-third rule" of Noyes for predicting outcomes could be improved: one-third of patients with ACL insufficiency will be able to compensate adequately and recover to athletic fitness, one-third will be able to compensate but must forego important activities, and the remaining third will develop complications and will probably have to undergo a reconstructive operation at some point in their life.

Nevertheless, a review of the current literature confirms the clinical experience that ACL insufficiency can produce significant functional disability, especially in young, active patients. Today the pendulum has swung back in favor of a more "aggressive" approach to these injuries. This has been due in part to progress in arthroscopic techniques, materials for ligament reconstruction, and other technical advances.

In 1979 Feagin characterized as "disastrous" the rush to market prosthetic replacements for the ACL. Today we know that the future of ACL surgery rests to a degree on the development of such materials, but that this must be paralleled by advances in the use of autologous and homologous grafts. Key questions remain to be answered regarding long-term wear and material fatigue in prosthetic cruciate ligaments.

Other important questions relate to rehabilitation and the use of splints and braces. What rehabilitation method is best for operatively and nonoperatively treated cases? What are the prophylactic and therapeutic benefits of bracing? Although a relatively greater degree of rolling and gliding occurs in the lateral knee compartment than medially, there is still no bracing device on the market whose design allows for this physiologic asymmetry.

The future will no doubt clarify and resolve many of these critical points. A more uniform method and "language" for the documentation of clinical results based on standardized criteria of functional disability will bring about a better understanding of the natural history of ACL insufficiency. Technical advances involving improved surgical fixation techniques, improved tensioning of the graft at operation, better graft selection and augmentation, more appropriate patient selection, and clearer guidelines for postoperative splinting and bracing and the conduct of postoperative physical therapy will do much to lower the morbidity of operatively and nonoperatively treated knees with ACL insufficiency.

References

Alm A, Ekström H, Gillquist J (1974) The anterior cruciate ligament. A clinical and experimental study on tensile strength, morphology, and replacement by patellar ligament. Acta Chir Scand [Suppl 445]

Alwyn Smith S (1918) The diagnosis and treatment of injuries to the crucial ligaments. Br J Surg 6: 176–189

Andrish JT, Wood CD (1984) Dacron augmentation in anterior cruciate ligament reconstruction in dogs. Clin Orthop 183: 298–302

Arnoczky SP, Warren RF, Minei JP (1985) Replacement of the anterior cruciate ligament using a synthetic prosthesis. An evaluation of graft biology in the dog. Am J Sports Med 14: 1–6

Arnoczky SP, Torzilli PA, Warren RF, Allen AA (1988) Biologic fixation of ligament prosthesis and augmentation. Am J Sports Med 16/2: 106–112

Arnold JA, Coker TP, Heaton LM et al. (1979) Natural history of anterior cruciate ligament tears. Am J Sports Med 7: 305–313

Augustine RW (1956) The unstable knee. Am J Surg 92: 380-388

Bach BR, Warren RF, Wickiewicz TL (1988) The pivot shift phenomenon: results and description of a modified clinical test for anterior cruciate ligament insufficiency. Am J Sports Med 16/6: 571-576

Battle WH (1900) A case after open section of the knee joint for irreducible traumatic dislocation. Clin Soc Lond Trans 33: 232-233

Bircher E (1921) Die Arthroendoskopie. Zentralbl Chir 48: 1460-1461

Bircher E (1922) Beitrag zur Pathologie und Diagnose der Meniscus-Verletzungen. Bruns Beitr Klin Chir 127: 239-250

Bosworth DM, Bosworth BM (1936) Use of fascia lata to stabilize the knee in cases of ruptured crucial ligaments. J Bone Joint Surg [Am] 18: 178-179

Brantigan OC, Voshell AF (1941) The mechanics of the ligaments and menisci of the knee joint. J Bone Joint Surg 23: 44

Burman MS, Finkelstein H, Mayer L (1934) Arthroscopy of the knee-joint. J Bone Joint Surg 16: 255-268

Campbell WC (1936) Repair of the ligaments of the knee joint. Surg Gynecol Obstet 62: 964-968

Campbell WC (1939) Reconstruction of the ligaments of the knee. Am J Surg 43: 473-480

Cerabona F, Sherman MF, Bonamo JR, Sklar J (1988) Patterns of meniscal injury with acute anterior cruciate ligament tears. Am J Sports Med 16/6: 603-609

Chick RR, Jackson AW (1979) Tears of the anterior cruciate ligament in young athletes. J Bone Joint Surg [Am] 60: 970

Clancy WG, Nelson DA, Reider B et al. (1982) Anterior cruciate ligament reconstruction using one-third of the patellar ligament, augmented by extraarticular tendon transfers. J Bone Joint Surg [Am] 67: 352-359

Cubbins WR, Callahan JJ, Scuderi CS (1937) Cruciate ligament injuries. Surg Gynecol Obstet 64: 218-225

Daniel D, Biden EN (1987) The language of knee motion. In: Jackson DW, Drez D (eds) The anterior cruciate deficient knee. Mosby, St Louis, pp 1-16

DeHaven KE (1980) Diagnosis of acute knee injuries with hemarthrosis. Am J Sports Med 8: 9-14

Dye SF (1988) An evolutionary perspective. In: Feagin JA (ed) The crucial ligaments. Diagnosis and treatment of ligamentous injuries about the knee. Churchill Livingstone, New York, pp 161-172

Eriksson E (1983) Ivar Palmer. A great name in the history of cruciate ligament surgery. Clin Orthop 172: 4-13

Feagin JA (1979) The syndrome of the torn anterior cruciate ligament. Orthop Clin North Am 10/1: 81-91

Feagin JA, Curl WW (1976) Isolated tear of the anterior cruciate ligament: 5-year follow up study. Am J Sports Med 4: 95-100

Feagin JA, Abbott HG, Rokus JR (1972) The isolated tear of the anterior cruciate ligament. J Bone Joint Surg [Am] 54: 1370

Felsenreich F (1937) Klinik der Kreuzbandverletzungen. Arch Klin Chir 179: 375-408

Fetto JF, Marshall JL (1980) The natural history and diagnosis of anterior cruciate ligament insufficiency. Clin Orthop 147: 29

Freiberger RH, Kaye JJ, Spiller J (1979) Arthrography. Appleton-Century-Crofts, New York

Galen C (1968) On the usefulness of parts of the body. May MT (trans). Cornell University Press, Ithaca/NY

Galway HR, Beaupré A, MacIntosh DL (1972) Pivot shift. A clinical sign of anterior cruciate ligament instability. J Bone Joint Surg [Br] 54: 763

Garrick JG (1988) Epidemiology of the ACL. In: Feagin JA (ed) The crucial ligaments. Diagnosis and treatment of ligamentous injuries about the knee. Churchill Livingstone, New York, pp 173-176

Gillquist J, Hagberg G, Oretorp N (1977) Arthroscopy in acute injuries of the knee joint. Acta Orthop Scand 48: 190-196

Girgis FG, Marshall JC, Monajem AL (1975) The cruciate ligaments of the knee joint. Anatomical, functional and experimental analysis. Clin Orthop 106: 216-231

Goetjes H (1913) Über Verletzungen der Ligamenta cruciata des Kniegelenks. Dtsch Z Chir 123: 221-289

Goodfellow J, O'Connor J (1978) The mechanics of the knee and prosthetic design. J Bone Joint Surg [Br] 60: 358-369

Grona WA, Muse G (1988) The effect of exercise on laxity in the anterior cruciate deficient knee. Am J Sports Med 16/6: 586-588

Harter RA, Osternig LR, Singer KM, James SL, Larson RC, James DC (1988) Long-term evaluation of knee stability and function following surgical reconstruction for anterior cruciate ligament insufficiency. Am J Sports Med 16/8: 434-443

Henche HR, Holder J (1985) Arthroskopie des Kniegelenks, 2. Aufl. Springer, Berlin Heidelberg New York

Hey Groves EW (1920) The crucial ligaments of the knee joint. Their function, rupture, and the operative treatment of the same. Br J Surg 7: 505-515

Hobson D, Torfason L (1974) Optimization of the four-bar knee mechanism — a computerized approach. J Biomech 7: 371-376

Hughston JC, Andrews JR, Gross MJ et al. (1976) Classification of knee ligament instability. Parts I and II. J Bone Joint Surg [Am] 58: 159-179

Jakob RP (1987) Pathomechanical and clinical concepts of the pivot shift sign. Semin Orthop 2/1: 9-17

Jakob RP, Stäubli H-U, Deland JT (1987) Grading the pivot shift. Objective tests with implications for treatment. J Bone Joint Surg [Br] 69: 294-299

Jones R, Smith A (1913) On rupture of the crucial ligaments of the knee and on fractures of the spine of the tibia. Br J Surg 1: 70-89

Kain CC, McCarthy JA, Arms S, Pope MA, Steadman RJ, Manske PR, Shively RA (1988) An in vivo analysis of the effect of transcutaneous electrical stimulation of the quadriceps and hamstrings on anterior cruciate ligament deformation. Am J Sports Med 16/2: 147-152

Kannus P, Jarvinen M (1987) Conservatively treated tear of the anterior cruciate ligament. J Bone Joint Surg [Am] 69: 1007-1011

Kennedy JC, Weinberg HW, Wilson AS (1976) The anatomy and function of the anterior cruciate ligament as determined by clinical and morphological studies. J Bone Joint Surg [Am] 56: 223-235

Kornblatt I, Warren RF, Wickiewicz TL (1988) Long-term follow up of anterior cruciate ligament reconstruction using the quadriceps tendon substitute for chronic anterior cruciate ligament insufficiency. Am J Sports Med 16/5: 444-448

Kreuscher PH (1925) Semilunar cartilage disease. A plea for early recognition by means of the arthroscope and early treatment of this condition. Int Med J 47: 290-292

Lemaire M (1967) Ruptures anciennes du ligament croisé antérieur du genou. J Chir (Paris) 93: 311-320

Lynch MA, Henning CE, Glick KR Jr (1983) Knee joint surface changes: long-term follow up of meniscus-tear treatments in stable anterior cruciate ligament reconstructions. Clin Orthop 172: 148-153

Mayo Robson AW (1903) Ruptured crucial ligaments and their repair by operation. Ann Surg 37: 716-718

McDaniel WJ Jr, Dameron JB Jr (1980) Untreated rupture of the anterior cruciate ligament. A follow up study. J Bone Joint Surg [Am] 62: 696

McPherson GK, Mendenhall HV, Gibbons DF et al. (1985) Experimental mechanical and histological evaluation of the Kennedy ligament augmentation. Clin Orthop 196: 186-195

Noyes FR, Grood ES (1976) The strength of the anterior cruciate ligament in humans and rhesus monkeys. Age-related and species-related changes. J Bone Joint Surg [Am] 58: 1074-1082

Noyes FR, McGinnes GH (1985) Controversy about treatment of the knee with anterior cruciate laxity. Clin Orthop 198: 61-76

Noyes FR, Bassett RW, Grood ES et al. (1980a) Arthroscopy in acute traumatic hemarthrosis of the knee: incidence of anterior cruciate tear and other injuries. J Bone Joint Surg [Am] 6: 687-695

Noyes FR, Grood ES, Butler DL, Malick M (1980b) Clinical laxity tests and functional stability of the knee. Biomechanical concepts. Clin Orthop 196: 84-89

Noyes FR, Matthews DS, Movar PA (1983a) The symptomatic anterior cruciate deficient knee. Part II: The results of rehabilitation, activity modification, and counseling on functional disability. J Bone Joint Surg [Am] 65: 163-174

Noyes FR, Movar PA, Mathews DS, Butler DL (1983b) The symptomatic anterior cruciate-deficient knee. Part I: The long term functional disability in athletically active individuals. J Bone Joint Surg [Am] 65: 154-162

Noyes FR, Butler DL, Grood ES, Zernicke RF, Hefzy M (1984) Biomechanical analysis of human ligament grafts used in knee-ligament repair and reconstruction. J Bone Joint Surg [Am] 66: 344-352

Odensten M, Tegnér Y, Lysholm J, Gillquist J (1983) Knee function and muscle strength following distal iliotibial band transfer for anterolateral rotary instability. Acta Orthop Scand 54: 924

Odensten M, Hamberg P, Nordin M, Lysholm J, Gillquist J (1985) Surgical or conservative treatment of the acutely torn anterior cruciate ligament. Clin Orthop 198: 87-93

O'Donoghue DH (1950) Surgical treatment of fresh injuries to the major ligaments of the knee. J Bone Joint Surg [Am] 32: 721-738

O'Donoghue DH (1977) An analysis of end results of surgical treatment of major injuries to the ligaments of the knee. J Bone Joint Surg [Am] 37: 1-13

O'Donoghue DH, Rockwood CA, Frank GR et al. (1966) Repair of the anterior cruciate ligament in dogs. II. J Bone Joint Surg [Am] 48: 503-519

Palmer I (1938) On the injuries to the ligaments of the knee joint. A clinical study. Acta Chir Scand 81 [Suppl 53]: 2-282

Paulos LE, France PE, Rosenberg TD, Jayaraman G, Abbott PJ, Jean J (1987) The biomechanics of lateral knee bracing. Parts I and II. Am J Sports Med 15: 419-439

Schutte MT, Dabazies EJ, Zimny ML, Happel LT (1987) Neural anatomy of the human anterior cruciate ligament. J Bone Joint Surg [Am] 69: 243-247

Snook GA (1988) The ACL: a historical review. In: Feagin JA (ed) The crucial ligaments. Diagnosis and treatment of ligamentous injuries about the knee. Churchill Livingstone, New York, pp 157-161

Solonen KA, Rokkanen P (1967) Operative treatment of torn ligaments in injuries to the knee joint. Acta Orthop Scand 38: 67

Sommer R (1937) Die Endoskopie des Kniegelenkes. Zentralbl Chir 64: 1692-1697

Stark J (1850) Two cases of ruptured crucial ligaments of the knee-joint. Edinb Med Soc 74: 267-271

Steadman JR (1983) Rehabilitation of acute injuries of the anterior cruciate ligament. Clin Orthop 172: 129-132

Tim KE (1988) Postsurgical knee rehabilitation. A five year study of four methods and 5381 patients. Am J Sports Med 16/5: 463-468

Turner NP, Turner IG, Jones CB (1987) Prosthetic anterior cruciate ligaments in the rabbit — a comparison of four types of replacement. J Bone Joint Surg [Br] 69: 312-316

Warren RF, Levy IM (1983) Meniscal lesions associated with anterior cruciate ligament injury. Clin Orthop 172: 32-37

Watanabe M, Takeda S, Ikeuchi H (1969) Atlas of arthroscopy, 2nd edn. Igako-Shoin, Tokyo

Wilke KH (1939) Endoskopie des Kniegelenkes an der Leiche. Bruns Beitr Klin Chir 169: 75-83

Wood GW (1985) Synthetics in anterior cruciate ligament reconstruction: a review. Orthop Clin North Am 16: 227-235

Anatomy and Biomechanics

Surgical Anatomy of the Knee Joint

E. B. Hunziker, H.-U. Stäubli, and R. P. Jakob

The knee is a trochoginglymoid joint that derives its physiologic joint play and its typical rolling-gliding mechanism of flexion and extension from its six degrees of freedom – three in translation and three in rotation. The translations of the knee take place on the anterior-posterior, medial-lateral, and proximal-distal (compression-distraction) axes. The rotational motions consist of flexion-extension, internal-external rotation, and abduction-adduction.

The knee joint derives its functional stability (1) from the three-dimensional geometry of the opposing articular surfaces of the distal femur and proximal tibia and (2) from the passive restraining action of the ligaments and meniscocapsular structures and the active restraining forces exerted by the musculotendinous units. Even when the cruciate ligaments are intact, the knee joint has a certain "play" determined by the constitutional quality of the ligaments and the three-dimensional configuration of the articular surfaces.

Generally, a translational motion of the knee is associated with some degree of rotation, and vice-versa. This "coupled motion" occurs, for example, when an anterior force is applied to a knee in 10° of flexion, producing a combined anterior translation (parallel anterior glide of the medial and lateral tibial plateaus) and internal rotation as the lateral tibial plateau moves farther forward, by several millimeters, than the medial plateau. Conversely, a posterior force (on a knee with an intact posterior cruciate ligament) produces a combined posterior translation and external rotation of the tibia with respect to the femur.

This physiologic joint play, consisting of coupled translation and rotation, depends on the angle of knee flexion. In the fully extended knee that has completed automatic terminal rotation, the tibia and femur are locked in place. When flexion is initiated, the joint becomes unlocked. As flexion proceeds, the degrees of rotational freedom increase, explaining why data on degrees of rotation are clinically important only when considered in relation to a known flexion angle.

Valgus-varus (abducting-adducting) forces act in the coronal plane. Normally, the fully extended knee joint cannot be opened by either a varus or valgus force. As the knee is progressively flexed, the degrees of freedom for varus and valgus motion increase. With the knee in 20° of flexion, a slight degree of valgus mobility (medial joint opening) can be demonstrated when the medial capsule and ligaments are intact. This valgus displacement at 20° flexion is a coupled motion consisting of abduction, medial distraction, lateral compression, and slight lateral translation of the tibia with respect to the femur. Additionally, this valgus motion can be tested in various positions of rotation, i.e., in neutral, internal, and external rotation.

The same considerations apply to varus testing in extension, which generally will not elicit lateral joint opening in the intact knee. An exception to this rule is genu varum, where 4–5 mm of varus opening can normally be demonstrated at 20° of knee flexion. Multiple degrees of freedom are involved in varus motion: adduction, medial compression, lateral distraction, medial translation, and a variable amount of internal or external rotation depending on the flexion angle.

If we now try to analyze the complex joint play of the knee and its coupled motions, we can measure the following normal ranges of motion starting from the neutral position. The physiologic range of knee flexion-extension is generally 10°-0°-145°. Internal and external knee rotation are flexion-dependent and are more constrained near extension than at higher flexion angles. Internal, neutral, and external rotation are stated in degrees as follows: The normal range of internal or external rotation in 20° of flexion is 15°-0°-35°. The physiologic degrees of freedom of knee motion are numerous and are generally coupled. The normal ranges of motion as well as the increased ranges of motion seen in pathologic states depend on the structural and functional integrity of the active and passive restraints and their compliance. The three-dimensional geometry of the bony elements and the configuration of the femoral condyles, of the tibial plateau with its pivot-like intercondylar tubercles, and of the patella, which is integrated into the extensor apparatus, act in concert with the intact capsuloligamentous apparatus, the menisci, and active muscular tension to guarantee the functional stability of the knee joint.

To facilitate a systematic description of the structural elements of the knee, it is convenient to divide the joint into four compartments. This division has proved to be very useful in clinical knee arthroscopy (Fig. 1): The medial compartment consists of the medial femoral condyle, the medial tibial plateau, the medial meniscus, and the medial capsule and ligaments. The lateral compartment consists of the lateral femoral condyle, the lateral tibial plateau, the lateral meniscus, and the lateral capsule and ligaments including the arcuate complex. The central compartment or "central pivot" encompasses the intercondylar notch, which contains the cruciate ligaments, the anterior and posterior intercondylar areas of the tibia (the distal sites of insertion of the cruciate ligaments), and the intercondylar eminences and tubercles. The femoropatellar compartment consists of the femoropatellar joint, the infrapatellar fat pad, the patellar ligament and quadriceps tendon, and the normally present medial and lateral patellar plicae and suprapatellar pouch.

The Medial Compartment

The medial compartment is subdivided into an anterior, middle, and posterior third (see Fig. 1).

Anterior Third

Overlying the joint capsule in the anterior third of the medial compartment is the vastus medialis muscle with its (almost) horizontal portion, the vastus medialis obliquus (Fig. 2), which exerts tension on the patella via the medial patellar retinaculum. Located about the medial patellar retinaculum are the origins of the medial longitudinal patellar retinaculum, which arises broadly between the patella, vastus medialis, and proximal attachment of the medial collateral ligament and passes distally to the upper tibia, where it inserts posterior to the pes anserinus and anterior and proximal to the attachment of the medial collateral ligament (Figs. 2, 3).

The insertion of the pes anserinus runs obliquely downward and backward on the anterior third of the tibia. The distal part of the medial longitudinal patellar retinaculum, close to the pes anserinus insertion, appears narrower than its fanlike origin (see Fig. 2). The fibers of both retinacula bridge the anterior portions of the joint. The origins of both include sheetlike fibers arising from the vastus medialis fascia and quadriceps tendon. This arrangement "dynamizes" (dynamically stabilizes) the retinacula, enabling them to function as active restraints in the anteromedial quadrant of the knee. Some fibers of the medial longitudinal patellar retinaculum originate in the medial collateral ligament, where they cannot be clearly distinguished from the fibers of that ligament.

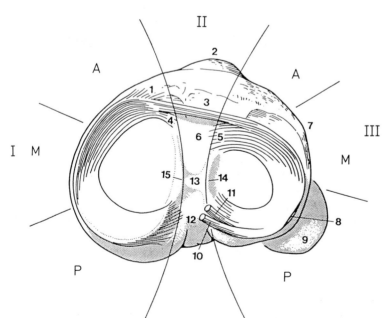

Fig. 1. Knee joint. Superior aspect of the tibial plateau and menisci

I Medial compartment with anterior (A), middle (M), and posterior third (P)
II Central pivot
III Lateral compartment with anterior (A), middle (M), and posterior third (P)
1 Anterodistal attachment of medial meniscus
2 Tibial tuberosity
3 Transverse ligament of the knee
4 Anterolateral attachment of medial meniscus in anterior intercondylar area
5 Anteromedial attachment of lateral meniscus in anterior intercondylar area
6 Anterior intercondylar area
7 Tubercle of Gerdy
8 Depression on meniscal border for popliteus tendon
9 Fibula
10 Posterior meniscofemoral ligament (of Wrisberg)
11 Anterior meniscofemoral ligament (of Humphry)
12 Posterior intercondylar area
13 Intercondylar eminence
14 Lateral intercondylar tubercle
15 Medial intercondylar tubercle

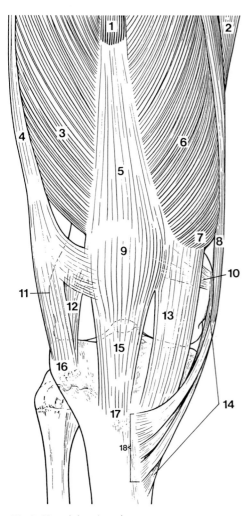

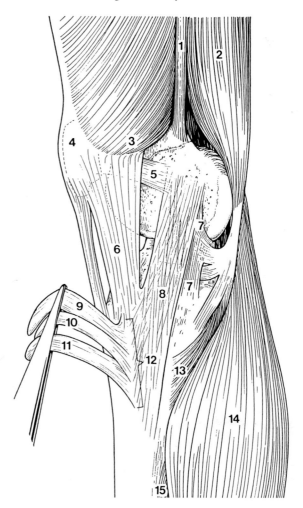

Fig. 2. Knee joint. Anterior aspect

 1 Rectus femoris muscle
 2 Gracilis muscle
 3 Vastus lateralis muscle
 4 Iliotibial tract
 5 Quadriceps tendon
 6 Vastus medialis muscle
 7 Vastus medialis obliquus muscle
 8 Sartorius muscle
 9 Patella
10 Medial patellar retinaculum
11 Lateral femoral epicondyle
12 Lateral longitudinal patellar retinaculum
13 Medial longitudinal patellar retinaculum
14 Medial collateral ligament
15 Patellar ligament
16 Tubercle of Gerdy
17 Tibial tuberosity
18 Pes anserinus

Fig. 3. Knee joint. Medial aspect

 1 Tendon of adductor magnus muscle
 2 Semimembranosus muscle
 3 Vastus medialis obliquus muscle
 4 Patella
 5 Medial transverse patellar retinaculum
 6 Medial longitudinal patellar retinaculum
 7 Posterior oblique ligament
 8 Medial collateral ligament
 9 Sartorius tendon
10 Gracilis tendon
11 Semitendinosus tendon
12 Pes anserinus
13 Popliteus muscle
14 Gastrocnemius muscle, medial head
15 Soleus muscle

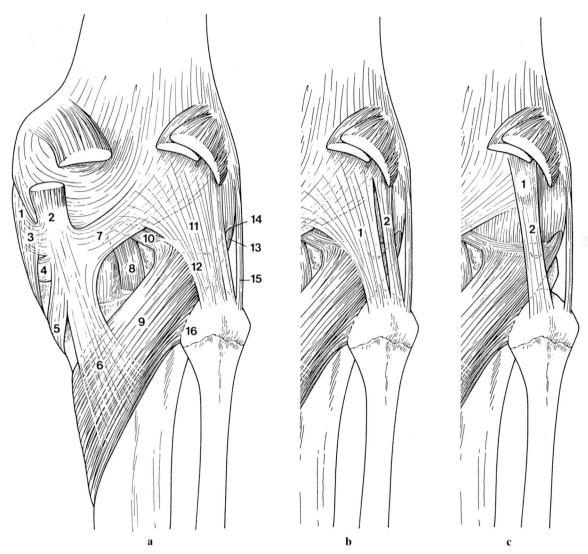

Fig. 4a–c. Knee joint. Posterior aspect

a *1* Posterior oblique ligament
2 Semimembranosus tendon
3 Semimembranosus tendon fibers inserting on the posterior oblique ligament
4 Pars reflexa of semimembranosus tendon
5 Semimembranosus tendon fibers inserting on the posteromedial tibia
6 Semimembranosus tendon fibers attached to the aponeurosis of the popliteus muscle
7 Semimembranosus tendon fibers attached to the oblique popliteal ligament
8 Posterior cruciate ligament
9 Popliteus muscle

10 Posterior meniscofemoral ligament
11 Arcuate popliteal ligament
12 Partial insertion of popliteus muscle on the arcuate popliteal ligament
13 Popliteus tendon (to lateral femoral condyle)
14 Popliteal hiatus
15 Lateral collateral ligament
16 Popliteus fibers inserting on the fibular head

b, c Variants of the arcuate popliteal ligament
b *1* Arcuate popliteal ligament
2 Short lateral collaeral ligament

c *1* Fabella
2 "Peroneofabellar" ligament of Vallois (fabellofibular ligament)

Fibers of this retinaculum also run posteriorly into superficial fascial layers, where they unite with pes anserinus tendons and then continue as a common sheath into the popliteal fasciae. Because of this arrangement, the retinaculum is additionally dynamized to a degree by the pes anserinus group. Finally, deep fibers of the medial longitudinal patellar retinaculum run posteriorly beneath the superficial fascia to enter the medial collateral ligament, some of the posterior fibers continuing on to blend with the semimembranosus tendon (Fig. 4). Thus the semimembranosus muscle likewise contributes to dynamizing the medial longitudinal patellar retinaculum, especially in the flexed knee. Both medial patellar retinacula also play a major role in the control of patellar tracking on the femur (avoidance of lateral deviation), the equalization of compressive stresses between the lateral and medial patellar surfaces, and the internal rotation of the tibia (via the vastus medialis obliquus and the patellar ligament).

The tendons of insertion of the pes anserinus (Figs. 2, 3; sartorius, gracilis, semitendinosus) exert a ligament-protecting action on the medial side of the joint in both flexion and extension owing to their superficial course. The pes anserinus is also an important muscle-controlled stabilizer of the medial side. Functionally, it represents a kind of active duplication of the medial collateral ligament.

Middle Third

In the middle third of the medial compartment (see Fig. 1), the medial collateral ligament is the dominant restraining structure deep to the tendinous layer of the pes anserinus group. The middle-third medial ligamentous elements of the "second layer" are more difficult to identify as separate structures than on the lateral side. This applies very much to the lateral expansions of the medial collateral ligament but not to the relation of the second layer to the third, next deeper layer, where the deep portion of the medial collateral ligament is structurally distinct from its superficial portion. The deep portion consists largely of femoromeniscal and meniscotibial fibers (i. e., the coronary ligament, in addition to direct femorotibial fibers; Fig. 5). Thus, the superficial layer of the medial collateral ligament is structurally separate from the medial meniscus and has no connection with it. This situation does not change until the posterior margin of the ligament, where its superficial and deep layers unite to form the posterior oblique ligament ("posterior medial collateral ligament").

The posterior oblique ligament is firmly attached to

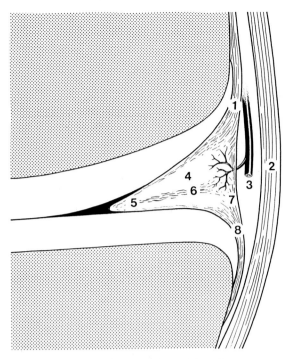

Fig. 5. Coronal section through the medial meniscus

1 Meniscofemoral fibers
2 Medial collateral ligament (superficial portion)
3 Blood vessels in the connective-tissue space between the meniscus and collateral ligament
4 Medial meniscus
5 Inner zone: hyaline cartilage
6 Middle zone: fibrocartilage, some hyaline cartilage centrally
7 Peripheral zone: stiff, fibrous connective tissue
8 Meniscotibial fibers

the posterior horn of the medial meniscus (see below and Figs. 2, 3).

The medial collateral ligament courses obliquely forward and downward from the distal femur to the proximal tibia (see Fig. 3). Its line of origin on the medial femoral condyle has a similar proximal-posterior to distal-anterior orientation. This is opposite to its oblique downward-and-backward line of insertion on the proximal tibia. The medial longitudinal patellar retinaculum and pes anserinus insert just anterior to the medial collateral ligament, paralleling its line of attachment.

The fiber structure of the medial collateral ligament shows a crossed arrangement that subdivides the ligament into "triangles." This causes portions of its fibers to come selectively under tension according to the position of the knee. (In internal rotation, for example, the posterior fibers of the triangles are taut, so it is normal for local variations of fiber tension to occur within the ligament.) This fiber arrangement "smooths out" changing forces such that, for example, the longest fibers are tense during flexion, whereas the shortest fibers are tense during extension. All the fibers are lax in moderate flexion, allowing for increased rotatory movements of the knee in that position.

Dividing the medial collateral ligament into thirds, it will be noted that its proximal third overlies the femur while its distal third overlies the proximal tibia. During flexion, which begins with a rolling motion of the femoral condyle, the anterior fibers move posteriorly over the femoral and tibial surfaces. Thus the ligament must be freely mobile in these regions (and over the medial meniscus) so that it can glide over the bony surfaces, and it must have no attachments with the deep layer.

The superficial fiber layers unite posteriorly with the deep fibers to form the posterior oblique ligament, which also receives an expansion from the semimembranosus tendon. Accordingly, superficial portions of the ligament are dynamized by the semimembranosus muscle, especially in positions of flexion. Other fiber attachments with the adductor magnus fascia and tendon contribute further to the "dynamization" of the medial collateral ligament. The connections with the vastus medialis muscle, chiefly via the medial longitudinal patella retinaculum, were mentioned previously. Passive, rigid attachments from bone to bone are found in the deeper portions of the ligament. Owing to the large proportion of dynamized superficial fibers, passive instabilities can be satisfactorily compensated by good muscular function. They also constitute a fiber population that can adapt to high-demand, high-performance situations.

Posterior Third

In the posterior third of the medial compartment (see Fig. 1), the fibers of the medial collateral ligament unite with those of the coronary ligament – i.e., the femoromeniscal and femorotibial fibers of the third layer – at the level of the posterior horn of the meniscus. Their union forms the posterior oblique ligament, which descends posteriorly from the medial femoral condyle to the posterior horn of the medial meniscus and thence to the upper tibia. The posterior oblique ligament is one component of the posteromedial corner of the knee, and thus part of the "semimembranosus corner," a functionally vital region that is quite distinct from the medial collateral ligament despite their close topographic relationship.

The posterior oblique ligament courses between the adductor magnus tendon and semimembranosus tendon. Structurally and functionally, it constitutes the key element of the semimembranosus corner. The semimembranosus muscle attaches to the posteromedial corner by five separate arms (Fig. 4). The first arm passes directly to the posterior oblique ligament (3 in Fig. 4a). The second arm ascends diagonally across the posterior capsule as the oblique popliteal ligament (7 in Fig. 4a), terminating laterally at the fabella or a corresponding site (see Fig. 4). Both of these insertions, which blend with the posteromedial capsule, make the semimembranous muscle the active stabilizer of the posteromedial corner. A third arm, the pars reflexa (4 in Fig. 4a), passes forward beneath the medial collateral ligament to the tibia, exerting a direct pull in flexion. A fourth arm inserts directly on the posteromedial aspect of the tibia (5 in Fig. 4a). A fifth and final expansion from the semimembranosus tendon blends with the aponeurosis of the popliteus muscle (6 in Fig. 4a). The five arms are distributed in such a way that at least one is tense in each position of flexion, applying traction in a direction that is appropriate for the given flexion angle. Superficial to the medial collateral ligament and posterior oblique ligament is a thin fiber layer that runs posteriorly and is dynamized by the vastus medialis. However, the principal dynamizing muscle of the medial corner is the semimembranosus, which stabilizes the knee posteromedially. The knee is stabilized anteromedially by an analogous arrangement in which the medial longitudinal retinaculum is dynamized by the vastus medialis. During the "screw home" mechanism in terminal extension, the semimembranosus corner is under maximal tension due to the associated posteromedial glide of the medial femoral condyle. In extension the semimembranosus muscle can expand its field of action and help to stabilize the entire medial side. In 90° of flexion, where its fibers pass from the tibia at a 90° angle, the semimembranosus performs the accessory functions of transmitting tension to loose capsuloligamentous fibers and stabilizing the knee against external rotation.

A structural element of the medial compartment that extends from the anterior to the posterior third is the medial meniscus (Figs. 1, 6). The medial meniscus appears relatively narrow in its anterior third. It attaches to the tibial plateau by a fiber bundle that projects anteriorly from the meniscus, and there is also a medial slip that anchors the anterolateral part of the meniscus to the anterior intercondylar area (see Fig. 1). The transverse ligament of the knee forms a fibrous bridge linking the anterior horns of the medial and lateral menisci (see Fig. 1). The medial patellomeniscal ligament passes from the anterior border of the medial meniscus to the patella. The meniscus is

Fig. 6. Knee joint. Superior aspect with intact capsule, muscles, and ligaments

1 Subcutaneous (subfascial) prepatellar bursa
2 Patella
3 Infrapatellar fat pad
4 Lateral collateral ligament
5 Popliteus tendon
6 Lateral meniscus
7 Biceps femoris muscle
8 Gastrocnemius muscle, lateral head
9 Plantaris longus muscle
10 Popliteal artery
11 Popliteal vein
12 Tibial nerve
13 Sural artery
14 Short saphenous vein
15 Sural nerve
16 Gastrocnemius muscle, medial head
17 Semitendinosus muscle
18 Semimembranosus muscle
19 Gracilis muscle
20 Sartorius muscle
21 Medial meniscus
22 Synovial membrane
23 Posterior meniscofemoral ligament
    (of Wrisberg)
24 Posterior cruciate ligament
25 Anterior meniscofemoral ligament
    (of Humphry)
26 Anterior cruciate ligament
27 Infrapatellar synovial plica
28 Alar plicae

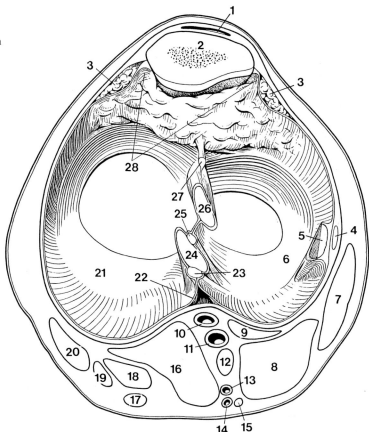

still quite narrow in the middle third of the medial compartment. At its outer border it has fibrous attachments with the femur (femoromeniscal fibers) and with the tibia (coronary ligament, see Fig. 5), but it has no attachments with the medial collateral ligament. In the posterior third of the medial compartment, the meniscus widens greatly toward the posterior horn. The femoromeniscal fibers and coronary ligament unite with the posterior oblique ligament, anchoring the posterior horn to that ligament. Fibers at the distal end of the posterior horn anchor it to the posterior intercondylar area. The posterior horn must be very strongly attached to the coronary ligament and anteromedial collateral ligament so that it can contribute to anteroposterior stability and perform its essential function as a site for the redirection of stress transfer ("braking wedge" to check anterior tibial displacement and posterior displacement of the femur). The posterior horn of the medial meniscus can function as a braking wedge only if the femoromeniscal portion of the posterior oblique ligament and the posterior horn itself are intact (so that the femoral condyle can ride upon it), and the semimembranosus attachment is undamaged (to preserve anteromedial rotatory stability). The anterior cruciate ligament (ACL) functions synergistically with the posterior oblique ligament, both coming under tension with anterior displacement of the tibia. Approximately 80% of ACL tears are associated with lesions of the medial ligaments (posterior oblique ligament, medial collateral ligament).

The Lateral Compartment

The lateral compartment of the knee (see Fig. 1) has a generally greater muscular stabilization than that on the medial side, but the passive restraints are less well developed. The relative predominance of dynamized structures relates to the large displacements that can occur on the lateral side during flexion (biceps, popliteus, tensor fasciae latae). As on the medial side, we subdivide the lateral compartment structurally into an anterior, middle, and posterior third (see Fig. 1). These regions will be discussed in that order.

Anterior Third

As in the medial compartment, the anterior third of the lateral compartment features a superficial lateral patellar retinaculum and lateral longitudinal patellar retinaculum (see Fig. 2). However, the vastus lateralis muscle does not extend as far distally as does the horizontal portion of the vastus medialis (vastus medialis obliquus). Thus, the origin of the lateral longitudinal patellar retinaculum is somewhat different from its medial counterpart. This contrast is heightened by the presence of the iliotibial tract, which runs lateral to the retinaculum (Fig. 7). Some of the iliotibial tract fibers terminate on the lateral femoral condyle, some pass to the patella, and the bulk continue on to the tubercle of Gerdy (see Figs. 2, 7). The lateral patellar retinaculum has numerous fibers of origin in the iliotibial tract region, which then pass to the patella. The longitudinal lateral patellar retinacular fibers originate from three different areas: some arise from the patella, some pass to the patella from the vastus lateralis and medial iliotibial tract, and some pass to the lateral femoral epicondyle or tibia (tubercle of Gerdy) from the lateral iliotibial tract. The longitudinal lateral patellar retinaculum inserts in the medial portion of the tubercle of Gerdy and in a medially adjacent area of the proximal tibia (see Fig. 7).

Both lateral patellar retinacula are dynamized by the vastus lateralis, tensor fasciae latea (iliotibial tract), and gluteus maximus muscles (iliotibial tract). The main function of the lateral retinacula is to direct femoropatellar tracking (avoiding medial deviation) and equalize compressive loads between the lateral and medial halves of the patella.

As noted earlier, the lateral retinacula are functionally linked to the iliotibial tract. Located in the anterior third of the lateral compartment, the iliotibial tract provides a very important active and passive lateral restraint. Although the iliotibial tract is considered part of the fascia lata and courses within it, some of the tract fibers originate from the lateral intermuscular septum (Fig. 8), and the superior portion of the tract is made tense by the tensor fasciae latae and gluteus maximus muscles. The iliotibial tract has terminal attachments with the femoral condyle proximally, the patella medially, and the tubercle of Gerdy distally (see Figs. 7, 8). It also blends with aponeurotic expansions from the tibialis anterior muscle. The "Kaplan fibers" attach the tract to the lateral femoral condyle (see Fig. 8). This arrangement causes a portion of the iliotibial tract to descend obliquely forward from the femur to the tibia (Fig. 9), analogous to the medial collateral ligament, and gives it the func-

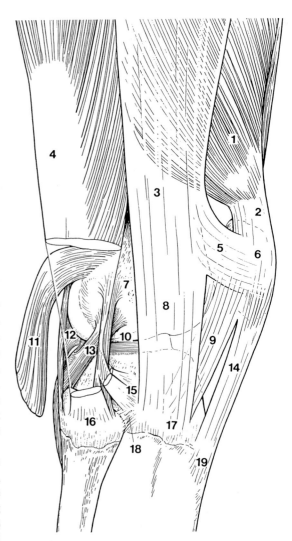

Fig. 7. Knee joint. Lateral aspect

 1 Vastus lateralis femoris muscle
 2 Quadriceps tendon
 3 Iliotibial tract
 4 Biceps femoris tendon
 5 Fibers from iliotibial tract to patella
 6 Patella
 7 Lateral femoral epicondyle
 8 Anterolateral femorotibial ligament
 9 Lateral longitudinal patellar retinaculum
10 Lateral collateral ligament
11 Lateral head of gastrocnemius muscle
12 Arcuate popliteal ligament
13 Popliteus tendon
14 Patellar ligament
15 Biceps tendon: tibial insertion
16 Biceps tendon: fibular insertion
17 Tubercle of Gerdy
18 Anterior ligament of fibular head
19 Tibial tuberosity

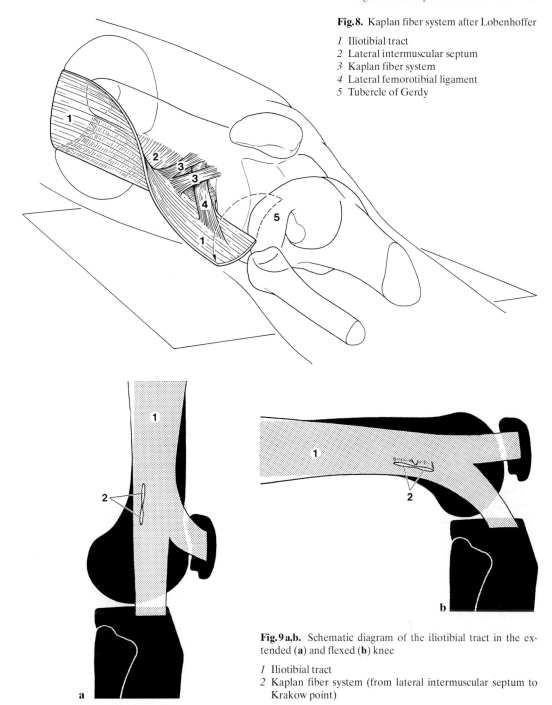

Fig. 8. Kaplan fiber system after Lobenhoffer

1 Iliotibial tract
2 Lateral intermuscular septum
3 Kaplan fiber system
4 Lateral femorotibial ligament
5 Tubercle of Gerdy

Fig. 9 a,b. Schematic diagram of the iliotibial tract in the extended (**a**) and flexed (**b**) knee

1 Iliotibial tract
2 Kaplan fiber system (from lateral intermuscular septum to Krakow point)

tional status of a "lateral femorotibial collateral ligament." Thus, its dynamized components terminate both on the lateral femoral condyle (Kaplan fiber complex to Krakow point) and on the proximal tibia (Gerdy tubercle). The passive fiber components, most of which are anterior and deep to the active fibers, establish a firm attachment between the lateral condyle and the tubercle of Gerdy. Thus, they are often referred to separately as the "anterolateral femorotibial ligament."

The iliotibial tract can act synergistically with two different muscle groups, i.e., with both the flexors and extensors of the knee. In the range between 0° and 40° of flexion, the tract runs anterior to the rotational axis (see Fig. 9) and thus supports the extensor muscles. With increasing flexion, it glides posteriorly

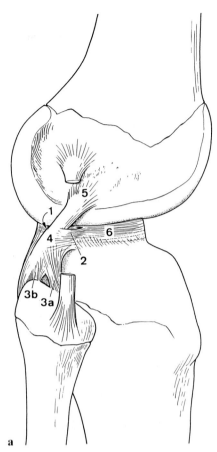

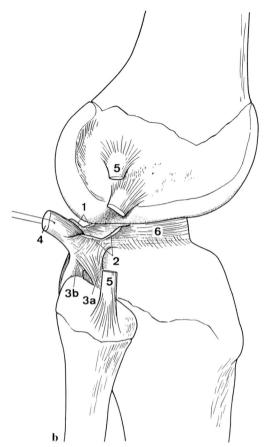

Fig. 10. a Right knee, lateral aspect (lateral collateral ligament resected). *1*, Posterosuperior popliteomeniscal fascicle; *2*, inferior popliteomeniscal fascicle; *3a*, popliteofibular fascicle, anterior part; *3b*, popliteofibular fascicle, posterior part; *4*, popliteus tendon; *5*, femoral attachment of popliteus tendon; *6*, lateral meniscus. **b** Popliteus tendon and popliteomeniscal fas-

cicle. Right knee, lateral aspect (popliteus tendon divided and retracted). *1*, Posterosuperior popliteomeniscal fascicle; *2*, inferior popliteomeniscal fascicle; *3a*, popliteofibular fascicle, anterior part; *3b*, popliteofibular fascicle, posterior part; *4*, popliteus tendon; *5*, lateral collateral ligament (resected); *6*, lateral meniscus. (From Stäubli and Birrer 1990)

over the lateral epicondyle (backward from the flexion axis), becoming a synergist of the flexor group when the flexion angle exceeds 40° (see Fig. 9) (movement of the iliotibial tract over the lateral femoral epicondyle plays an important role in the occurrence of the pivot shift phenomenon). The iliotibial tract functionally assists anterolateral rotatory stability while stabilizing the knee against lateral gapping (varus stress). It thus stabilizes the lateral tibial plateau in a way that keeps it from gliding anteriorly during rotational motions. This enables the iliotibial tract to perform very important femorotibial joint functions in addition to its role as a lateral restraint to varus stress. In clinical cases of residual varus instability, a good stabilizing effect is achieved by advancing the iliotibial tract insertion posteriorly and distally on the tibia (Fig. 10a, b).

The joint capsule forms the next deeper layer in the

anterior (and middle) third of the lateral compartment. Here the capsule consists of the synovial investment and, lacking reinforcement by ligamentous fibers, is very distensible. Only the fibers of the lateral patellomeniscal ligament (of Panzat) pass (as in the medial compartment) from the lateral meniscal border (most arising at the level of the middle and anterior thirds) to the patella, and sometimes they may be integrated into the anterior capsule. This ligament functions mainly as a receptor for the reflex stabilization of femoropatellar and femorotibial movements (analogous to the medial meniscopatellar ligament). Thus, the anterior portion of the deep capsule on the lateral side remains freely mobile with respect to the iliotibial tract. It is often permeated by fat and generally blends anteriorly with the infrapatellar fat pad. It is always firmly adherent to the border of the lateral meniscus. As on the medial side, fibers of the transverse ligament of the knee pass from the anterior horn of the lateral meniscus to the opposite side.

Middle Third

Structurally and functionally, the middle and posterior thirds of the lateral compartment (see Fig. 1) are closely interrelated. Most of their structural elements show a hierarchical arrangement from front to back or vice-versa.

The most superficial structure in this region is the broad tendon of the biceps muscle, which runs downward and forward in the lateral portion of the posterior third to insert on the head of the fibula. Trauma frequently causes a bony avulsion of the tendon (see Fig. 7), or excessive muscular exertion may dislocate the fibular head. The biceps tendon also inserts on the tibia via expansions that pass superficial and deep to the lateral collateral ligament. The fibular attachment of the biceps tendon splits into a posterior portion (main portion of fibular insertion) and an anterior portion (middle insertion of the biceps tendon together with the fibular collateral ligament). The two anterior, tibial insertions bypass the lateral collateral ligament on either side, the deeper expansion known also as the "anterior ligament of the proximal tibia" (see Fig. 7). The biceps femoris muscle is an important stabilizer against varus angulation in the extended knee and against internal rotation in the flexed knee. In particular, its short head is a direct antagonist to the popliteus muscle (and thus to internal rotation). Besides being an important external rotator, the muscle is also a flexor owing to its position behind the flexion axis. If the posterolateral tendinous expansions of the biceps are severed along with the iliotibial tract anteriorly, only the fibular collateal ligament is left laterally and, posterolaterally, the popliteus tendon and posterolateral collateral ligament.

The lateral collateral ligament descends obliquely backward from the femoral condyle to the fibular head (see Fig. 7). It is considerably smaller than the medial collateral ligament and, unlike the latter, is readily identifiable as a separate structure. It contributes to passive stabilization of the lateral side while also functioning as a synergist to the posterior cruciate ligament (PCL).

Deep to and completely separate from the lateral collateral ligament is the popliteus tendon, which arises from the lateral femoral condyle and descends posteriorly to unite with the popliteus muscle belly in the posterior third of the lateral compartment. As in the anterior third, the underlying joint capsule is very delicate and is not fused with other collagenous structural elements. Even more significant, it has no anatomic connections with the lateral meniscus, whose border is freely mobile in the middle third of the lateral compartment.

Posterior Third

The posterior third of the lateral compartment (see Fig. 1) is dominated structurally and functionally by the posterolateral corner, also called the "popliteus corner" owing to the major functional importance of the popliteus muscle in this region.

On examining the superior portion of the posterolateral corner, we find superficially the fibers of the oblique popliteal ligament (which incorporates semimembranosus tendon fibers). The ligament fibers may terminate in a fabella (see Fig. 4c) or, if a fabella is not present, they continue laterally upward toward the origin of the lateral head of the gastrocnemius. Thus, both the oblique popliteal ligament and the fabella are linked structurally and functionally to the lateral gastrocnemius tendon (see Fig. 4). The deep tendon plate of this muscle additionally forms the joint capsule in this area. Distal to the fabella, the joint capsule and gastrocnemius tendon continue as separate structures, i.e., as two separate layers. When present, then, the fabella forms the end point for the oblique popliteal ligament (as a diagonal expansion from the semimembranosus tendon) and for the slips of the main gastrocnemius tendon. The arcuate ligament, a tendinous expansion from the popliteus muscle, terminates at the fabella from below, as does the fabellofibular ligament of Vallois (see Fig. 4c). These terminations highlight the role of the fabella as a nodal point for stress transfer (even though it is present in only about 20% of the population).

The arcuate ligament arches from the posterolateral tibia and fibular head to the middle of the joint capsule. Some of its fibers project to the fabella, but it also receives tendinous fibers from the popliteus muscle (whose tendon of origin is thus divided), enabling the muscle to exert tension on the ligament as far as the fabella. The deep portion of the arcuate popliteal ligament is attached to the posterior horn of the lateral meniscus along with fibers of the popliteus tendon (see Fig. 10a, b, inferior and superior popliteomeniscal fascicles), enabling the popliteus muscle to retract the meniscus actively during flexion as the femoral condyle rolls posteriorly.

The fabellofibular ligament (of Vallois) passes from the fabella to the fibular head (see Fig. 4c). It is often described as part of the arcuate complex. Owing to its inferolateral attachment on the fibular head, it helps to neutralize posterolateral muscle forces (gastrocnemius and popliteus tendons) by transmitting them to the fabella (where the tensile forces intersect). A "short lateral collateral ligament" is occasionally present as an anatomic variant (see Fig. 4 b).

The popliteus muscle, the dominant structure posteroinferiorly, initially runs parallel to the arcuate popliteal ligament from the posteromedial tibial surface (see Fig. 4). After giving off its main tendons to the arcuate popliteal ligament complex and the posterior horn of the lateral meniscus, the popliteus continues laterally upward and forward. This tendinous portion of the popliteus muscle pursues a deeper course, its tendon passing beneath the arcuate ligament to enter the popliteal hiatus and then coursing over the lateral part of the upper tibia, below the lateral collateral ligament, to reach the lateral femoral condyle (see Fig. 7). Its tendon in this region is still approximately pencil-thick. Besides its attachments to the arcuate ligament, lateral meniscus (see Fig. 10) and femur, the popliteus also has direct, deep tendinous attachments with the posterior joint capsule.

This region of the capsule is strengthened by fibers sometimes termed the "posterolateral collateral ligament." These fibers enter the capsule like a ligament, running almost parallel to the popliteus tendon, attach to the posterior horn of the lateral meniscus, and pass from there to the tibia. Thus, the posterior capsule (unlike the anterior two-thirds) is always reinforced by firm femorotibial attachments in the lateral compartment. The most important active stabilizer of the posterolateral corner is the popliteus muscle with its various deep attachments.

Ruptures of the popliteus tendon can be reconstructed by a "popliteus bypass" (see Fig. 25, p. 488) in which a strip of biceps tendon, for example, is mobilized and fixed to the lateral femoral condyle.

The posterior segment of the lateral meniscus is directly attached to the posterior capsular wall, the popliteus tendon, and the arcuate popliteal ligament (site of predilection for tears or avulsions). The popliteus actively retracts the lateral meniscus during flexion so that it is not caught beneath the "wheel" of the femoral condyle. The popliteal hiatus, moreover, gives the meniscus the free space necessary for its high mobility (accounting for the low incidence of tears in that area). The popliteus tendon itself, coursing to its femoral insertion site, is completely separate from the lateral meniscus in the popliteal hiatus. Two separate ligamentous attachments anchor the posterior horn of the lateral meniscus in the "central pivot." The posterior meniscofemoral ligament (of

Wrisberg) anchors the meniscus to the posterior intercondylar area of the tibia, while the anterior meniscofemoral ligament (of Humphry) attaches the front part of the posterior horn to the rear portion of the anterior intercondylar area (see Figs. 1, 6).

The lateral compartment, then, possesses a relatively weak passive restraint system compared with the medial compartment: the anterolateral femorotibial ligament, the lateral collateral ligament, and the passive elements of the popliteus corner. Active stabilization is decidedly predominant and is provided by the dynamized portion of the iliotibial tract (tensor fasciae latae, gluteus maximus), the biceps femoris muscle, and the popliteus muscle. The latter is the major active stabilizer of the posterolateral corner, as it completely dynamizes the arcuate complex, moves the lateral meniscus posteriorly (together with the posterior capsule), and stabilizes the knee with a deep tendon attached to the lateral femoral condyle. (It also rotates the tibia medially in the flexed knee.)

Accordingly, we find symmetrical, functionally linked triads of structures on the posteromedial and posterolateral sides of the joint: medially the posterior horn of the medial meniscus, the posterior oblique ligament, and the semimembranosus muscle; laterally the posterior horn of the lateral meniscus, the arcuate complex, and the popliteus muscle. Further symmetry exists with respect to synergistic functions. The inner posteromedial ligaments correlate functionally with the ACL (combined tears in approximately 80%), and the posterolateral corner with the PCL (again, combined tears in approximately 80%).

The Central Pivot

The dominant structures of the central pivot are the anterior and posterior cruciate ligaments (see Figs. 1, 6). Both ligaments dictate the shape of the femoral condyles and the kinematic laws of articular motions. The anterior third of the central pivot, bounded essentially by the intercondylar area of the tibia and the intercondylar notch of the femur, contains the sites of attachment of the medial and lateral menisci and the transverse ligament of the knee (described above). Between these structures, the tibial attachment of the ACL occupies a relatively large portion of the anterior intercondylar area (Figs. 6, 11 a). In the extended knee, the ACL ascends steeply through the intercondylar notch to its femoral origin, which is located far back on the medial aspect of the lateral condyle. In hyperextension the ACL engages against the vault of the intercondylar notch at a grooved site called

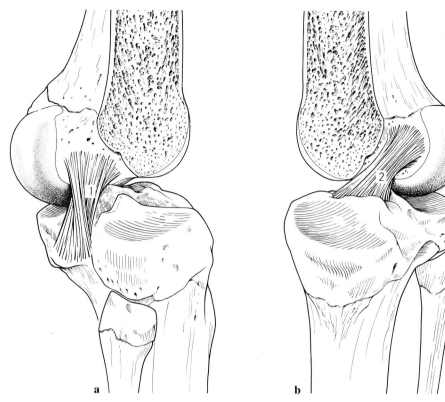

Fig. 11. a Knee joint. Anteromedial aspect (femur sawed open, medial portion removed). *1*, Anterior cruciate ligament. **b** Knee joint. Posterolateral aspect (femur sawed open longitudinally, lateral portion removed). *2*, Posterior cruciate ligament

"Grant's notch." The ligament may angulate at Grant's notch and may even tear as extension draws it more tightly into the notch. Generally having the shape of a pointed arch, Grant's notch is also a measure of the width of the ACL. A medially adjacent, flat, round arch receives the PCL when the knee is flexed. As flexion progresses, the ACL increasingly assumes a horizontal position. It relates most closely to the PCL at the site where the ligaments cross, directly above the vascular pedicle.

The ACL stabilizes the tibia against anterior displacement. Other structural elements that function synergistically in this regard are the semimembranosus corner and the anterolateral femorotibial ligament. Approximately one-third of the capacity for anterior stabilization resides in the ACL, and approximately two-thirds in the other two structural elements (an isolated tear of the ACL thus leaves about two-thirds of this capacity intact). The maximum load-bearing capacity of the ACL, like that of the medial collateral ligament, is only about 40 kg. However, the structure of the ACL is such that it almost never transmits stresses through the whole of its substance; rather, different portions of its fibers (see

Fig. 11 a, b) are stressed selectively during certain motions and in certain joint positions. The anteromedial fibers are most heavily stressed when the knee is near extension, and the posterolateral fibers at greater degrees of flexion. The intermediate fibers stabilize against internal rotation, during which the cruciate ligaments coil around each other.

The ACL derives its total blood supply from a single small artery (from its origin on the femur to its insertion on the tibia). This vessel unites the ACL with the PCL at their site of crossing, directly above the vascular pedicle. At its sites of origin and insertion, small blood vessels enter the ACL from the subcortical (osseous) network, but these vessels supply only the attachment sites and cannot nourish the whole ligament.

Both cruciate ligaments have a common anterior synovial investment. So despite their intraarticular location, both are extrasynovial. The common synovial investment has its origin on the cruciate "central pivot," where the middle genicular artery also gives off its branches. The PCL is far better endowed in terms of blood supply, as it receives four branches from the middle genicular artery that are distributed over its entire length. Able to support a stress of approximately 80 kg before tearing, it has far greater structural strength than the ACL (see Fig. 11b).

The PCL originates from a broad area on the medial aspect of the medial femoral condyle, passing downward and backward to a very low insertion site on the posterior intercondylar area of the tibia. The PCL lies relatively flat in extension and rears up during flexion, though it is not jeopardized by impingement on the anterior rim of the intercondylar notch. By becoming vertical with flexion, the PCL becomes the pivot point for knee rotation and thus can exert a significant rotational stabilizing effect. Its only synergist in flexion is the quadriceps femoris muscle. Its synergists in extension, with orientations similar to that of the PCL, are the posterior oblique ligament and the posteromedial capsule (concomitant lesions of both are common with trauma).

Like its counterpart, the PCL consists of three different fiber bundles that are subjected to different loads in different joint positions. The posteromedial fibers are most tense in extension, where they function as a restraint to hyperextension (they insert far back in the intercondylar area). The central and anterolateral fiber bundles are most tense in moderate and full flexion (they insert in the lateral part of the posterior intercondylar area, close to the lateral meniscus).

Among other functions, the PCL serves as a posterior restraint, though in internal rotation this function can be partially taken over by the meniscofemoral ligaments of Humphry and Wrisberg, which are taut in that position (see Figs. 1, 6). (These structures can mask posterior instability in the internally rotated knee.) From its medial side, the PCL receives connecting fibers from the posterior horn of the medial meniscus, giving the meniscus a partial insertion on that ligament.

As noted earlier, the PCL increasingly assumes the function of the central pivot in the sharply flexed knee. At small and moderate flexion angles, the intercondylar eminence of the tibia functions as the essential pivot of the knee (see Fig. 1). This structure is covered by a thick, strong cartilage layer that apposes to the medial surfaces of the femoral condyles, which likewise are cartilage-covered. The posterior portion of the meniscal cartilage, distinguished by its hardness, thickness, and lack of compliance, can function as a counterpart to the intercondylar eminence. The "pivotal" function of the eminence at moderate flexion angles is very important for guiding the articular surfaces under varus, valgus, and rotatory stresses and for the absorption of compressive forces. Meanwhile the peripheral joint apparatus is very lax in intermediate flexion, which further accentuates the

central guide function of the intercondylar eminence. If the outer collateral ligaments become disrupted, incidentally, the cruciate ligaments can protect the joint from varus or valgus stresses by functioning as "internal" collateral ligaments for the individual femoral condyles.

Another important function of the cruciate ligaments is their guidance of the terminal "screw home" mechanism of the knee. This automatic terminal rotation is caused by the position of the cruciate ligaments and also by the unequal lengths of the femoral condyles. The shorter length of the lateral condyle causes it to ride up on the tibial plateau earlier than the medial condyle (Fig. 11) and complete its rolling motion, while the longer medial condyle continues to roll.

The Femoropatellar Compartment

The central structure of the femoropatellar articulation is the patella, a sesamoid bone which, though movable, provides a fixed point of attachment for ligaments and tendons. Analogous to the fabella in the posterolateral corner on the flexor side, the patella forms a nodal point for forces transmitted from multiple directions: longitudinal tensile forces via the quadriceps tendon and patellar ligament, and transverse tensile forces via the meniscopatellar ligaments and transverse retinacula (see Fig. 2). Thus, the function of the patella depends entirely on the action of the quadriceps femoris muscle. The proximal part of the patella is embedded in the quadriceps tendon; hence it is completely extraarticular and does not have an articular surface (Fig. 12). The intraarticular space extends far upward beneath the patellar apex and quadriceps tendon, along the anterior femoral surface, in the form of the suprapatellar pouch. The inferior articular surface of the patella does not articulate smoothly with the trochlea of the femur over its entire surface, in either flexion or extension. In particular, the medial facet of the patella, with its exceptionally thick layer of articular cartilage and irregularly shaped surface ("odd facet"), is poorly congruent with the medial flank of the femoral trochlea. Occasionally this incongruity creates a free space between the articular surfaces, which generally is occupied by a protruding synovial fold that appears to contribute to a more uniform stress distribution (Figs. 6, 11). The lateral articular facet of the patella is reasonably congruent with the lateral flank of the trochlea. In extension the patella articulates solely with the femoral patellar surface, but in full flexion the descent of the patella additionally opposes it to

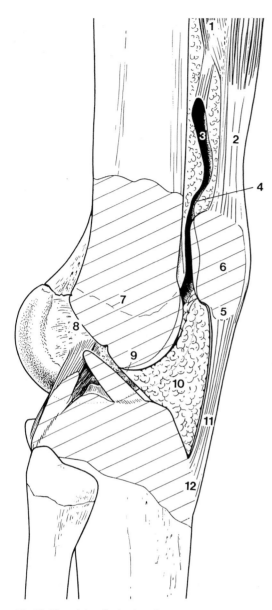

Fig. 12. Knee joint. Sagittal section

1 Fibers of vastus intermedius muscle
2 Quadriceps tendon
3 Suprapatellar pouch
4 Synovial plica
5 Patellar apex
6 Patella
7 Distal femoral epiphyseal plate (closed)
8 Roof of intercondylar notch (Blumensaat's line)
9 Infrapatellar synovial plica
10 Infrapatellar fat pad
11 Patellar ligament
12 Tibial tuberosity

the condylar portion of the femorotibial joint. The "limiting groove" (sulcus terminalis) demarcates the femoral patellar surface, with its relatively high rims (especially laterally), from the region of femorotibial articulation. This groove appears morphologically as a conspicuous depression in the femoral articular cartilage. As this area lacks the delimiting medial and lateral rims that constrain patellar motion within the trochlea, it is the site of predilection for lateral patellar subluxation (in approximately 30° flexion with a rotatory stress). Generally this subluxation is not associated with chondro-osseous flake fractures due to the lack of mechanical resistance on the lateral side. However, flakes may be sheared from the patellar ridge or the condylar border itself when the patella subsequently reduces over the high lateral rim of the trochlea in the extended knee.

The distal end of the patella, like its proximal end, is embedded in ligamentous tissue (see Fig. 12) – the patellar ligament. Posterior to these structures is the heavily vascularized infrapatellar fat pad with its alar plicae projecting into the sides of the joint space (see Fig. 6). It is held in place by the patellar ligament, the bilateral longitudinal retinacula, and the infrapatellar synovial plica, an unpaired central structure that passes posterosuperiorly to the roof of the intercondylar notch.

The movements of the patella are subject to fine control mechanisms in which the ligaments between the patella and meniscus play a significant role (receptor functions: medial and lateral patellomeniscal ligaments). These ligaments explain, for example, why the clinical picture of medial patellar chondropathy is virtually identical to that of medial meniscal damage. The function of the patellofemoral joint is completely dependent on the function of the quadriceps femoris muscle. It is mainly the action of this muscle that drives patellar gliding within the trochlea. This action places greater pressure on the lateral flank of the condyle than on the medial flank because the main vector of the quadriceps femoris muscle is directed laterally (Q angle). This causes a slight posterior displacement of the lateral femoral condyle, accompanied by internal rotation of the tibia. The vastus medialis and vastus medialis obliquus muscles act as antagonists to these forces and can draw the patella medially. High patellar contact pressure against the lateral femoral condyle also occurs in association with angulation and external rotation, where the vastus medialis obliquus again exerts an antagonistic action. Conversely, patellar pressure against the medial femoral condyle increases during angulation in internal rotation, the vastus lateralis exerting a compensatory antagonistic pull. In positions of neutral rotation, both the medial and lateral vastus muscles function equally as agonists and antagonists, resulting in constant pressure changes on the various patellar contact surfaces in the medial, lateral, proximal, and distal directions.

Normal patellar movements rely on the differentiated action of various portions of the quadriceps femoris muscle. Slight disturbances in this complex functional sequence lead rapidly to decompensation of the finely balanced system. This particularly applies to the medial joint facet, where even mild decompensation can rapidly lead to abnormalities of nutrition and diffusion.

Menisci

The menisci make a significant contribution to weight bearing, shock absorption, joint stability, and lubrication of the joint surfaces. Their structural integration into the capsuloligamentous system was analyzed earlier in our description of the individual compartments of the knee. Their histologic structure is non-homogeneous, the menisci consisting of three different types of tissue whose boundaries blend together. The heterogeneity of the meniscus is most apparent in cross section, where the outer portion is seen to consist of a stiff, fibrous connective tissue that contains nerve endings and has a copious blood supply (see Fig. 5). The middle portion consists mainly of fibrocartilage with a variable fiber density. The central tissue is predominantly hyaline and thus contains fewer fibers and blood vessels than the more fibrous and more vascular tissue near the surfaces. The inner portion of the meniscus consists of pure (avascular, noninnervated) hyaline cartilage (see Fig. 5).

Special importance is ascribed to the fiber architecture of the menisci. The outer portions are partially integrated into the capsuloligamentous system (see Fig. 5). The meniscal fiber systems display an arcade arrangement of the individual fiber tracts, with their base directed toward the joint interior. The fibers are parallel in the outer zone (approximately one-third) and more radial in the inner zone (Fig. 5). The chemical composition of the different meniscal segments varies considerably, with collagen types I and III predominating in the fibrous connective tissue of the outer third. Collagen types V and VI are also present. Other constituents, quantitatively less abundant but still functionally significant, are elastin and the proteoglycans. The hyaline cartilage of the inner zone consists largely of type II collagen and proteoglycans. Also present are minority collagens (e.g., types V, IX,

XI) as well as various matrix proteins such as link protein and tenascin.

The middle third is histologically and chemically diverse, with defined topographic gradients that produce corresponding changes from the superficial to the deep portions of the meniscus.

Joint Capsule and Synovium

The structure of the joint capsule shows marked local variations. At some sites it is fused with the periarticular ligament system to form a very strong, mechanically stable layer; at others the capsule consists only of the delicate synovial membrane with adjacent fibrofatty tissues.

The synovium (synovial membrane, stratum synoviale) consists of two morphologically distinct tissues. One, called the intima, is the superficial cell layer lining the joint cavity. Epithelial in character, this layer varies from 3 to 4 cells in thickness. However, the general mass of cells is perforated by frequent gaps that open directly into the subintimal, loose fibrous connective tissue, which contains abundant lymphatic and blood capillaries and numerous scattered fat cells.

The cells of the synovial intima do not synthesize a continuous basement membrane that would separate the epithelioid intima from the subintimal connective tissue. Three morphologically distinct synovial cell types have been identified in the intima: type A (also called type M for "macrophage-like"), whose cytoplasm contains a very prominent Golgi apparatus, many vacuoles and lysosomal vesicles, but little rough endoplasmic reticulum. Long cellular processes are common. Type B cells (also called type F for "fibroblast-like") contain an abundance of rough endoplasmic reticulum but few vacuoles, lysosomal vesicles, and Golgi lamelli. Cell processes tend to be poorly developed. A mixed cell type (sometimes called AB) also has been described. The synovial cells are responsible for the production of hyaluronic acid, glycosaminoglycans, and some of the glycoproteins in the synovial fluid. With their abundant microvesicles, they also have the ability to phagocytize particulate matter from the synovial fluid – a capability ascribed chiefly to the M cells.

A significant portion of the proteins in synovial fluid pass from the subintimal connective tissue directly through the intercellular clefts into the synovial fluid. Many of these proteins are micromolecular plasma proteins, which can diffuse through the many fenestrated capillary walls from the blood plasma into the intercellular space of the subintimal connective tissue. Free nerve endings generally are not found in the subintimal space, although there are autonomic nerve fibers passing to the adventitia of the blood vessels. In deeper layers more distant from the intima, the collagenous fiber component of the subintima increases (stratum fibrosum), imparting a ligament-like character to the joint capsule and providing the capsule with numerous pain-conducting nerve fibers in addition to blood vessels. This layer establishes frequent structural contacts with the periarticular ligaments, producing a very heavy reinforcement in some areas of the capsule.

The authors thank Mr. Hans Holzherr, Audiovisual Department (AUM), University of Bern and Inselspital Bern, for providing the excellent drawings used in this chapter.

References

Fabbriciani C, Oransky M, Zoppi U (1982) Il legamento popliteo arcuato e le sue varianti. J Sports Traumatol 4: 171

Fuss FK (1989) Anatomy of the cruciate ligaments and their functions in extension and flexion of the human knee joint. Am J Anat 184/2: 165

Ghadially FN (1983) Fine structure of synovial joints. Butterworths, London

Grood ES (1984) Meniscal function (review). Adv Orthop Surgery: 193–197

Ham AW, Cormack DH (1979) Histology. Lippincott, Philadelphia Toronto

Henry AK (1973) Extensile exposure. Churchill-Livingstone, London

Hoppenfeld S, de Boer P (1984) Surgical exposures in Orthopaedics. The anatomical approach. Lippincott, Philadelphia

Kaplan EB (1958) The iliotibial tract. J Bone Joint Surg [Am] 40: 817–832

Kaplan EB (1961) The fabellofibular and short lateral ligaments of the knee joint. J Bone Joint Surg [Am] 43: 169

Kieffer DA, Curnow RJ, Southwell RB, Tucker WF, Kendrick KH (1984) Anterior cruciate ligament arthroplasty. Am J Sports Med 12/4: 301–312

Lobenhoffer P, Posel P, Witt S, Piehler J, Wirth CJ (1987) Distal femoral fixation of the iliotibial tract. Arch Orthop Trauma Surg 106: 285–290

Müller We (1982) Das Knie. Springer, Berlin Heidelberg New York

Müller We, Biedert R, Hefti F, Jakob RP, Munzinger U, Stäubli H-U (1988) OAK knee evaluation. A new way to assess knee ligament injuries. Clin Orthop 232: 37–50

Odensten M (1984) Treatment of the torn anterior cruciate ligament. Linköping University Medical Dissertations No 177

Oretorp N (1978) On the diagnosis and treatment of meniscus and ligament injuries in the knee. Linköpings Trycheri, Linköping

Rauber A, Kopsch F (1987) Anatomie des Menschen, Bd 1: Bewegungsapparat. (Hrsg B Tillmann, G Töndury) Thieme, Stuttgart

Seebacher JR, Inglis AE, Marshall JL, Warren RF (1982) The structure of the posterolateral aspect of the knee. J Bone Joint Surg [Am] 41: 536

Stäubli H-U, Birrer S (1990) The popliteus tendon andits fascicles at the popliteal hiatus: Gross anatomy and functional arthroscopic evaluation with and without anterior cruciate deficiency. J Arthroscopy 6, 3, 209–220

Stäubli H-U, Jakob RP, Noesberger B (1981) Die posterolaterale Knieinstabilität, Helv Chir Acta 48: 693–696

Stäubli H-U, Jakob RP, Noesberger B (1986) Diagnostik der hinteren Kreuzbandinsuffizienz: Wertigkeit der extensionsnahen hinteren Schubladenphänomene. Z Unfallchir Versicherungsmed Berufskr 79: 85

Terry GC, Hughston JC, Norwood LA (1986) The anatomy of the iliopatellar band and iliotibial tract. Am J Sports Med 14: 39–45

Töndury G (1970) Angewandte und topographische Anatomie. Thieme, Stuttgart

Woo SLY, Buckwalter JA (eds) (1987) Injury and repair of the muscoloskeletal soft tissues. American Academy of Orthopedic Surgeons. Park Ridge/IL

The Popliteus Muscle

C. Fabbriciani and M. Oransky

Given the major significance of posterolateral structures in reconstructive surgery of the knee ligaments, it is important to have a precise understanding of their anatomy.

Because the nomenclature and morphology of anatomic descriptions of the arcuate popliteal ligament vary in classic anatomical textbooks (Weitbrecht 1742; Macalister 1875; Gruber 1875; Krause 1897; Dujarier 1905; Vallois 1914; Kaplan 1961), it is important to analyze and properly name the various morphologic variants that are encountered.

Regarding the popliteus muscle, which is the most important structure of the posterolateral capsuloligamentous complex, Gruber performed an important anatomic study of that muscle in 1875, while Fürst published a landmark monograph in the early part of this century (1903).

Although the terminal expansions of the popliteus muscle had been represented in early anatomic drawings (Heitzman 1890, Fig. 1), they were not accurately described. The popliteus muscle was subsequently forgotten for more than half a century before it was "rediscovered" in the mid-19th century (Last 1950; Lovejoy and Harden 1971).

The Popliteus Muscle

The popliteus muscle, occupying the deepest layer of the popliteal region, is the only monoarticular muscle of the knee joint. It is adherent anteriorly to the posterior surface of the tibia. The muscle fibers, which have an overall triangular shape, are covered posteriorly by the aponeurosis of the direct tendon of semimembranosus (Fig. 2). These muscular fibers originate from the medial side just behind the medial collateral ligament and semimembranosus tendon to which the fibers are strictly attached. These fibers terminate in a complex aponeurotic structure that we divide into 3 sections (capsular, meniscal, fibular) and in a strong tendon. An understanding of this important aponeurotic structure helps us to understand the original function of the popliteus muscle. The popli-

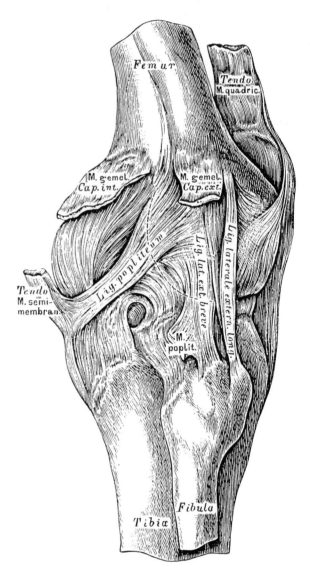

Fig. 1. Anatomic drawing showing the popliteus expansions on the fibular head (popliteofibular fibers). (From Heitzmann 1890)

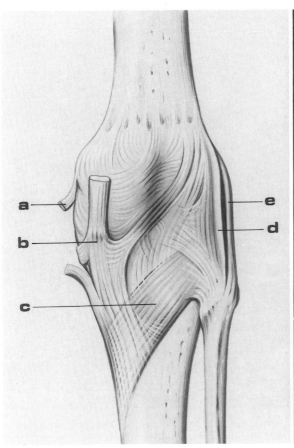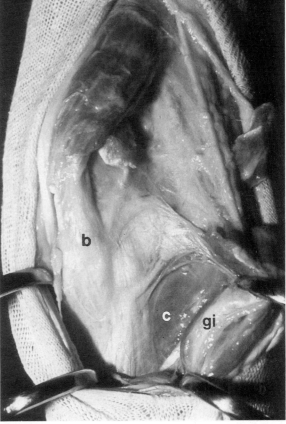

Fig. 2. Popliteal lozenge dissection with the medial head of the gastrocnemius *(mg)* divided and displaced laterally. The muscle belly of the popliteus is seen *(c)* covered medialy by the apo-neurosis of the semimembranosus muscle *(b)*. *a*, Medial collateral ligament; *d*, arcuate popliteal ligament; *e*, lateral collateral ligament

teal capsular fibers, of minor importance, form the most superficial layer of the aponeurotic expansion of the popliteus muscle.

The expansion of the lateral meniscus forms the popliteal meniscal fibers, which various authors (Last 1950; Kaplan 1961; Lovejoy 1971) have described without providing a complete and detailed description. To make it easier to understand these attachments to the lateral meniscus, we have divided them into 2 bundles – superior and inferior – in addition to a structure that we call the inferolateral bundle.

The popliteal fibular fibers form the inferior portion of the popliteus expansion. These fibers are usually very strong and attach to the fibular head behind the lateral collateral ligament (Fig. 3).

The Popliteus Tendon

The tendon of the popliteus is a continuation of its muscular fibers. It initially passes inferior to the posterolateral border of the tibia and sometimes may occupy a groove. The tendon is strong and is oval in cross section. At its origin, the tendon is covered by the popliteal arcuate ligament, to which it is firmly attached. The popliteus tendon provides the dynamic support for the arcuate popliteal ligament. The tendon enters the capsule and crosses the lateral surface to the lateral meniscus, to which it is attached by the popliteomeniscal fibers. These fibers terminate at the popliteal hiatus, where the tendon is separate from the meniscus (Fig. 3). A small bursa (superior popliteal recess) that communicates with the articular cavity is sometimes found between the popliteus tendon and the lateral collateral ligament. The tendon passes obliquely around the lateral condyle, where it crosses beneath the lateral collateral ligament and inserts

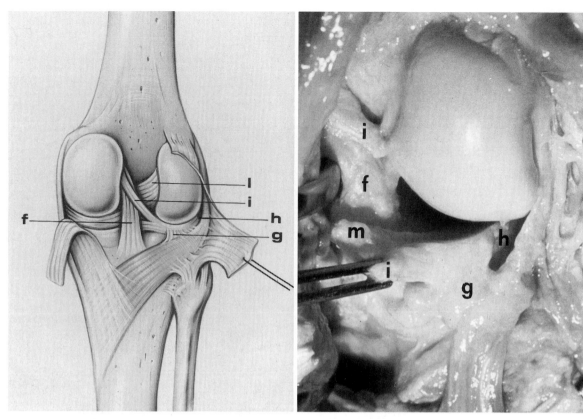

Fig. 3. In this dissection the posterior horn of the lateral meniscus has been detached, showing the sectioned insertions of the ligaments of Wrisberg *(i)* and Humphry *(m)*. The inferior popliteomeniscal fibers are seen *(g)*. The popliteal hiatus *(h)* delineates the popliteus tendon from the lateral meniscus and from the popliteomeniscal fibers. *f*, Posterior cruciate ligament

slightly in front of the anterior margin of the ligament. When the knee is flexed, the popliteus tendon lies within a groove called the popliteal sulcus. In the extended knee, the tendon shifts to another groove called the "sulcus statarius" (Fürst 1903).

The popliteus tendon plays a major functional role. Best known as an internal rotator of the tibia, the popliteus is equally important, along with the ACL, as a passive restraint to external rotation. It also exerts an anti-varus force, which is greatest in extension and decreases with flexion. The popliteus muscle is insignificant as a flexor, as indicated by electromyographic studies and by the proximity of the rotational axes of the femoral condyles to the femoral attachment of the popliteus tendon in the extended knee.

Popliteal Capsular Fibers

These fibers originate on the posterior surface of the musculotendinous part of the popliteus muscle. After a short distance (1 cm), the fibers insert into the distal part of the lateral condylar capsule. Muscular con-traction, then, exerts tension on the posterolateral capsule.

Popliteomeniscal Fibers

The expansion of the popliteal muscle aponeurosis to the lateral meniscus constitutes the popliteomeniscal fibers, which were first described by Last (1950) as a single fascia performing a specific functional role. This fibrous structure is about 2.0–2.5 cm wide and terminates on the posterior horn of the lateral meniscus. To see the fibers clearly, it is necessary to detach the popliteus tendon from the femoral condyle and fold back the tendon: 2 different fasciae can be seen. The superior fascia, which we call the superomedial bundle, inserts on the free superior border of the meniscus. The second, called the inferolateral bundle, inserts laterally on the lateral meniscus. The borders of both fasciae define the entrance of the popliteal bursa (Figs. 4,5). When the anterior horn of the lateral meniscus is detached as far as the popliteal hiatus and turned back 90°, one can see that the

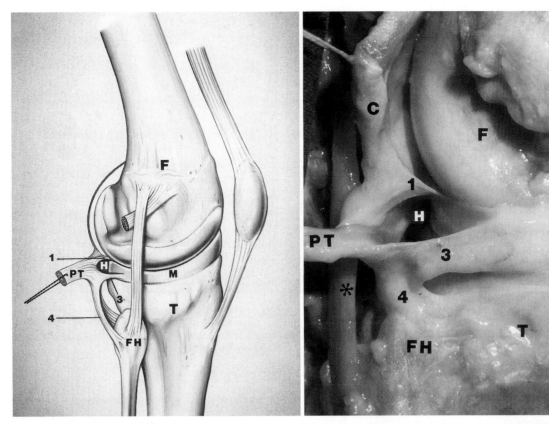

Fig. 4. In this dissection the popliteus tendon *(PT)* has been detached from the femoral condyle and reflected to expose all the expansions of the tendon to the meniscus *(M)*, capsule *(C)*, and fibular head *(FH)*. *1*, Superior popliteomeniscal fibers; *3*, lateral inferior popliteomeniscal fibers; *4*, popliteofibular fibers; *asterisk* lateral peroneal sciatic nerve; *T*, tibia; *F*, lateral femoral condyle; *H* popliteal hiatus. The lateral collateral ligament has been removed

superomedial bundle is composed of 2 separate bundles: 1 superior and 1 inferior. The superior fibers originate from the posterior surface of the popliteus tendon and terminate mainly on the superior part of the posterior horn of the meniscus. The inferior fibers originate from the anterior surface of the popliteus tendon and pass to the inferior border of the posterior horn of the lateral meniscus (Fig. 6). This anatomical arangement of the popliteomeniscal fibers results in an oblique, medial-to-lateral fiber path that runs from the inferior border of the meniscus to the superior border where it terminates, delimiting the popliteal hiatus. This path follows that of the popliteus muscle and tendon.

Along with the popliteomeniscal fibers, the popliteus muscle plays an important role in the active control of the lateral meniscus by exerting a posterior traction on the meniscus. This prevents the meniscus from being crushed between the tibia and femur and coordinates the sliding of the meniscus with the rotation and sliding of the condyle. The posterior traction and the posterior displacement of the meniscus also exert traction on the meniscofemoral ligaments of Wrisberg and Humphry.

The ligaments of Wrisberg and Humphry have not been widely described in the literature. They originate on the superior border of the posterior horn of the lateral meniscus. The Humphry ligament passes anteriorly to the PCL, while the ligament of Wrisberg passes posteriorly. Both insert on the medial aspect of the medial femoral condyle. The ligament of Wrisberg was first described by Weitbrecht in 1742. Unlike the ligament of Humphry, we consistently found this ligament in our dissections. It is important to note, however, that its morphology is highly variable. The 2 basic forms are cordlike and fan-shaped. The latter type has a large area of insertion on the meniscus and then tapers into one or more fascicles that terminate on the medial condyle. As mentioned, the Humphry ligament is weaker and less commonly found than the ligament of Wrisberg. It is firmly attached to the anterior surface of the PCL, from which it is sometimes difficult to separate by dissection (Fig. 7).

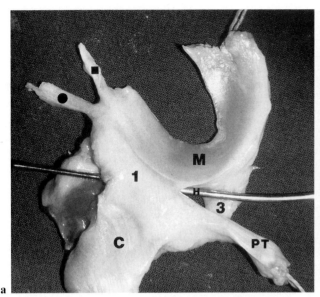
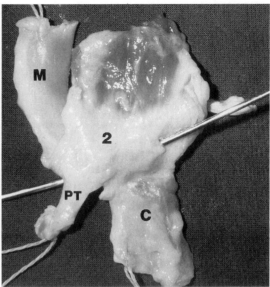

Fig. 5a,b. Dissection of the lateral meniscus and popliteus muscle. **a** The broad attachment of the superior fibers of the posterior popliteomeniscal fibers *(1)* can be seen. A probe has been inserted between the superior and inferior popliteomeniscal fiber layers. *3* Inferolateral popliteomeniscal fibers.

b Reverse view of the preparation in **a**, showing the inferior popliteomeniscal fibers *(2)*. *PT*, Popliteus tendon; *black circle*, ligament of Wrisberg; *black square*, ligament of Humphry; *C*, posterior joint capsule

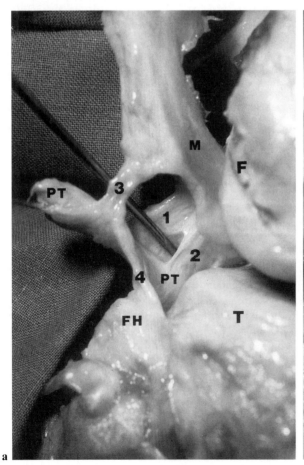
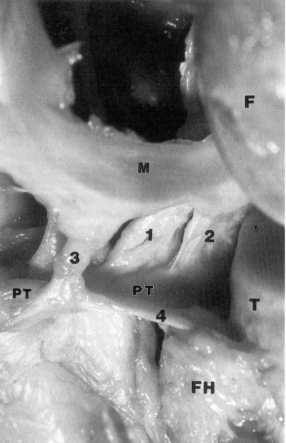

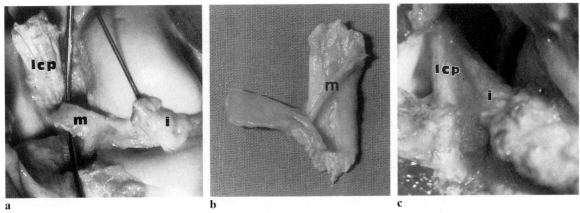

Fig. 7a–c. Dissection of the ligaments of Wrisberg and Humphry. **a** Wrisberg's ligament is sectioned and suspended by a suture. The posterior cruciate ligament *(PCL)* is sectioned and folded back at its tibial insertion, exposing Humphry's liga- ment *(m)*. **b** Anterior view of the PCL and the posterior horn of the lateral meniscus, including Humphry's ligament. **c** The PCL covered by the synovial membrane. The large size of Wrisberg's ligament can be seen

Popliteofibular Fibers

Despite their anatomic and functional importance, the popliteofibular fibers have been ignored in anatomy texts and described only fleetingly in scientific journals, except for the publication of Lovejoy and Harden in 1971. These fibers constitute the inferior expansion of the popliteus muscle; they insert on the anteromedial part of the fibular head, and a small group may also insert on the tibia. The popliteofibular fibers are situated deep and lateral to the arcuate popliteal ligament. Rectangular in shape and approximately 2 cm long and slightly more than 2 cm in width, the popliteofibular fibers are the only ligamentous fibers that attach to bone (Fig. 8). The fibers' free medial border, together with that of the popliteomeniscal fibers, forms an archlike structure over the bursa of the popliteus muscle. They perform an extremely importantfunctional role. These fibers are involved in controlling external tibial rotation and recurvatum and in maintaining proper positioning of the popliteus tendon. We have found that the selective experimental sectioning of the popliteofibular fibers is sufficient to cause posterolateral laxity. The role of the fibers in checking external tibial rotation is confirmed by the fact that, with flexion and external rotation of the knee, the fibers become maximally tense while the lateral collateral ligament becomes lax. Conversely, the popliteofibular fibers become lax when the knee is internally rotated.

The Popliteal Bursa

From the popliteal hiatus, a portion of the synovial membrane of the knee joint is reflected outward to follow the proximal part of the popliteus tendon and terminates between the meniscal and fibular expansions and the posterior surface of the tibia (inferior popliteal recess or popliteal bursa). The bursa is bounded superiorly by the popliteomeniscal fibers, posteriorly by the popliteus tendon, and inferiorly by the popliteofibular fibers. On its anterior aspect, the popliteal bursa rests against the posterior surface of the tibia and part of the posterior wall of the lateral meniscus. Its fundus is defined by an archlike structure (previously described) formed by the free border of the popliteomeniscal fibrs and the free border of the popliteofibular fibers (Fig. 9).

Anatomic Variants of the Popliteus Muscle

An unusual morphologic variant of the popliteus muscle consists in a duplication of the muscle belly. This variant was first described in 1687 by Hieronymus Fabricius. In 1875 Gruber found what he called the "musculus popliteus biceps" in 8 of 250 dis-

◁

Fig. 6. a Dissection demonstrating the 2 planes of the popliteomeniscal fibers, the superior *(1)* and the inferior *(2)*. A probe has been inserted between them. *3*, Inferolateral popliteomeniscal fibers; *PT*, popliteus tendon. **b** Detail of **a**. *M*, Lateral meniscus; *T*, tibia; *F*, femoral condyle; *FH*, fibular head

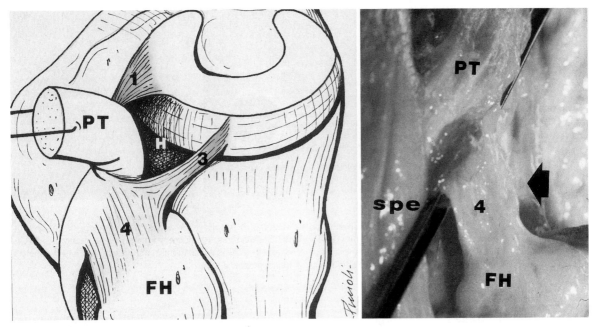

Fig. 8. Dissection of the popliteofibular fibers *(4)*, which pass from the popliteus tendon *(PT)* to the fibular head. *1,* Superior popliteomeniscal fibers; *3,* inferolateral popliteomeniscal fibers

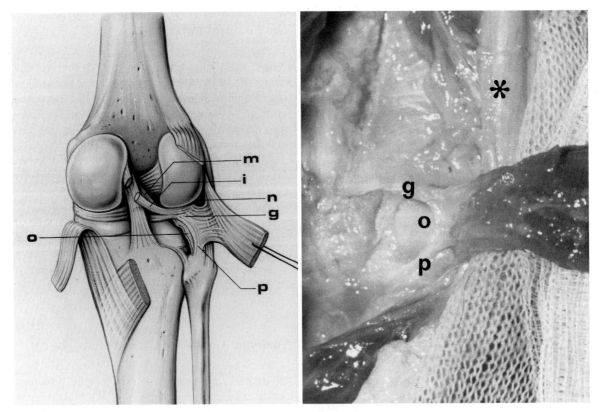

Fig. 9. The belly of the popliteus muscle has been sectioned and retracted laterally, and the popliteal bursa has been opened *(o).* The free medial border of the popliteomeniscal fibers *(g)* and of the popliteofibular fibers form an archlike structure. *asterisk* Peroneal nerve; *i,* Wrisberg's ligament; *m,* Humphry's ligament; *n,* popliteal hiatus

sections (3.2%) and described 3 morphologic types (Fig. 10 a). In our 40 dissections, we observed this variant in 1 case (2.5%) (Fig. 10 b).

The Arcuate Ligament

The other component of the posterolateral corner of the knee is the "arcuate complex." Descriptions of this complex in anatomy texts are sketchy and imprecise and often differ from one another, creating. Also, the nomenclature used is often arbitrary, even though the Nomina Anatomica recognizes only the term "arcuate popliteal ligament." The discordance of descriptions and nomenclature can be partially explained by the extreme anatomic variability of the arcuate popliteal ligament.

The arcuate popliteal ligament is defined as the structure that runs from the posterolateral condylar capsule, below the insertion of the lateral gastrocnemius tendon, distally to the posterior aspect of the fibular head, passing above the popliteus tendon, to which it is attached. We do not believe that a true internal arch of the arcuate popliteal ligament exists, even though it is described in some anatomy texts (Testut).

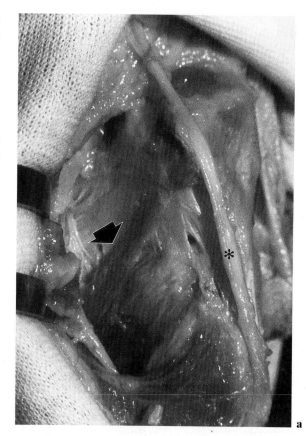

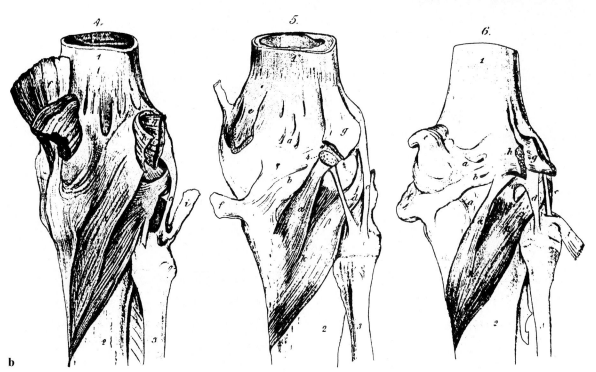

Fig. 10. a Morphologic types of the "popliteus biceps" (after Gruber 1875). **b** The *arrow* indicates the presence of an accessory popliteus muscle belly; * popliteal nerve. In drawing 5, *a*, fabellofibular ligament; *d*, fabella; in drawing 6, *d*, arcuate popliteal ligament

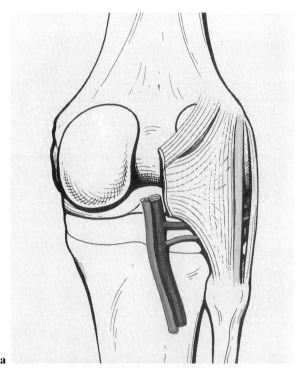

Fig. 11. a Drawing of the arcuate popliteal ligament. The most lateral portion is thicker than the rest of the ligament. The inferolateral genicular artery and vein always pass below the arcuate ligament. **b** The *arrow* indicates the path of the vessels under the arcuate ligament. *c*, Popliteus muscle; *ge*, proximal insertion of the lateral head of the gastrocnemius muscle. **c** Thickened lateral border of the arcuate popliteal ligament *(arrow)*. *c*, Popliteus muscle

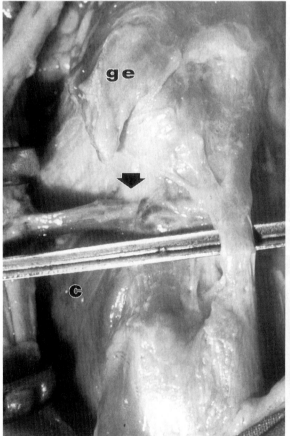

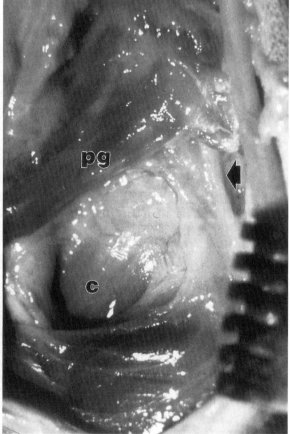

What has been incorrectly described as the "internal arch" is actually composed of the articular capsule and the popliteal capsular fibers located anterior to the plane of the external arch.

To give an accurate anatomic description of the arcuate ligament complex, we must distinguish the findings on the basis of the presence or absence of the fabella sesamoid bone in the knee.

Knees Without a Fabella

The fabella was absent in the 92% of our dissections. Two types of arcuate ligament can be distinguished in this situation. In the first group, which is more common, the arcuate ligament has a morphology similar (except for the internal arch) to that commonly described in anatomy texts. The ligament, which is highly variable, has a thickened external border along its entire length. Although Kaplan described the inferior lateral genicular artery and vein as passing above the arcuate ligament, these vessels actually pass below it (Fig. 11). In several cases the arcuate ligament consists of a very thin band of fibrous tissue that does not have the morphologic or structural characteristics of a ligament. The second group includes a less common morphologic variant in which the lateral aspect of the arcuate ligament is more developed and differentiated to form a cordlike ligamentous structure distinct from the arcuate ligament itself (Fig. 12), which we believe to be the same as the "short lateral collateral ligament" described by Weitbrecht in 1742. The term "short lateral collateral ligament" does not designate an autonomous structure of the posterolateral corner; rather, it is a thickening of the capsule which forms the arcuate ligament. We understand the "short lateral ligament" to mean the thick portion of the capsule that forms the lateral border of the popliteal lozenge (Vallois 1914).

The short lateral collateral ligament originates at the lateral condylar capsule and inserts on the fibular head behind the lateral collateral ligament. The anterior surface of the ligament blends with the underlying capsule, while the posterior surface is well-defined and laterally delineates the popliteal lozenge. In our specimen we observed that the inferior genicu-

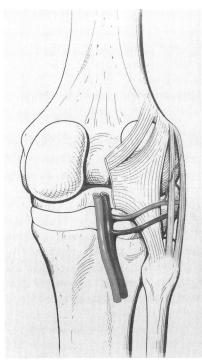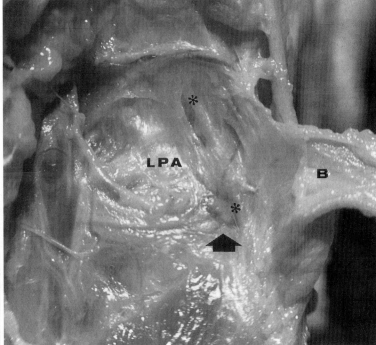

Fig. 12. Occasional finding in which the most lateral part of the arcuate popliteal ligament separates to form a separate "short lateral collateral ligament." In this case the inferolateral genicular vessels pass above the arcuate ligament and below the short lateral collateral ligament. In the dissection showing the popliteus biceps muscle (b), the arcuate popliteal ligament (LPA) is firmly attached to the underlying capsule. Lateral to it is a separate fibrous band. * Short lateral collateral ligament. The path of the vessels (arrow) is shown

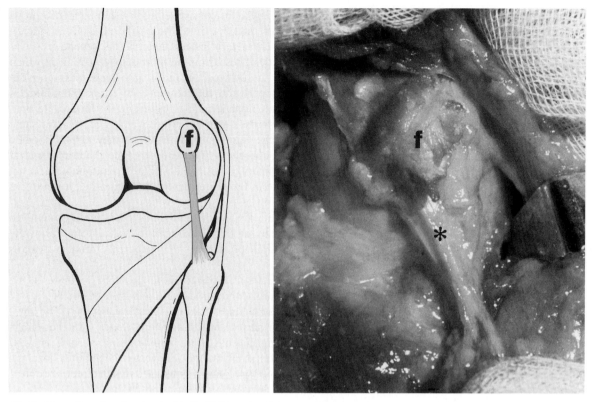

Fig. 13. Knee dissection showing the fabella *(f)*. Note the thickness of the fabellofibular ligament (*) when a bony fabella is present

late vessels ran above the arcuate ligament and below the short lateral collateral ligament. This route of the genicular vessels is different from that observed in the first group and thus serves to distinguish the arcuate popliteal ligament from the short lateral collateral ligament.

Knees With a Fabella

When the fabella is present (8% of our cases), the arcuate popliteal ligament is a strong structure whose morphology resembles that of the lateral collateral ligament. This ligament was first described by Gruber in 1875; his report included a very accurate drawing of the ligament and fabella (Fig. 10), which he called the "ligament genu externum posticum." This structure corresponds to the fabellofibular ligament since it runs from the fabella to the fibular head, passing, like the arcuate ligament, above the popliteus tendon. It should be emphasized that the fabellofibular ligament is a variation of the arcuate popliteal ligament and does not coexist with the arcuate ligament itself. We should remember that the fabella is situated at the origin of the lateral head of the gastrocnemius muscle on the condylar capsule. The fabella originates from a a fragment of the fibular head that becomes detached during the descent of the primitive femoroperoneal articulation (Fürst 1903; Pearson 1921).

The fabellofibular ligament was also described by Dujarier (1905) as an autonomous structure, which he called the fibular sesamoid ligament This structure was studied more thoroughly by Kaplan in 1961. The fabellofibular ligament is a true ligament only when an osseous fabella is present (Figs. 13, 14a). If the fabella is cartilaginous or fibrocartilaginous (of small size), the ligament is very thin or absent (Fig. 14b). The inferior lateral geniculate vessels pass below the fabellofibular ligament (Fig. 14). In comparative anatomy, the fibular sesamoid ligament is described as a distinct entity only in lower vertebrates. In primates such as the orangutan, the fibular sesamoid ligament tends to be less distinct and integrated with the underlying capsule, being represented at that level by the arcuate popliteal ligament. In summary, the arcuate popliteal ligament is extremely variable from one individual to the next. Also, the limits of the differences characterizing variants are debatable.

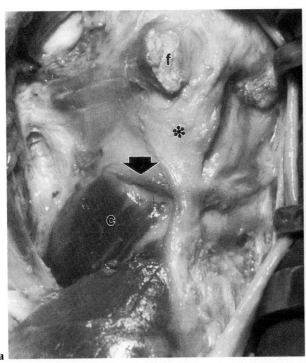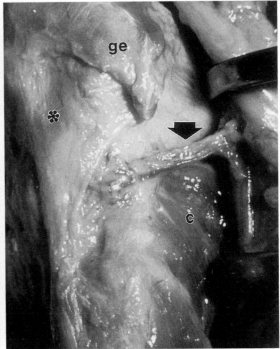

a   b

Fig. 14a,b. Dissections of the fabellofibular ligament. Note the course of the inferolateral artery and vein below the ligament *(arrow)*. **b** A fibrocartilaginous fabella is associated with a weaker fabellofibular ligament (*). *ge*, Lateral head of gastrocnemius; *c*, popliteus muscle; *f*, fabella

The functional significance of the arcuate popliteal ligament in man is poorly understood, mainly because for many years the ligament has been considered an accessory structure of little importance. Undoubtedly, its functional role is difficult to interpret (in our opinion, the functional role is less important than its morphologic role); but when the fabellofibular ligament is present, the functional role must be considered in a different light. The fabellofibular ligament, whose fibers are under maximum tension in hyperextension, has a large cross section and represents a structural component which most likely reinforces the posterolateral corner of the knee during hyperextension. It is reasonable to assume that this ligament may have a primary role in the passive limitation of hyperextension and external rotation, implying that the knee with an osseous fabella has a stronger posterolateral corner structure.

Embryogenesis

The embryogenesis of the human knee joint has been described in several studies (Henke and Reyher 1874; Kazzander 1894; Fürst 1903; Gray and Gardner 1950; Haines 1953; Kaplan 1955; Gardner and O'Rahilly 1968). Despite the number of articles, little attention has been given to the development and fetal morphology of the connections between the popliteus tendon, fibula, and lateral meniscus. To confirm our anatomic observations, we studied human embryos and fetuses ranging from 20 to 140 mm in crownrump length.

Results

In early developmental stages (Haines 1953) the tibia is situated beneath the medial femoral condyle. In the 13-mm fetus the fibula is located under the lateral condyle, but there is still a considerable distance between them. At a later stage (18 mm) (Haines 1953), the tibia is already under both femoral condyles, and the fibular head has almost reached its definitive position near the tibia. At this stage Haines observed that there is a cellular connection between the popliteus tendon and the fibular head. The tibia elongates faster than the fibula, which results in a marked descent of the fibula with respect to the femur and tibia. The different rates of elongation between the tibia and fibula cause an elongation of the connections between the tendon, femur, and fibula. In the 30-mm

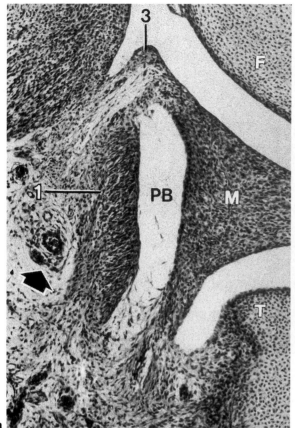

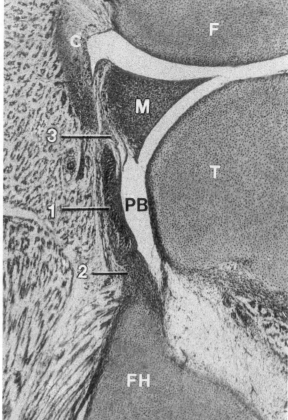

Fig. 15a,b. Lateral view of the knee of a 10-week human fetus (crown-rump length 66 mm), sagittal plane. The cavitation process is almost complete. *F*, Femur; *T*, tibia; *M*, meniscus; *FH*, fibular head. **a** Lateral section showing the superior popliteomeniscal fibers *(3)*, which insert into the superior border of the meniscus *(M)*. *1*, Popliteus tendon; *PB*, popliteal bursa; *arrow* indicates the inferolateral genicular artery and vein (H & E, × 200). **b** Sagittal section through the posterior horn of the lateral meniscus, where the popliteomeniscal fibers unite with the middle third of the posterior wall of the meniscal posterior horn. The inferior pole of the popliteus tendon *(1)* is attached to the fibular head by a ligamentous structure *(2)* representing the popliteofibular fibers. The popliteal bursa *(PB)* is seen anterior to the popliteus tendon and its attachments with the meniscus *(3)* and fibula *(2)*. *C*, Capsule (H & E, × 100)

fetus (8 weeks), the knee joint has a shape similar to that of the adult knee.

The process of cavitation begins during the 10th week of embryonic development. The intraarticular synovial mesenchyme and the mesenchyme that separates the popliteus tendon from the lateral meniscus develop numerous vacuoles due to an increase in the amount of ground substance between cells. The cellular elements rarefy and separate but remain in contact through thin fibrillary extensions. The enlargement of the space between cells and their degeneration form the articular cavities. As it happens, the first cavity to be formed in the knee joint is located in the suprapatellar pouch and is called the porta. Another cavity, the popliteal bursa, forms in the mesenchymal layer between the popliteus tendon and the lateral meniscus. The popliteal bursa is bounded at the top by a cellular fascicle that connects the popliteus tendon with the meniscus; these are the popliteomeniscal fascicles (Fig. 15). The popliteal bursa is bounded at its base by another thick connection between the tendon and the fibular head; these are the popliteofibular fibers (Figs. 15, 16). This connection is a thick band composed of closely packed cells with interconnecting collagen fibrils located between them as in other ligaments.

Understanding how the cavitation process develops the popliteal bursa and how its expansion is limited by the connections of the popliteal tendon with the meniscus and fibular head has helped to demonstrate that, by the 10th week of gestation, the popliteomeniscal fibers and the popliteofibular ligament are already distinct and easily recognizable structures in the human fetus. By the 16th week of development,

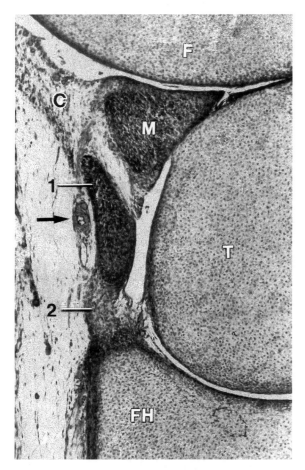

Fig. 16. Lateral view of the knee of a 10 1/2-week human embryo (crown-rump length 62 mm), sagittal plane. Median section through the posterior horn of the lateral meniscus. The cavitation process appears to be less advanced than in Fig. 15. The popliteofibular fibers *(2)* unite the inferior pole of the popliteus tendon *(1)* with the fibular head. *C*, Capsule; *M*, posterior horn of lateral meniscus; *F*, femur; *T*, tibia. The site of the arcuate ligament in adults is marked by a lax areolar tissue posterior to the inferolateral genicular vessels *(arrow)*

the connections between the popliteus tendon, lateral meniscus, and fibular head are fully formed.

In our embryologic study, we were unable to observe the arcuate ligament. The space corresponding to its adult location (behind the popliteus tendon and inferior geniculate vessels) was occupied by loose areolar tissue (Fig. 16). We found neither the fabella nor its cartilaginous nuclei.

References

Basset DL (1962) A stereoscopic atlas of human anatomy. The lower extremity. Section VII; 190-2, 191-1, 191-5, 195-2, 196-1

Dujarier C (1905) Anatomie des membres. Steinheil, Paris

Fabbriciani C, Oransky M, Zoppi U (1982a) Il legamento popliteo arcuato e le sue varianti. Ital J Sports Traumatol 4/3: 171-177

Fabbriciani C, Oransky M, Zoppi U (1982b) Il muscolo popliteo: studio anatomico. Arch Ital Anat Embriol 87/3: 203-217

Fürst CM (1903) Der Musculus popliteus und seine Sehne. Acta Regiae Societatis Physiographicae Lundensis E. Malström Boktrycheri Lund

Gardner E, O'Rahilly R (1968) The early development of the knee joint in staged human embryos. J Anat 102/2: 289-299

Gray DJ, Gardner E (1950) Prenatal development of the human knee and superior tibiofibular joint. Am J Anat 86: 235-288

Gruber W (1875) Über den Musculus Popliteus Biceps. Arch Anat Physiol Wiss Med: 599-605

Haines RW (1953) The early development of the femoro-tibial and tibio-fibular joints. J Anatomy 87: 192-206

Heitzmann C (1890) Anatomia Umana Descrittiva e Topografica, 5. ed. Vienna

Henke W, Reyher R (1874) Studien über die Entwicklung der Extremitäten des Menschen, insbesondere der Gelenkflächen. Sitzungsber Akad Wiss Math Naturw Klasse 70: 217-273

Kaplan EB (1955) The embryology of the menisci of the knee joint. Bull Hosp Jt Dis 16: 111-124

Kaplan EB (1961) The fabello fibular and short lateral ligaments of the knee joint. J Bone Joint Surg [Am] 43: 169-179

Kaplan EB (1975) Surgical approach to the lateral (peroneal) side of the knee joint. Surg Gynecol Obstet 104: 346

Kazzander G (1894) Sullo Sviluppo dell'articolazione del ginocchio. Monitore Zool Ital 5: 220-235

Krause T (1879) Handbuch der Menschlichen Anatomie, 3. Aufl. Hannover

Last RJ (1950) The popliteus muscle and lateral meniscus. J Bone Joint Surg [Br] 32: 93-99

Lovejoy JF, Harden TP (1971) Popliteus muscle in man. Anat Rec 169: 727-730

Macalister A (1875) Additional observations on muscular anomalies in human anatomy. Trans Roy Ir Acad 25

O'Rahilly R (1975) The development of joints. Ir J Med Sci 4: 456-461

O'Rahilly R, Bossy J, Müller F (1981) Introduction à l'étude des stades embryonnaires chez l'homme. Bull Assoc Anat 65: 141-234

Oransky M, Canero G, Maiotti M (1989). The embryonic development of the posterolateral structures of the knee. Anat Rec 225: 347-354

Pearson K, Davin AG (1921) On the sesamoids of the knee joint. Biometrika 13: 133

Seebacher JR, Inglis AE, Marshall JL, Warren RF (1982) The structure of the posterolateral aspect of the knee. J Bone Joint Surg [Am] 64: 536-541

Testut JL (1911) Traité d'anatomie humaine. Doin, Paris

Vallois HV (1914) Étude anatomique l'articulation du genou chez les primates. L'Abeille, Montpellier (thèse)

Weitbrecht J (1742) Syndesmologia sive Historia Ligamentorum Corporis Humani quam Secundum Observations Anatomicas Concinnavit. Typographia Academiae Scientiorum, Petropoli

Structural Molecules in Articular Cartilage, Tendons, and Ligaments

E.B. Hunziker

The numerous functions of the knee joint are based on a finely coordinated interaction of diverse elements of the locomotor system, including the articular cartilage, tendons, and ligaments. These tissues owe their unique biomechanical properties to the presence of specific macromolecules in the extracellular space, their organization into higher-order structural units, and the interactions among them. The macro- and supramolecular organization of the extracellular matrix in these tissues remains under cellular control throughout the life of the individual. This is of crucial importance as it relates to the ongoing "transformation and renewal" of tissues and to possible regenerative processes.

Our goal in this chapter is to present a brief overview of the principal extracellular structural molecules that make up the articular cartilage, tendons, and ligaments. Reference will be made to the functional implications of the molecular and supramolecular patterns of structural organization in these tissues as we currently understand them. The macromolecules that are most abundant in cartilage tissue are the proteoglycans and collagens. These are accompanied by many types of smaller matrix molecule, most notably glycoproteins. Tendons and ligaments are composed chiefly of collagens, with relatively small amounts of proteoglycans and matrix molecules. In the sections that follow, these classes of molecule will be individually discussed, and the functional aspects of their arrangements and interactions in cartilage, tendons, and ligaments will be explored.

Proteoglycans

Formerly known as mucopolysaccharides, proteoglycans are giant molecules having molecular weights of several million daltons. They consist of a central protein filament (core protein), which in the case of cartilage proteoglycans may be approximately 200–400 nm in length (Fig. 1). The protein constituent has two globular units at its N-terminal end, one of which contains a binding site specific for hyaluronic acid. A single globular domain may occur at the C-terminus, but it is not consistently observed. Various types of polymeric carbohydrate are covalently bonded to sites along the core filament. In cartilage proteoglycans, these consist mostly of chondroitin sulfate glycosaminoglycans (Fig. 2), whose numerous sulfate groups are present in dissociated form at physiologic pH. This gives the proteoglycan molecule a very high number and spatial density of fixed, negatively charged (ionized) groups. The chondroitin sulfate (CS) glycans (approximately 40–60 nm in length) appear to be distributed over the full length of the core filament, showing a slightly lower density toward the N-terminal end. Another glycan, keratan sulfate (KS), tends to be more abundant along that segment.

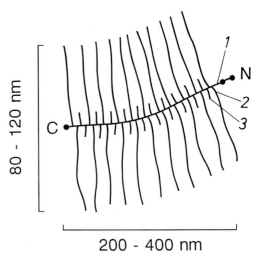

Fig. 1. Schematic diagram of a cartilage proteoglycan molecule (monomer). The molecule ranges from 200 to 400 nm in length, from 80 to 120 nm in transverse diameter. The central protein filament (core protein) *(1)* has two globular units at its N-terminus, which contains a binding site for hyaluronic acid. The opposite, C-terminal end has only one globular domain. Attached to the core filament are more than 100 long glycosaminoglycan chains *(2)* (mainly chondroitin and keratan sulfates), which possess a high density of anionic groups (see Fig. 2). These strands radiate away from the core protein, giving the proteoglycan molecule a "bottle brush" form. The long glycan chains include more than 100 oligosaccharides *(3)*, which are bound covalently to the core protein

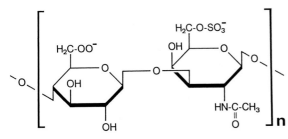

Fig. 2. Schematic diagram of a polymerization unit (disaccharide) from the chondroitin sulfate side chain of a cartilage proteoglycan molecule. The disaccharide pictured is the polymer unit of a chondroitin-6-sulfate glycan. Note the fixed anionic groups (COO^-, SO_4)

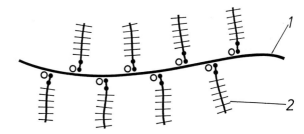

Fig. 4. Schematic diagram of a proteoglycan aggregate. Numerous proteoglycan monomers *(2)* bind at their N-terminal ends to a hyaluronic acid filament *(1)*. These bonds are stabilized by link proteins *(circles)* (= glycoproteins of the cartilage matrix)

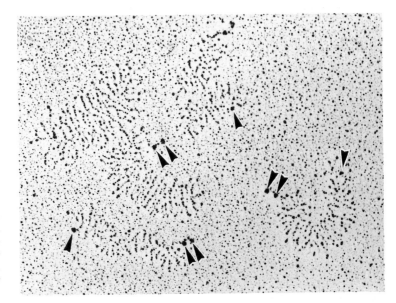

Fig. 3. Electron micrograph of proteoglycan monomers. *Double arrows:* N-terminal ends with two globular domains. *Single arrows:* C-terminal ends with one globular domain. (With kind permission of M. Paulsson and M. Mörgelin, Biocenter Basel)

An average of about 100 glycans (CS and KS) are attached to one core protein, so thousands of firmly bound negative charges are present within a single proteoglycan molecule.

An equally large number of oligosaccharide chains are attached to the core protein (via oxygen or nitrogen binding). These short-chain elements are evenly distributed over the length of the core protein filament (Fig. 1). Electron microscopic studies of isolated proteoglycan molecules have confirmed this structural model (Fig. 3). The proteoglycan molecules (PG) themselves are referred to as PG subunits or PG monomers, because their binding sites for hyaluronic acid enable them to attach to hyaluronate filaments, leading to the formation of giant molecular assemblies called proteoglycan aggregates (Figs. 4–6).

The PGs that occur in connective tissue, tendons, and ligaments are generally much smaller than cartilage PGs. They may contain only two or three glycan side chains, as in dermatan sulfate PG (which also occurs in very young cartilage tissue and plays a role in cartilage regeneration). There are also membrane-bound PGs, whose core protein filament has a hydrophobic segment that permits their attachment, say, to the plasma membrane of a cell.

Collagens

All collagen molecules consist of three polypeptide chains twisted into a helix. The collagen triple helix is synthesized intracellularly and released in a soluble form, procollagen, into the extracellular space. During the intracellular synthesis of the procollagen pre-

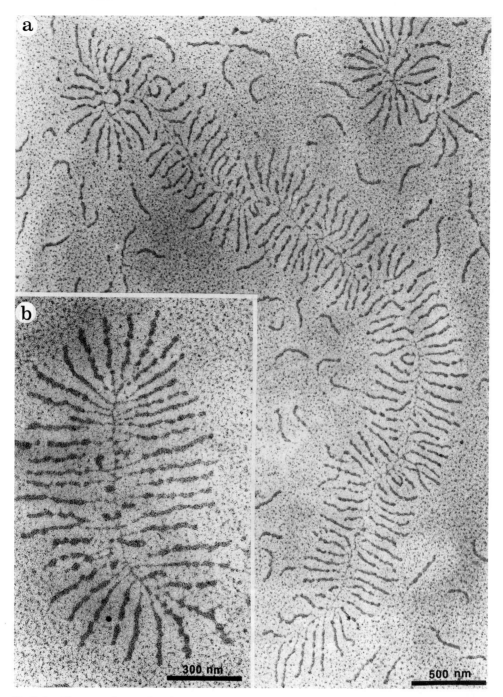

Fig. 5 a,b. Electron micrographs of proteoglycan aggregates. The individual proteoglycan monomers appear as long, dense strands because glycan chains precipitate onto the core proteins during preparation. (From Buckwalter and Rosenberg 1988)

cursor peptides, in which every third amino acid is a glycine and which is also very rich in proline, these peptides are hydroxylated to a high degree (with formation of hydroxyproline and hydroxylysine) before they assemble to form the triple-helical procollagen molecules. These molecules are semirigid linear elements, approximately 280–300 nm in length, with reg-

istration peptides at their C- and N-terminal ends. They are still water-soluble and are secreted in that form into the extracellular space. Outside the cell, procollagen peptidases cleave off the terminal registration peptides to form the true collagen molecules (formerly called tropocollagen). These molecules can polymerize to form collagen fibrils (Fig. 7); this ap-

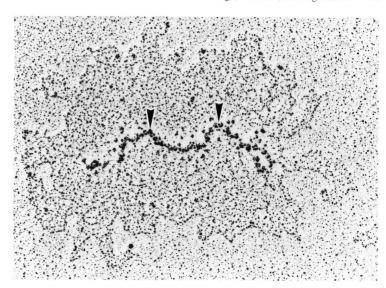

Fig. 6. Electron micrograph of a proteoglycan aggregate after (heavy-metal) rotary shadowing with platinum-carbon in a high vacuum. The central hyaluronic acid filament is saturated with (dark) globular domains *(arrows)* of the hyaluronic acid-binding N-terminal ends of the proteoglycan monomers. The numerous glycan chains of the monomers are not precipitated and form an interdigitating pattern, though they are not clearly visible as separate chains. (From Mörgelin et al. 1988)

plies, however, only to certain species of collagen molecule (see below).

The collagen molecules within the fibrils are arranged in a parallel configuration in which adjacent fibrils are staggered from one another by about one-quarter of their length (see Fig. 7). This leads to the presence of gaps among the fibrils, which can be utilized for microscopic visualization. Specifically, we can stain these gaps with contrast material (heavy metal salts) so that the collagen fibrils exhibit a typical cross-striation or "banded" pattern (period 64 nm) when viewed by electron microscopy (Fig. 8 a–d). Once fibril formation in the extracellular tissue space is completed, the collagen molecules in the fibrils additionally undergo a chemical cross-linking in which the individual polypeptide chains in the collagen triple helix are cross-linked and the collagen molecules within the fibrils are covalently cross-linked one to the other. These chemical modifications influence the biomechanical properties of the collagen fibrils, the most notable effect being an increase in their resistance to tensile loading.

Fifteen different types of collagen have been described to date, these being derived from at least 25 different gene products. The different types of triple-helical collagen molecule are distinguished by specific polypeptide chains, which differ qualitatively in their amino acid sequences. There are also quantitative differences that involve marked variations in the lengths of the triple-helical molecules of the different collagen species. Nonfibrillary collagens may contain non-triple-helical (e.g., linear or globular) protein segments in addition to their triple-helical components, and glycosaminoglycan chains can attach to the molecule (Fig. 9).

The fibril-forming collagens – types I, II, III, V, and XI – comprise a structurally homogeneous group. They all possess triple-helical collagen domains that are approximately 300 nm in length and relatively inflexible. All are synthesized in a precursor state (i.e., as a procollagen triple helix) and are secreted by the cells in that form.

The marked structural similarities among the different collagen types explain why antisera produced against a specific collagen type show a high degree of cross-reactivity with other types. Nor are we surprised by evidence that there are no "pure" collagen fibrils composed of only one type of molecule, but that the collagen fibrils represent copolymers composed of multiple collagen species (see Fig. 8 a–d).

It has been shown, for example, that the "type I collagen-containing" fibrils of the cornea also contain type V collagen, and thus that type I collagen merely forms the predominant constituent of the corneal fibrils. Type V appears to occur only in the interior of the fibrils and not on their surface. The banded collagen fibers in general appear to be composed of more than one collagen type. The genetic heterogeneity of the fibril-forming collagens most likely represents an important biological adaptation for the regulation of fibrillogenesis in vivo.

Hydroxylated procollagen
precursor peptides

Procollagen (soluble) with
registration peptides

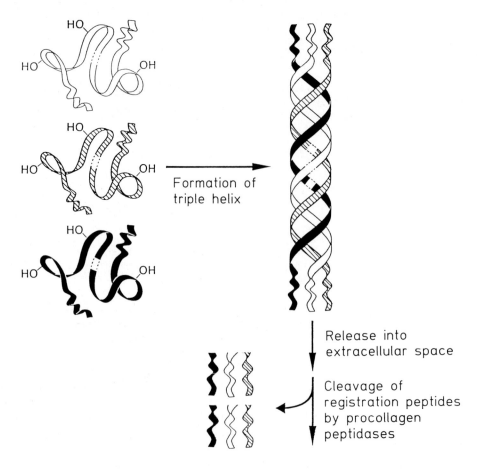

Formation of
triple helix

Release into
extracellular space

Cleavage of
registration peptides
by procollagen
peptidases

Collagen molecule

Aggregation

Collagen fibrils

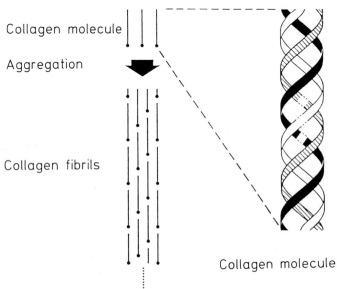

Collagen molecule

Fig. 7. Schematic diagram of collagen synthesis, polymerization and fibrillogenesis. The procollagen precursor peptides are synthesized intracellularly in the rough endoplasmic reticulum, where their hydroxylation also commences. Three polypeptide chains assemble into a triple helix to form the procollagen molecule; this likewise occurs in the endoplasmic reticulum. The procollagen molecules carry terminal registration peptides, which give them the property of water solubility. Following release of the procollagens into the extracellular space, the registration peptides are split off from the procollagen molecules by procollagen peptidases. With this step, the true water-insoluble collagen molecule is formed. Types I, II, III, V, and XI collagen molecules can polymerize by this pattern (aggregate) to form fibrils

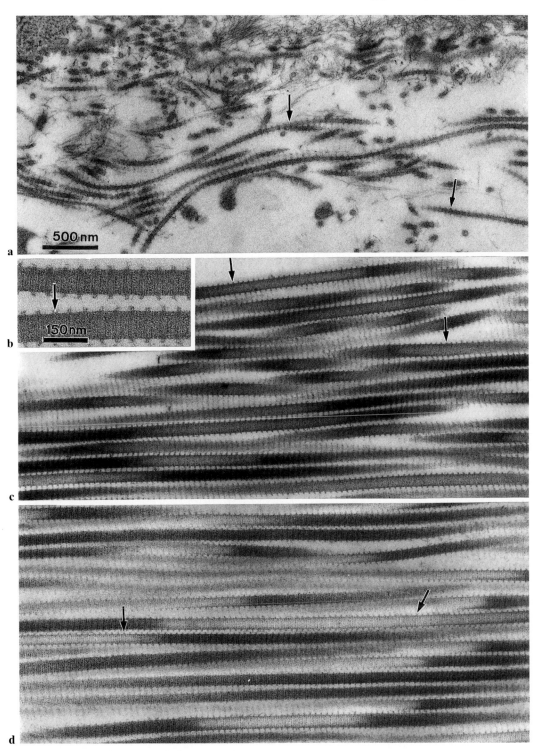

Fig. 8 a–d. Transmission electron micrographs of type I collagen fibrils. Codistribution of type I and type III collagen in various tissues. Monoclonal IgM antibody molecules *(arrows)* against type III collagen are visualized on collagen fibrils composed predominantly of type I collagen; this signifies copolymeriza- tion processes during fibrillogenesis. **a** Collagen in neonatal dermis. **b** Plantar surface toe skin of 14-year-old. **c** Back skin of 11-year-old. **d** Thigh skin of 14-year-old. (From Keene et al. 1987a)

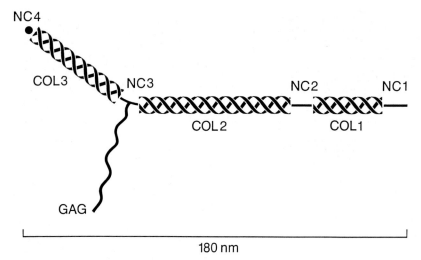

Fig. 9. Schematic diagram of a type IX collagen molecule. Approximately 180 nm in length, the molecule consists of three triple-helical collagen segments (*COL1, COL2, COL3*) and four noncollagenous protein segments (*NC1, NC2, NC3, NC4*). The NC3 region appears to form a flexible site at which the molecule generally becomes "kinked." A glycosaminoglycan chain (GAG) also attaches to that site, giving the collagen molecule "proteoglycan" properties. The NC4 region is present at the N-terminal end as a globular domain

Another example is the tendon collagens, in which the fibrils are assembled into higher-order units, or fibers, and are composed chiefly of type I collagens. Immunohistochemical studies have shown that type III collagen is also uniformly present on the tendon fibrils (Fig. 10a–e). This is surprising because previous studies using biochemical isolation techniques were unable to demonstrate type III collagen in tendons. The finding of type III collagen provided further evidence that fibrils generally are composed of two or more distinct collagen species. The implication of these findings is that fibrillogenesis is a highly complex process and that each of these collagen types is probably responsible for a specific regulatory task.

Similarly, the fibrillary collagen in cartilage consists chiefly of type II collagen, which is very similar structurally to type I. But type II also appears to copolymerize with other collagen types, as evidenced by the finding of type XI collagen in the interior of the fibrils. Type XI collagen probably performs a regulatory task by determining the ultimate lateral dimension (thickness) attained by fibrils during fibrillogenesis. The type XI collagen molecule is structurally analogous to type V collagen, with only minor differences.

In addition to types II and XI, cartilage tissue also contains type IX collagen. In contrast to the fibril-forming collagens (I, II, III, V, XI), all of which have a similar structure (triple helical, approximately 300 nm long), the triple-helical component of type IX collagen is only about 180 nm in length and is interrupted by two nonhelical segments (see Fig. 9). Another difference is the presence of a single chondroitin sulfate glycosaminoglycan chain covalently attached to a nonhelical segment. Type IX collagen binds to the surface of cartilage collagen fibrils (Figs. 11, 12) and appears to be more abundant at sites of fibril crossing. The association of type IX collagens with the cartilage collagen fibrils is such that the triple-helical segment (near the C-terminus) is parallel to the fiber axis whereas the N-terminal segments and the glycan chain are oriented perpendicular to the fibril (see Figs. 11, 12). The glycan chain may appose to the fibril surface or may stand away from it (see Fig. 11).

None of the foregoing cartilage collagens are present in tendon or ligamentous tissues, which consist predominantly of the type I and type III triple-helical fiber-forming collagens (see Fig. 10). The ultimate fibril diameter attained during fibrillogenesis does not appear to be regulated by the presence or absence of a specific collagen type, as in the case of the cartilage collagen fibrils. It appears to depend, rather, on the quantitative ratio in which the type I and type III collagens are secreted during fibril polymerization. Thus, the specific properties of the collagen triple helix can directly influence the process of fibrillogenesis in some circumstances. Type IX collagen does not exist in tendons or ligaments, but there is a collagen, type XII, that assumes an analogous function in those tissues. It appears to bind to the surface of fibrils, but only those containing types I and III (or type V collagen, which is not discussed here). Type

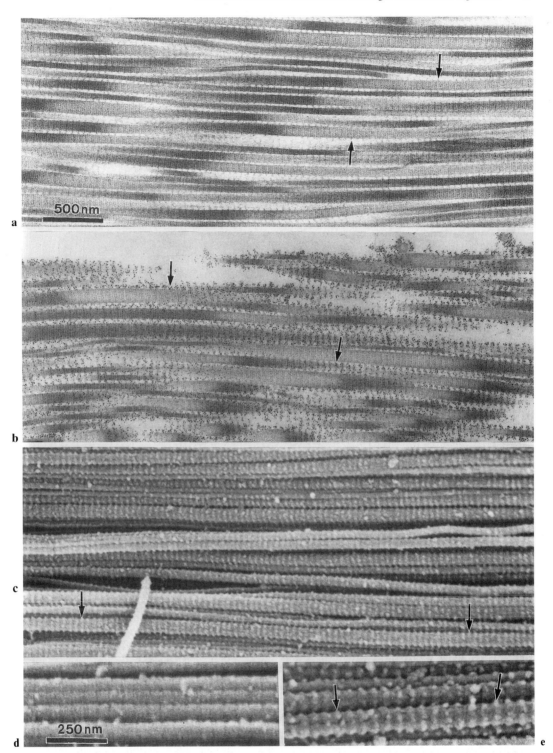

Fig. 10a–e. Immunolocalization of type III collagen in human tendon tissue (analogous to Fig. 8a–d). Achilles tendon specimens from 77- to 80-year-old subjects were incubated with monoclonal anti-type III collagen antibody (IgM). **a, b** Transmission electron micrographs. Collagen fibrils in **a** are decorated with IgM *(arrows)*. **b** Fibril-decorating IgM molecules labeled with colloidal gold particles *(black spots* along fibrils). **c, d, e** Scanning electron micrograph. **c, e** Anti-type III collagen IgM molecules *(arrows)* decorate tendon collagen fibrils (type I collagen). **d** Control tendon without (IgM) antibody. (From Keene et al. 1987a)

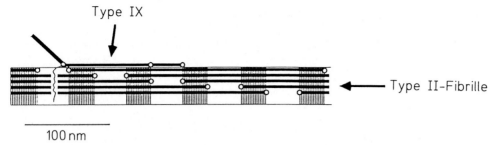

Fig. 11. Schematic diagram of surface association of type IX collagen with type II collagen fibrils in cartilage tissue. The segments COL1, COL2, NC1, and NC2 are apposed to the fibril surface. The remaining segments (COL3, NC4) stand away from the fibril at the flexible NC3 segment. The glycan chain probably apposes to the fibril as well. (From van der Rest and Mayne 1988)

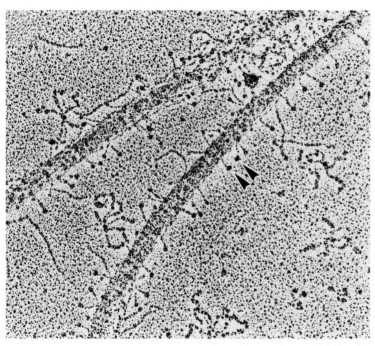

Fig. 12. Electron micrograph of fibrillary cartilage specimen visualized by rotary shadowing. Type IX collagen molecules are seen along the fibril surfaces, some of them standing away from the fibril. For clarity, they are labeled *(black dots)* with anti-type IX collagen antibody *(arrowheads)*. (With kind permission of Dr. L. Vaughan, ETH, Zürich)

XII collagen has only recently been detected in tendon tissue, and its functional significance remains unclear. Type VI collagen is another type that can occur in association with fibrillary cartilage surfaces, though it can also occupy interfibrillary spaces in the form of larger polymers (Fig. 13).

Thus, the mixing ratio of different collagen types is a critical factor regulating fibrillogenesis and determining the ultimate fibril diameter (and probably its biomechanical properties as well). A significant biological influence is also exerted by the enzymes that cleave registration peptides from the procollagen molecules. In all fibril-forming collagens, the C-terminal registration peptides must be removed before fibrillogenesis can take place. But the N-terminal registration peptides may remain in place for a longer time or may be only partially cleaved by the specific procollagen peptidases before fibrillogenesis begins. This circumstance, plus the fact that the kinetics of this cleavage reaction generally proceeds at a slower rate than that for the C-terminal peptides, gives the reaction a regulatory role in fibrillogenesis. As long as N-terminal registration peptides remain attached in significant quantities, the collagen molecules appear to be able to form only fibrils having a small transverse diameter.

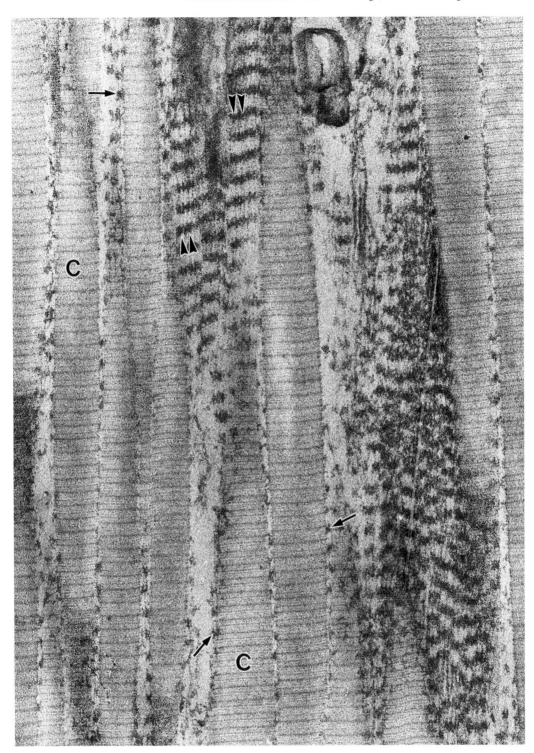

Fig. 13. Longitudinal section through a rat tail tendon, electron micrograph. Numerous type I collagen fibrils *(C)* are decorated with type VI collagen *(arrows)*. Type VI collagen also occupies part of the collagen interspaces *(arrowheads)*, displaying a coarsely periodic (100-nm) signal. (From Bruns et al. 1986)

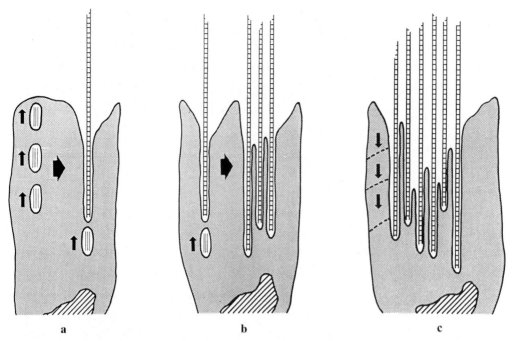

Fig. 14 a–c. Schematic diagram of collagen fibrillogenesis in extracellular compartments of tendon tissue. **a** Secretory vacuoles containing procollagen molecules align tandemly within the cells and fuse with the cell surface and with adjacent vacuoles. This leads to the development of long, narrow recesses, the fibril-forming compartments. **b** The lateral fusion of multiple fibril-forming compartments leads to the development of large "bundle-forming" compartments. Collagen fibrils are added to the fibril bundles by the continued fusion of fibril-forming compartments with bundle-forming compartments. **c** Large bundle-forming compartments fuse laterally with other compartments as the intervening cytoplasm is retracted. As indicated by the *dotted lines* and *arrows*, large processes between adjacent cells are also retracted, permitting the coalescence of large fiber aggregates between fibroblasts. (From Birk and Trelstad 1986)

Collagen fibrillogenesis, then, is controlled at the cellular level both by a posttranslational modification of the molecules and by the synthesis and secretion of different collagen types and different procollagen-modifying enzymes. A direct cellular action on fibrillogenesis, moreover, is illustrated by tendon collagen fibrillogenesis, in which fibrils are assembled in topographically defined directions into fibril bundles, which in turn are assembled into fibers or large (macro) aggregates (Figs. 14–16). These processes take place in well-defined extracellular compartments, which appear electron microscopically as deep, narrow invaginations in the plasma membrane of the tendon fibroblasts (see Figs. 15, 16). The cells, then, control collagen fibrillogenesis in three ways:

- At the intracellular level by the posttranslational modification and simultaneous synthesis of various collagen types
- At the extracellular level by the secretion of a specifically defined enzyme matrix for fibrillogenesis (and the simultaneous secretion of different collagen types)

- By a topographic effect achieved through compartment formation in the plasma membrane

Thus, the cell exerts complete control over the quality of the fibril and fiber structure and their orientation.

Matrix Molecules

This class of molecule consists almost exclusively of glycoproteins. By themselves, they do not perform a direct structure-defining function, but they can play an important role through their effect on various structural proteins.

A major representative of this group is the link protein. The function of link proteins is to stabilize the proteoglycan aggregates. In this capacity they interact directly with hyaluronic acid filaments and with proteoglycan core proteins via specific binding sites (see Figs. 4–6). It is possible that they facilitate the postulated interactions of proteoglycan molecules with collagen fibrils.

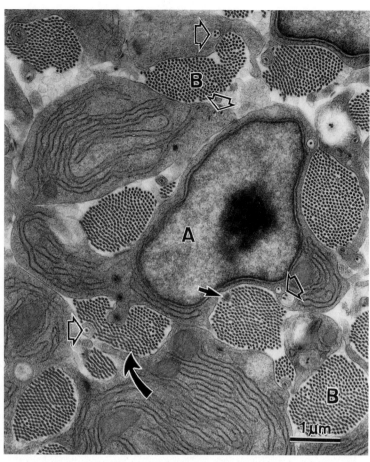

Fig. 15. Electron micrograph: transverse section through a collagen-forming fibroblast. *A* Cell nucleus; *B* numerous fibril bundles closely associated with the compartment-forming cell membrane. *Open arrows:* narrow recesses (compartments) in which the processes of fibrillogenesis occur. *Curved arrow:* cytoplasmic processes that separate the bundle-forming compartments. *Short, black arrow:* elastin-associated microfilaments. These are commonly seen at the surface of fibril bundles. (From Birk and Trelstad 1986)

Chondronectin and chondrocalcin are two other matrix glycoproteins whose functions remain unclear. Chondronectin may be involved in the interaction of the chondrocyte membrane with collagen fibrils; chondrocalcin may play a role in the induction of cartilage matrix mineralization.

Only trace amounts of proteoglycans are present in tendons and ligaments (<1% dry weight). Some elastin is present in these tissues (up to 5% dry weight) but does not occur in cartilage. Tendons and ligaments also contain fibronectin and other glycoproteins that have not been specifically analyzed.

Molecular Organization of the Cartilage Matrix

Articular cartilage derives its distinctive functional properties – resiliency, durability, ability to distribute loads and glide smoothly against an opposing surface – entirely from its intercellular substance, or cartilage matrix, which makes up approximately 90% of the articular cartilage. Cartilage tissue is devoid of nerve fibers, blood vessels, and lymphatics.

Cartilage matrix is composed chiefly of water (60%–80%), and it is the water molecules that give the cartilage tissue its essential biomechanical properties. To perform these functions, the tissue water must be present in a "bound" form so that it is not simply extruded by mechanical loading. Nature solves this problem in a unique way: by the incorporation of proteoglycan molecules. These polyanionic giant mole-

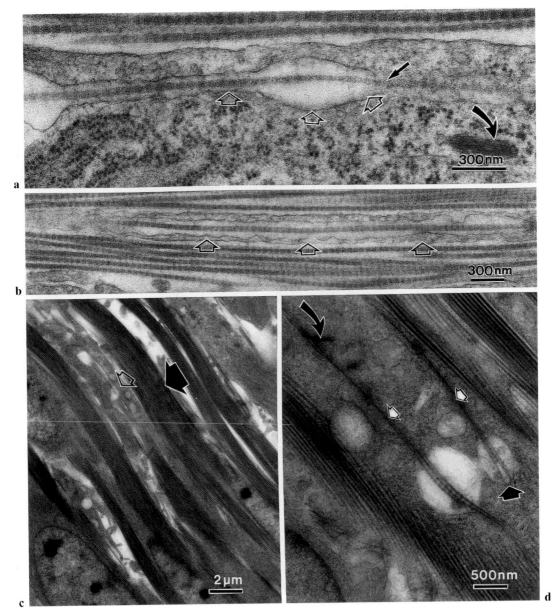

Fig. 16 a–d. Electron micrographs of a collagen-forming tendon fibroblast. **a** A narrow cytoplasmic recess (fibril-forming compartment), cut in longitudinal section, contains a single collagen fibril *(solid arrow)*. The recess is membrane delimited and contains a dilated portion with wavy borders *(open arrows)*. Secretory vacuoles *(curved arrow)* are often associated with these regions. **b** Fibril-forming compartment, cut longitudinally as in **a**. The delimiting membranes still appear wavy *(open arrows)*, probably due to the fusion of several secretory vacuoles. **c** High-voltage electron micrograph showing portions of four adjacent fibroblasts. *Open arrow:* numerous secretory vacuoles. *Solid arrow:* larger fibril bundles in close association with the cell membrane. **d** High-voltage electron micrograph. *Open arrows:* fibril-forming recesses (compartments). *Solid arrow:* hairpin loop in a collagen fibril within a recess. *Curved arrow:* narrow secretory vacuole. (From Birk and Trelstad 1986)

cules are released by the cartilage cells into the matrix in a greatly underhydrated state, and thus at an extremely high concentration. The many anionic groups give these molecules a tremendous water binding capacity, and if placed into a pure aqueous solution they would undergo a massive expansion to 6–8 times their original volume. In cartilage, however, the molecules are held in a collagen fibril network that is extremely fine in the superficial layers (tangential zone) and prevents the proteoglycans from escaping into the joint cavity. The constant resting pressure (expansion pressure) exerted by the hydrophilic proteoglycans is transmitted to the essentially noncompliant collagen fiber network, keeping it in a state of tension. It is this unique interaction between two matrix macromolecules, the proteoglycans and the collagen fibrils, together comprising about 20%–40% of the fresh tissue weight, which gives the articular cartilage its distinctive properties.

When weight-bearing forces act upon a joint, water may temporarily be extruded from the matrix. This increases the degree of underhydration of the articular cartilage, which in turn increases its resistance to further compression. As this occurs, the countless bound anionic groups of glycosaminoglycans (see Fig. 2) pack more closely together, giving rise to electrical repulsive forces that increasingly inhibit further compression of the cartilage. Another immediate consequence of the reversible water loss is a massive increase in the relative concentration of free counterions (cations: Ca^{2+}, Na^+, K^+, etc.), thereby raising the osmotic pressure and progressively opposing further water shifts (and further compression). The following mechanisms are available, then, for counteracting gross biomechanical forces on the macromolecular level:

- Macromolecular interactions (proteoglycan trap in the collagen fibril network)
- Physicochemical forces (increasing expansion pressure and osmotic pressure)
- Electrical repulsion (increasing negative charge density)

The resting pressure of the cartilage matrix (expansion pressure, osmotic pressure), incidentally, is very high and is on the order of 2–3 atm (0.2–0.3 MPa).

The complex but strictly defined structural organization of the matrix molecules is under cellular control and is very sensitive to interference by external factors (such as trauma, changes in the physiologic load pattern, etc.). Once locally disrupted, the unique ultrastructural, chemical, and physical characteristics of the cartilage matrix are extremely difficult to restore. The regeneration of cartilage tissue, if it occurs at all, generally results in a functionally inferior tissue such as fibrocartilage. The permanent regeneration of articular cartilage is very rarely observed. Even with supportive therapy, physicians have been unable to effect a complete cure in terms of restoring the articular cartilage.

Molecular Organization in Tendons and Ligaments

The molecular structural organization of tendons and ligaments is designed essentially for the transmission or neutralization of tensile forces. Fresh tissue is composed mainly of water (60%–70%), which performs no specific biomechanical function per se (unlike the water in cartilage). The mechanical functions are performed by collagen (high tensile strength), which accounts for 70%–80% of the tissue dry weight. Type I collagen is far more abundant than type III collagen (approximately 90% and 10%, respectively). Minority collagens such as types V, VI, and XII also occur. The tendon and ligament collagens have an estimated half-life of 300–500 days. Although the proteoglycans account for less than 1% of the tissue dry weight, they appear to play a major functional role through their specific interactions with the collagen fibrils. It is unclear whether they also perform a regulatory function in fibrillogenesis and in the control of fibril diameters.

Elastin generally accounts for less than 5% of the dry weight of ligaments. Its functional significance is poorly understood. There are also a number of glycoproteins (such as fibronectin) whose precise functions remain obscure.

The high resistance of ligaments and tendons to tensile loading and to stretch ($< 5\%$) are based largely on the specific properties of collagen. Collagen molecules (1–2 nm in diameter) associate to form microfibrils (3–4 nm); these combine into subfibrils (10–20 nm), from which fibrils (50–500 nm) are formed. The fibrils in turn assemble into collagen fibers approximately 0.5–3 µm in diameter.

Besides the (probably specific) proteoglycan-collagen interactions described above, the functions of ligaments and tendons are critically influenced by the degree of collagen glycosylation and by collagen cross-linking. The latter process occurs in the extracellular space after formation of the fibrils and fiber systems. These systems are constructed by the fibroblasts in accordance with a spatially controlled pattern. The tendons and ligaments are prime examples of the cellular control function of directional or defined fibril synthesis (see Figs. 15, 16), as noted above. In regenerative processes, this requires that the cells, too, align in accordance with prevailing lines of force, and they seem to have the ability to do this. Although cell forms and cellular density can vary considerably from ligament to ligament, the cells consistently determine the direction of the collagen fibril arrangement with very high precision. As a rule, various populations of fibrils coexist within the same ligament. In the anterior cruciate ligament, for example, there is a preponderance (< 85%) of thin collagen fibrils (i.e., fibrils < 100 nm in diameter). In tendons, this population is markedly reduced (< 55%) in favor of larger-diameter fibrils.

The mean fibril diameter correlates poorly with the mechanical properties of a ligament. A more useful parameter is the size of the subpopulation of fibrils with a smaller (< 100 nm) or larger diameter. This is illustrated by the significant increase in the subpopulation of small fibrils (80–100 nm), with an associated increase in mechanical strength, which is effected therapeutically by specific ligament training. This is accomplished, however, at the cost of a slight reduction in stiffness. A predominant synthesis of small-diameter fibers is also seen initially in regenerative processes, which depend basically on an adequate vascular supply.

References

Birk DE, Trelstad RL (1986) Extracellular compartments in tendon morphogenesis: Collagen fibril, bundle, and macroaggregate formation. J Cell Biol 103: 231–240

Birk DE, Fitch JM, Babiarz JP, Linsenmayer TF (1988) Collagen type I and type V are present in the same fibril in the avian corneal stroma. J Cell Biol 106: 999–1008

Bruns RR, Press W, Engvall E, Timpl R, Gross J (1986) Type VI collagen in extracellular, 100-nm periodic filaments and fibrils: Identification by immunoelectron microscopy. J Cell Biol 103: 393–404

Buckwalter JA, Rosenberg LC (1988) Electron microscopic studies of cartilage proteoglycans. Electr Microsc Rev 1: 87–112

Burgeson RE (1988a) Do banded collagen fibers contain two or more collagen types? ISI Atlas of Science/Biochemistry 1/1: 88–91

Burgeson RE (1988b) New collagens, new concepts, Ann Rev Cell Biol 4: 551–577

Carney SL, Muir H (1988) The structure and function of cartilage proteoglycans. Physiol Rev 68/3: 858–910

Dublet B, van der Rest M (1987) Type XII collagen is expressed in embryonic chick tendons. J Biol Chem 262/36: 17727–17727

Dublet B, Dixon E, de Miguel E, van der Rest M (1988) Bovine type XII collagen: amino acid sequence of a 10 kDa pepsin fragment from periodontal ligament reveals a high degree of homology with the chicken 1(XII) sequence. FEBS Lett 233/1: 177–180

Evered D, Whelan J (eds) (1986) CIBA Foundation Symposium 124. Functions of the proteoglycans. Wiley, Chichester

Eyre DR, Wu JJ, Apone S (1987) A growing family of collagens in articular cartilage: Identification of 5 genetically distinct types. J Rheumatol 14/14: 25–27

Eyre DR, Dickson IR, van Ness K (1988) Collagen crosslinking in human bone and articular cartilage. Age-related changes in the content of mature hydroxypyridinium residues. Biochem J 252: 495–500

Fleischmajer R, Perlish JS, Olsen BR (1987) The carboxyl-propeptide of type I procollagen in skin fibrillogenesis. J Invest Dermatol 89/2: 212–215

Goetinck PF, Stirpe NS, Tsonis PA, Carlone D (1987) The tandemly repeated sequences of cartilage link protein contain the sites for interaction with hyaluronic acid. J Cell Biol 105: 2403–2408

Grant WT, Sussman MD, Balian G (1985) A disulfide-bonded short chain collagen synthesized by degenerative and calcifying zones of bovine growth plate cartilage. J Biol Chem 264: 3798–3803

Hascall VC (1981) Proteoglycans: structure and function. In: Ginsburg V, Robbins P (eds) Biology of carbohydrates, vol 1. Wiley, Chichester, pp 1–48

Hay ED (ed) (1982) Cell biology of extracellular matrix. Plenum, New York London

Heinegård D, Larsson T, Sommarin Y, Franzen A, Paulsson M, Hedbom E (1986) Two novel matrix proteins isolated from articular cartilage show wide distributions among connective tissues. J Biol Chem 261/29: 13866–13872

Hørslev-Petersen K, Pedersen LR, Bentsen KD et al. (1988) Collagen type IV and procollagein type III during granulation tissue formation: a serological, biochemical, immuno-histochemical and morphometrical study on the viscose cellulose sponge rat model. Eur J Clin Invest 18:352–359

Huber S, Bruckner P, van der Rest M, Rodriguez E, Winterhalter KH, Vaughan L (1986) Identification of the type IX collagen polypeptide chains. J Biol Chem 261/13: 5965–5968

Kapoor R, Sakai LY, Funk S, Roux E, Bornstein P, Sage EH (1988) Type VIII collagen has a restricted distribution in specialized extracellular matrices. J Cell Biol 107: 721–730

Keene DR, Sakai LY, Bächinger HP, Burgeson RE (1987a) Type III collagen can be present on banded collagen fibrils regardless of fibril diameter. J Cell Biol 105: 2393–2402

Keene DR, Burgeson RE, Sakai LY, Lunstrum GP, Morris NP (1987b) Type VII collagen forms and extended network of anchoring fibrils. J Cell Biol 104: 611–621

Kimura T, Yasui N, Wakitani S, Araki N, Ono K (1988) Type IX and type II collagens are coordinately expressed during chick limb development. Biomed Res 9/4: 319–324

Kuettner KE, Schleyerbach R, Hascall VC (eds) (1985) Workshop Conference Hoechst-Werk Albert, Wiesbaden. Articular cartilage biochemistry. Raven Press, New York

Kuijer R, van de Stadt RJ, de Koning MHMT, van der Korst JK (1985) Influence of constituents of proteoglycans on type II collagen fibrillogenesis. Collagen Rel Res 5: 379–391

Mayne R, Burgeson RE (eds) (1987) Biology of extracellular matrix: A series. Structure and function of collagen types. Acad. Press, Orlando/FL

Mayne R, von der Mark K (1983) Collagens of cartilage. In: Hall BK (ed) Cartilage, vol 1: Structure, function, and biochemistry. Acad Press, Orlando/FL

Mörgelin M, Paulsson M, Hardinghaus T, Heinegard D, Engel J (1988) Cartilage proteoglycans: Assembly with hyaluronate and link proteins as studied by electron microscopy. Biochem J 253: 175–185

Müller-Glauser W, Bruckner P, Humbel B, Glatt M, Sträuli P, Winterhalter KH (1986) On the role of type IX collagen in the extracellular matrix of cartilage: Type IX collagen is localized to intersections of collagen fibrils. J Cell Biol 102: 1931–1939

Paulsson M, Mörgelin M, Wiedemann H et al. (1987) Extended and globular protein domains in cartilage proteoglycans. Biochem J 245: 763–772

Poole AR (1986) Proteoglycans in health and disease: structures and functions. Biochem J 236: 1–14

Poole AR, Pidoux I, Reiner A, Rosenberg L (1982) An immunoelectron microscope study of the organization of proteoglycan monomer, link protein, and collagen in the matrix of articular cartilage. J Cell Biol 93: 921–937

Poole AR, Pidoux I, Reiner A, Choi H, Rosenberg LC (1984) Association of an extracellular protein (chondrocalcin) with the calcification of cartilage in endochondral bone formation. J Cell Biol 98: 54–65

Ruoslahti E (1988) Structure and biology of proteoglycans. Ann Rev Cell Biol 4: 229–255

Schmid T, Linsenmayer TF (1985) Developmental acquisition of type X collagen in the embryonic chick tibiotarsus. Dev Biol 107: 373–381

Smith GN jr, Brandt KD, Williams JM (1987) Effect of polyanions on fibrillogenesis by type XI collagen. Collagen Rel Res 7: 17–25

Trelstad RL, Birk DE, Silver FH (1982) Collagen fibrillogenesis in tissues, in solution and from modeling: A synthesis. J Invest Dermatol 79/1: 109s–112s

van der Rest M, Mayne R (1987) Type IX collagen. In: van der Rest M, Mayne R (eds) Structure and function of collagen types. Academic Press, Orlando/FL

van der Rest M, Mayne R (1988) Type IX collagen proteoglycan from cartilage is covalently cross-linked to type II collagen. J Biol Chem 263/4: 1615–1618

Wight TN, Mecham RP (eds) (1987) Biology of extracellular matrix: A series. Biology of proteoglycans. Academic Press, Orlando/FL

Functional Anatomy of the Cruciate Ligaments

N. F. Friederich and W. R. O'Brien

The cruciate ligaments are the nucleus of knee joint kinematics (We. Müller 1977). In addition, they are the primary restraints to anterior-posterior translation of the tibia (Butler et al. 1980). Their momentary biomechanical efficiency depends on the flexion angle of the knee joint, because their functional angle of insertion on the tibial plateau varies with the degree of knee flexion.

If the tibia is held vertically while the knee is moved from extension through flexion, the line of insertion of the anterior cruciate ligament (ACL) relative to the tibial plateau becomes increasingly acute, thereby increasing the biomechanical efficiency of the ligament as a restraint to anterior tibial translation. By contrast, the posterior cruciate ligament (PCL) becomes less biomechanically efficient as the knee flexes because its fibers assume a more vertical orientation.

Besides the angle of insertion, the relative biomechanical efficiency of the cruciate ligaments in restraining anterior or posterior tibial translation also depends on how many of the fibers are taut at a given point in time.

A century ago, advanced concepts on the mechanics of the knee joint had already been developed on the basis of extensive anatomic studies (Meyer 1853; Strasser 1917; Weber and Weber 1836; Zuppinger 1904).

The cruciate ligaments can be represented functionally on the sagittal plane by a crossed four-bar linkage (Bradley et al., personal communication; Goodfellow and O'Connor 1978; Huson 1974; Kapandji 1970; Kummer and Yamamoto 1988; Menschik 1974a,b, 1975; Montgomery et al. 1988; Müller 1977; Strasser 1917). The cruciate ligaments intersect at the crossing point P of the four-bar linkage, which is the "instant center" of knee rotation (Frankel et al. 1971; Gerber and Matter 1983; Kinzel et al. 1972). This point is located on the transverse flexion axis. The location of P can be redefined for every rigid joint mechanism (Goodfellow and O'Connor 1978; Müller 1977; Reuleaux 1876). This model is not without its critics, however (Blankevoort et al. 1986; Crowninshield et al. 1976; Huiskes et al. 1984). Some authors (Dye 1987) have conducted paleo-ostologic studies based on the model of the four-bar linkage. Various mathematical models have been developed on the basis of the crossed four-bar linkage (Kummer and Yamamoto 1988; Wismans et al. 1980), while other mathematicians have attempted to model the ligaments without any reference to a four-bar linkage (Sidles et al. 1988).

In 1974 and 1975 Menschik described the "Burmester curve" for the knee joint, a roughly figure-of-eight curve consisting of two third-order curves called the "vertex cubic" (tibia) and the "pivot cubic" (femur) (Fig. 1). A ligament that has its origin on the pivot cubic of the knee will be isometric (maintain a constant length and tension during knee motion) if it passes through the instant center of rotation and inserts at the corresponding point on the vertex cubic. The cruciate ligaments, collateral ligaments, popliteus tendon, and anterolateral femorotibial ligaments basically conform to this model (Menschik 1974a, b, 1975, 1988; Müller 1977).

In reality, all the fibers in a knee ligament cannot fit on the isometric points of the Burmester curve. *Only a limited number* of fibers can directly interconnect the isometric points on the curve. The remaining "nonisometric" fibers are arranged strategically according to a well-defined pattern so they can be "recruited" by tension in situations where the ligament is less biomechanically efficient or is subjected to increased loads.

The surgical reconstruction of the ACL or PCL with an autograft, allograft, or synthetic substitute represents an attempt to reestablish physiologic joint stability and kinematics (Cabaud et al. 1980; Clancy et al. 1982, 1983; Hoogland and Hillen 1982). Unfortunately, even the most sophisticated surgical procedures now available cannot duplicate the complex spatial arrangement of the individual cruciate ligament fibers. The goal of the surgeon, therefore, should be to duplicate the *function* of the deficient ligament.

It has been postulated that the cruciate ligaments are isometric, pivoting about the ideal isometric points (Menschik 1974b, 1988). This implies that cruciate li-

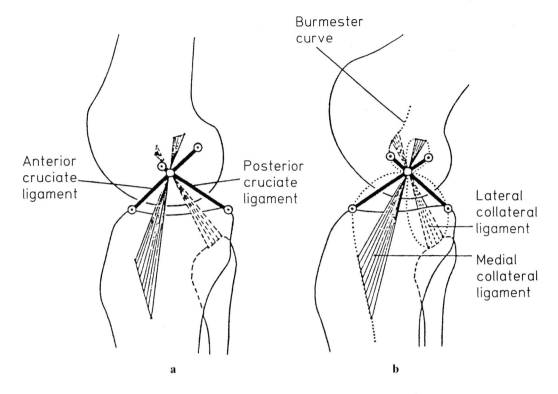

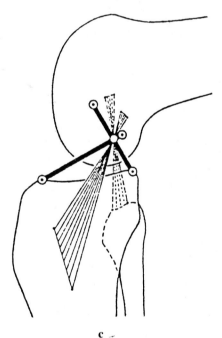

Fig. 1 a–c. Schematic representation of the ligaments in full extension (**a**), 43° flexion (**b**), and 90° flexion (**c**). (Modified from Müller 1982)

gament substitutes, too, should be positioned so that they pivot about the isometric points of the deficient ligament. In this way the function of the ligament could theoretically be restored, even if its exact anatomy is not.

If a cruciate ligament substitute is not positioned isometrically, the distance between the femoral and tibial pivot points will vary during knee motion (Butler et al. 1988; Graf et al. 1987; Hasenpflug et al. 1985; Hefzy et al. 1987; Lew and Lewis 1978; Penner et al. 1986; Sidles et al. 1988; Trent et al. 1976). This causes the substitute to become taut through certain flexion arcs and slack (with associated joint laxity) through other arcs (Montgomery et al. 1988; van Dijk 1983; van Dijk et al. 1979; Wang et al. 1973).

The results and conclusions presented here are based on a series of 11 experiments performed on a total of 122 cadaveric knees from January, 1987, to October, 1988. The purpose of the investigation was to gain further understanding of the structural design of the cruciate ligaments and of factors important in duplicating ligament function during reconstructive surgery. We shall describe the methods used and present a summary of the results. On the basis of our results, we shall propose a *theory of functional isometry* for the cruciate ligaments.

ACL

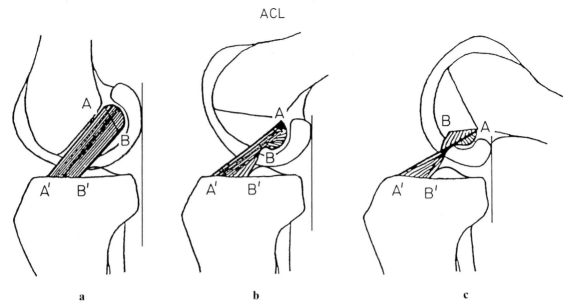

a   b   c

Fig. 2a–c. Tension patterns in the ACL during knee motion. **a** All the fibers are taut in extension. **b** When the knee is flexed, the anterior fibers maintain the greatest tension. In full flexion, the ligament twists upon itself (**c**). When a load acts upon the ACL, the anterior fibers become taut first, followed by the more posterior fibers

Anatomy

Gross fiber anatomy and tension patterns were investigated in the cruciate ligaments of 40 fresh, unprepared cadaveric knee joints (20 per ligament, age 22–79 years) that were deep-frozen immediately postmortem. The studies covered a complete range of motion from 5° hyperextension to 135° flexion while various external forces were applied: anterior-posterior translation of the tibia, varus-valgus angulation, and internal-external rotation. Individual cruciate ligament fibers were meticulously dissected to determine their course from femoral origin to tibial insertion. The relative position of the individual fibers within the ligament as a whole was ascertained.

Anterior Cruciate Ligament (Fig. 2)

In the extended knee, the ACL consists of multiple parallel fibers with clearly identifiable sites of proximal and distal attachment. Fibers arising from the more superior portion of the femur insert anteriorly on the tibia, while fibers arising more inferiorly insert farther back. Fibers arising posteriorly from the femur insert medially on the tibia; those arising anteriorly insert laterally. Fibers originating at the center of the ligament remain central throughout their course. The anterior fibers are the longest, the fiber length decreasing steadily in the anterior-to-posterior direction. In the extended knee all the ACL fibers are parallel, and all are under complete, uniform tension. When the knee is flexed from full extension, the anterior edge of the ACL serves as a *rotational axis* for the ligament as it becomes twisted upon itself. As flexion increases, the ACL fibers become increasingly less tense, the slackness progressing in an inferior-to-superior direction in the area of the femoral origin and in a posterior-to-anterior direction in the area of the tibial insertion. Similar findings were reported by the Weber brothers in 1836.

In the absence of an externally applied force, the majority of ACL fibers are lax in the fully flexed knee. Even a minimal anteroposterior tibial translating force will cause the fibers to become tense. As the applied force is increased, the fiber tension radiates progressively from anterior to posterior within the ligament.

Posterior Cruciate Ligament (Fig. 3)

The PCL also exhibits a simple parallel fiber arrangement that is most apparent in the fully flexed knee. Fibers arising from the anteroinferior portion of the femur insert anteromedially on the tibia, while fibers originating posteroinferiorly insert posteromedially, and central fibers remain centralized over the course

PCL

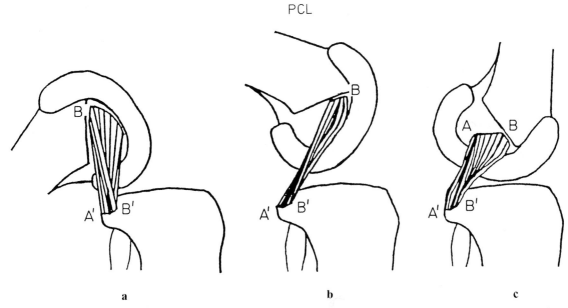

a   b   c

Fig. 3 a–c. Tension patterns in the PCL during knee motion. All the fibers are tense in flexion (**a**). The posterior oblique bundle (A–A') remains the most tense when the knee is extended

of the ligament. In most cases inspection of the ligament will reveal a distinct fiber bundle passing obliquely across the posterior surface of the PCL. It originates from the posterosuperior portion of the anatomic femoral attachment and inserts posterolaterally on the tibial attachment of the PCL. We call this bundle the "posterior oblique bundle," which consistently has the longest fibers within the PCL. The length of the PCL fibers progressively decreases anteromedially from the posterior oblique bundle.

In the fully flexed knee with no load applied, all the PCL fibers are under a constant, uniform tension. As the knee is extended from full flexion, the posterior oblique bundle serves as a rotational axis for the PCL, and fiber slackness progresses methodically from anteromedially to posterolaterally, i.e., toward the posterior oblique bundle. With the knee in full extension, most of the PCL fibers are slack, and only the posterior oblique fibers are tense. If the tibia is subluxated posteriorly with the knee partially flexed, the fibers become progressively tense starting from the posterior oblique bundle and proceeding anteromedially.

Meniscofemoral Ligaments (of Humphry and Wrisberg)

An early description of the meniscofemoral ligaments was published by Poirier and Charpy in 1911. We found that both meniscofemoral ligaments were present in the majority of specimens examined (Last 1948). Other investigators such as Last (1948), Schabus (1988), and van Dommeln (1989) reported similar findings, whereas others found both ligaments coexisting with far less frequency (Brantigan and Voshell 1946; Heller and Langman 1964).

The anterior meniscofemoral ligament (of Humphry) originates anteroinferior to the attachment of the PCL on the medial femoral condyle and inserts on the posterior horn of the lateral meniscus. The ligament of Humphry is easily distinguished from the true PCL. It follows a more oblique course (medial-to-lateral descent) than the PCL fibers, which are oriented more vertically in the fully flexed knee.

The posterior meniscofemoral ligament (of Wrisberg) originates directly posterior to the attachment of the PCL on the medial femoral condyle and inserts on the posterior horn of the lateral meniscus. Like its anterior counterpart, the ligament of Wrisberg is easily distinguishable from the PCL. Its oblique, medial-to-lateral descent carries it over the posterior portion of the PCL.

Isometry of the Anatomic Attachment Sites

Data on the isometry of the attachment sites and specific subdivisions of the cruciate ligaments were obtained in a total of 8 knee joint specimens (4 for each ligament). The entire tibial insertions were removed along with an intact block of bone. Sutures (Novolen no. 3) were passed through drill holes in the bone block, and the attachment was replaced at its original site. The sutures were passed through a tunnel drilled in the tibia and attached to a pneumatic isometer (Synthes, USA) that exerted a constant tension on them. Under a primary tension of 30 N, the "length changes" of the cruciate ligament were measured over the range from 5° hyperextension to 135° flexion. After these measurements, the tibial insertion bone blocks were further subdivided:

– In the 4 specimens for study of the ACL, 2 blocks were cut into anterior and posterior halves, and 2 were divided so that they contained the anteromedial (20%) and the posterolateral (80%) fiber bundles.
– In the 4 specimens for study of the PCL, 2 were cut into anterior and posterior halves, and 2 so that they contained the 2 posterior oblique fibers (5%) and the remaining bulk of the ligament (approximately 95%). The "length changes" were determined for each bone block, starting from full extension and progressing through the full range of motion. Care was taken that the blocks were in their original anatomic positions before the measurements were made.

The measured "length changes" are *not* synonymous with "elongation" of the anatomic cruciate ligaments but reflect the fact that certain portions of the cruciate ligaments are slack at certain flexion angles. These portions were made tense with the Synthes isometer at all flexion angles, and the change in the distance between the femoral and tibial attachments was read from the isometer to determine the relative amount of fiber slackness throughout the arc of flexion.

Anterior Cruciate Ligament

The whole ACL and all its subdivisions showed a "length increase" (tension increase) during knee extension.
The ACL as a whole, and its posterolateral bundle alone, demonstrated a "length increase" of 7.5 mm from full flexion to full extension. The anteromedial bundle was the most isometric component, experiencing a length increase of only 2 mm. The anterior half

of the ACL was more isometric than the posterior half (4 mm vs. 10 mm). Indeed, isometry showed a progressive anterior-to-posterior decrease within the ligament.

Posterior Cruciate Ligament

The whole PCL and all its major subdivisions demonstrated a "length increase" (tension increase) during knee flexion.
The whole PCL and the 95% posterior bulk subdivision demonstrated an initial length decrease of 1.0 mm over the first 10° of knee flexion from the fully extended position, followed by a steady length increase of 6 mm until the full 135° of flexion was reached. The posterior oblique bundle was the most isometric, showing a 0.4-mm length increase during the last 10° of extension with no additional length or tension changes from 10° to 135° flexion. The posterior half of the ligament was more isometric than the anterior half (4 mm vs. 8 mm of length change). Thus, the posterior oblique bundle was the most isometric subdivision, with isometry progressively decreasing in the anterior direction.

Isometry of the Fiber Attachments

Seven key fibers per cruciate ligament were carefully dissected from 10 cadaveric knees (5 specimens per ligament). Holes 2 mm in diameter were drilled through the femoral origins and corresponding tibial insertions of these fibers, and no. 3 Novolen sutures were passed through each of the fiber attachment sites. The changes in the distance between the femoral origins and tibial insertions were determined with the Synthes pneumatic isometer using a primary tension of 30 N. Measurements were performed over the complete range of joint motion.

Anterior Cruciate Ligament (Fig. 4, Table 1)

The greatest distance between the femoral and tibial attachment sites was measured in the fully extended knee for all 7 fibers.
The anterior fibers were the longest and were nearly isometric, showing a maximum distance change of only 0.2 mm (in the last 10° of extension). The average distance between the attachment sites decreased with the anterior-to-posterior increase of nonisometry within the ACL.

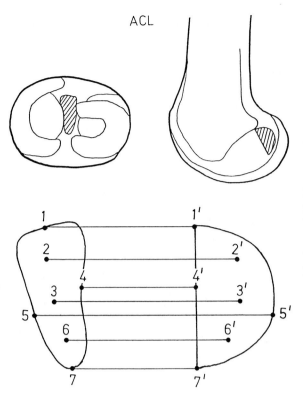

ACL

Fig. 4. Fiber paths in the anterior cruciate ligament from the femoral origin *(right)* to the tibial insertion *(left)*. Fiber *1* corresponds to the anterior border of the anterior cruciate ligament. Fiber *3* is central, and fiber *7* corresponds to the posterior border of the anterior cruciate ligament

Table 1. Isometricity of anterior cruciate ligament fibers. The fiber numbers correspond to those in Fig. 4

Fiber	Maximum distance between the femoral and tibial attachments in mm (average for 5 knees)	Average distance change in flexion (%)
1	37	< 1
2	34	–18
3	31	–28
4	26	–25
5	32	–30
6	27	–35
7	24	–41

The distance between the femoral and tibial attachments of the *central* fibers increased by an average of 28% from flexion to extension, compared with 41% measured for the shortest and least isometric *posterior* fibers.

Posterior Cruciate Ligament (Fig. 5, Table 2)

For 6 of the 7 fibers tested, the measured distance between the attachment sites was greatest when the knee was in full flexion. The one exception was the posterior border of the posterior oblique bundle, which was the longest and most isometric fiber. Measured over a complete range of joint motion, the distance between the femoral and tibial attachments increased by 0.2 mm in the final 10° of extension and showed no change between 10° and 135° of flexion.

Progressing anteromedially within the PCL, we found that the distance between the femoral and tibial attachments steadily decreased with an associated increase of nonisometry. Central fibers underwent an average 31% distance increase during flexion, while the least isometric anteromedial fiber

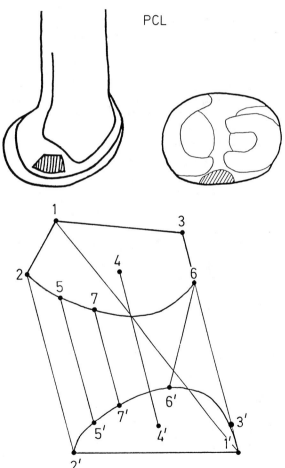

PCL

Fig. 5. Fiber paths in the posterior cruciate ligament from the femoral origin *(above)* to the tibial insertion *(below)*. Fiber *1* corresponds to the posterior oblique bundle, fiber *4* to a central fiber, and fiber *7* to the anteromedial fibers of the posterior cruciate ligament

Table 2. Isometricity of PCL fibers. The fiber numbers correspond to those in Fig. 5

Fiber	Maximum distance between the femoral and tibial attachments in mm (average for 5 knees)	Average distance change in flexion (%)
1	41	<1
2	30	−21
3	35	−25
4	35	−31
5	32	−40
6	32	−44
7	28	−53

(and the shortest) underwent an average distance change of 53%.

Zones of Isometry

Zones of isometry for the cruciate ligament attachments were studied in 38 knee joints (20 for the ACL, 18 for the PCL). The cruciate ligament to be investigated was excised, leaving its counterpart intact. A no. 3 Novolen suture was passed through 2-mm holes

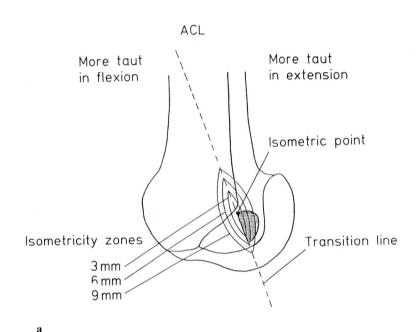

a

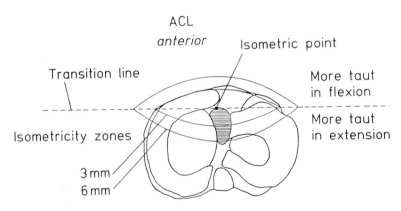

b

Fig. 6. a Femoral zones of isometry for the ACL, with the tibial isometric point as a reference. The anatomic area of origin is *shaded*. The anterior limit of the anatomic origin lies on the transition line. Fibers attached posterior to that line become taut during extension. Fibers (pseudofibers) attached anterior to that line would become taut during flexion. **b** Tibial zones of isometry for the ACL, with the femoral isometric point as a reference. The anatomic area of insertion is *shaded*. The anterior limit of the anatomic attachment of the ACL lies on the transition line. Fibers inserting posterior to that line become taut during extension. Fibers (pseudofibers) inserting anterior to the line would become taut during flexion

drilled in the femur and tibia and attached to the pneumatic tension isometer. Measurements were performed over a complete range of flexion-extension.

Combinations of 21 femoral and 13 tibial positions were measured for the ACL, and combinations of 20 femoral and 9 tibial positions for the PCL.

The drill holes were mapped according to their relation to the anatomic cruciate attachments. In each knee we identified the positional combinations that were associated with the smallest length changes (isometric positions). We defined a combination as isometric if the corresponding length change was 0.3 mm or less.

Anterior Cruciate Ligament (Fig.6)

The best isometric combination was observed for the attachments of the most anterior fibers of the ACL, i.e., the fibers passing from the anterosuperior border of the femoral origin to the anteriior border of the tibial insertion.

With the tibial isometric point as a reference, the anterior border of the anatomic femoral attachment corresponded to the *femoral transition line*. Points *posterior* to the transition line showed a *tension increase during knee extension*, while "pseudofibers" (no. 3 Novolen) which we attached *anterior* to that line showed a *tension increase during knee flexion*.

With the femoral isometric point as a reference, that the anterior border of the tibial insertion corresponded to the *tibial transition line*. Fibers inserting *posterior* to the transition line showed a *tension increase during knee extension*, while "pseudofibers" (no. 3 Novolen) attached *anterior* to that line showed a *tension increase during knee flexion*. The greater the distance from the isometric point and the transition line, the greater the degree of nonisometry. When the femoral or tibial reference point was shifted anteriorly or posteriorly, the corresponding point had to be shifted in reciprocal fashion to restore some degree of isometry. However, we were unable to locate a second point that was truly isometric if one isometric point was abandoned.

From any point within either anatomic attachment of the ACL, the opposite anatomic attachment was always in a zone of increased tension during knee extension, verifying the observation that all fibers of the ACL become more tense during knee extension.

Posterior Cruciate Ligament (Fig. 7)

The best isometric combination was observed for the attachments of the "posterior oblique bundle." A transition line was identified as for the ACL. With the tibial isometric point as a reference, the *femoral transition line* ran along the posterior border of the anatomic origin of the PCL. Fibers attached *anterior* to the transition line underwent a *tension increase during knee flexion*, while the "pseudofibers" (no. 3 Novolen) attached *posterior* to that line showed a *tension increase during extension*.

With the femoral isometric point as a reference, the posterior border of the anatomic tibial insertion corresponded to the *tibial transition line*. Points located *anterior* to that line showed *increased tension during knee flexion*, while Novolen "pseudofibers" attached *posterior* to the transition line showed *increased tension in extension*.

Relocation of either reference point required reciprocal movement of the opposite attachment to improve isometry. However, ideal isometric placement could not be achieved if the attachment deviated from either isometric point.

From any point within either anatomic attachment of the PCL, the opposite anatomic attachments were always in zones of increased fiber tension during knee flexion, verifying our observation that PCL fibers demonstrate increased tension during knee flexion.

On the Theory of Functional Isometry

The foregoing results provide a basis for postulating a theory of functional isometry of the cruciate ligaments (Friederich et al. 1989 a, 1988). The cruciate ligaments achieve *functional isometry* by forming a "crossed four-bar linkage" for the femorotibial articulation. Fibers spanning the isometric points of each cruciate ligament function as the (rigid) links in the crossed four-bar linkage and as the rotational axis for the ligament during flexion-extension. These "most isometric" fibers are always the first to be recruited when the ligament becomes taut. The remaining "nonisometric" fibers are strategically placed such that they can be "progressively recruited" from a slack state as increased biomechanical demands arise.

This theory differs from other proposed models, some of which regard the cruciate ligaments as consisting of 2 or 3 bundles (Brantigan and Voshell 1941; Furman et al. 1976; Gollehon 1987; Haines 1941; Lew and Lewis 1985; Norwood and Cross 1979; Odensten

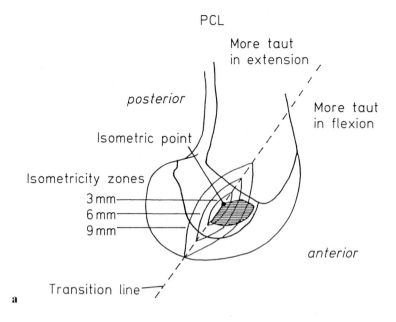

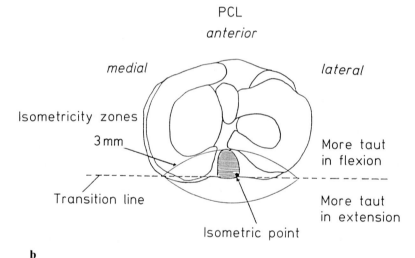

Fig. 7. a Femoral zones of isometry for the PCL, with the tibial isometric point as a reference. The anatomic area of origin is *shaded*. The posterior limit of the anatomic origin lies on the transition line. Fibers originating anterior to that line become taut during flexion. Fibers (pseudofibers) attached posterior to that line would become taut during extension. **b** Tibial zones of isometry for the PCL, with the femoral isometric point as a reference. The anatomic area of insertion is *shaded*. The posterior limit of the anatomic insertion lies on the transition line. Fibers inserting anterior to that line become taut during flexion. Fibers (pseudofibers) inserting posterior to the line would become taut during extension

and Gillquist 1985; Sidles et al. 1988; van Dommelen and Fowler 1989). Instead, we propose a concept of homogeneous structures with a design permitting relative isometry of some fibers with progressive fiber recruitment depending on the instantaneous biomechanical demands.

Anterior Cruciate Ligament

The ACL is most efficient biomechanically in the fully flexed knee, where it assumes an acute angle relative to the tibial plateau. As the knee is extended, the ACL becomes progressively less efficient due to its less acute angle of insertion. An increasing number of cruciate ligament fibers must be recruited in anticipation of a potential anterior translation of the tibia. The most isometric anterior fibers of the ACL are recruited first, the less isometrically placed posterior fibers becoming tight later, e.g., when the knee reaches full extension or when large anterior translating forces are applied.

The anterior edge of the ACL is the isometric link that provides the low-load function to determine the kinematics of the joint. The more posterior fibers serve as a strength reserve for high-load situations.

Posterior Cruciate Ligament

The PCL is most efficient biomechanically in the fully extended knee, where it inserts on the tibial plateau at a more acute angle. As flexion increases, the PCL assumes a more vertical orientation, and its efficiency is reduced. This means that more fibers must be recruited to resist posterior translation of the tibia. The posterior oblique bundle of the ligament is the isometric link that determines joint kinematics. The anterior bulk of PCL fibers provide a strength reserve and are recruited progressively when increased biomechanical demands are placed on the ligament.

Isometry of Cruciate Ligament Substitutes

In vitro reconstructions of the cruciate ligaments furnished data on the isometry of combinations of different femoral and tibial placements of the ligament substitute. Fifty-four anterior cruciate reconstructions and 17 posterior cruciate reconstructions were performed using patellar tendon grafts. In all reconstructions the isometry of the graft was measured with a pneumatic isometer (Synthes, USA) from full extension to 135° of flexion.

The ACL grafts had a cross-sectional area of 10 mm and were placed through drill holes (tunnels) 10 mm in diameter. The corresponding values for the PCL grafts were 12 mm.

Seven different femoral and 4 tibial attachment sites were studied for the ACL reconstructions. The femoral positions for the graft were designated as extreme anterior, anterosuperior, central, and over the top. Three over-the-top troughs were also studied (anterior, anteroinferior, inferior). The tibial positions for the graft were designated as over the front, anterior, central, and posterior. (The positions of the drill holes were designated according to the position of the overdrilled guide wire relative to the anatomic attachments.)

Five different femoral and 5 tibial attachment sites were investigated for the PCL reconstructions. The

femoral placements were designated as extreme superior, extreme posterior, posterosuperior, central, and inferior. The tibial placements were designated as anterior, central, posterolateral, over the back, and a modified over-the-back placement using an anterior trough.

The graft position was considered to be isometric if the isometer indicated less than 0.5 mm of length change over the full range of joint motion. An isometric position could be achieved only when the Kirschner wires for the femoral origin and tibial insertion were centered on the aforementioned isometric points.

As we were able to predict from the model of the crossed four-bar linkage, the degree of nonisometry increased as the graft was moved away from the isometric position. Relocating the femoral or tibial attachment site anteriorly or posteriorly required a reciprocal posterior or anterior shift of the corresponding attachment site to improve isometry. However, moving either the femoral or the tibial placement away from the isometric point prevented ideal isometric tracking in both cruciate reconstructions.

Anterior Cruciate Ligament (Fig. 8, Table 3)

An isometric femoral attachment could be achieved in two ways: by placing the drill hole at the antero-superior border of the anatomic origin of the ACL ("isometric point"), or by using a modified over-the-top trough directed anteroinferiorly. Both placements yielded the same values. The two positions differ only in the less acute angle of the over-the-top substitute relative to the femoral attachment compared with the tunnel technique. This has theoretical advantages, some of which have been confirmed experimentally, in terms of reducing crimp of the substitute fibers (Montgomery 1988).

An isometric tibial insertion site was achieved by placing the drill hole so that the anterior edge of the hole was directly posterior to the posterior border of the medial meniscus anterior horn, avoiding injury to the meniscotibial fibers or transverse ligament.

Grafts placed in the center of the anatomic attachment sites were not isometric. This has been verified by other authors (Sapega 1989; Schabus 1988). Measured from full flexion to full extension, the distance between the femoral and tibial attachments increased by an average of 5.9 mm in the centrally positioned grafts.

The least isometric position was obtained by routing the graft over the top of the femur without a trough and attaching it to the posterior portion of the ana-

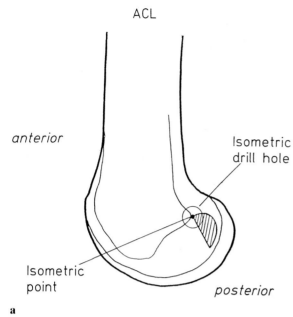

ACL

anterior

Isometric drill hole

Isometric point

posterior

a

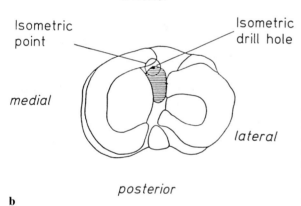

ACL

anterior

Isometric point

Isometric drill hole

medial

lateral

posterior

b

tomic insertion site on the tibia. From full flexion to full extension, the distance between the attachment sites increased by 16 mm in a graft positioned in this way.

Posterior Cruciate Ligament (Fig. 9, Table 4)

Isometric placement was achieved by centering the Kirschner guide wire on the isometric points of the posterior oblique bundle. An isometric femoral attachment for the PCL graft could be achieved by centering the guide wire on the posterosuperior border of the anatomic area of origin. The isometric tibial attachment was located on the posterolateral border of the anatomic area of insertion or through a drill hole by using a modified over-the-back trough approximately 6 mm deep.

Grafts placed at the centers of the anatomic areas of origin and insertion were not isometric, the distance between the femoral and tibial attachments increasing by an average of 6.1 mm from full flexion to full extension.

◁

Fig. 8. a Isometric femoral position of an ACL substitute. The drill hole or modified over-the-top trough is centered at the anterosuperior border of the anatomic area of attachment. **b** Isometric tibial position of the ligament substitute. The drill hole is centered on the anterior border of the anatomic area of insertion, so that the anterior edge of the drill hole is just posterior to the anterior horn of the medial meniscus

Table 3. Isometry of the ACL substitute (average "length change" over the full range of knee motion, stated in millimeters)

		Femoral position[a]						
		Extreme anterior	Antero-superior	Central	Over the top	Over-the-top with anterior trough	Over-the-top with antero-inferior trough	Over-the-top with inferior trough
Tibial position[a]	Over the front	–	– 2,2	–	–	–	–	–
	Anterior	– 8,4	+ 0,4	+ 5,2	+ 5,3	± 4,1	+ 0,5	+ 4,3
	Central	± 3,7	+ 4,4	+ 5,9	+ 8,3	± 5,5	+ 4,0	+ 5,9
	Posterior	± 7,0	+ 6,3	+ 9,5	+ 16,3	± 13,7	+ 11,2	–

[a] In relation to the anatomic insertion
+ = "Length increase" in extension
− = "Length increase" in flexion
± = Transitional "length changes": increase and decrease, total excursion

Table 4. Isometry of the PCL substitute (average "length change" over the full range of knee motion, stated in millimeters)

Tibial position[a]		Femoral position[a]				
		Extreme superior	Extreme posterior	Postero-superior	Central	Inferior
Tibial position[a]	Over-the-back	–	–	+ 2,7	–	–
	Over-the-back, anterior trough	–	–	+ 0,4	–	–
	Posterolateral	+ 4,5	–	– 0,4	– 3,2	– 5,6
	Central	+ 5,4	–	– 3,7	– 6,1	– 6,9
	Anterior	–	± 5,8	–	–	– 8,2

[a] In relation to the anatomic insertion
+ = "Length increase" in extension
– = "Length increase" in flexion
± = Transitional "length changes": increase and decrease, total excursion

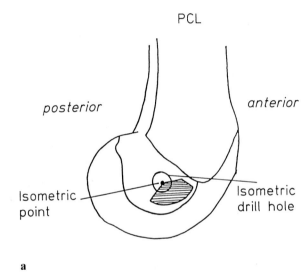

PCL

posterior   anterior

Isometric point — — Isometric drill hole

a

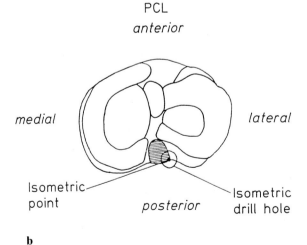

PCL
anterior

medial   lateral

Isometric point — — Isometric drill hole
posterior

b

Fig. 9. a Isometric femoral position of a PCL substitute. The drill hole is centered on the posterosuperior border of the anatomic area of attachment. **b** Isometric tibial position of the substitute. The drill hole or modified over-the-back trough is centered on the posterolateral border of the anatomic insertion

Clinical Relevance

At first sight, our experimental findings appear to differ from previously published studies (Butler et al. 1988; Daniel et al. 1987; de Lange et al. 1983; Graf et al. 1987; Grood et al. 1983; Grood et al, personal communication; Hassenpflug et al. 1985; Hefzy et al. 1986, 1987; Sidles et al. 1988). On closer scrutiny of the published results, however, we find that they correlate well with our own. Though they do not state them explicitly, some studies point implicitly to the same conclusions that can be drawn from our investigations (Sapega 1989, Schabus 1988).

The significance of our study lies in the accuracy of the measurements, the precision of our instruments (prototypes of pneumatic isometers), and the careful documentation of various fiber positions in relation to *anatomic* reference points at the cruciate ligament attachments. Given the diversity in the shape and size of knee joints, stating data in millimeters is of little practical value (Girgis et al. 1983). We believe that all knees are designed to fit basic laws of nature, but on different size scales.

A key finding of our anatomic studies was that the cruciate ligament fibers have an essentially parallel arrangement and that their tension radiates within the ligament itself according to a strictly defined pattern. These findings conflict with the "bundle" architecture postulated by other authors, for which we were unable to find an anatomic or functional correlate (Odensten and Gillquist 1985; Weber and Weber 1836). More recent histologic studies appear to support this hypothesis to some degree on the basis of neural supply (proprioceptivity) (Haus and Refior 1987, 1988).

Present-day surgical techniques do not permit the surgeon to duplicate the *anatomy* of the cruciate ligaments. The goal, rather, must be to reproduce the *function* of the deficient ligament. In cruciate ligament reconstructions performed in cadaveric knees, a definite correlation was found between the isometric position of the guide wire and the isometric values of the substitute that was positioned by overdrilling the wire (Friederich and O'Brien et al. 1989b). The anatomic structure of the cruciate ligaments creates *functionally* isometric conditions owing to the fact that the nonisometric fibers are under low tension in joint positions where they would otherwise interfere with normal knee kinematics. Our results did not confirm the concept of placing the drill holes eccentrically, as some authors have proposed (Clancy et al. 1982, 1983).

Our data pertain only to the placement of the ligament substitute. We did not investigate the effects of biological fixation and remodeling. In theory, functional forces acting on the cruciate ligament graft may stimulate remodeling processes, resulting in a "recruitment" of graft fibers like that occurring in the natural ligament.

It should be noted that the isometric placement of an ACL substitute necessitates enlargement of the intercondylar notch (anterior notch plasty). The tibial insertion is positioned far anteromedially in an isometric reconstruction (O'Brien et al. 1987), leading to impingement of the graft against the anterior and anterolateral portion of the intercondylar notch – hence the need to enlarge the notch. However, enlarging the notch anteriorly to more than 16 mm can lead to significant patellofemoral crepitation. Thus, a tradeoff must be made between an ideal isometric placement of the graft and the avoidance of intercondylar notch impingement.

In full extension the PCL engages upon the posterior roof of the intercondylar notch. An isometrically positioned graft may impinge against the posterior outlet of the intercondylar notch, so a rationale also exists for notch plasty in posterior cruciate reconstructions.

Other studies of ours (O'Brien et al. 1989) underscore the importance of the precise isometric placement of the cruciate ligament substitute in order to:

– Minimize loading of the substitute during knee motion
– Reestablish physiologic joint kinematics
– Restore physiologic joint stability
– Prevent excessive loading of the graft in the early postoperative period

Our research was funded by generous contributions from the Maurice E. Müller Foundation in Bern and the Stipend Fund of the Swiss Society for Orthopedics (SGO).

References

Blankevoort L, Huiskes R, de Lange A (1986) Helical axes along the envelope of passive knee joint motion. Trans Orthop Res Soc 11: 410

Brantigan OC, Voshell AF (1941) The mechanics of the ligaments and menisci of the knee joint. J Bone Joint Surg [Am] 23: 44–66

Brantigan OC, Voshell AF (1946) Ligaments of the knee joint. The relationship of the ligament of Humphry to the ligament of Wrisberg. J Bone Joint Surg [Am] 28: 66–67

Butler DL, Noyes FR, Grood ES (1980) Ligamentous restraints to anterior-posterior drawer in the human knee. A biomechanical study. J Bone Joint Surg [Am] 62: 259–270

Butler DL, Martin ET, Kaiser AD, Grood ES, Chun KJ, Sodd AN (1988) The effects of flexion and tibial rotation on the 3-D orientations and lengths of human anterior cruciate ligament bundles. Trans Orthop Res Soc 13: 59

Cabaud HE, Feagin JA, Rodkey WG (1980) Acute anterior cruciate ligament injury augmented repair. Experimental studies. Am J Sports Med 8: 395–401

Clancy WG Jr, Nelson DA, Reider B, Narechana RG (1982) Anterior cruciate ligament reconstruction using one-third of the patellar ligament augmented by extra-articular tendon transfers. J Bone Joint Surg [Am] 64: 352–359

Clancy WG Jr, Shelbourne KD, Zoellner GB, Keene JS, Reider B, Rosenberg TD (1983) Treatment of knee joint instability secondary to rupture of the posterior cruciate ligament. Report of a new procedure. J Bone Joint Surg [Am] 65: 310–322

Crowninshield R, Pope MH, Johnson RJ (1976) An analytical model of the knee. J Biomech 9: 397–405

de Lange A, van Dijk R, Huiskes R (1983) Three-dimensional experimental assessment of knee ligament length patterns in vitro. Trans Orthop Res Soc 8: 10

Dye SF (1987) An evolutionary perspective of the knee. J Bone Joint Surg [Am] 69: 976–983

Frankel VH, Burstein AH, Brooks DB (1971) Biomechanics of internal derangement of the knee: Pathomechanics as determined by analysis of the instant center of motion. J Bone Joint Surg [Am] 53: 945–962

Friederich NF, O'Brien WR (1989b) Isometricity measurements in anterior cruciate ligament reconstruction. Vortrag AOSSM Annual Meeting, Las Vegas, NE

Friederich NF, O'Brien WR, Müller We, Henning CE (1989a) Anterior cruciate ligament fiber tension patterns during knee motion. Proceedings of the 6th ISK Congress. Am J Sports Med 17: 699

Friederich NF, O'Brien WR, Müller We, Henning CE, Jackson RW (1988) Functional anatomy of the cruciate ligaments and their substitutes. Part II: The posterior cruciate ligament. Vortrag, 3. ESKA-Kongress Amsterdam

Furman W, Marshall JL, Girgis FG (1976) The anterior cruciate ligament. A functional analysis based on postmortem studies. J Bone Joint Surg [Am] 58: 179–185

Gerber C, Matter P (1983) Biomechanical analysis of the knee after rupture of the anterior cruciate ligament and its primary repair. An instant-center analysis of function. J Bone Joint Surg [Am] 65: 391–399

Girgis FG, Marshall JL, Al Monajem ARS (1983) The cruciate ligaments of the knee joint. Clin Orthop 106: 216–231

Gollehon DL, Torzilli PA, Warren RF (1978) The role of the posterolateral and cruciate ligaments in the stability of the human knee. J Bone Joint Surg [Am] 69: 233–242

Goodfellow J, O'Connor J (1978) The mechanics of the knee and prosthesis design. J Bone Joint Surg [Br] 60: 358–369

Graf B, Simon T, Jackson DW (1987) Isometric placement of substitutes for the anterior cruciate ligament. In: Jackson DW, Drez D'Jr (eds) The anterior cruciate deficient knee. Mosby, St. Louis, pp 102–113

Grood ES, Hefzy DL, Butler WJ (1983) On the placement and the initial tension of anterior cruciate ligament substitutes. Trans Orthop Res Soc 9: 145

Haines RW (1941) A note on the actions of the cruciate ligaments of the knee joint. J Anat 75: 373

Hassenpflug J, Blauth W, Rose D (1985) Zum Spannungsverhalten von Transplantaten zum Ersatz des vorderen Kreuzbandes. Zugleich ein Beitrag zur Kritik an der „over-the-top"-Technik. Unfallchirurg 88: 151–158

Haus J, Refior HJ (1987) A study of the synovial and ligamentous structure of the anterior cruciate ligament. Int Orthop 11: 117–124

Haus J, Refior HJ (1988) Zur Anatomie und Histologie des vorderen Kreuzbandes. Orthop Prax 5: 296–298

Hefzy MS, Grood ES, Lindenfeld TL (1986) The posterior cruciate ligament: A new look at length patterns. Trans Orthop Res Soc 11: 128

Hefzy MS, Grood ES, Noyes FR (1987) ACL intra-articular reconstruction: Factors affecting the region of most isometric attachments. Trans Orthop Res Soc 12: 267

Heller L, Langman J (1964) The meniscofemoral ligaments of the human knee. J Bone Joint Surg [Br] 46: 307–313

Hoogland T, Hillen B (1984) Intra-articular reconstruction of the anterior cruciate ligament. Clin Orthop 185: 197–202

Huiskes R, Blankvoort L, van Dijk R, de Lange A, van Rens TJG (1984) Ligament deformation patterns in passive knee-joint motions. Adv Bioeng: 53–54

Huson A (1974) The functional anatomy of the knee joint. The closed kinematic chain as a model of the knee joint. In: Ingwersen OS (ed) The knee joint: Recent advances in basis research and clinical aspects. Excerpta Medica, Amsterdam, pp 163–168

Kapandji IA (1970) The physiology of the joints, vol 2: Lower limbs, 2nd edn. Churchill-Livingstone, London, pp 72–135

Kinzel GL, Hall AS, Hillberry BM (1972) Measurement of the total motion between two body segments 1. Analytical development. J Biomech 5: 93–105

Kummer B, Yamamoto M (1988) Morphologie und Funktion des Kreuzbandapparates des Kniegelenks. Arthroskopie 1: 2–10

Last RJ (1948) Some anatomical details of the knee joint. J Bone Joint Surg [Br] 30: 683–688

Lew WD, Lewis JL (1978) A technique for calculating in vivo ligament lengths with application to the human knee joint. J Biomech 11: 365–377

Menschik A (1974a) Mechanik des Kniegelenkes. 1. Teil. Z Orthop 112: 481–495

Menschik A (1974b) Mechanik des Kniegelenkes. 3. Teil. Sailer, Wien

Menschik A (1975) Mechanik des Kniegelenkes. II. Teil. Schlußrotation. Z Orthop 113: 388–400

Menschik A (1988) Biometrie. Springer, Berlin Heidelberg New York Tokyo

Meyer H (1853) Die Mechanik des Kniegelenkes. Arch Anat Physiol Wiss Med: 497–547

Montgomery RD, Milton JL, Terry GC, McLeod WD, Madson N (1988) Comparison of over-the-top and tunnel techniques for anterior cruciate ligament replacement. Clin Orthop 231: 144–153

Müller We (1977) Verletzungen der Kreuzbänder. Zentralbl Chir 102: 974–981

Müller We (1982) Das Knie. Form, Funktion und ligamentäre Wiederherstellungschirurgie. Springer, Berlin Heidelberg New York Tokyo

Norwood LA, Cross MJ (1979) Anterior cruciate ligament: Functional anatomy of its bundles in rotatory instabilities. Am J Sports Med 7: 23–26

O'Brien WR, Henning CE, Eriksson E (1987) Femoral intercondylar notch impingement on anterior cruciate ligament substitutes. Vortrag, 13th Annual Meeting AOSSM, Orlando/FL

O'Brien WR, Friederich NF, Müller We, Henning C (1989) Functional anatomy of the cruciate ligaments and their substitutes. Scientific Exhibit, 56th Annual Meeting AAOS, Las Vegas

Odensten M, Gillquist J (1985) Functional anatomy of the anterior cruciate ligament and a rationale for reconstruction. J Bone Joint Surg [Am] 67: 257–262

Penner DA, Daniel DM, Wood P (1986) An in vitro study of anterior cruciate ligament graft orientation and isometry. 12th Annual Meeting AOSSM, Sun Valley/CA

Poirier P, Charpy A (1911) Traité de l'anatomie humaine, Masson, Paris, pp 1892–1904

Reuleaux F (1876) The kinematics of machinery: Outlines of a theory of machines. Kennedy ABW (ed and transl) Macmillan, New York

Sapega AA, Moyer RA, Schneck C, Goldstein S, Komaiahiranya N (1989) The biomechanics of intra-operative „isometry" testing during anterior cruciate ligament reconstruction. Trans Orthop Res Soc 14: 130

Schabus R (1988) Die Bedeutung der Augmentation für die Rekonstruktion des vorderen Kreuzbandes. Acta Chir Aust [Suppl 76]

Sidles JA, Larson RV, Garbini JL, Downey DJ, Matson FA (1988) Ligament length relationships in the moving knee. J Orthop Res 6/4: 593–610

Strasser H (1917) Lehrbuch der Muskel- und Gelenksmechanik. Springer, Berlin

Trent PS, Walker PS, Wolf B (1976) Ligament length patterns, strength, and rotational axes of the knee joint. Clin Orthop 117: 263–270

van Dijk R (1983) The behaviour of the cruciate ligaments in the human knee. Dissertation, University of Nijmegen, The Netherlands

van Dijk R, Huiskes R, Selvik G (1979) Roentgen stereophotogrammetric methods for the evaluation of the three-dimensional kinematic behaviour and cruciate ligament length patterns of the human knee joint. J Biomech 12: 727–731

van Dommelen BA, Fowler PJ (1989) Anatomy of the posterior cruciate ligament. A review. Am J Sports Med 17: 24–29

Wang CJ, Walker PS, Wolf B (1973) The effects of flexion and rotation on the length patterns of the ligaments of the knee. J Biomech 6: 587–596

Weber W, Weber E (1836) Mechanik der menschlichen Gehwerkzeuge. Dieterich, Göttingen

Wirth CJ, Artmann M (1974) Verhalten der Roll-Gleitbewegung des belasteten Kniegelenks bei Verlust und Ersatz des vorderen Kreuzbandes. Arch Orthop Unfallchir 78: 356–361

Wismans J, Veldpaus F, Janssen J (1980) A three-dimensional mathematical model of the knee-joint. J Biomech 13: 677–685

Zuppinger H (1904) Die aktive Flexion im unbelasteten Kniegelenk. Bergmann, Wiesbaden

Anatomy and Biomechanics of the Anterior Cruciate Ligament: A Three-Dimensional Problem

R. Huiskes and L. Blankevoort

The cruciate ligaments perform the contrasting functions of permitting motion of the articular surfaces on the one hand, and restraining their motion on the other by offering resistance to certain forces. The excessive restraint of mobility leads to functional disability and unphysiologic loading of the ligaments, whereas deficient restraint leads to instability. The anterior cruciate ligament (ACL) plays a critical role in the performance of this task. This role is determined entirely by the anatomic configuration of the ligament attachments and the mechanical properties of the ligament itself. In turn, the mechanical properties of the ACL depend on its three-dimensional collagenous structure. These interdependencies are of clinical importance. In knee laxity tests, for example, an attempt is made to assess the function of the ACL and diagnose the severity of lesions on the basis of observed or elicited joint motion. In reconstructions of the ACL, an attempt is made to repair the lesion to the degree that normal motion restraint is reestablished. In both cases the geometry of the ACL attachments and the mechanical properties of the ligament affect the overall mechanical behavior of the knee joint in a manner that can be utilized diagnostically and therapeutically. However, the situation is complicated by the fact that the ACL does not exert this effect in isolation but in concert with the articular geometry and the other ligaments of the knee. Thus, the relationship between the morphology and function of the ACL operates within a complex system of structures that influence one another.

For the scientist faced with a system as complex as the knee, the primary task is to create order out of apparent chaos. One way to do this is to develop a "model," i.e., a simplified description or reflection of a complex reality which makes certain aspects of this reality comprehensible and manageable. A familiar example is the "four-bar linkage" (Fig. 1), which models the cruciate ligaments as rigid links having mobile attachments to the femur and tibia (Strasser 1917; Menschik 1974; Huson 1974; Müller 1982). Basic assumptions in this model are that the cruciate ligaments experience little or no strain during knee motion and that they are represented mechanically by linear elements in one plane. The correctness of these assumptions is less important than the usefulness of the model, i.e., whether the model enhances our understanding of the relationship between form and function, and whether it offers an explanation for the phenomena observed. And indeed, the model accomplishes this reasonably well (Müller 1982). It explains the shape of the articular surfaces (at least in reasonable approximation on the sagittal plane), and it explains why the rotational axis for knee flexion, which the model represents as the point where the bars intersect, is not rigidly attached to the tibia or femur. It also offers an explanation for the resistance

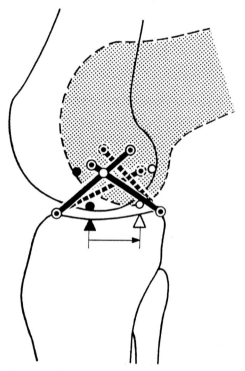

Fig. 1. Model of the knee as a four-bar linkage in the sagittal plane. The anterior and PCLs are represented by rigid bars that are connected to the tibia and femur by hinges. In all degrees of flexion, the instant center of rotation coincides with the point of intersection of the cruciate ligament bars. The constraining action of the cruciate ligaments causes the femur to roll backward on the tibia with increasing flexion. (From Müller 1982)

that the anterior and posterior cruciate ligaments offer especially to anterior and posterior drawer motion, and it explains the posterior translation of the femur relative to the tibia during flexion. However, the model does not describe the phenomenon of knee laxity, the role of the collateral ligaments, or internal-external rotation of the knee in the transverse plane. If we are to comprehend and describe the functional role of the ACL in greater detail, we must approach it as a three-dimensional problem. This requires that we first investigate the physiologic mobility of the knee joint in three dimensions.

Freedom of Motion of the Knee

The passive freedom of motion of the knee is investigated by mounting amputated or cadaveric knee joint specimens in an apparatus that permits the joint to be moved incrementally through designated flexion angles while leaving other tibial motions with respect to the femur unconstrained (Fig.2) (Blankevoort et al. 1988). This apparatus can exert axial forces, AP forces, or torques (torsional moments) upon the joint (Fig.3). The three-dimensional motions that are elicited by the applied load are analyzed using techniques of roentgen stereophotogrammetric analysis (RSA) (Selvik 1974; Huiskes et al. 1985b; de Lange et al. 1985; Blankevoort et al. 1988). For this purpose the bones are marked with radiopaque tantalum pellets, and radiographs are taken from two directions in each joint position (Fig.4). Digitized and computer analyzed, these films can yield very precise data on the position of the tibia with respect to the femur in

relation to a given starting position (unloaded extension). Multiple sequential positions serve to simulate a joint movement.

These experiments (Blankevoort et al. 1988) have shown that joint motion in one plane or in one direction is almost invariably associated with motion in another plane or direction. That is, translational motions in the three anatomic directions (proximal-distal, anterior-posterior, medial-lateral) tend to be coupled with rotational motions in the three anatomic planes (sagittal, transverse, frontal). The experiments further show that the degree of coupling depends greatly on the external load. An example is shown in Fig.5. When the joint is flexed in the unloaded condition, practically no tibial rotation occurs. But if a (small) axial force is applied to the joint, internal tibial rotation does occur during flexion (Fig.5a). A (small) anterior force on the tibia likewise leads to internal rotation during flexion, while a posterior force leads to external rotation (Fig.5b). Small internal and external torques exerted on the tibia lead to internal and external rotation, respectively, during knee flexion (Fig.5c).

This load dependence of the kinematic coupling between flexion and tibial rotation is caused by an extremely low ligamentous restraint to rotation (Fig.6). We can conceptualize this lack of restraint as a freedom of rotatory motion whose excursion limits are defined by threshold torques of, say, $+/-3$ Nm (Fig.6). The knee, then, can be modeled as a mechanism with two degrees of freedom, flexion and tibial rotation, within the limits defined by internal and external torques of 3 Nm (see Fig.5c).

This (qualitative) kinematic model provides an explanation for the observed sensitivity to external

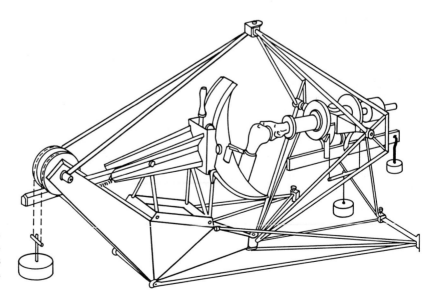

Fig.2. Motion and loading apparatus for the quasistatic kinematic testing of the knee joint, as used by Blankevoort et al. (1988). (From Blankevoort et al. 1988)

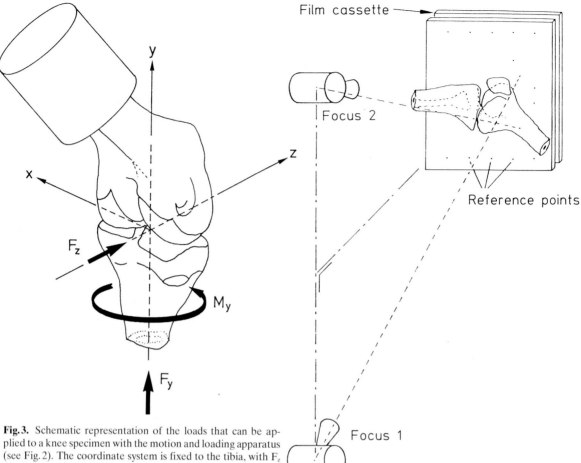

Fig. 3. Schematic representation of the loads that can be applied to a knee specimen with the motion and loading apparatus (see Fig. 2). The coordinate system is fixed to the tibia, with F_z representing the a.p. force, F_y the axial force, and M_y the torque. (From Blankevoort et al. 1988)

Fig. 4. Schematic representation of the experimental setup for roentgen stereophotogrammetric analysis (RSA). The knee specimen is positioned in front of a reference plate and X-ray cassette. In each joint position the specimen, with its affixed tantalum markers, is X-rayed by two roentgen tubes, and a calibration process is used to determine the spatial position of the X-ray focal spots and the spatial relationship between the tantalum reference markers and the laboratory coordinate system. The spatial positions of the markers can be reconstructed following digitization of the films. A series of successive joint positions simulate a movement, whose kinematic parameters can be determined from the positions of the markers. (From Blankevoort et al. 1988)

loads (Fig. 5 a,b): An axial force produces a small, internally directed torque that results from the shape of the articular surfaces, and which causes the tibia to rotate toward the internal limit of rotation (screw motion). Forces in the a. p. and p. a. direction likewise produce small torques that result in internal or external rotation. Torques are also exerted by the quadriceps muscle group during walking and running (Fig. 7), and this, combined with the axial force of the foot strike, produces internal rotation. As the envelope of rotatory motion becomes smaller with decreasing flexion, the joint approaches its internal limits (Fig. 7), ultimately resulting in a combination of extension and external rotation. This "screw home" phenomenon, then, is not just caused by passive joint properties but occurs exclusively in conjunction with an external load. The phenomenon does not occur during extension of the unloaded joint (see Fig. 5 a).

Thus, the three-dimensional kinematic model of the knee as a mechanism with two degrees of freedom

implies that the actual motion pathway within the envelope of motion depends on the external load. This further implies that the joint axes are not uniquely defined. As Fig. 8 demonstrates, pure flexion without tibial rotation occurs about a horizontal axis, while pure rotation without flexion occurs about a vertical axis. If the actual motion is a combination of flexion and rotation, its axis will be oblique to the horizontal and frontal planes.

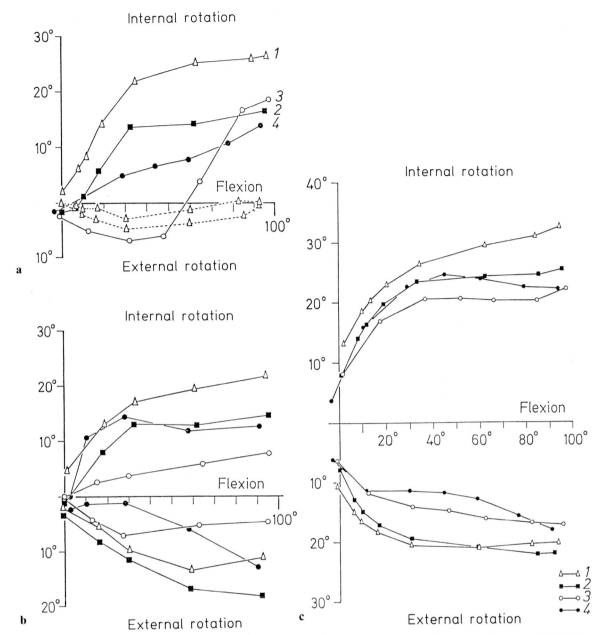

Fig. 5a–c. Tibial rotation versus flexion angle for various external loads in 4 knee joint specimens. **a** *Dashed lines:* 2 motion sequences in unloaded specimens. (The other 3 specimens showed similar responses.) *Solid lines:* motion pattern in 4 different specimens with an imposed axial load F_y of 300 N. **b** The motion pattern with an anterior load F_z of 30 N shows internal tibial rotation during flexion, while the motion pattern with a posterior load F_z of -30 N shows external rotation (4 different specimens). **c** Internal rotation occurs with a torque M_y of 3 Nm, external rotation with a torque M_y of -3 Nm (4 different specimens). If the knee is viewed as having 2 degrees of freedom, flexion and tibial rotation, and the excursion limit of tibial rotation is defined as $+/-$ 3 Nm, then the inner and outer curves describe the envelope of knee motion. (From Blankevoort et al. 1988)

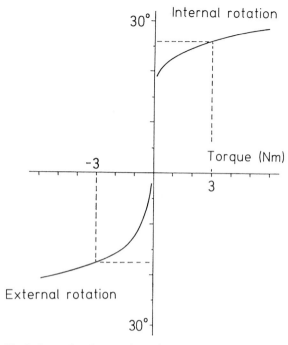

Fig. 6. Internal and external rotation versus torque at a fixed flexion angle of 25° (result for a representative specimen). Threshold torques of +/−3 Nm are arbitrarily defined as the limits of excursion for tibial rotation. (From Blankevoort et al. 1988)

The accuracy of the RSA method makes it possible to calculate the joint axes for specific flexion movements (Blankevoort et al. 1990). One result of this approach is shown in Fig. 9, where the internal and external limits of the motion are defined in terms of +/−3 Nm of torque. We find that the axes of the motion pathways are indeed different for both of these loads. The initially oblique course of the axes in the frontal plane reflects the strong internal or external rotation occurring for that pathway. But the final axes (at approximately 40°–90° of flexion) are almost horizontal, indicating that the motion consists of almost pure flexion. The oblique course of the axes in the transverse plane means that flexion and tibial rotation are coupled with some degree of valgus or varus rotation. The visible posterior displacement of the axis in this plane is comparable to the corresponding posterior shift of the instant center in the anatomic four-bar model and the "roll-back" of the femur upon the tibia. On examining the results, we are struck by the fact that over both (outermost) motion pathways along the limits of the motion envelope, the axes always pass through the region between the femoral attachments of the cruciate ligaments. Thus, while they do not pass through the intersection of "bars" as in the two-dimensional anatomic four-bar linkage model, they still appear to be determined largely by the configuration of the cruciate ligaments.

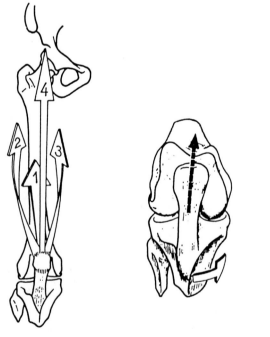

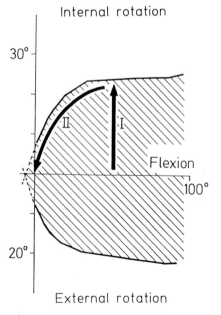

Fig. 7. The quadriceps muscles exert a small internal torque on the tibia, resulting in internal rotation (I). When the knee is extended, quadriceps contraction directs the motion pathway along the internal limits of the envelope of motion. As the en-velope of motion dwindles, the knee is forced into external rotation (II). This can account for the "screw home" phenomenon, or compulsory external rotation of the tibia in terminal extension

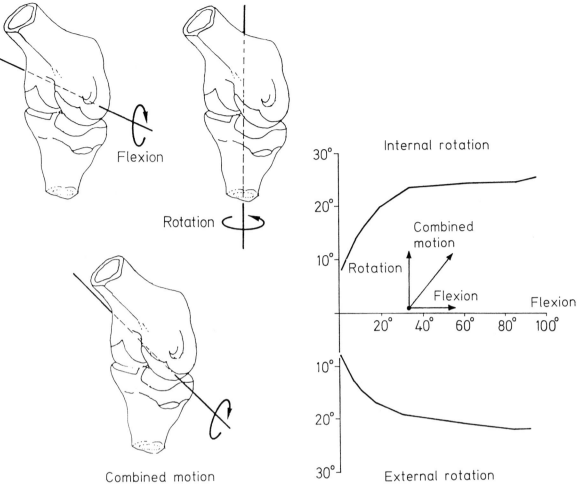

Fig. 8. Schematic representation of the axes of knee motion (helical axes) *(left)* for various motions within the envelope of knee motion *(right)*. The instantaneous axes are not uniquely defined. Pure flexion generally occurs about horizontally di- rected axes, and pure tibial rotation about vertically directed axes. Coupled flexion and rotation have axes directed obliquely to the anatomic planes

In summary, we can regard the knee joint as a mechanism with two independent degrees of freedom, flexion and tibial rotation, within a limited envelope of motion. During each combination of motions and along each motion pathway within this envelope, small translations (in 3 directions) coupled with flexion and rotation occur in addition to varus-valgus rotation. For motions along the limits of the envelope of motion, flexion likewise is coupled with tibial rotation. This is the coupling for which the ligaments, acting in concert with articular geometry, perform their specific task. By extending to the limits of the envelope of motion, the ligaments can exert forces that offer resistance to external loads and constrain further motion. The coupling, then, results from an internal balance of forces to which each ligament makes its own contribution. To isolate and analyze

the role of a single ligament in this mechanism, force analyses must be performed. Clearly, our results show that we are dealing with an essentially three-dimensional problem that is made even more complex by the irregular geometric configuration of the anatomic structures.

A schematic representation of this problem is shown in Fig. 10. Knee motion occurs as the result of a combination of internal and external forces. The motion strains the ligaments, stretching them outside the envelope of motion. Depending on the mechanical and geometric properties of the ligaments, this strain gives rise to forces that in turn contribute directly or via the articular surfaces to the internal forces, and thus to the motions of the joint members. This means that we are dealing with a feedback control mechanism. Before proceeding to analyze this system in its

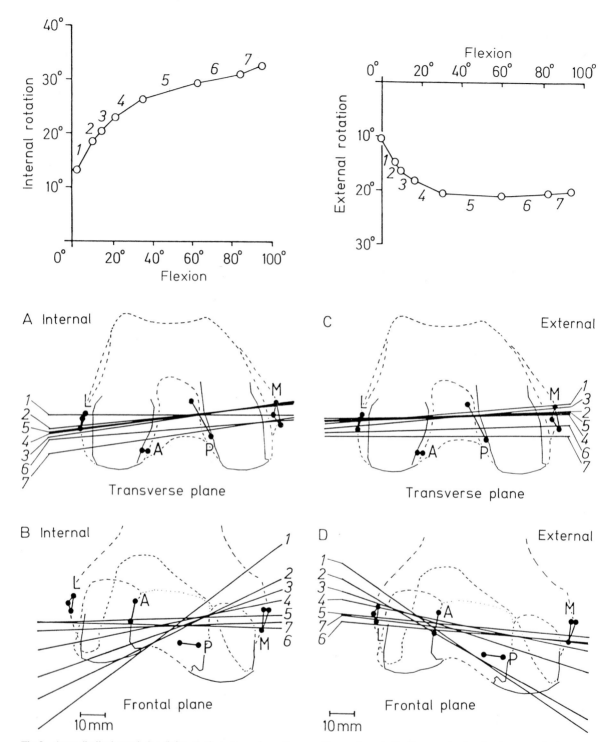

Fig. 9. Axes (helical axes) for finite motion steps along the limits of internal rotation *(left column)* and along the limit of external rotation *(right column)*. Each axis is shown projected onto two anatomic planes, the transverse and frontal, together with markers indicating anatomic structures, articular geometry, and ligament attachments (*A* ACL, *P* PCL, *L* lateral collateral ligament, *M* medial collateral ligament). Each axis is numbered according to the motion step in the graph

entirety, especially in terms of the role of the ACL, we shall first investigate the relationship between knee motion, typical ligament length changes, and ligament forces.

Mechanical Properties of the ACL

As Fig. 10 demonstrates, a ligament exerts its function by elongating. The force produced by this elongation depends on the mechanical properties of the ligament. These properties can be measured in vitro with a mechanical test rig (Noyes and Grood 1976; Butler et al. 1986; Woo et al. 1983; van Rens et al. 1986) that records displacement (strain) as a function of applied load. An example is shown in Fig. 11 (Meijer et al. 1987). In this experiment a bone-ligament-bone specimen was mounted such that the ligament was able to align in the direction of the applied force. The resulting stress-strain curve is nonlinear, especially in its initial portion where a very small force produces a relatively large elongation. In this region the ligament does not offer much resistance despite the relatively large strain. It is believed that this phenomenon relates to the unfolding and aligning of the collagen fibers (Butler et al. 1983). As loading proceeds, the strain resistance (the stiffness of the ligament) progressively increases until the curve becomes (almost) linear due to the increased number of taut collagen fibers and their elastic properties. As the load increases further, rupture begins to occur in isolated fibers and finally involves the whole ligament, represented by the "frayed" curve segment in Fig. 11.

It should be noted at this point that collagenous structures are viscoelastic in their behavior rather than purely elastic. One consequence of this is that the stress-strain curve is dependent on the loading rate. With rapid (impact) loading, the ligament exhibits greater stiffness than with a slowly incremental load.

As stated earlier, ligament stiffness and thus the amount of force exerted by the elongating ligament depends on the number of tense collagen fibers. This number is small in the initial stage (see first portion of curve in Fig. 11) but then gradually increases to the total maximum number present in the ligament, which in turn relates to the ligament thickness. The process whereby increasing numbers of fibers become tense is called "recruitment." It is essential to have a correct understanding of this process, because it determines the effect of a ligament, such as the ACL, on knee function for a given collagen density and given collagen properties. Recruitment is a complex process, especially in the ACL, which has a complicated three-dimensional structure in which the collagen fibers do not exhibit a strictly parallel arrangement. This is illustrated in Fig. 12, which shows the result of a new technique developed for the geometric measurement and numerical description of the three-dimensional collagenous structure of the knee ligaments (Meijer et al. 1989).

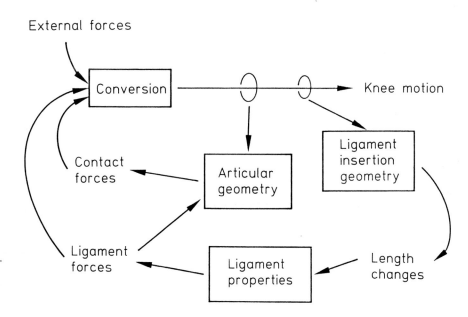

Fig. 10. Schematic representation of the mechanical interactions among the articular structures of the knee

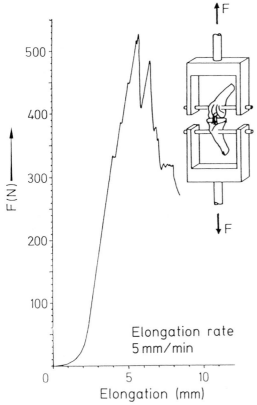

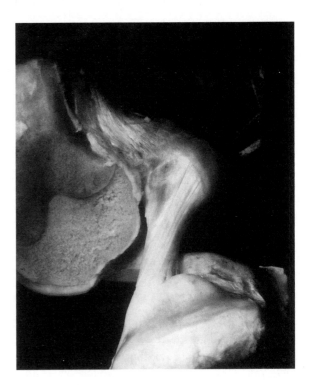

Fig. 11. Tensile test curve of an ACL in a canine knee (bone-ligament-bone specimen with drawing of experimental setup). The specimen was elongated at a prescribed rate, and the associated force was recorded. (From Meijer et al. 1987)

Recruitment of the ACL

Recruitment is the process that determines the relationship between knee movements and typical ligamentous length changes (see Fig. 10), which in turn determine the forces that are developed and thus the restraining action of the ACL. To study this process, a technique was developed that permitted typical ligament length changes to be determined during motion measurements (van Dijk et al. 1979; van Dijk 1983; Blankevoort et al. 1991a). Following the RSA experiments, the attachment sites of the cruciate ligaments were marked with small tantalum pellets (Fig. 13). The RSA technique was again used to measure these markers in the bone segments so that the distances between the individual pairs of markers could be reconstructed during the various motion experiments. In this case each of the cruciate ligaments was described by 2 lines (Fig. 13): the anterior portion of the ACL (A–B), the posterior portion of the ACL

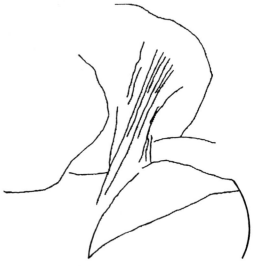

Fig. 12. Sample result of the technique of Meijer et al. (1988) for determining the three-dimensional fiber pattern of ligament bundles. Photographs taken from several directions are analyzed to reconstruct the three-dimensional course of the fiber bundles. *Above* is a photo from the series, from which the reconstruction *(below)* was prepared. (From Meijer et al. 1989)

(C–D), and the anterior (E–F) and posterior (G–H) portions of the posterior cruciate ligament (PCL).

Figure 14 shows an example of these mathematical reconstructions for 5 flexion angles in the frontal and sagittal projections (van Dijk 1983). These reconstructions convey a vivid impression of the changes in

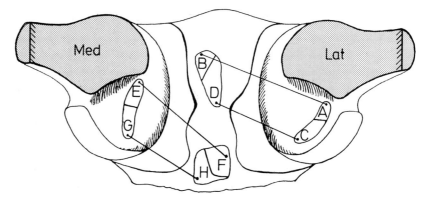

Fig. 13. Schematic representation of the technique for marking the cruciate ligament attachments to measure length changes in the cruciate ligament fiber bundles. Two fiber bundles in each cruciate ligament are identified, and their tibial and femoral attachments are marked with tantalum pellets. The spatial posi- tions of the markers *(A–H)* are then determined using roentgen stereophotogrammetric analysis. With this technique, the distance between each pair of markers can be determined for each measured joint position (van Dijk 1983). See text for further explanation

Fig. 14. see p. 102

the configuration of these ligaments during knee flexion. The only interpretation of these findings is that each position of flexion is associated with the recruitment of different fiber bundles in the ligaments. Also, both projections demonstrate that the mechanical effects of the ligaments are not restricted to one plane. Figure 15 shows the associated length changes in the fiber bundles during flexion in relation to their length in the control state (0° flexion). We see that the anterior bundles of both cruciate ligaments elongate while the posterior bundles shorten. In terms of fiber recruitment, this means that the posterior portions of both ligaments make no functional contribution during flexion. This can also be demonstrated in anatomic specimens (Fig. 16a–c) (van Dijk 1983).

Besides flexion, tibial rotation also influences the recruitment of the fiber bundles. For each position of flexion, the ACL bundles were found to be elongated in internal rotation and shortened in external rotation. The same applies to the posterior bundle of the PCL, whereas the opposite is true for the anterior bundle (Blankevoort et al. 1991a). The length changes associated with tibial rotation, however, are not very large compared with the length changes in flexion.

Apparently the recruitment of the ACL fiber bundles within the envelope of motion depends chiefly on the position of joint flexion and is limited to the anterior portion of the ligament. It may be that the application of excessive anterior forces or internal torques would recruit more of the ligament fibers, but the degree to which this is true remains unknown.

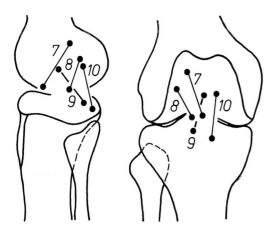

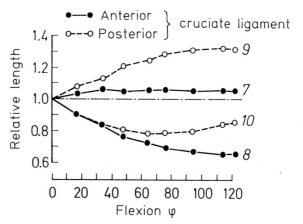

Fig. 15. Relative cruciate ligament length changes versus flexion angle in a single knee specimen. The distance between the ligament markers during flexion is related to the distance in the reference position of extension. *7,* Anterior bundle of ACL; *8,* posterior bundle of ACL; *9,* anterior bundle of PCL; *10,* posterior bundle of PCL. (From Huiskes et al. 1985b)

Projections on the frontal plane (xy)

Projections on the midsagittal plane (yz)

$\phi = 0$ $\phi = 16,6$ $\phi = 44,8$ $\phi = 59,6$ $\phi = 86,6$

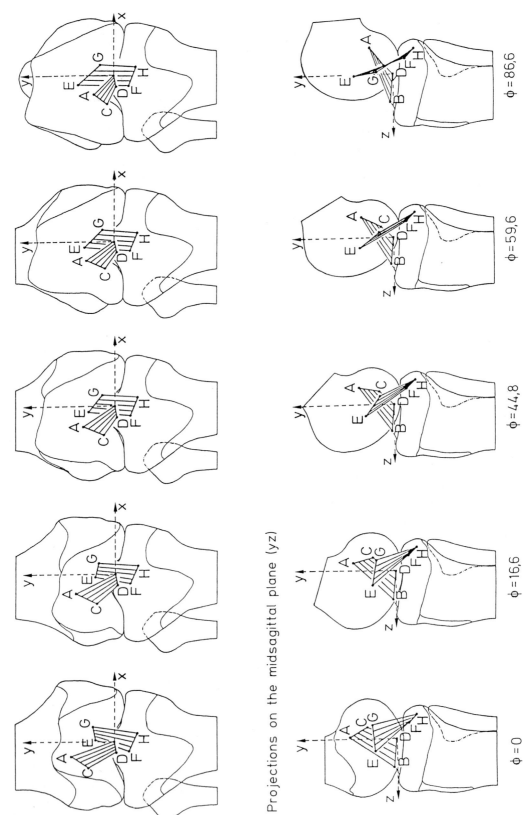

Fig.14. Sample reconstructions of the spatial orientations of the cruciate ligaments for 5 knee positions, projected onto the frontal and sagittal planes. Right knee of a 16-year-old. φ = Flexion angle. (From van Dijk 1983)

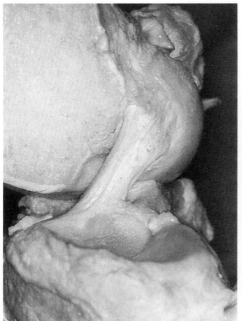
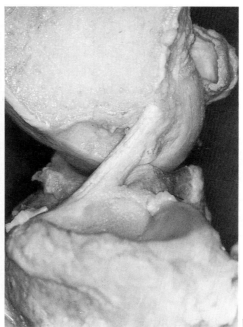
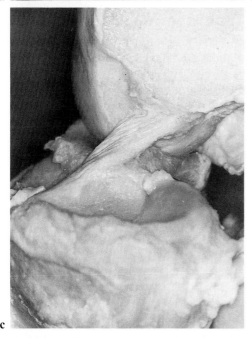

Fig. 16a–c. ACL, medial aspect. **a** Full extension. The posterior bundle is taut. **b** Moderate flexion. The posterior bundle is lax, as indicated by the folds in the posterior edge of the ligament. **c** In complete flexion the anterior bundle is very tense, while the femoral attachment of the posterior bundle is rotated in front of the attachment of the anterior bundle, and the posterior bundle is completely lax. (From van Dijk 1983)

Role of the ACL in the Play of Forces

The above technique for the investigation of fiber recruitment yields information on the portion of the ligament that can exert force in a given position, and it provides some indication of the direction of the force. The magnitude of this force remains unknown, however, because nothing is known about the relationship between force and length change in the recruited portion. Nor do we have definite information about the reference strain of the ligament. In other words, we can measure the *relative* length change but not the length change with respect to an absolute zero point (see Fig. 11). Thus, a force analysis is the only means available for understanding the system outlined in Fig. 10 and investigating the effect of the ACL on knee function. To perform a force analysis in a system as complex as the knee joint, it was necessary to develop computer simulation models (Wismans et al. 1980; Andriacchi et al. 1983; Essinger 1986; Blankevoort et al. 1991 b; Blankevoort and Huiskes 1991). Computer simulation models essentially consist of systems of equations, based on mechanical laws, that incorporate the relevant properties of the individual joint structures. Some degree of schematization is required so that these properties can be mathematically described. The model used by us (Blankevoort et al. 1991 b; Blankevoort and Huiskes 1991) has a three-dimensional character and employs realistic repre-

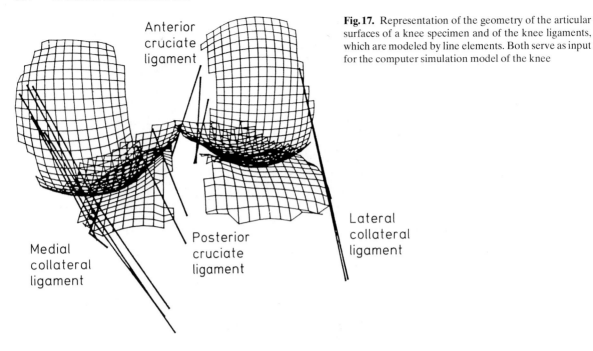

Fig. 17. Representation of the geometry of the articular surfaces of a knee specimen and of the knee ligaments, which are modeled by line elements. Both serve as input for the computer simulation model of the knee

sentations of the articular surface geometry of the femur and tibia (Fig. 17) as measured in a number of knee specimens using a specially developed stereophotogrammetric technique (Huiskes et al. 1985 a). The model allows for some deformability in the contact zone between the articular surfaces. The menisci are not represented in the model due to a lack of basic theoretical data. Experiments have shown, however, that the menisci have little effect on motion patterns in the intact knee joint (Huiskes et al. 1985 b). The ligaments are represented by a number of nonlinear, elastic line segments with the properties shown in Fig. 11. The ACL is modeled as consisting of 3 lines, the PCL as consisting of 2. The input data for the simulation model consist of the successive flexion angles and external load configuration. The following data are available as output: the successive three-dimensional equilibrium states of the joint (tibial rotation, varus-valgus rotation, and translation in the 3 directions), the locations of the femorotibial contact zones, the contact forces, the ligament strain values, and the ligament forces. Because this is a very complex model and some quantities (such as the stiffness curve of the modeled ligaments and their primary tension) are not precisely known, use of the model requires continuous checking against experimental findings. So far it has been found that the results of motion experiments can be simulated quite accurately with this model (Blankevoort et al. 1991 b). Of course, the model yields much more information than experiments, especially in terms of the forces that develop in the joint.

As an example, let us consider a simulation experiment in which the joint is flexed 20°, and internal and external torques are applied to the joint so that the tibia rotates from $+30°$ to $-30°$ (Blankevoort and Huiskes 1988). The model can calculate, among other things, the forces in the modeled ligaments, the contact forces, and the relative contribution of these forces to the equilibrium of forces and moments. Figure 18 shows sample results in which the calculated forces in the modeled ACL and PCL are plotted as a function of tibial rotation. These data clearly depict the recruitment of the ACL during internal rotation. The forces computed in the modeled collateral ligaments indicate that the lateral collateral ligament is a restraint only to external rotation, while the medial collateral ligament restrains both external and internal rotation. These results are consistent with the experimental findings of Ahmed et al. (1987), who estimated the ligament forces from measurements with "buckle transducers" (Lewis et al. 1982). But here again, the model provides additional information. The external torque is held in balance by the sum of the moments produced by the transverse components of the ligament forces and the moments produced by the transverse components of the contact forces. The contact forces in turn are produced indirectly by the tension of the ligaments, as shown in Fig. 10. The model can calculate the relative contributions of both these effects, the direct effect of ligament resistance and the indirect effect via the contact surfaces. The result, shown in Fig. 19, clearly indicates that the contributions of both effects are approximately equal, es-

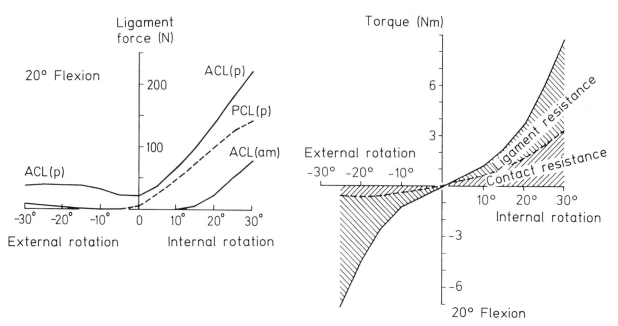

Fig. 18. Forces in the cruciate ligaments during internal and external rotation of the knee for a fixed flexion angle of 20°, determined by simulation with a mathematical knee model. *PCL (p)* posterior portion of PCL, *ACL (p)* posterior portion of ACL, *ACL (am)* anteromedial portion of ACL. (From Blankevoort and Huiskes 1988)

Fig. 19. Torque versus internal and external knee rotation for a fixed flexion angle of 20°, and distribution of the torque over 2 mechanisms of resistance, determined by simulation with a mathematical knee model. (From Blankevoort and Huiskes 1988)

pecially in internal rotation. Thus, through its indirect effect on articular contact forces, the ACL functions as a much more important restraint to internal rotation than one would expect from its anatomic configuration and the forces that develop in the ligament.

This analysis offers a prime example of the potential importance of simulation models, which can be used to investigate an almost limitless number of fundamental questions. A second example that further illustrates the complex role of the ACL concerns the problem of "isometric" cruciate ligament reconstructions. This simulation experiment (Blankevoort and Huiskes 1987) focused on the effect of nonisometric placement of the ligament, which was mathematically modeled by 2 nonlinear elastic lines. The joint was flexed in the unloaded condition, and all the foregoing kinematic and mechanical quantities were recomputed. Primary attention was given to the length changes in the anterior and posterior components of the ACL as the knee moved through flexion. As had been found in the experiments described above, the study showed that the anterior portion of the ACL elongates during flexion, while the posterior portion shortens (Fig. 20). Another simulation was run to learn how the lengths would change if the femoral attachment were placed 5 mm farther anteriorly or pos-

teriorly. These results, also shown in Fig. 20, indicate that advancing the ligament anteriorly causes the ligament to undergo greater elongation, while moving the ligament posteriorly causes it to undergo greater shortening. These results, which agree with the experimental findings of Hefzy and Grood (1986) and Sidles et al. (1988), suggest that placing the ligament too far anteriorly in an ACL reconstruction could expose the ligament to excessive forces and restrict joint mobility. Placing the ligament too far posteriorly could lead to instability. Such a conclusion is frequently drawn in the literature, due in part to the fact that it is intuitively clear. It should be noted, however, that our analyses, like those of Hefzy and Grood (1986) and Sidles et al. (1988), were based on identical motion paths. Thus, while the analysis included the elongation imposed on the ligament by the knee motion, it did not take into account the feedback effect on the motion pathway due to the altered force pattern caused by transposing the ligament attachment (see Fig. 10).

This led us to perform a second experiment in which the actual alternative reconstructions were simulated. A separate simulation was run for each configuration. The results indicate that the length changes caused by the altered ACL attachments are less dramatic than one might have thought based on the al-

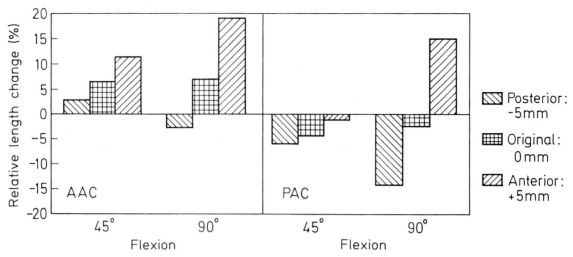

Fig. 20. Anticipated effect of AP transposition of the femoral attachment of the ACL on relative length changes in the modeled *AAC* (anterior part of ACL) and *PAC* (posterior part of ACL) for 2 identical positions of flexion in a simulated knee, where the transposition is not actually carried out. The relative length changes are shown relative to the length in the extended knee. (After Blankevoort and Huiskes 1987)

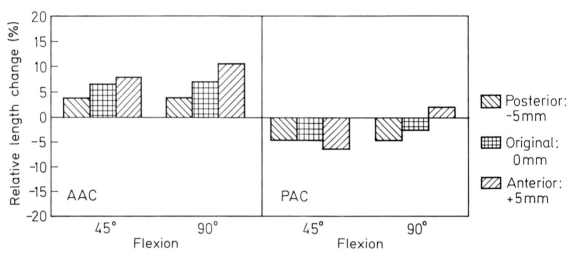

Fig. 21. Effect of an *actual* variation in the a.p. placement of the femoral attachment of the ACL on relative length changes in *AAC* (anterior part of ACL) and *PAC* (posterior part of ACL) for 2 identical positions of flexion in a simulated knee. (After Blankevoort and Huiskes 1987)

teration of typical ligament length changes noted in the previous experiment (Fig. 21). The reasons for this discrepancy can be read directly from the diagram in Fig. 10: A change of insertion geometry alters the pattern of forces via the mechanical properties of the ligament, which in turn alters the course of the movement. The change in the motion pattern chiefly affects a.p. translation (Fig. 22): An anterior femoral attachment of the ACL causes an anterior displacement of the femur with respect to the tibia – perhaps as much as 3.5 mm at large flexion angles. This results

from the decreased length of the ligament, which holds the femur more anteriorly on the tibia during flexion. A posterior femoral attachment gives the femur a greater freedom of posterior motion during flexion, allowing the PCL to pull the femur backward. Of course, the altered motion pattern also affects the strain values in the PCL. These increase to a maximum of 3.5% relative to the initial situation. Thus, the system partially "corrects" for the effects of the altered biomechanical environment of the ACL by altering the pathways of joint motion, giving rise

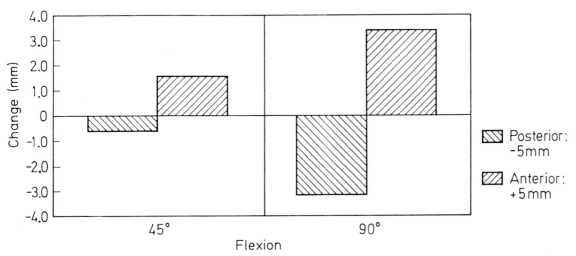

Fig. 22. Change in the a.p. position of the femur relative to the tibia caused by varying the a.p. placement of the femoral attachment of the ACL for 2 identical positions of flexion in a simulated knee. (After Blankevoort and Huiskes 1987)

to different strain values in the remaining ligaments.

This does not mean that a nonanatomic reconstruction of the ACL is desirable, because it could very well have adverse effects in terms of knee laxity and the stresses that develop in the ligament. We may conclude, though, that the sensitivity of the joint to deviations of ligament placement is less than is occasionally believed (and reported). Above all, however, this example gives us greater insight into the functional relationship between the ACL and the other anatomic structures of the knee. This means that the effects of cruciate ligament lesions and reconstructions are very difficult to appreciate in an isolated analysis. The use of simulation models is practically indispensable for an integral analysis.

Discussion and Conclusions

The functional analysis of the ACL is a three-dimensional problem. Two-dimensional anatomic models such as the four-bar linkage are useful for obtaining a general appreciation of the primary effects of motions in one anatomic plane. But for a more detailed analysis, the knee must be conceptualized as a three-dimensional system in which mechanical feedback plays an important role. Because the behavior of the knee and the role of the ligaments and articular surfaces happen within the context of a play of forces, analytical methods are necessary to comprehend and interpret the results of experiments. The computer simulation model discussed here is an example of

this. Although it is not perfect, use of this model for the simulation of experiments offers greater insight into the relevant phenomena than can be gained from experimental results alone.

The knee joint derives its complexity from its complicated anatomic structure and mechanical properties as well as from its three-dimensional laxity and the kinematic coupling between its degrees of freedom. Conceptually, the joint can be regarded as a mechanism with 2 independent degrees of freedom. The ligaments restrain mobility and produce kinematic couplings in both a direct sense and an indirect sense via the articular surfaces. In the process, a ligament does not function as a unit but as a complex of collagen fibers that are recruited as required. This recruitment process has considerable clinical significance in both the diagnosis and repair of ligamentous injuries. Thus, a fiber bundle damaged by a tear is not recruited, and an incorrectly positioned fiber bundle will not be recruited at the appropriate time.

Drawer tests are unquestionably useful for the evaluation of the ACL, especially when they can be documented and quantified with the aid of an instrumented test device (Daniel et al. 1985; Edixhoven et al. 1987, 1989). An example of an instrumented drawer tester is shown in Fig. 23. However, these devices are based on the concept of the knee as a two-dimensional mechanism, and they are most effective for testing the fibers that must be recruited in selected positions of flexion and tibial rotation. For a more exacting diagnosis of partial tears of the ACL, additional test methods are required. Perhaps this could be accomplished by developing methods based on the recruitment mechanism described above and

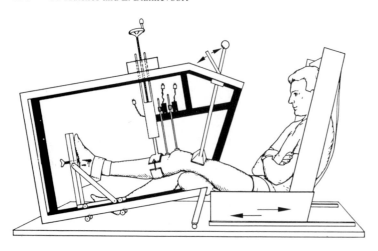

Fig. 23. Instrumented drawer tester of Edix-hoven et al. (1987)

the indirect effect that the ACL exerts on the limits of knee motion via the articular surfaces. The function of the ligament should be approached as a three-dimensional problem, even in laxity tests.

One of the very few acknowledgments of this basic concept in the clinical diagnosis of ligamentous injuries is the pivot shift test (Galway et al. 1972), an essentially three-dimensional test that is difficult to perform and quantitate. The pivot shift test is an important component of a quantitative biomechanical analysis that respects the three-dimensional character of ligamentous function.

Even in discussions of "anatomic" reconstructions of the ACL, the two-dimensional four-bar linkage model is implicitly used as a reference. Often this disregards the fact that an alternative ligament results in an alternative recruitment pattern, which in turn alters the characteristics of joint motion through mechanical feedback within the joint as a whole. The extent of this process depends in turn on the condition of the PCL and collateral ligaments.

The finding that the function of the ACL is far more complex than is often assumed on the basis of simple anatomic models, while scientifically interesting, is of no immediate clinical benefit in itself. This chapter, then, is concerned more with defining the problem than offering a solution. Nevertheless, it would be very useful to approach the injured ACL as a three-dimensional problem in the development of diagnostic techniques, therapeutic procedures, and diagnostic and therapeutic instruments.

References

Ahmed AM, Hyder A, Burke DL, Chan KH (1987) In-vitro ligament tension pattern in the flexed knee in passive loading. J Orthop Res 5: 217–230

Andriacchi TP, Mikosz RP, Hampton SJ, Galante JO (1983) Model studies of the stiffness characteristics of the human knee joint. J Biomech 16: 23–29

Blankevoort L, Huiskes R (1987a) The effects of ACL substitute location on knee joint motion and cruciate ligament strains. Orthop Trans 11/2: 350

Blankevoort L, Huiskes R (1988) The interaction between articular geometry and cruciate ligament function in the knee joint. Proceedings of the sixth meeting of the European Society of Biomechanics, University of Bristol, England

Blankevoort L, Huiskes R (1991) Ligament-bone interaction in a threedimensional model of the knee. J Biomech Eng 113: (in press)

Blankevoort L, Huiskes R, Lange A de (1988) The envelope of passive knee joint motion. J Biomech 21: 705–721

Blankevoort L, Huiskes R, de Lange A (1990) Helical axes of passive knee-joint motions. J Biomechanics 23: 1219–1229

Blankevoort L, Huiskes R, de Lange A (1991a) Recruitment of knee joint ligaments. Biomech Eng 113: 94–103

Blankevoort L, Kuiper JH, Huiskes R, Grootenvoer HJ (1991b) Articular contact in a three-dimensional model of the knee. J Biomechanics 24: (in press)

Butler DL, Stouffer DC, Wukusick PM, Zernicke RF (1983) Analysis of non homogeneous strain response of human patellar tendon. ASME Biomechanics Summer Symposium 1983, American Society for Mechanical Engineers, New York, pp 129–132

Butler DL, Kay MD, Stouffer DC (1986) Comparison of material properties in fascicle-bone units from human patellar tendon and knee ligaments. J Biomech 19: 425–432

Daniel DM, Malcolm LL, Losse G, Stone ML, Sachs R, Burks R (1985) Instrumented measurement of anterior laxity of the knee. J Bone Joint Surg [Am] 67: 720–726

Dijk R van (1983) The behavior of the cruciate ligaments in the knee. Dissertation, University of Nijmegen

Dijk R van, Huiskes R, Selvik G (1979) Roentgen stereophotogrammetric methods for the evaluation of the three-dimensional kinematic behavior and cruciate ligament length patterns of the human knee joint. J Biomech 12: 727–731

Edixhoven P, Huiskes R, Graaf A de (1989) Anteroposterior drawer measurements in the knee using an instrumented test device. Clin Orthop 247: 232–242

Edixhoven P, Huiskes R, Graaff R de, Rens TJG van, Slooff TJ (1987) Accuracy and reproducibility of instrumented knee-drawer tests. J Orthop Res 5: 378–387

Essinger JR (1986) NEJ: a numerical model for the investigation and the analysis of knee prostheses. Dissertation, École Polytechnique Féderale de Lausanne

Galway RD, Beaupré A, MacIntosh DL (1972) Pivot shift: a clinical sign of symptomatic anterior cruciate ligament insufficiency. J Bone Joint Surg [Br] 54: 763–764

Hefzy MS, Grood ES (1986) Sensitivity of insertion loctions on length patterns of anterior cruciate ligament fibers. J Biomech Eng 108: 73–82

Huiskes R, Kremers J, Lange A de, Woltring HJ, Selvik G, Rens TJG van (1985a) Analytical stereophotogrammetric determination of three-dimensional knee-joint geometry. J Biomech 18: 559–570

Huiskes R, Dijk R van, Lange A de, Woltring HJ, Rens TJG van (1985b) Kinematics of the human knee joint. In: Berme N, Engin AE, Correia da Silva KM (eds) Biomechanics of normal and pathological human articulating joints. Nijhoff, Dordrecht Boston Lancaster, pp 165–188

Huson A (1974) Biomechanische Probleme des Kniegelenks. Orthopädie 3: 119–126

Lange A de, Kauer JMG, Huiskes R (1985) Kinematic behavior of the human wrist joint: a Roentgen-stereophotogrammetric analysis. J Orthop Res 3: 56–64

Lewis JL, Lew WD, Schmidt J (1982) A note on the application and evaluation of the buckle transducer for knee ligament force measurement. J Biomech Eng 104: 125–128

Meijer RCMB, Huiskes R, Kauer JMG (1987) Mechanische Belastung im Sport. In: Huiskes R (Hrsg) Biomechanica — Aspekte des Bewegungsapparats. Stafleu, Alphen aan den Rijn Brussel, S 9–27

Meijer RCMB, Huiskes R, Kauer JMG (1989) A stereophotogrammetric method for measurements of ligament structure. J Biomech

Menschik A (1974) Mechanik des Kniegelenks, Teil 1. Z Orthop 112: 481–495

Müller We (1982) Das Knie. Springer, Berlin Heidelberg New York

Noyes FR, Grood ES (1976) The strength of the anterior cruciate ligament in humans and rhesus monkeys. J Bone Joint Surg [Am] 58: 1074–1082

Rens TJG van, Berg AF van den, Huiskes R, Kuypers W (1986) Substitution of the anterior cruciate ligament: a long-term histologic and biomechanical study with autogenous pedicled grafts of the iliotibial band in dogs. J Arthroscopic Rel Surg 2: 139–154

Selvik G (1974) A Roentgen stereophotogrammetric method for the study of the kinematics of the skeletal system. Dissertation, University of Lund

Sidles JA, Larson RV, Garbini JL, Downey DJ, Matsen III FA (1988) Ligament length relationships in the moving knee. J Orthop Res 6: 593–610

Strasser H (1917) Lehrbuch der Muskel- und Gelenkmechanik. Springer, Berlin

Wismans J, Veldpaus F, Janssen J, Huson A, Struben P (1980) A three-dimensional mathematical model of the knee-joint. J Biomech 13: 677–685

Woo SL-Y, Gomez MA, Seguchi Y, Endo CM, Akeson WH (1983) Measurement of mechanical properties of ligament substance from a bone-ligament-bone preparation. J Orthop Res 1: 22–29

Significance of Anatomy and Biomechanics

W. Hackenbruch

The extremely close link between anatomy (form) and biomechanics (function) has long been recognized but was brought most forcibly into current awareness by the studies of Müller (1983, 1987). The discoveries of recent years on the biomechanics of the ligaments and the diagnosis and treatment of ligamentous knee injuries have prompted further investigations on *anatomy* as well. By the same token, recent discoveries in anatomy have had an impact on clinical practice and especially the operative reconstruction of ligaments. The ligaments about the joints perform essentially mechanical tasks. To understand this function, it is important to define origins and insertions, which can explain the course of a ligament and its relationship to the center of rotation of the knee. This qualitative problem has been largely solved for the anterior cruciate ligament (ACL) in the sagittal plane (Menschik 1974). The angle of the ACL relative to the femoral and tibial axes and to the posterior cruciate ligament (PCL) in the sagittal plane changes as the knee moves through flexion. This has been well documented in the cadaveric knee (Hertel 1980) by marking the origins and insertions of the cruciate ligaments with screw heads and studying the course of the ligaments on radiographs taken in various flexion angles (Fig. 1). The broad areas of attachment of the ACL on the femur and tibia lead to variations in the tension pattern and course of the twisted ligament fibers in different positions.

Attempts have been made in anatomic studies to define the origin and insertion of the ACL in mathematically precise terms (Girgis et al. 1975; Odensten and Gillquist 1984; Wagner and Schabus 1982). Most of these studies were done with the object of designing guides for drilling the bone tunnels in ACL reconstructions. These drill guides are useful only for a statistically average population of knees. They are of

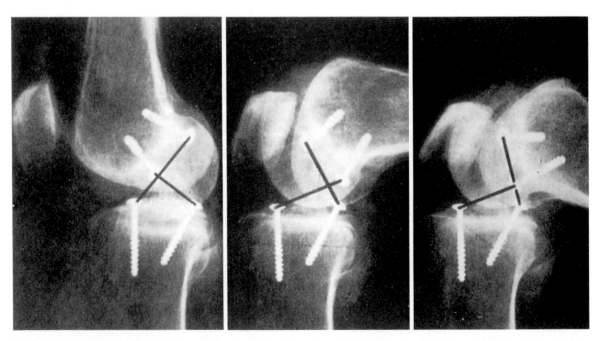

Fig. 1. Orientations of the cruciate ligaments in approximately 120°, 90°, and 0° flexion. The origins and insertions are marked with screw heads. The angle between the two cruciate ligaments, the ligaments and femur, and the ligaments and tibia varies with the angle of knee flexion. (From Hertel 1980)

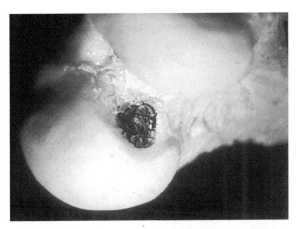

Fig. 2. This photo shows the large area of femoral attachment of the ACL on an anatomic specimen. Note that the area of attachment is located far posteriorly at the cartilage-bone junction

limited use at best in knees with a small or very large radius of the femoral condyles.

Special attention should be given to the proximal attachment of the ACL, which is located far back on the femoral condyle at the chondro-osseous junction (Fig. 2). This is an important anatomic fact, for one of the most common errors in ACL reconstructions is faulty placement, a mistake frequently seen at re-

operation. The proximal attachment is often placed too far anteriorly, an error that unfortunately is perpetuated in recent illustrations published in respected journals (Eady et al. 1982). In the example shown (Fig. 3a), the ACL was reattached far in front of the cartilage-bone junction, forming a right angle to the tibial plateau in approximately 80° of flexion. The ligament should form an approximately 30° angle to the plane of the tibial plateau in that position (Fig. 3b).

Virtually nothing has been published on the angle of the ACL on the *frontal plane*, yet this angle is important surgically in terms of locating the optimum proximal and distal sites of attachment. Visualization of the ACL on the frontal plane clearly shows that a simple "over-the-top" proximal attachment does not conform to anatomy. The angle can be stated both in relation to the PCL and in relation to the axis of the tibial or femoral shaft. As in the sagittal plane, the angle of the ligament on the frontal plane changes with the position of knee flexion.

Prompted by the studies of Hertel (1980), we used screw heads to mark the centers of the proximal and distal cruciate ligament attachments in cadaveric knee joints so that we could document radiographically the course of the ACL in various positions of flexion. The ligament angles measured at 2 charac-

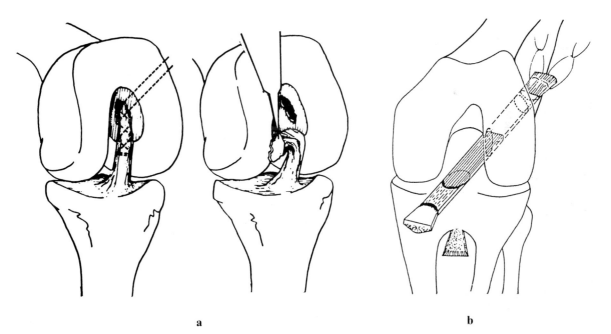

a   b

Fig. 3. a These drawings (from Eady et al. 1982) give a *wrong* impression of the course of the ACL. The proximal attachment is too anterior; this would inevitably lead to restricted motion or retearing. **b** Schematic representation of the correct course of the ligament in approximately 80° flexion. The ACL forms an angle of about 30° with the tibial plateau in the sagittal plane, not 90° as shown in **a**. Neither is the course of the ligament in **a** correctly portrayed in the frontal plane. (From Hackenbruch and Henche 1981)

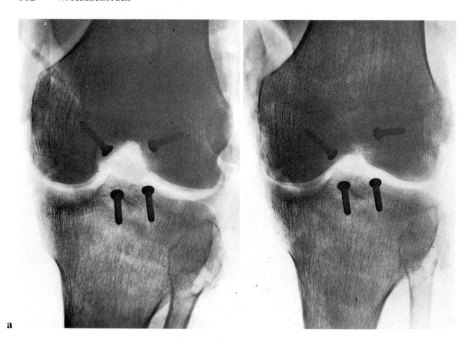

a

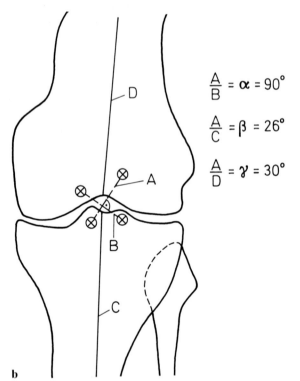

$$\frac{A}{B} = \alpha = 90°$$

$$\frac{A}{C} = \beta = 26°$$

$$\frac{A}{D} = \gamma = 30°$$

b

Fig. 4. a Radiographs of a knee joint in 10° flexion on the AP plane (cadaveric knee). Screw heads mark the centers of the cruciate ligament attachments. In 10° flexion the ACL forms a 90° angle with the PCL, a 26° angle with the tibial axis, and a 30° angle with the femoral axis. In 45° flexion of the same knee (tunnel view), the ACL forms an angle of 95° with the PCL, 28° with the tibial axis, and 32° with the femoral axis. Thus, all the angles increase with the angle of knee flexion. **b** Schematic drawing of the radiographs, with the angles drawn in. α Angle between ACL and PCL, β angle between ACL and tibial axis, γ angle between ACL and femoral axis. The slight deformity of the cadaveric knee (0° axis) should be noted

teristic flexion angles (10° and 45°) are shown in Fig. 4. Greater flexion angles interfere with radiographic visualization due to superimposition of the bony femur.

The frontal-plane view of the cruciate ligaments gives a good impression of the width of the intercondylar notch, which usually is narrowed by a lateral osteo-phyte in the chronically anterior cruciate-deficient knee. The osteophyte must be removed at recon-struction to avoid angulation of the graft in the ex-tended knee (notch plasty). A more precise geo-metric definition of the intercondylar notch and its minimum width are controversial and are a subject of current research. While an accurate knowledge of the origin and insertion tells us something about the overall status of the ACL, it says nothing about the course of the individual fibers. The concept of the ACL as consisting of 3 fiber bundles (anteromedial, intermediate, posterolateral) offers a simplified explanation for the variable course of the ligament (Wagner and Schabus 1982) but can only hint at its structural complexity, which involves a spiralization of the fibers and fiber bundles (Fig. 5). The "bundle anatomy" concept has been largely discarded in recent years (Odensten and Gillquist 1984). Based on our own operative and arthroscopic experience, about 20% of ACLs have a palpable or visible cleft separating the ligament into an anteromedial and posterolateral bundle. The division into 2 bundles may have some clinical significance in partial ruptures, but these lesions can only be diagnosed arthroscopically. The individual cruciate ligament fibers show an approximately parallel arrangement in the extended knee, while in flexion they become twisted and alter their course. This fact is sobering for the surgeon attempting to reconstruct the ACL, for even with the best operating technique, he can do no better than approximate the ligament geometry.

Like most ligaments, the cruciate ligaments conform in their course to the laws of isometry. The principle of isometry has long been recognized, and its relevance to operative repairs of the ACL has been tested in thread models (Artmann and Wirth 1974). The problems of isometry are a subject of ongoing research (see also the chapter by Friederich and O'Brian, p. 78 ff.).

Besides its course, the length of the ACL also has been investigated (Alm 1974; Girgis et al. 1975; Odensten and Gillquist 1984), and marked discrepancies have been reported. Odensten and Gillquist found a length of 31 mm, a thickness of 5 mm, and a volume of 2.3 ml. However, as the twisted course of the ligament would suggest, even simple length measurements pose considerable difficulties, because different fibers in the same ligament must have different lengths in different joint positions. Thus, data reported in the literature represent no more than statistical averages.

The cruciate ligaments are intraarticular but extrasynovial. This results from the embryonic development of the cruciate ligaments from a sagittal mesenchymal fold that enters the knee joint from behind, carrying with it a synovial covering. This also explains why the cruciate ligaments derive their blood supply from a branch of the middle genicular artery. The synovial membrane that ensheaths the cruciate ligaments contains abundant vessels from the middle genicular artery. These vessels, along with small terminal branches of the medial and lateral inferior genicular arteries, form a synovial plexus that has connections with the infrapatellar fat pad. The synovial vessels form a periligamentous (perifibrillary) plexus that pierces the ligaments with fine transverse branches and anastomoses with an intraligamentous vascular network. The intraligamentous vessels are oriented longitudinally and run parallel to the collagen bundles. The sites of ligament attachment on the femur and tibia do not contribute significantly to the blood supply of the cruciate ligaments. The connection of the synovial plexus from the infrapatellar fat pad is significant, however. The blood supply comes from an infrapatellar transverve anastomosis between the medial and lateral inferior genicular arteries. All the vessels are subject to anatomic variations, particularly the arterial supply route via the infrapatellar fat pad. The PCL, owing to its proximity to the main artery (medial inferior genicular), receives a more copious blood supply than the ACL, and this influences their rates of healing (Arnoczky 1987; Arnoczky et al. 1979). When examined by light microscopy, the ACL shows a rigid collagenous structure with a parallel, undulating arrangement of the collagen fibers. Its electron microscopic appearance is similar (Hackenbruch and Schmiebusch 1985), the general morphology suggesting habitual exposure to multiaxial loads (Fig. 6). The ligament consists of type 1, α-1, and α-2 collagen fibers (Rovere and Adair 1983). (See the chapter by Hunziker, p. 62 ff., for a more detailed structural description.)

Despite an abundance of research data, anatomic questions remain. Free nerve endings and corpuscles

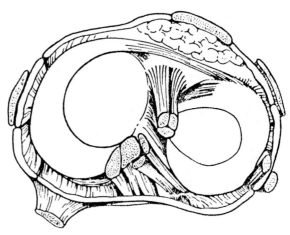

Fig. 5. Transverse section through a right knee joint, 1 cm above the meniscal plane. The individual bundles of the anterior (and posterior) cruciate ligament are clearly visible on the schematic drawing (anteromedial, intermediate, posterolateral). (From Wagner and Schabus 1982)

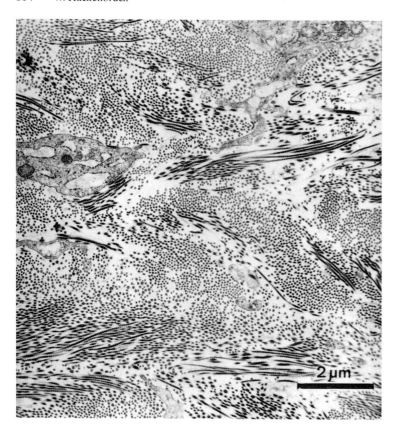

Fig. 6. Electron micrograph of an ACL. The tissue sample was taken during meniscectomy in a 63-year-old male with a clinically stable knee and a grossly healthy ACL. Note the regular fibril arrangement and homogeneous ultrastructure with signs of multiaxial loading

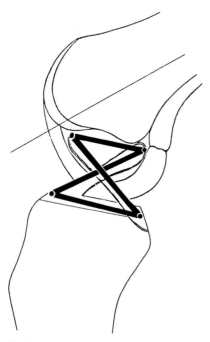

Fig. 7. Schematic representation of the four-bar linkage model of the cruciate ligaments. The large areas of attachment of the three-dimensional ligaments are reduced to simple points in the two-dimensional model. (From Hackenbruch and Henche 1981)

have been demonstrated in the middle third and proximal attachment of the ACL (Cerulli 1986, personal communication). Further reserach is needed to determine whether these structures provide a definitive explanation for proprioceptive control.

Finally, the numerous anatomic variations have not yet been explained, although they probably stem from a correlation between the geometry of the cruciate ligaments and the radius of the femoral condyles.

From our knowledge of anatomy, we can speculate about *function*. In describing the ACL, we must also mention the PCL because both are arranged in the pattern of a four-bar linkage on the sagittal plane (Fig. 7) (Menschik 1974). In this past, this model has provided a useful simplification of geometry and function, as it reduces a complex three-dimensional problem to two dimensions. The three-dimensional model of Müller (1987) is based on the concept that the cruciate ligaments and intercondylar eminence together form a pedestal or "central pivot." The flattened femoral condyles in the model can roll and glide on the tibial plateau, while the cylindrical central pivot permits their simultaneous rotation (Fig. 8). Modern biomechanics, with its physical and electronic aids, has led to ongoing progress in the descrip-

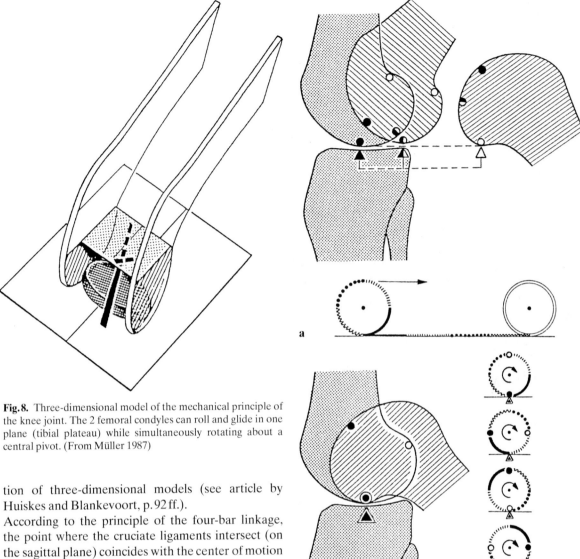

Fig. 8. Three-dimensional model of the mechanical principle of the knee joint. The 2 femoral condyles can roll and glide in one plane (tibial plateau) while simultaneously rotating about a central pivot. (From Müller 1987)

tion of three-dimensional models (see article by Huiskes and Blankevoort, p. 92 ff.).

According to the principle of the four-bar linkage, the point where the cruciate ligaments intersect (on the sagittal plane) coincides with the center of motion for each joint position. In theory, the attachments of the peripheral ligaments can be derived under isometric conditions. Besides defining the center of motion, the four-bar linkage can aid in explaining the maximum range of motion as well as the rolling-gliding and posterior movement of the femur on the tibia during flexion (Fig. 9). Both the center of motion and the area of femorotibial contact move backward with flexion. As a result, the center of rotation also depends on the position of knee flexion under physiologic conditions, though this fact is frequently disregarded. The dependence of the physiologic center of rotation on flexion angle is mirrored by an even more pronounced change in the pathologic center of rotation in the unstable knee. As a result, the pathologic center of rotation for a given type of instability (e.g., anteromedial or anterolateral rotatory instability) cannot be precisely defined. We can only de-

Fig. 9 a, b. Schematic representation of pure rolling (**a**) and pure gliding (**b**) of the femur upon the tibial plateau. A pure rolling motion would carry the femur past the posterior edge of the tibia in maximum flexion. With pure gliding the femur would impinge on the posterior rim of the tibia at about 110° of flexion. Only a combination of rolling and gliding yields the natural motion sequence with posterior displacement of the femur and motion axis during flexion (see also Fig. 1)

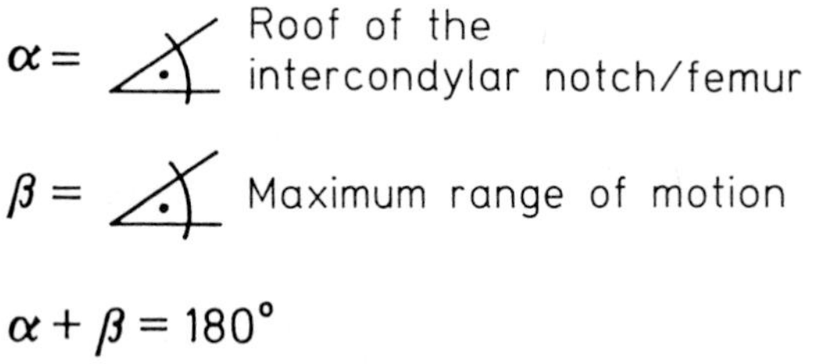

$$\alpha = \text{∠}\quad \text{Roof of the intercondylar notch/femur}$$

$$\beta = \text{∠}\quad \text{Maximum range of motion}$$

$$\alpha + \beta = 180°$$

Fig. 10. Mathematical relationship of the angle between the roof of the intercondylar notch and femoral axis and the maximum range of knee motion

scribe an area within which the center of rotation is located and is free to move (Hackenbruch and Henche 1981). The center can be defined as a unique point only for an individual knee positioned at a designated flexion angle.

The angle formed by the roof of the intercondylar notch with the femoral shaft axis has an important bearing on the range of knee motion. Normally this angle is 40°, and its complement, 140°, represents the maximum range of knee motion. This mathematical relationship is shown in Fig. 10. Thus, if the roof of the intercondylar notch formed a 90° angle, the maxi-

mum range of motion (complementary angle) would be 90°, consisting of 45° flexion and 45° hyperextension (Fig. 11). It should be added that the validity of this formula is limited in a strictly mathematical sense, and that it holds only for angles α in the range from 0° to 90°.

Besides essentially anatomic and quantitative functional descriptions, qualitative problems are still largely unresolved. We still know little about the rupture strength of the ACL. Some studies have been done in cadaveric knees and experimental animals (Noyes and Grood 1976), but many questions remain unanswered. Further research is needed to determine whether the flexion of the joint or the ligament rupture speed obey specific laws in terms of the type and location of tears.

Pathomechanics deals with disturbances of biomechanics, which usually are secondary to injury of the ACL. The most common pathologic situation is ACL insufficiency caused by a rupture. This leads to loss of anterior stability in the knee and to anterior translation of the proximal tibia. The altered rolling-gliding mechanism ultimately leads to subluxation, which occurs in the lateral compartment due to predisposing anatomic factors. The joint exhibits a dynamic sub-

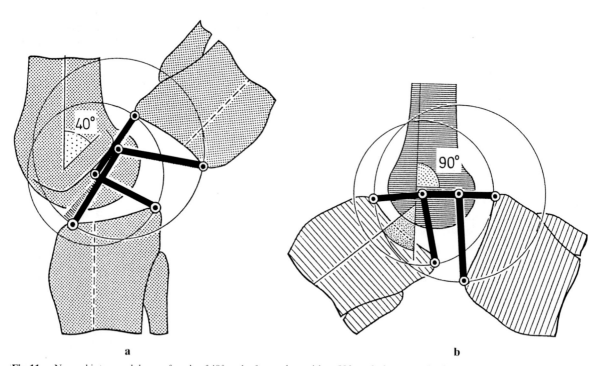

a   b

Fig. 11. a Normal intercondylar roof angle of 40° to the femoral axis. The ACL is parallel to the intercondylar roof in maximum extension (0°), the PCL in maximum flexion (140°). The parallel course of the ligaments in the two extreme positions represents the absolute limit of motion, corresponding to a total range of joint motion of 140° (180°–40°). **b** Hypothetical case

with a 90° angle between the intercondylar roof and femoral axis. Here the ACL is parallel to the intercondylar roof at about 45° of hyperextension, the PCL at about 45° of flexion. The total range of knee motion is only 90° (180°–90°). (From Müller 1983)

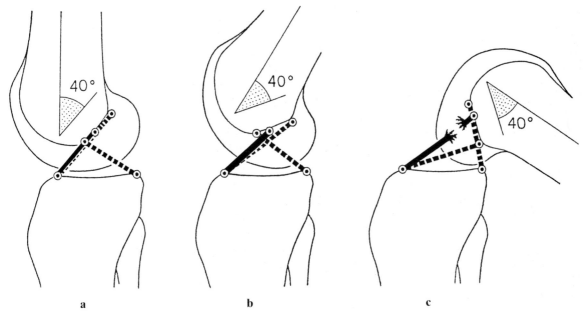

Fig. 12. Schematic representation of the faulty proximal reattachment of an ACL *(solid line)*. Too anterior in its placement, the ligament will either limit flexion to about 60° or will rupture due to insufficient length if flexion beyond that point is attempted. (From Müller 1982)

luxation snap that is pathognomonic for ACL insufficiency (see chapter by Jakob and Stäubli, p. 157 ff.). The anterior translation of the upper tibia (anterior drawer in various degrees of flexion) also depends on the stability of the peripheral capsuloligamentous structures, or "secondary restraints." The subluxation snap, combined with the instability, can lead to the further loosening of synergistic ligamentous structures (iliotibial tract, semimembranosus corner) with associated lesions of the cartilage and menisci.

The pathognomonic subluxation snap cannot always be elicited in acute injuries or even more chronic ones, and the rest of the clinical examination does not always yield a definite, let alone quantitative evaluation of the insufficiency. This has led to increasing reliance on arthroscopy as a diagnostic tool. Even partial tears of the ACL can be diagnosed by this method, providing significant advantages in terms of differential therapeutic decision making. Other imaging techniques (CT, MRI, ultrasound) have been somewhat disappointing in this regard; nor has the quantitative assessment of joint instability (arthrometry) achieved much practical importance for routine clinical use.

A surgically untreated rupture of the ACL with loss of continuity will inevitably lead to insufficiency, since for anatomic reasons a lesion of this type cannot heal conservatively. With loss of continuity, the torn fibers of the ACL hang loosely in the joint. By con-

trast, the torn ends of peripheral ligaments are held in apposition by adjacent tissues, and even a complete rupture can heal without surgery. Rotatory instabilities (anteromedial and anterolateral with lesions of the ACL) may develop, depending on primary damage or secondary insufficiency of the secondary restraints, and can vary greatly in degree. The pathologic center of rotation in these cases depends both on the degree of the instability and the position of knee flexion and thus can be accurately defined only for an individual case and a specified flexion angle.

The ACL is subject to pathomechanical problems other than insufficiency. One of the most common is faulty placement of the ligament attachment during a repair or reconstruction. This leads to a disturbance of isometry, which in turn leads to limitation of motion or loosening of the ligament (Fig. 12). Similar problems result from intercondylar eminence fractures that heal with malunion (Fig. 13). Angular deformities about the joint following fractures, especially in the sagittal plane (bony recurvatum or antecurvatum), lead to a mechanically incompetent ligament insertion, resulting in cruciate ligament insufficiency or restricted motion (Fig. 14).

Secondary pathomechanical sequelae for the ACL can result from disturbances of the secondary restraints or of periarticular muscles. Insufficiency of the secondary restraints or PCL can lead to loosening of the ACL as surely as loss of muscular function

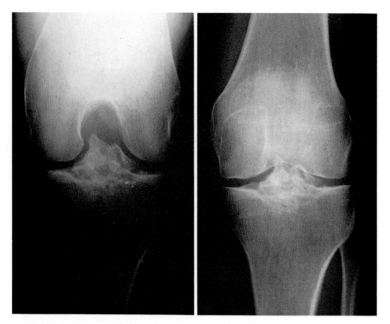

Fig. 13. Radiographs of a 20-year-old woman with a conservatively treated, malunited intercondylar eminence fracture. She presented clinically with instability and limited motion. ACL insufficiency secondary to osseous deformity

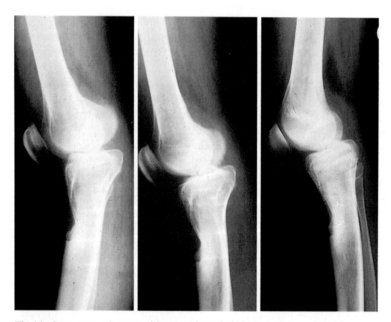

Fig. 14. Osseous recurvatum with approximately 20° of angular deformity. The normal 10° posterior inclination of the tibial plateau is replaced by a 10° anterior slope. Radiographs of a 17-year-old male following proximal tibial traction with epiphyseal plate injury, sequelae to childhood femoral fracture. Bony deformity has led to malposition of the distal cruciate ligament attachments, causing elongation and insufficiency

about the knee (e.g., in poliomyelitis). It should be noted in this regard that the hamstrings are the synergists of the ACL, while the quadriceps group is its antagonist. The mechanical effect and force of these muscles naturally depend on the lever arm and thus on the angle of knee flexion. Total meniscectomy, too, can secondarily affect the ACL through the attendant loss of stability. In a broader sense, all diseases that compromise neuromuscular coordination can lead to functional instability and eventual pathomechanical disturbances of the ACL.

A knowledge of anatomy is essential for the diagnosis and treatment of capsuloligamentous injuries in the knee, especially those involving the ACL. In the diagnostic evaluation of these injuries, the examiner should always describe the anatomic lesions in "quantitative" terms (e.g., a partial rupture of the ACL with a complete rupture of the medial collateral ligament). This increases diagnostic precision and helps to define the therapeutic approach. By contrast, a diagnosis of "anterior instability" says nothing about the precise anatomic lesion and has no specific therapeutic implications. Isometry, blood flow, and neuromuscular control are essential factors in the anatomy of the ACL.

References

Alm A (1974) On the anterior cruciate ligament. Med Dissertation, Linköping University

Arnoczky SP (1987) The vascularity of the anterior cruciate ligament and associated structures. In: Jackson DW, Drez D (eds) The anterior cruciate deficient knee. Mosby, St. Louis, p 27

Arnoczky SP, Rubin RM, Marshall JL (1979) Microvasculature of the cruciate ligaments and its response to injury. An experimental study in dogs. J Bone Joint Surg [Am] 61: 1221-1229

Artmann M, Wirth CJ (1974) Untersuchung über den funktionsgerechten Verlauf der vorderen Kreuzbandplastik. Z Orthop 112: 160-165

Cerulli G, Ceccarini A, Alberti PF, Caraffa A, Caraffa G (1988) Mechanoreceptors of some anatomical structures of the human knee. In: Müller We, Hackenbruch W (eds) Surgery and Arthroscopy of the knee. Springer, Berlin Heidelberg New York Tokyo, pp 50-54

Eady JL, Cardenas CD, Sopa D (1982) Avulsion of the femoral attachment of the anterior cruciate ligament in a seven-year-old child. J Bone Joint Surg [Am] 64: 1376-1378

Girgis FG, Marshall JL, Monajem ARS (1975) The cruciate ligaments of the knee joint. Anatomical, functional and experimental analysis. Clin Orthop 106: 216-231

Hackenbruch W, Henche HR (1981) Diagnostik und Therapie von Kapselbandläsionen am Kniegelenk. Eular, Basel

Hackenbruch W, Schmiebusch H (1985) Arthroskopische Kontrollen und elektronenmikroskopische Untersuchungen nach vorderer Kreuzbandrekonstruktion. Z Orthop 123: 601

Hertel P (1980) Verletzung und Spannung von Kniebändern. Hefte Unfallheilkd 142: 1-94

Menschik A (1974) Mechanik des Kniegelenkes, Teil 1. Z Orthop 112: 481-495

Müller We (1983) The knee. Form, function and ligament reconstruction. Springer, Berlin Heidelberg New York Tokyo

Müller We (1987) Kniegelenk: normale und pathologische Mechanik. In: Witt AN, Rettig H, Schlegel KF (Hrsg) Orthopädie in Praxis und Klinik. Thieme, Stuttgart, S 7

Noyes FR, Grood ES (1976) The strength of the anterior cruciate ligament in humans and rhesus monkeys. Age related and species related changes. J Bone Joint Surg [Am] 58: 1074-1082

Odensten M, Gillquist J (1984) Functional anatomy in anterior cruciate ligament surgery. J Bone Joint Surg [Am]: 67: 257-262

Rovere GD, Adair DM (1983) Anterior cruciate-deficient knees: A review of the literature. Am J Sports Med 6: 412-419

Wagner M, Schabus R (1982) Funktionelle Anatomie des Kniegelenkes. Springer, Berlin Heidelberg New York

OAK Knee Documentation and Evaluation

OAK Knee Evaluation: A New Way to Assess Knee Ligament Injuries

We. Müller, R. Biedert, F. Hefti, R. P. Jakob, U. Munzinger, and H.-U. Stäubli

In the past, attempts were made to facilitate the understanding of knee instabilities using a system of clinical examination and a description of classifications. Different emphasis was put on the relation of the detected abnormal femorotibial motion and the corresponding structural damage. Hughston et al. (1976) worked on a classification system in which the posterior cruciate ligament (PCL) was the rotational center of the knee. If the PCL was ruptured, straight instability had occurred; if the PCL was intact, rotational instability had occurred. In working with this system over the past 10 years, the authors have learned that not every case can be attributed arbitrarily to one of the three groups.

In 1980 Hertel showed that even after cutting the anterior cruciate ligament (ACL) alone, the axis of rotation left the center of the knee. It became located more peripherally and did not coincide any more with the PCL. This implied that the resulting abnormal knee motion was a combined rotation and translation.

There is, however, no doubt that the main merit of the Hughston et al. classification was the stimulation of compartmental understanding of combined instabilities (anteromedial, anterolateral, posterolateral rotation instability). Assessment of knee instability implies assessment of the corresponding structural deficits. Methods of treatment would not be based on symptoms alone, but on a direct reconstruction of the injured ligaments.

In Europe during the 1970s, Trillat et al. (1978) from Lyon, France, presented cadaver experiments to study abnormal knee motion. These sequential ligament-cutting studies led to the production of a film by Noesberger and Paillot (1976) measuring increased abnormal knee motion according to various combinations of structural defects (Fig. 1). Since then, there have been many papers describing sequential cutting studies in cadaver knees and demonstrating specific types of instabilities (e. g., Kennedy and Fowler 1971; Trickey 1984 a, b; Hertel 1980; Jakob et al. 1981 a; Fabbricciani et al. 1982; Noyes et al. 1983).

The idea for developing a new system to document and classify knee instabilities gradually evolved from

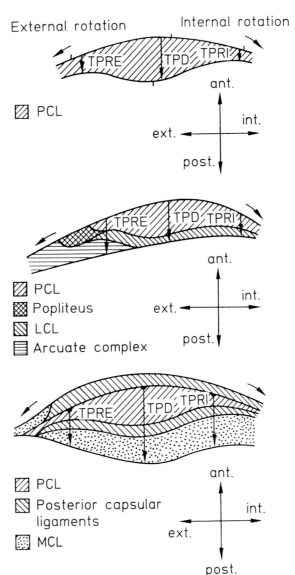

Fig. 1. Increasing posterior instability depending on the number of divided ligaments. *TPRE*, posterior drawer in external rotation; *TPD*, posterior drawer in neutral position; *TPRI*, posterior drawer in internal rotation. *Top*, isolated division of PCL *(LCP)*. *Middle*, Sequential division of PCL, popliteus, lateral collateral *(LLE)*, and arcuate ligaments. *Bottom*, Sequential division of PCL, posterior capsular ligament (lig. caps. post.), and medial collateral ligament *(LLI)*. (Drawing by J. M. Paillot, from Chambat 1978)

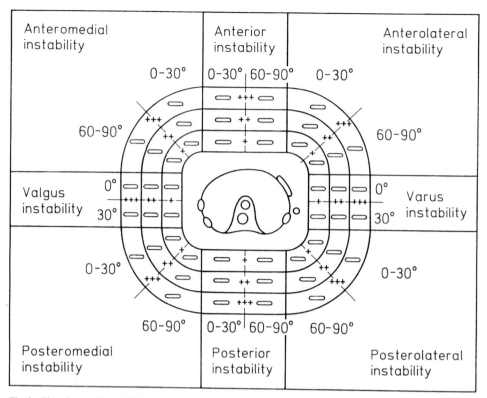

Fig. 2. First form of the Müller diagram. The various instabilities were tested and registered in the Lachmann position and in flexion

the basic work contributed by the OAK group. In 1978 the various types of knee instabilities were registered visually on a documentation sheet. In 1982 the first schematic format was presented at an OAK meeting by Müller (Fig. 2). This format was based on the "shells" concept of instability. In 1985 the two senior authors refined the system to be released for investigatory purposes among the members of the OAK group. Figure 3 represents the 2-year practical experience of the OAK group after analyzing and refining the data sheet continuously (Figs. 3, 4). The exchange of thoughts with other groups confirmed the group's ideas.

Generally accepted kinematic and biomechanical models of normal and abnormal knee motion are prerequisites to perceive the underlying pathology. Suntay et al. (1983) have shown that a system with six degrees of freedom can be applied to the knee joint to describe specific knee motion patterns. There are basically three rotational and three translational axes of the knee joint. The three rotational axes are extension/flexion, internal/external rotation, and varus/valgus angulation. The three translational axes are anterior/posterior, medial/lateral, and distraction/compression (telescoping).

Measurements of pathological motion such as the extent of subluxation can be described in millimeters of translation or in symbols of + (3–5 mm), + + (6–10 mm), + + + (10–15 mm), or more (more than 16 mm). Theoretically they can also be described as degrees of rotation. Because there is no pure rotational or pure translational motion, the authors have agreed to express themselves in a compromise of millimeters of translation as observed on a lateral stress roentgenogram. For example, a maximal anterior drawer of the tibia will produce a combination of an anterior translation and a few degrees of internal rotation.

The goal of the measurements is to register the greatest possible motion between the tibia and the femur. As translation and rotation are always occurring as coupled motions, clinical tests should take place in an unconstrained manner. The examiner should guide the knee on the path of its greatest laxity to assess the limit of the envelope of motion (Noyes et al. 1983). It is self-evident that such a system has evolved from earlier thinking, in which a given clinical test was meant to detect one injured ligament. Because of the complexity of the capsuloligamentous apparatus, the detection of the envelope of motion will comprise

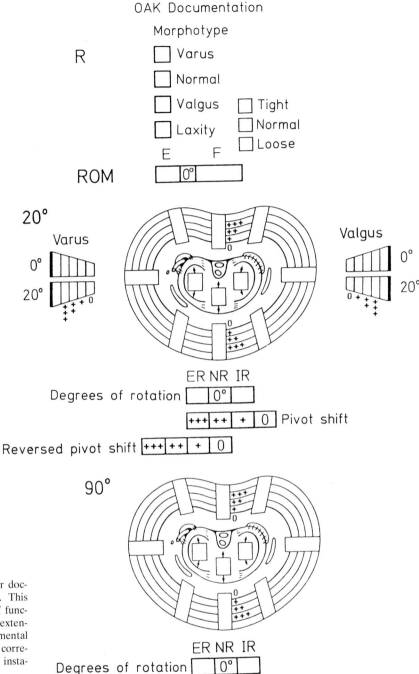

Fig. 3a,b. The OAK diagrams for documentation of knee instabilities. This format represents the synopsis of functional knee stability testing near extension and near flexion. Compartmental displacements are visualized in the corresponding squares of the shell of instability. **a** Right knee. **b** see p. 126

damage to primary and secondary restraints, mainly in chronic instabilities (Noyes et al. 1983).

Under the dynamic tests (true and reversed pivot shift), the pattern of motion occurs so quickly that detection of the maximal extent of translation and rotation is difficult. Here, uncoupling this motion can be useful to measure and grade the intensity of dynamic phenomena. This information can also be gained for therapeutic implications (Jakob et al. 1981b).

In the practical example, the maximal unconstrained anterior and posterior displacement of each compartment (including the midline area of the tuberosity) is estimated and recorded in millimeters or plus symbols. For manual proprioceptive training and teaching, an artificial knee joint simulator in the Lachmann position (between 0° and 15° of knee flexion) has been introduced.

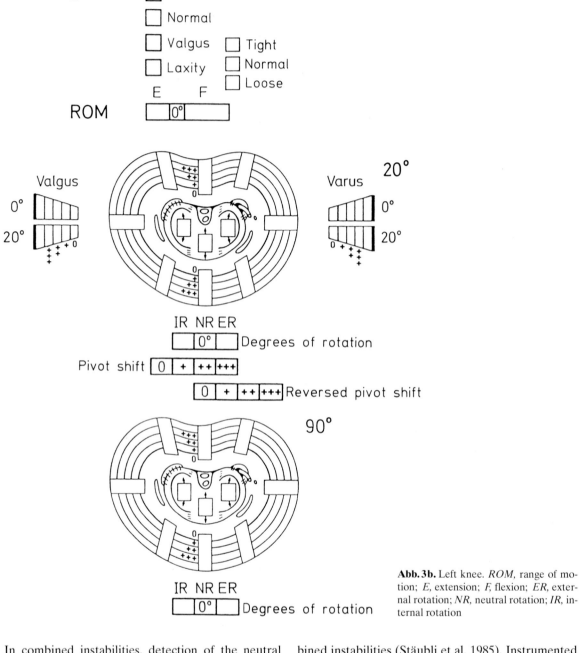

OAK Documentation

Morphotype

L
☐ Varus
☐ Normal
☐ Valgus   ☐ Tight
☐ Laxity   ☐ Normal
                      ☐ Loose

                E   F
ROM   [|0°|]

Valgus   Varus   **20°**
0°   0°
20°   20°

                    IR NR ER
                [|0°|] Degrees of rotation

Pivot shift [0 | + |++|+++]

                    [0 | + |++|+++] Reversed pivot shift

                    90°

                    IR NR ER
                [|0°|] Degrees of rotation

Abb. 3b. Left knee. *ROM*, range of motion; *E*, extension; *F*, flexion; *ER*, external rotation; *NR*, neutral rotation; *IR*, internal rotation

In combined instabilities, detection of the neutral point between anterior and posterior displacement is extremely difficult if not impossible. The square fields in the center of the knee diagram are marked in such instances to register the maximal anteroposterior motion (Figs. 3, 4). A possible solution to overcome this difficulty is offered by the technique of stress roentgenography, a technique that the authors use routinely in clinical work-ups to evaluate combined instabilities (Stäubli et al. 1985). Instrumented techniques have been evaluated by some of the authors, but they have not given the same consistency of results as accurate clinical measurement and stress roentgenography.

Once all the data have been collected, the instability can be classified. Here, the system of compartmental displacement described by Hughston et al. (1976) and recommended by the American Orthopedic Society

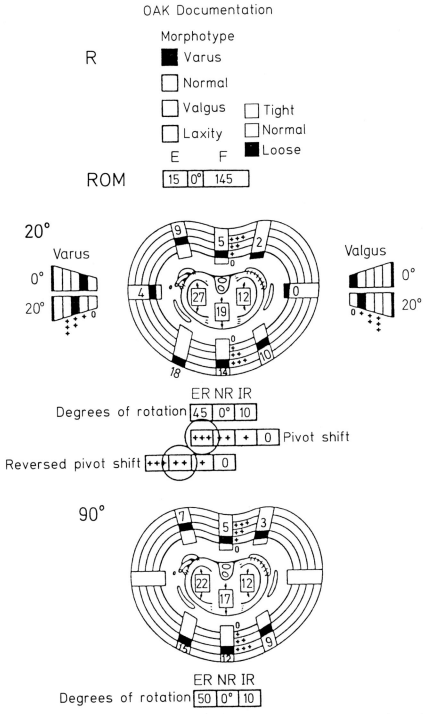

Fig. 4a. Documentation of a chronic ACL-deficient knee. The morphotype is a varus alignment with increased constitutional laxity. The passive range of motion measures 15°–0°–145° for extension/flexion. There is a varus opening in extension coded + in the corresponding square at 0° measuring + + in 20°. There is no valgus opening in extension but a + medial opening in 20° of flexion marked in the corresponding square of the medial bar. The measured anterior and posterior displacements of the medial and the lateral tibial plateaus are marked in the corresponding squares at 20° and 90° of flexion. The average anterior displacement measures 14 mm near extension and 12 mm near flexion. The mean posterior displacement measures 5 mm near extension and near flexion. The total sagittal displacement measures 19 mm in extension and 17 mm in flexion. The 4-mm lateral translation during valgus stress testing is marked in the corresponding square. The degrees of femorotibial rotation are marked near extension and near flexion. The dynamic signs, i.e., the pivot shift and the reversed pivot shift, are then graded according to their severity. **b** See p. 128

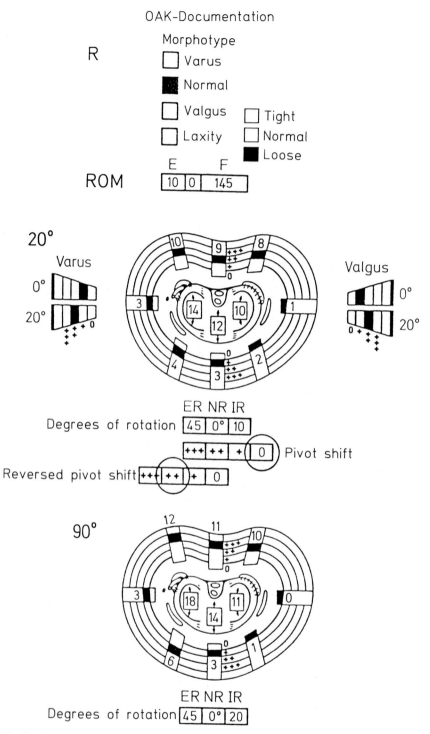

Fig. 4b. Documentation of a chronic PCL-deficient knee. There is a normal standing alignment in the frontal plane with normal laxity. There is a varus opening of + in extension and of + + in 20° of flexion. The posterior displacement of the lateral tibial plateau measures 10 mm near extension and 12 mm near flexion. The posterior displacement of the medial tibial plateau measures 8 mm near extension and 10 mm near flexion. There is a 3-mm lateral translation during stress valgus testing. The femorotibial rotation measures 45°–0°–10° near extension and 45°–0°–20° near flexion. The pivot shift is negative. The reversed pivot shift is graded + +, reflecting a posterolateral structural deficit

for Sports Medicine (AOSSM) is helpful (antero-medial/anterolateral, posterolateral/posteromedial). Because a marked anterolateral instability is always connected with an anteromedial instability, the term "global anterior instability" is used. Posterior in-stability is most marked in neutral and/or external rotation of the tibia and is then determined as "posterior/posterolateral" with the posteromedial component being discrete.

An accurate clinical assessment and analysis of the functional deficit is of high diagnostic value. The di-agnostic synthesis aims at the determination of struc-tural deficits and lost primary and secondary re-straints.

One of the goals of clinicians and biomechanists is to analyze the material from the literature and develop a generally accepted syllabus. Only when this is com-pleted will the clinician be fully equipped to apply reconstructive surgical techniques according to sound biomechanical principles.

Methods

Assessment of Constitutional Laxity

Prior to assessing functional knee stability, the degree of constitutional joint laxity has to be evaluated. Clinical signs of multidirectional shoulder laxity, ap-parent cubitus valgus with hyperextension of the elbow joint, radiocarpal laxity of the wrist joint, sagit-tal laxity of the metacarpophalangeal joint of the thumb, and increased dorsiflexion of the metacarpo-phalangeal joint of the index finger are tested in the upper extremity.

Hyperextension and hyperflexion of the knee joint, increased anteroposterior laxity in the sagittal plane with discrete ACL and PCL endpoints, as well as in-creased external and internal tibial rotation are char-acteristic signs of increased constitutional laxity of the knee joint. Frequently a hypermobile, high-riding patella is associated with increased constitutional knee joint laxity. The constitutional laxity is coded as tight, normal, or loose (Fig.3).

Analysis of the Morphotype

The morphotype is evaluated in the one-leg standing position in the frontal plane for varus or valgus, in the sagittal plane for recurvatum or antecurvatum, and in the horizontal plane for internal or external femoral and tibial torsion.

Coding the Passive Range of Motion

Passive knee motion (extension/flexion axis) is coded according to Debrunner (1982) and Russe et al. (1972). The neutral position in the sagittal plane in regard to the flexion/extension axis is the position of the anatomic standing alignment of the femur and of the tibia. While describing passive knee motion, the degree of hyperextension is coded first. Then the passive knee motion reaches the neutral or zero posi-tion at zero degrees of flexion. In a normal individual, the passive physiological range of motion measures an average of 10° of hyperextension and 145° of flex-ion. This passive range of motion is coded as follows: extension–neutral–flexion, i.e., 10–0–145 (Fig.5a).

Coding an Extension Deficit

If there is an extension deficit, the zero position is not reached. An extension deficit measuring 10° com-pared with the neutral position is coded as follows: extension–neutral–flexion: involved knee (0–10–145)/noninvolved knee (10–0–145). This represents 20° of extension loss compared with the normal side.

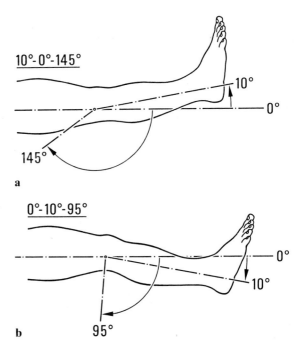

Fig.5a,b. Passive range of motion: knee extension/flexion axis. Knee flexion documented using the Debrunner (1987) conven-tion (neutral–zero method). **a** Normal passive range of motion. **b** Coding an extension and flexion deficit

Coding a Combined Extension and Flexion Deficit

If there is a combined extension deficit measuring 10° in respect to the neutral position and a flexion deficit of 50°, the passive range of motion is coded as follows: extension–neutral–flexion: involved knee (0–10–95)/noninvolved knee (10–0–145). Compared with the noninvolved knee, there are 20° of extension loss and 50° of flexion loss (Fig. 5 b).

Coding the Passive Range of Rotation

The neutral position in regard to the internal/external tibial rotational axis in the horizontal plane represents the unconstrained position of the tibia in respect to the femur. The degrees of internal and external tibiofemoral rotation depend upon the flexion angle at which passive internal and external tibial rotation are measured. In the fully extended (hyperextended) position, there is no tibial rotation. With an increasing flexion angle, a passive range of internal/external tibiofemoral rotation with discrete or altered endpoints is measured. This passive external/external tibial rotation is coded as follows: internal/external rotation 15–0–35 at 20° and 20–0–45 at 70° of knee flexion (Figs. 3, 4, 6).

Coding an Increase of Tibial Rotation

At 10° increase of external tibial rotation at 20° of knee flexion is coded as follows: internal–neutral–external rotation 15–0–55 involved and 15–0–35 noninvolved.

Coding a Decrease of Internal Rotation

Five degrees of decreased internal rotation and 20° of decreased external tibial rotation are coded as follows: internal/external rotation 10–0–25 involved and 15–0–45 noninvolved.

Clinical Assessment of Functional Knee Stability

The functional stability of the knee joint is the result of active and passive forces controlling knee motion under physiological loading conditions. This functional stability is provided by the threedimensional geometry of the articulating surfaces, by the passive restraining forces of the ligaments and meniscocapsular structures, and by the active forces of the musculotendinous units.

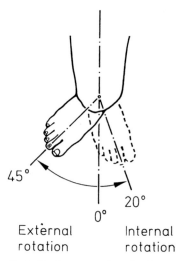

Fig. 6. Passive range of motion: knee external/internal rotation axis

Constrained or Nonconstrained Functional Assessment of Knee Stability

Basically two kinds of clinical tests can be applied to a knee joint, i.e., a constrained or a nonconstrained test. In a constrained test, the knee is held in a specific position, i.e., the knee flexion angle and the femorotibial rotational angle are defined. In a nonconstrained test, combined moments are applied to a knee joint in a given position to enhance the development of a combined abnormal knee motion, consisting of combined compartmental displacements. The degree of abnormal knee motion depends upon constitutional laxity factors, test conditions, magnitude and direction of applied forces, and severity of structural defects resulting from a given injury.

Assessment of Functional Knee Stability: The Structural Approach. In an injured knee joint, the functional assessment of a structural deficit is a major problem. According to the three translational and three rotational axes of the knee joint, specific reproducible clinical tests have to be performed. These clinical tests represent force couples applied to an individual knee joint in a well-defined test position. Ideally a single specific clinical test should reproduce the abnormal knee motion resulting from an isolated ligamentous injury. Although this concept might be true in an experimental set-up of restrained measurements or in progressive cutting studies, it must be questioned when an examiner is confronted with an acute or chronic knee injury.

Functional Assessment of Knee Stability in the Frontal Plane. Straight varus–valgus laxity stress tests are performed in 0° of knee flexion (i.e., in extension) with the tibia constrained in neutral rotation. These constrained varus and valgus laxity tests in extension are supplemented by varus and valgus stress tests in 20° of knee flexion with the tibia constrained in neutral rotation. In the same position varus and valgus stress tests are then performed with a few degrees of unconstrained external and internal tibial rotation.

Injuries of the Tibial Collateral Ligament and of the Medial Part of the Meniscocapsular Structures. Generally, isolated complete ruptures of the tibial collateral ligament are rare. An abduction/external rotational injury, for instance, may lead to a functional deficit of the tibial collateral ligament (TCL) of the posterior oblique ligament (POL) and of the deep medial meniscocapsular structures. The resulting abnormal knee motion is a coupled abduction, lateral translation, and increased rotation of the tibia in respect to the femur if an unconstrained abduction stress is applied to the tibia in 20° of knee flexion. The examining conditions in this specific injury pattern should include the best isolated test to document a specific structural defect: either (1) a valgus stress test in 20° of knee flexion and neutral rotation of the tibia to test for a tibial collateral ligament insufficiency, or (2) a valgus stress test in 20° of knee flexion and a few degrees of external rotation of the tibia to test the integrity of the tibial collateral ligament and of the middle one third of the medial meniscocapsular ligament and a valgus stress test in 20° of knee flexion and few degrees of internal rotation of the tibia to test the integrity of the tibial collateral ligament and of the posterior oblique ligament.

Injuries of the Fibular Collateral Ligament and of the Arcuate Ligament Complex. To diagnose a lateral ligamentous defect, an adduction or varus stress test in 0° and 20° of knee flexion is performed. In the varus stress test at 20° of knee flexion and neutral rotation of the tibia, the fibular collateral ligament is tested. In the varus stress test with a few degrees of external rotation of the tibia, the fibular collateral ligament, the middle third of the lateral capsular ligament, and the tendoaponeurotic fibrous connections of the popliteus tendon unit are tested. The varus stress test in 20° of knee flexion and internal rotation of the tibia is testing the arcuate ligament complex, the middle third of the lateral capsule, and the iliotibial tract as well as parts of the tendoaponeurotic portions of the popliteus tendon. An increase in external rotation in 20° of knee flexion is diagnostic of a functional deficit of the arcuate ligament complex.

Medial and Lateral Tibial Translation. In severe chronic instabilities, medial or lateral tibial translations can be observed. These translations can be estimated by palpation of the lateral or medial step-off during valgus and varus stress testing. The estimated values in millimeters or + symbols are now registered in the corresponding squares of the OAK documentation format (Figs. 3, 4).

Functional Assessment of Knee Stability in the Sagittal Plane. Comparing the injured with the noninjured knee, the increased abnormal knee motion in the sagittal plane is assessed near extension, i.e. between 0° and 20° of knee flexion, and near knee flexion, i.e., between 70° and 90° of knee flexion. As for the sagittal stability, anteroposterior compartmental displacements are assessed in millimeters. Thus a grading system measuring medial and lateral compartmental anteroposterior displacements is used.

Abnormal Anterior Knee Motion

Prior to performing any instability test, it is critical to note the presence of a posterior sag sign in flexion and near extension. If the posterior sag sign is not appreciated before the different drawer tests are performed, a false-positive anterior drawer test is misinterpreted as an ACL injury.

Clinical Tests to Diagnose Anterior Subluxation

Let us now consider the clinical assessment of abnormal anterior knee motion patterns resulting from a partial to a complete ACL insufficiency with concomitant medial and lateral meniscocapsular injuries.

When testing for a functionally competent ACL in the Lachmann position (i.e., between 0° and 15° of knee flexion), an anterior force is applied to the proximal tibia. The resulting physiological joint play near extension consists of a minimal coupled anterior translation and internal rotation of the tibia in respect to the femur. This coupled motion is increased in a partial ACL tear. A small amount of increased anterior translation of the medial tibial plateau can be palpated. The predominant increase of motion, however, is an anterior displacement of the lateral tibial plateau, resulting in increased combined anterior translation and internal rotation of the tibia.

In a complete intraligamentous ACL rupture, an increase of the anterior translation of both the medial and the lateral tibial plateaus can be assessed visually or by manual proprioception. The most important clinical test to detect this isolated ACL lesion is the Lachman test, e.g., the anterior drawer test in extension and in a few degrees of internal rotation of the tibia. The corresponding dynamic sign to detect this isolated functional deficit of the ACL is a trace positive pivot shift in internal rotation (grade I pivot shift). If there is an additional medial and posteromedial injury, the anterior translation of the medial tibial plateau will increase proportionally to the severity of the structural deficit, whereas the anterior displacement of the lateral tibial plateau will still exceed the one of the medial compartment according to the concomitant structural deficit of the iliotibial tract and of the arcuate ligament complex. The resulting abnormal knee motion is a significant combined anterior translation and internal rotation of the tibia. The clinical tests detecting this combined abnormal anterior knee motions are the Lachman test measuring + +, the anterior drawer test near flexion measuring + +, and a positive pivot shift in neutral rotation (pivot shift grade II). With severe or chronic global anterior subluxation, the resulting abnormal knee motion is a severe combined anterior translation and internal rotation of the tibia. The clinical signs describing this severe abnormal anterior knee motion are a + + + Lachman sign, a + + + anterior drawer, and a positive pivot shift in external rotation (grade III pivot shift) (Jakob et al. 1981b).

If there is an additional severe posterolateral capsular injury with a functional deficit of the popliteus tendon, a marked combined anterolateral/anteromedial and posterolateral displacement will be elicited. The clinical tests to detect these abnormal motion patterns are a positive pivot shift in external rotation (pivot shift grade III) and a reversed pivot shift (grade II). In addition, there is an increased passive external rotation in 20° of knee flexion (Fig. 4a; Jakob et al. 1981a).

Abnormal Posterior Knee Motion

Because of gravity a posterior sag sign near flexion and near extension may be present in a relaxed individual.

Clinical Tests to Diagnose Posterior Subluxation

If an anteroposterior (AP) force is applied to a stable knee with an intact PCL, there is a coupled posterior translation and external rotation of the tibia in respect to the femur. The amount of this physiological joint play depends on the magnitude of the applied AP force (the greater the AP force, the greater the resulting posterior displacement), the morphotype, and the constitutional laxity.

In a partial tear of the PCL there is an increased compartmental posterior displacement when the knee is tested in 20° of knee flexion. With a complete isolated PCL rupture there is a marked combined posterior displacement of the medial and lateral tibial plateaus. A combined injury of the PCL and of the posteromedial structures will result in a combined posterior translation and internal rotation of the tibia. The increased posteromedial displacement of the medial plateau can be palpated anteriorly by a loss of the step-off between the anterior margin of the medial femoral condyle and the anterior margin of the medial tibial plateau. The clinical tests to detect a complete PCL tear are (1) the posterior sag sign in 20° and 70° of flexion with the active reduction of posterior tibial subluxation and (2) a posterior drawer near extension and in 70° of flexion with an altered posterior end point.

In a PCL rupture with an additional significant posterolateral meniscocapsular injury, the resulting abnormal knee motion is a combination of a posterior translation and of an increased external rotation of the lateral tibial plateau. Visually or by palpation an increased loss of the physiological step-off between the anterior margin of the lateral femoral condyle and the anterior margin of the lateral tibial plateau is detectable.

The dynamic phenomenon to detect posterior/posterolateral instability is demonstrated with the reversed pivot shift sign. The reversed pivot shift sign is graded as + in the constitutionally lax individual. It is graded as + + with a moderate and as + + + with a marked posterolateral subluxation (Fig. 4b).

All the estimated values of sagittal instability are registered in the corresponding squares of the OAK format (Figs. 3, 4).

The synopsis of all the clinical data representing the sum of all structural defects is then documented schematically on the OAK functional knee stability format (Figs. 4).

References

Chambat P (1978) Les ruptures isolées du L.C.P. In: Trillat A, Dejour H, Bousquet G (éds) Chirurgie du Genou, 3èmes Journées Lyon, Septembre 1977. Simep, Villeurbanne, p 47

Debrunner HU (1982) Orthopädisches Diagnostikum. Thieme, Stuttgart

Fabbriciani C, Oransky M, Zoppi U (1982) Il muscolo popliteo: Studio anatomico. Arch Ital Anat Embryol 87: 203

Hefti F, Gächter A, Jenny H, Morscher E (1982) Replacement of the anterior cruciate ligament. A comparative study of four different methods of reconstruction. Arch Orthop Trauma Surg 100: 83

Hertel P (1980) Verletzungen und Spannung von Kniebändern. Hefte Unfallheilkd 142: 1–94

Hughston JC, Andrews JR, Cross MJ, Moschi A (1976) Classification of knee ligament instabilities. Part I. The medial compartment and cruciate ligaments. J Bone Joint Surg [Am] 58: 159

Jakob RP, Hassler H, Stäubli HU (1981 a) Observations on rotatory instability of the lateral compartment of the knee: Experimental studies on the functional anatomy and the pathomechanism of the true and the reversed pivot shift sign. Acta Orthop Scand 52: 191

Jakob RP, Stäubli HU, Deland JT (1981 b) Grading the pivot shift. Objective test with implications for treatment. J Bone Joint Surg [Br] 69: 294

Kennedy JC, Fowler RJ (1971) Medial and anterior instability of the knee. J Bone Joint Surg [Am] 53: 1257

Lukianov AV, Gillquist J, Grana WA, DeHaven KE (1987) An anterior cruciate ligament (ACL) evaluation format for assessment of artificial or autologous anterior cruciate reconstruction results. Clin Orthop 218: 167

Lysholm J, Gillquist J (1982) Evaluation of the knee ligament surgery results with emphasis on use of a scoring scale. Am J Sports Med 10: 150

Marshall JL, Fetto JF, Botero PM (1977) Knee ligament injuries. A standardized evaluation method. Clin Orthop 123: 115

Müller We (1982) Das Knie. Springer, Berlin Heidelberg New York

Müller We, Biedert R, Hefti F, Jakob RP, Münzinger U, Stäubli HU (1988) OAK Knee evaluation. A new way to assess knee ligament injuries. Clim Orthop 232: 37–50

Noesberger B, Paillot JM (1976) Biomécanique du genou (film). Springer, Berlin Heidelberg New York

Noyes FR, Grood ES, Suntay WJ, Butler DL (1983) The three dimensional laxity of the anterior cruciate deficient knee as determined by clinical laxity tests. Iowa Orthop J 3: 32

Russe O, Gerhardt Y, King P (1972) An atlas of examination. Standard measurements and documentation in orthopedics and traumatology. Huber, Bern

Stäubli HU, Jakob RP, Noesberger B (1985) Anterior-posterior knee instability and stress radiography. A prospective biomechanical analysis with the knee in extension. In: Perren SM, Schneider E (eds) Biomechanics. Current interdisciplinary research. Nijhoff, The Hague, pp 397–402

Suntay WJ, Grood ES, Butler DL, Noyes FR (1983) Error analysis of a system for measuring three-dimensional motion. ASME Transactions J Biomech Eng 105: 127

Tegner Y, Lysholm J (1985) Rating systems in the evaluation of knee ligament injuries. Clin Orthop 198: 43

Trickey EL (1984a) Acute ligamentous injuries. In: Jackson JP, Waugh W (eds) Surgery of the knee-joint. Chapman & Hall, London, pp 151

Trickey EL (1984b) Chronic ligamentous injuries. In: Jackson JP, Waugh W (eds) Surgery of the knee-joint. Chapman & Hall, London, pp 172–191

Trillat A, Dejour H, Bousquet G (éds) (1978) Chirurgie du genou. 3èmes Journées Lyon, Septembre 1977. Simép, Villeurbanne

Evaluation of Knee Ligament Injuries: The OAK and IKDC Forms

F. Hefti, T. Drobny, W. Hackenbruch, W. C. Kipfer, P. Holzach, R. P. Jakob, We. Müller, and H.-U. Stäubli

The Swiss Orthopedic Knee Study Group (Ortho-paedische Arbeitsgruppe Knie = OAK) decided in 1984 to develop a prospective evaluation sheet for the clinical assessment of acute and chronic knee in-stabilities. A small group of junior members was formed to undertake this task.

Prerequisites

The group first defined the features of an "ideal" evaluation and documentation system:

- It should cover all relevant findings.
- It should allow objective documentation.
- Evaluation should not be arbitrary.
- A good result cannot be simulated by adding up points for findings that have nothing to do with the patient's knee problem.
- The patient's knee problem should be apparent from an evaluation of the findings.
- The patient's preinjury activity level should be taken into account.
- The form should be easy to fill out, without a long introduction.
- The form should brief (not more than one page) so that it will be convenient to use under practical conditions.
- The system should be computer-compatible.
- It should allow documentation on a broad basis so that the largest possible volume of statistically rele-vant data can be compiled.

It is naturally impossible to satisfy all these require-ments without making some compromises. There are two major problems that need to be addressed: the scope of the documentation form and the objectivity of the recorded findings.

The practical utility of an evaluation form is greatly influenced by its scope. One of the first evaluation systems for knee instabilities was developed by Mar-shall et al. (1977). Though short and easy to read, this form has some significant drawbacks, most notably the potential for awarding a relatively high numerical score to a knee that still has serious problems (e. g., an extension deficit). Thus, the Marshall system has tended to overrate results in studies where it was used (Hefti et al. 1982).

In 1982, Lysholm and Gillquist presented a new rating system. It was a modification of Larson's "rating-sheet for knee function." In this system a total of 100 points were given to a perfectly normal knee. Function was evaluated better than with the Marshall score. The drawback was, however, that the distribution of points for various items was arbitrary and the result was reported only as a total score that did not reveal the specific problem of the knee. It also did not solve the problem that a low score in only one area could be hidden in a satisfactory total score, even if the persisting problem in that area were sig-nificant.

In 1985 Tegner and Lysholm published a new activity grading scale where work and sports activities were graded numerically as a complement to the func-tional score. The various activities were graded in 11 levels, where the highest level (10) was "compete-titive sports – soccer in national elite" and the lowest level (0) was "sick leave or disability because of knee problems." The Tegner system of activity levels is widely used as an addition to knee rating systems for comparison between preinjury and postoperative ac-tivities.

Perhaps the most comprehensive documentation sys-tem was proposed by Lukianov et al. (1987). Fifteen pages in length, this system represents a synthesis of the known evaluation systems of Marshall et al. (1977) and Lysholm and Gillquist (1982). A similarly complex system is also used by Noyes in Cincinnati (Noyes et al. 1989, 1991). Though feasible in the US, a 15-page form would not be practical in Europe given the current infrastructure of our hospitals; we lack the full-time "clinical research fellows" that are available to US physicians. For this reason we have developed a convenient, concise, one-page form that is still comprehensive enough to satisfy most of the above requirements.

Another problem concerns the objective recording of findings. The evaluation of a knee instability depends very strongly on the subjective impression and personal experience of the examiner. Even the grading of an anteroposterior drawer as $+$ (< 5 mm), $++$ (5–10 mm), or $+++$ (> 10 mm) is subject to large individual variations. With some practice, however, the examiner can make reasonably precise and reproducible estimates of anteroposterior displacement that are accurate to within a few millimeters.

There are electronic instruments on the market that claim to enhance the precision of instability measurements, but they are not without problems. First, they are costly. Second, use of the instruments is time-consuming and poorly suited for routine work. Third, numerous errors can arise in the use of these very sensitive devices. It is even recommended that one person should be designated as the permanent operator of the device in order to obtain uniform, reliable measurements. Asides from these drawbacks, the devices can measure only pure anteroposterior displacement. End-point resilience, rotatory laxity, and lateral subluxation phenomena (pivot shifts) must still be assessed manually (Daniel et al. 1985; Edixhoven et al. 1989; Forster et al. 1989; Andersson and Gillquist 1990; Barber et al. 1990; Wroble et al. 1990).

The Genucom, a computer-controlled system for measuring knee instability, has been developed in Canada. While the manufacturer claims that the device can measure instability in all directions and positions of flexion, including pivot shifts, with very high accuracy, it remains to be seen how the system will perform in practice. Again, initial experience points to considerable "consumer"-dependent variations leading to an inconsistent reproduction of measured values. In any case, the cost of the system, at approximately US\$ 50 000, will prohibit its widespread use regardless of its quality. Like other devices, the Genucom must be operated by trained personnel, so an appropriate infrastructure would be required. This poses yet another obstacle to its general clinical use (McQuade et al. 1989).

For these reasons we have chosen not to prescribe instrumented measurements for our workup: the measurements may be clinical, instrumented or radiographic. Any method can be chosen, but it must be noted which method was applied.

The OAK Form

The OAK form, introduced in 1985, is used preoperatively to evaluate chronic instability (more than 4 weeks postinjury) and for recording postoperative results. It is not used preoperatively for fresh injuries. The form consists of one page divided into four sections:

1. Documentation
2. Determination of the activity level (three levels).
3. Scoring section with parameters for four problem areas (symptoms, range of motion, ligament examination and functional tests)
4. Evaluation section

This form introduced a new and comprehensive way of assessing the injured knee. The final result is not only based on a total score, but each problem area is evaluated separately. All items have the same score (5 points). For the evaluation of the four areas, the missing points are decisive. Thus each problem area has the same significance. An overall score of more than 90 points is rated "excellent," 81–90 points "good," 71–80 points "fair," and 70 points or less "poor." In each category, 0–4 missing points is rated "excellent," 5–9 missing points "good," 10–14 missing points "fair," and more than 14 missing points "poor." The overall result, however, cannot be better than the result in the poorest category. Thus, if for example the range of motion is only "fair," the overall result cannot be better than "fair" even if the total score would imply a "good" result.

The OAK knee ligament evaluation form is shown in Fig. 1 (Müller et al. 1988; Hefti et al. 1990). It has been widely used in German-speaking countries and in several follow-up studies. In 1991 Fink and Hoser compared the OAK scoring system with the Marshall and Lysholm scores. They stated that with the OAK score the average ratings of the patients were lower than with the two other systems, but that the OAK score provided more realistic results. Our own experience brought similar findings. The advantage of the OAK system certainly is that a poor result in one area cannot be hidden by a high average score in all the other areas.

The IKDC (International Knee Documentation Committee) Form

In 1987, an international group was founded by the chairman of the OAK group, Werner Müller, and John Feagin from the American Orthopedic Society of Sports Medicine (AOSSM) to set standards for terminology, documentation, and evaluation of knee ligament instabilities. The most prominent knee surgeons from America and Europe were invited to join the group. AOSSM and the European Society

CATEGORIES:

A = pain/swelling   B = ROM/strength
C = stability   D = function

POINTS (category):

CRITERION:	SCORE:	A	B	C	D	total

HISTORY:

pain	(5=no;3=rare;2=frequ.;0=severe)					
swelling	(5=no;3=rare;2=frequ.;0=always)					
gving way (true)	(5=no;3=rare;2=frequ.)					
work	(5=full;3=part.;1=change;0=unable)					
sports	(5=unlim.;3=limit.;1=maj.limit.;0=unable)					

GENERAL FINDINGS AT EXAMINATION:

effusion / swelling	(5=no;3=minim.;1=moder.;0=severe)					
tenderness	(5=no;3=minim.;1=moder.;0=severe)					
diff. circumfer. thigh	(5=no;3=2cm.;1=>2cm)					
extension deficit (passive)	(5=no;3=5°;1=10°;0=>10°)					
flexion (passive)	(5=free;3=>120°;1=>90°;0=<90°)					

INSTABILITY:

anterior drawer	(5=no;4=+;2=++;0=+++)					
posterior drawer	(5=no;4=+;2=++;0=+++)					
Lachman	(5=no;4=+;2=++;0=+++)					
lateral (in 30° flexion)	(5=no;4=+;2=++;0=+++)					
medial (in 30° flexion)	(5=no;4=+;2=++;0=+++)					
pivot shift	(5=no;3=uncertain.;0=pos.)					
reversed pivot shift	(5=neg.;0=pos.)					

FUNCTIONAL TESTS:

lateral hop on one leg	(5=free;3=difficult;1=not possible)					
kneeflexion on one leg	(5=free;3=difficult;1=not possible)					
duck-walking	(5=free;3=difficult;1=not possible)					

	A	B	C	D	total
I. MAXIMUM NUMBER OF POINTS IN EACH CATEGORY TOTAL	20	20	35	25	100
II. ACTUAL NUMBER OF POINTS IN EACH CATEGORY TOTAL (IIA+IIB+IIC+IID)					
III. MISSING POINTS IN EACH CATEGORY (IA–IIA;IB–IIB;IC–IIC;ID–IID)					

Fig. 1. Knee ligament evaluation form of the Swiss "Orthopaedische Arbeitsgruppe Knie" (OAK)

for Knee Surgery and Arthroscopy (ESKA). The group was named the International Knee Documentation Committee (IKDC). The current members of the group are: A. Anderson, W. G. Clancy, K. E. DeHaven, P. J. Fowler, J. Feagin, E. S. Grood, F. R. Noyes, G. Terry, P. Torzilli, R. F. Warren (AOSSM); P. Chambat, E. Eriksson, E. Gillquist, F. Hefti, R. Huiskes, R. Jakob, B. Moyen, We. Müller, H.-U. Stäubli, and A. VanKampen (ESKA). This group worked for 4 years on a standard evaluation form that should obtain international acceptance and should be the minimum requirement for any evaluation of results for publication.

The IKDC Knee Ligament Standard Evaluation Form (Fig. 2) is again a one-page form that includes a documentation section, a qualification section (see below), and a evaluation section. The basic principles of the OAK form are incorporated in this new form, but the four problems areas of the OAK form are supplemented by three additional areas. The form can be used pre- and postoperatively and at follow-up. The minimum follow-up time for short-term results has been defined as 2 years, for medium-term results 5 years, and for long-term results 10 years.

The documentation section is for recording the patient's name, birth date, record number, date of examination, examiner, date of injuries, date of surgery,

GROUPS (PROBLEM AREA)	QUALIFICATION WITHIN GROUPS				GROUP QUALIF.
	A: normal	B: nearly norm.	C: abnormal	D:sev. abnorm.	A B C D
1. PATIENT SUBJECTIVE ASSESSMENT					
How does your knee function?	normally	nearly norm.	abnormally	sev. abnorm.	
On a scale of 0 to 3 how does your knee affect your activity level?	0	1	2	3	▢▢▢▢
2. SYMPTOMS					
(absence of significant symptoms, at highest activity level known by patient)					
No pain at activity level	I	II	III	IV or worse	
No swelling at activity level	I	II	III	IV or worse	
No partial giving way at activity level	I	II	III	IV or worse	
No complete giving way at activity level	I	II	III	IV or worse	▢▢▢▢
3. RANGE OF MOTION					
Lack of extension (from zero anatomic)	<3°	3–5°	6–10°	>10°	
△ lack of flexion	0–5°	6–15°	16–25°	>25°	▢▢▢▢
4. LIGAMENT EXAMINATION		3 to 5mm or	6 to 10mm		
△ Lachman (in 25°. flex.)	–1 to 2mm	–1 to –3mm	or <–3mm	>10mm	
idem (alternative measurement, optional)	–1 to 2mm	3–5 /–1 to–3mm	6–10/<–3mm	>10mm	
Endpoint: firm soft					
△ total a.p.transl. in 70° flex.	0 to 2mm	3 to 5mm	6 to 10mm	>10mm	
idem (alternative measurement, optional)	0 to 2mm	3 to 5mm	6 to 10mm	>10mm	
△ post. sag in 70° flex.	0 to 2mm	3 to 5mm	6 to 10mm	>10mm	
△ med. joint opening (valgus rotation)	0 to 2mm	3 to 5mm	6 to 10mm	>10mm	
△ lat. joint opening (varus rotation)	0 to 2mm	3 to 5mm	6 to 10mm	>10mm	
Pivot shift	neg.	+ (glide)	++ (clunk)	+++ (gross)	
△ reversed pivot shift equal(neg.)	equal(pos.)	slight	marked	gross	▢▢▢▢
5. COMPARTMENTAL FINDINGS					
△Crepitus patellofemoral	none/equal	moderate	painful	severe	
△Crepitus medial compartment	none	moderate	painful	severe	
△Crepitus lateral compartment	none	moderate	painful	severe	
6. HARVEST SITE PATHOLOGY					
Tenderness, irritation, numbness	none	slight	moderate	severe	
7. X–RAY FINDINGS (DEGENERATIVE JOINT DISEASE)					
Patellofemoral cartilage space	normal	> 4mm	2–4mm	< 2mm	
Medial compartment cartilage space	normal	> 4mm	2–4mm	< 2mm	
Lateral compartment cartilage space	normal	> 4mm	2–4mm	< 2mm	
8. FUNCTIONAL TEST					
△One leg hop (percent of opposite side)	90–100%	76–90%	50–75%	<50%	
FINAL EVALUATION					▢▢▢▢

Fig. 2. Knee ligament evaluation form of the International Knee Documentation Committee (IKDC)

cause of injury, time interval from injury to surgery, side involved, type of examination (without or under anesthesia), diagnosis, surgical procedure, status of the menisci, and morphotype.

Next, the preinjury, pretreatment, and present activity levels have to be recorded. Four activity levels are defined: (I) jumping, pivoting, hard cutting, football, soccer; (II) heavy manual work, skiing, tennis; (III) light manual work, jogging, running; and (IV) sedentary work, activities of daily living.

The major part of the sheet includes the qualification section. It is called "qualification" section and not "scoring" section, because no scores are given, as figures for qualification are always arbitrary, especially if the maximum score varies for each item. Each parameter is qualified as "normal," "nearly normal," "abnormal," or "severely abnormal." This description is less subjective and emotional than "very good," "good," "fair," and "poor." No knee and no knee function can be better than normal, and it is rather doubtful whether any operated knee can ever be "normal" again.

The parameters are incorporated in eight problem areas. To the four areas of the original OAK form (symptoms, range of motion, ligament examination, and functional tests) have been added four more areas (subjective assessment, compartmental findings, harvest site pathology, and x-ray findings). These must be documented, although the evaluation is still based on four problem areas.

For subjective assessment the patient answers two questions: "How does your knee function?" This can be answered with "normally," "nearly normally," "abnormally," and "severely abnormally." The second question, "On a scale of 0 to 3, how does your knee affect your activity level?" the patients answers with a figure between 0 and 3. This answer should clarify whether the activity level has decreased for reasons not related to the knee.

Symptoms are closely related to one's activity level. The patient should be asked what is the highest activity level at which he could use his knee without having one of the specific symptoms (pain, swelling, or partial or complete giving way), even if he does not usually perform these activities. For example, if the patients answers that he could jump or cut or play soccer without pain, even if he usually does not do these things, he is qualified as "normal." This method of investigation should solve the problem that patients often do not have symptoms, because they avoid activities that could provoke them. On the other hand, some patients may have a normal knee, but as they have a low activity level, they might score poorly in other rating systems.

Clinical findings are evaluated in comparison with the (healthy) opposite side. In case of an abnormal opposite knee, the findings are compared with presumed normal values.

Range of motion is documented with the neutral–zero method. Three figures are filled in for flexion/zero-point/hyperextension. For example, 150° flexion, 10° hyperextension = 150/0/10; 150° flexion, full extension = 150/0/0; 150° flexion, 20° flexion contracture = 150/20/0. The lack of extension is qualified. In contrast to all other parameters, lack of extension is not compared to the opposite (healthy) side but to anatomic zero. The reason is that the members of the committee did not want to give a bad qualification to a knee that reaches zero extension but does not hyperextend abnormally (as the opposite knee). This point will, of course, be subject of further discussion. Lack of extension of more than 5° from anatomic zero is qualified as abnormal. Lack of flexion, on the other hand, is compared with the op-

posite side. A difference of more than 15° is qualified as abnormal.

Ligament examination includes anteroposterior translation tests in 25° and 70° flexion, posterior sag, medial and lateral joint opening, pivot shift, and reversed pivot shift. The anteroposterior translation tests can be carried out manually, as an instrumented examination (e. g., with KT-1000), or with x-rays. The quality of the endpoints should be marked. Any displacement (anteroposterior translation, posterior sag, or valgus/varus rotation) of more than 5 mm more than on the (healthy) opposite side is qualified as abnormal. In addition, a knee that demonstrates 3 mm or more less anteroposterior translation than the opposite (healthy) knee (i. e., that is too tight) is also qualified as abnormal. Also, for qualification as normal or nearly normal, both endpoints must be firm. The pivot shift test is normal if it is negative, nearly normal in the presence of a glide, abnormal when a clunk is found, and severly abnormal if the knee demonstrates gross shifting. The reversed pivot shift is normal if it is equal to that of the opposite knee (a healthy knee can also demonstrate a slight reversed pivot shift), abnormal in the presence of marked shift, and severely abnormal gross shifting occurs.

Compartmental findings are clinical signs of osteoarthritis. Crepitus should be palpated in the patellofemoral, medial, and lateral compartments. It is normal when absent, nearly normal when moderate, abnormal when painful, and severely abnormal when painful and audible.

Harvest site pathology must be documented if an autologous graft has been used. The qualifications are none, slight, moderate, and severe.

X-ray findings also address degenerative joint disease. The joint (cartilage) space is measured in the patellofemoral, medial, and lateral compartments. It is normal with a width of more than 4 mm. It is nearly normal when there are minimal changes (e. g., small osteophytes, slight sclerosis or flattening of the femoral condyle) without narrowing. It is abnormal with a width of 2–4 mm, and severely abnormal if it is less than 2 mm.

Only one functional test is included in the form: The one-leg hop test. The percentage of the score of the opposite side gives the qualification (90 % or more = normal, 76 %–90 % nearly normal, 50 %–75 % abnormal, less than 50 % severely abnormal).

The four problem areas subjective assessment, symptoms, range of motion, and ligament examination are evaluated for the group qualification. The worst qualification within the group gives the group qualification. The worst group qualification finally gives the final evaluation. If the knee is abnormal in any of the problem areas, it cannot be a normal knee. For chronic knees it is also possible to evaluate the sum of levels of improvement or deterioration of all groups compared with the preoperative evaluation. The problem areas compartmental findings, harvest site pathology, x-ray findings, and function must be documented. They do not affect the final qualification.

The IKDC form has passed the process of clinical testing. It is a short and concise form that is easy to fill in and can be ordered from the members of the committee. It represents the minimum standard for evaluation and documentation that is required for any publication of results of treatment of knee ligament injuries in qualified journals.

References

Andersson C, Gillquist J AD (1990) Instrumented testing for evaluation of sagittal knee laxity. Clin Orthop 256: 178–184

Barber SD, Noyes FR, Mangine RE, McCloskey JW, Hartman WAD (1990) Quantitative assessment of functional limitations in normal and anterior cruciate ligament deficient knees. Clin Orthop 255: 204–214

Daniel DM, Stone ML, Sachs R, Malcom L (1985) Instrumented measurement of anterior knee laxity in patients with acute anterior cruciate ligament disruption. Am J Sports Med 13: 401–407

Edixhoven P, Huiskes R, de Graaf R AD (1989) Anteroposterior drawer measurements in the knee using an instrumented test device. Clin Orthop 247: 232–242

Fink C, Hoser C (1991) Die Ruptur des vorderen Kreuzbandes. Eine Langzeituntersuchung operative versus konservative Therapie. Dissertation, Universitätsklinik für Unfallchirurgie der Universität Innsbruck

Forster IW, Warren Smith CD, Tew M AD (1989) Is the KT 1000 knee ligament arthrometer reliable? J Bone Joint Surg [Br] 71: 843–847

Hefti F, Gaechter A, Jenny H, Morscher E (1982) Replacement of the anterior cruciate ligament. A comparative study of four different methods of reconstruction. Arch Orthop Traumatol Surg 100: 83–94

Hefti F, Drobny T, Hackenbruch W, Kipfer W, Holzach P (1991) Dokumentation und Evaluation von Knieinstabilitäten. In: Jakob RP, Stäubli HU (eds) Kniegelenk und Kreuzbänder. Springer, Berlin Heidelberg New York, pp 138–144

Larson R (1972) Rating sheet for knee function. In: Smillie I (ed) Diseases of the knee joint. Churchill-Livingstone, Edinburgh, pp 29–30

Lukianov AV, Gillquist J, Grana WA, DeHaven K (1987) An anterior cruciate ligament (ACL) evaluation format for assessment of artificial or autologous anterior cruciate reconstruction results. Clin Orthop 218: 167–180

Lysholm J, Gillquist J (1982) Evaluation of knee ligament surgery results with special emphasis on use of a scoring scale. Am J Sports Med 10: 150–154

Marshall JF, Fetto JF, Botero PM (1977) Knee ligament injuries. A standardized evaluation method. Clin Orthop 123: 115–129

McQuade KJ, Sidles JA, Larson RV (1989) Reliability of the Genucom Knee Analysis System. A pilot study. Clin Orthop 245: 216–219

Müller W, Biedert R, Hefti F, Jakob RP, Munzinger U, Stäubli HU (1988) OAK knee evaluation. A new way to assess knee ligament injuries. Clin Orthop 232: 37–50

Noyes FR, Barber SD, Mooar LA AD (1989) A rationale for assessing sports activity levels and limitations in knee disorders. Clin Orthop 246: 238–249

Noyes FR, Mooar LA, Barber SD (1991) The assessment of work related activities and limitations in knee disorders. Am J Sports Med 19: 178–188

Tegner Y, Lysholm J (1985) Rating system in the evaluation of knee ligament injuries. Clin Orthop 198: 43–49

Wroble RR, Van Ginkel LA, Grood ES, Noyes FR, Shaffer BL (1990) Repeatability of the KT 1000 arthrometer in a normal population. Am J Sports Med 18: 396–399

Diagnosis, Pathomechanics, and Pathomorphology of Anterior Cruciate Ligament Insufficiency

Diagnosis of Acute Tears of the Anterior Cruciate Ligament, and the Clinical Features of Chronic Anterior Instability

B. Noesberger

In an acutely injured or chronically unstable knee, the correct diagnosis of anterior cruciate ligament (ACL) insufficiency is based on the mechanism of the injury as recalled by the patient, clinical stability testing, and diagnostic arthroscopy. The most commonly injured ligament of the knee joint is the ACL. Diagnosis is not a simple matter. Noyes et al. (1978) report that in 103 patients with chronic symptomatic anterior instability, the first examining physician correctly diagnosed a torn anterior cruciate ligament in only 7 cases – truly a disturbing statistic. The slightest suspicion of a torn anterior cruciate ligament should prompt us to exhaust all available means to establish a diagnosis within 1 week.

For surgeons who advocate the early treatment of certain types of tear, whether by direct repair or reconstruction, a rapid diagnosis is essential so that the optimum timing for surgical treatment is not missed. By 2 weeks postinjury, reparative processes are so far advanced that a delayed operation offers little chance of success. An accurate, correct diagnosis is equally important for surgeons who favor a conservative approach. It informs the patient and also motivates him to undergo intense rehabilitation and modify his activities. A laissez-faire attitude can have serious consequences (see chapter by Stäubli and Jakob, p. 237 ff.).

Mechanism of Injury

The causative mechanisms of anterior cruciate ligament injuries have been described by Palmer (1938), Abbot et al. (1944), and Kennedy et al. (1974). Perhaps the most common mechanism involves a combination of flexion, abduction, and external rotation. This produces a typical pattern of injury that O'Donoghue (1970) called the "unhappy triad": concomitant tears of the anterior cruciate ligament, joint capsule, and medial collateral ligament. Kennedy et al. (1974) found that a tear of the anterior cruciate ligament combined with other capsular and ligamentous ruptures could result from abduction and external rotation, hyperflexion, and from the clinically rare direct blow to the tibia from behind.

Our hospital serves an area in Switzerland that is known for its skiing resorts. Here we have noticed a change in the frequency, pattern, and mechanism of knee injuries during the past 3–4 years. We are seeing fewer tears of the ACL combined with injuries of the collateral ligaments. This is not to say that patients are consistently presenting with "isolated" ACL tears, for there is a relatively high incidence of associated injuries in the form of small medial or lateral meniscocapsular ruptures and/or chondral fractures. Benedetto et al. (1984) of Innsbruck, who probably saw a patient population similar to ours, found that only 28.4% of cases presenting clinically as an "isolated" ACL rupture actually had an isolated tear by arthroscopy. In 20.3% there was a coexisting meniscal tear, another 20% had a flake fracture, and 17% had both.

Woods and Chapman (1984) addressed the question of the frequency of reproducible posterior meniscocapsular tears accompanying a rupture of the ACL. Some 230 patients with a positive Lachman test were examined under general anesthesia and then by arthroscopy.

A medial and/or lateral posterior meniscocapsular tear was found in 27.7% of patients with an acute ACL rupture and in 29.5% of patients with chronic anterior instability.

The mechanisms producing an "isolated" rupture are diverse. In 1974 Kennedy et al. cited an internal twist of the tibia as a causative mechanism for an isolated ACL tear. This can occur, for example, when the skis become crossed during skiing. When the tibia rotates internally, tension is placed upon the ACL. If the internal rotational movement is abrupt and places the lateral meniscus on severe stretch, the meniscus may tear at its periphery. Marked anterolateral displacement of the tibia at this time can produce an accompanying rupture of the anterior third of the lateral capsule. If this part of the capsule is avulsed from the upper tibia with a flake of bone, then an AP radiograph of the knee will show the characteristic "Segond fragment" (Segond 1979) adjacent to the lateral tibial plateau, providing indirect evidence of an ACL tear.

If a skier is stopped abruptly due to the accidental tripping of a defective ski brake, the ACL can be actively ruptured by the sudden, massive contraction of the quadriceps. The same mechanism can occur when a ski racer "lies" on his skis while leaning back with the torso (Figueras et al. 1987). Again, the active quadriceps effort needed to restore the skier to an upright position can rupture the cruciate ligament. An extreme case occurred in a volleyball-playing gymnastics teacher who reported feeling a "pop" in her knee on jumping upward. We later confirmed an isolated rupture of the ACL at operation.

Radiographic Examination

Every freshly injured joint requires a minimum of 2 radiographic views on 2 planes to ensure the detection of concomitant injuries. The internal knee lesion may produce a hemarthrosis manifested radiographically by the appearance of a blood-fat layer. An avulsion fracture of the lateral capsule (Segond's fracture) signifies a possible lesion of the ACL, as does a bony avulsion of the intercondylar eminence.

Stressradiographs, while not necessary to assess medial joint space opening, still are often useful for scientific motion studies in the sagittal plane. In joints with coexisting anterior and posterior drawer laxity, stressradiographs help to determine the precise extent of the anterior and posterior displacement.

Medial joint opening greater than 4 mm signifies a rupture of the medial collateral ligament. A positive anterior drawer sign is declared if there is more than 3 mm of anterior displacement. Jacobsen (1977) found that pathologic joint opening as measured by stressradiography had a predictive value of 100% with regard to a torn medial collateral ligament, while pathologic anterior displacement had a 98% predictive value with regard to a rupture of the ACL. The predictive value of a negative drawer test was 96%. An ACL rupture may not produce a positive drawer sign if the synovial sack is intact or if tibial displacement is obstructed by an incarcerated bucket-handle fragment of meniscus. This blockage effect can even be demonstrated under anesthesia. Partial tears of the ACL, moreover, generally cannot be detected radiographically. It has been reported that an isolated tear of the anteromedial part of the ligament produces a mild instability in flexion, while damage to the posterolateral part renders the knee unstable near extension.

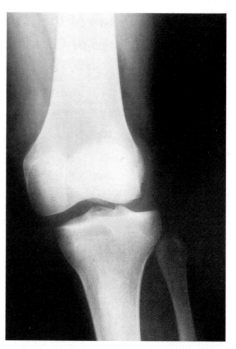

Fig. 1. Lateral displacement (lateral translation) of the tibia, even by a few millimeters, is possible only in a dislocated knee. This condition implies rupture of both cruciate ligaments and one collateral ligament along with the peripheral capsule

Nielson et al. (1984) found that partial division of the ACL produced no demonstrable instability aside from a slight increase of internal rotation in the flexed knee. We measured the drawer mobility of the slightly flexed knee joint in a prospective comparative study performed in 135 patients under peridural anesthesia (Stäubli et al. 1983b). In joints with a ruptured ACL, we measured a significant anterior displacement of the lateral condyle of 17.7 +/− 3.3 mm with respect to normal. An incarcerated bucket handle fragment reduced the anterior displacement by an average of 6 mm, even under anesthesia.

One diagnostic refinement is to check for lateral displacement of the tibia relative to the femur, even if it is only a few millimeters (Fig. 1). This lateral translation implies a rupture of the ACL as part of a knee dislocation. Figure 1 shows a slight lateral translation of the tibial plateau with a slight concomitant widening of the joint space. This type of motion is possible only if both cruciate ligaments and at least one collateral ligament are ruptured.

Neutral Position of the Knee Joint in the Sagittal Plane

The neutral position of a knee joint is clearly defined when the cruciate ligaments are functionally sound. But with any degree of anteroposterior instability, identification of the neutral position is not easy. In a knee with posterior instability, for example, even an experienced examiner will have difficulty detecting an anterior drawer by clinical examination alone. With the knee flexed 90°, the tibia will sag posteriorly under its own weight when posterior instability is present. When the tibia is pulled forward, it will travel an abnormally long distance from the posterior to the anterior drawer position. Drawing on the work of Jacobsen (1976), we devised a modified radiographic measuring technique (Fig. 2) in which neutral tibial rotation is defined as the neutral or starting position. The angle of knee flexion is immaterial. The reference points are the most posterior points on both tibial condyles and the corresponding femoral condyles. A line is drawn through these points parallel to the axis of the tibial shaft. In the normal, stable knee, both points should lie on the same line. But if pathologic drawer displacement is present, the lines will be separated by a measurable distance. The distance from the back of the tibial plateau to the line through the posterior border of the femoral condyles is measured. This can be done using the same criteria as in the Lachman test. Stäubli has refined the technique by performing separate measurements for the lateral and medial femoral condyles and the lateral and medial tibial plateaus, which are distinguished by their size and shape (Fig. 3). This makes it possible to determine the separate amounts of displacement in the medial and lateral compartments. Typical distinguishing features on the femur are its "limiting groove," the greater sagittal diameter and the larger radius of the posterior portion of the lateral condyle.

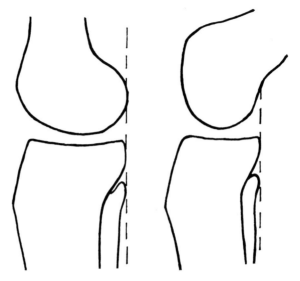

Fig. 2. The reference points for the radiographic measurement of drawer displacement are the most posterior borders of the tibial condyles and corresponding femoral condyles. In a stable knee that is neutrally positioned, a line through the points runs parallel to the axis of the tibial shaft

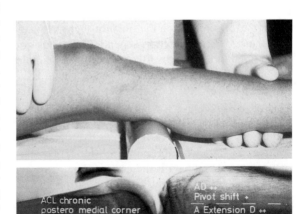

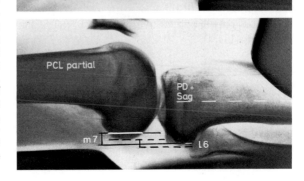

Fig. 3. a Radiographic test for drawer displacement near extension. For anterior drawer testing, an 8-cm roll is placed beneath the upper tibia. The femur and tibia are pressed downward with a force of about 15 kg, causing the tibial plateau to be pushed forward. For posterior drawer testing, the roll is placed beneath the distal femur, and the proximal tibia is pressed downward. **b** Radiograph demonstrating 18 mm anterior displacement of the lateral and medial tibial condyles. The patient, with chronic anterior instability, has a 2 + anterior drawer, a 1 + pivot shift, and a 2 + Lachman test. **c** Radiograph demonstrating slight posterior subluxation – 7 mm on the medial side and 6 mm on the lateral side – caused by a concomitant partial tear of the PCL

(b)

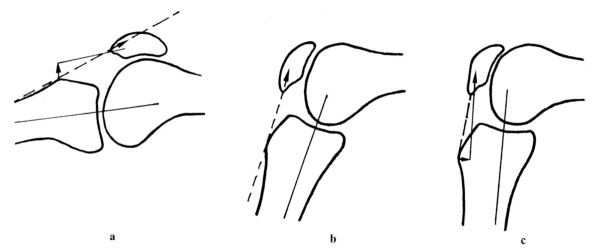

Fig. 4 a–c. The quadriceps neutral position of Daniels et al. (1983). **a** The line of force of the patellar tendon is directed anteriorly relative to the force of joint compression, causing a net forward-displacing force to act on the tibia. **b** In 70° flexion the lines of patellar tendon force and joint compression are parallel. The active quadriceps drawer is zero. **c** In 90° flexion the patella is posterior to the tibial tuberosity, so quadriceps contraction exerts a posteriorly directed force on the tibia

On the tibia, the lateral plateau is convex and has a steep posterior slope. Another way to define the neutral position of the knee is by the quadriceps neutral method of Daniel et al. (1983), which employs an active quadriceps drawer test. Active quadriceps contraction exerts a force on the tibia through the patellar ligament whose direction depends on the position of the tibial tuberosity. In 30° of flexion, for example, the more anterior position of the patella relative to the tuberosity causes a net anterior force to act on the tibia. As flexion increases, the femur moves backward on the tibia, altering the direction of the patellar ligament. At about 70° of flexion, active quadriceps contraction causes no anterior or posterior displacement of the tibia, even if the cruciate ligaments are absent. In this "quadriceps neutral" position, the active quadriceps drawer displacement is zero. If the posterior cruciate ligament (PCL) is torn, the weight of the lower leg causes the tibia to subluxate backward, leading to a posterior angulation of the patellar tendon. If the quadriceps is now contracted, it will pull the tibia forward. The quadriceps neutral position can serve to distinguish between anterior and posterior laxity in patients with tears of both cruciate ligaments (Fig. 4).

Acute Posttraumatic Symptoms

The symptoms of an acute rupture of the ACL are indistinguishable from internal knee injuries that do not involve the cruciate ligament. An audible pop or tear at the time of injury, an unsteady feeling causing the patient to fall to the ground, pain in the popliteal fossa, a joint effusion appearing within 2 h, and painful limitation of motion are usually present with an anterior cruciate tear but are equally common with other internal knee derangements. Even patients with tears of the medial collateral ligament and ACL may still be able to ski back to the valley station. Patients tend initially to discount the severity of their trauma, especially in noncontact injuries. Odensten (1984) reports that two-thirds of injuries occur in contact sports, although Noyes et al. (1980b) and our own records indicate that two-thirds of ACL ruptures are sustained in noncontact types of sport.

Acute Posttraumatic Hemarthrosis

Noyes et al. (1980b) found a partial or complete tear of the ACL in 72% of acutely injured knees with hemarthrosis and clinically negligible instability. Acute hemarthrosis usually develops within 2 h of injury and generally is quite distinct from the nonhemorrhagic effusion that slowly develops over about a 24-h period. The extent of the hemarthrosis is highly variable and correlates poorly with the extent and location of the injury. Gillquist et al. (1977) found a 59% incidence of ACL ruptures in joints with acute posttraumatic hemarthrosis. We agree with these authors that a patient with acute posttraumatic hemarthrosis should be considered to have a severe ligamentous injury until proven otherwise. This proof can be established only by examination under anesthesia and by arthroscopy. If we find an injury that does not require operative treatment, the knowledge gained enables us to counsel the patient about the precautionary measures he must take to promote the healing of a partially torn ACL. Simonsen et al. (1984) investigated the diagnostic accuracy of the clinical examination in 118 acutely knee-injured patients with hemarthrosis and/or clinical suspicion of a ligament injury. Clinical examination as well as examination under anesthesia yielded a large number of false-positive and false-negative diagnoses, especially concerning lesions of the ACL and menisci. Of patients without hemarthrosis who showed clinical evidence of a ligament instability, 66% had a subclinical hemarthrosis and the same percentage incidence of cruciate ligament tears as the overall series. This led the authors to conclude that arthroscopy should be used rather freely in patients with acute knee injuries, especially when hemarthrosis exists.

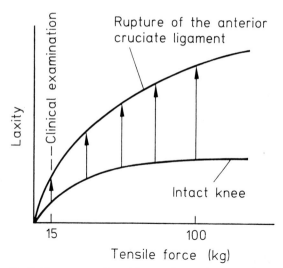

Fig.5. The curves, adapted from a diagram by Noyes (1980a), show how the degree of joint laxity increases with the applied force. The forces used for clinical stability testing are much smaller than the forces that act on the knee in many types of sport. This accounts for the potential discrepancy between mild clinical findings and profound disability for athletics. The difference between the injured and intact knee is very small when the drawer test is performed in 90° flexion with a tensile force of 15 kg

Symptoms of Chronic Injury

The chronic stage of injury to the ACL is characterized by frequent episodes of limb collapse or "giving way." The resulting disability is particularly apparent during athletics but also affects the activities of daily living, including ordinary walking. Any twisting motion of the knee with the foot planted can precipitate giving way as an expression of anterolateral instability. The episode itself is painful and is followed by swelling (usually hemarthrosis) and stiffness that persist for a few days. No further pain is experienced until the next giving-way episode occurs. Each new episode can damage the articular cartilage or menisci, which in turn can affect the symptomatology. The initial unsteadiness becomes less apparent, while pain on weight bearing and osteoarthritic symptoms become more prominent. A careful evaluation of the symptoms usually gives an indication of whether the shear forces resulting from the anterior cruciate tear have produced secondary degenerative changes in the cartilage and menisci, which Galway et al. (1972) referred to as the "ACL syndrome."

Effect of Applied Forces on Degree of Laxity

Even the most experienced examiner can recall instances where lesions of the ACL were not detected by clinical examination. Such lesions are missed be-

cause the manual forces that are applied for clinical testing are relatively small. Joint laxity, however, depends on the magnitude of the forces applied. The forces typically used for clinical anterior drawer testing are from 5 to 10 kg. Noyes et al. (1980a) showed that laxity becomes more pronounced as greater force is applied. This means that the difference in drawer mobility between an intact ACL and a torn ligament is slim or even negligible with clinical testing (Fig.5). When the knee is tested under general anesthesia, muscular tension about the joint is eliminated, and a more obvious positive test is generally obtained. Any effusion or hemarthrosis reduces laxity and should always be percutaneously aspirated so that a meaningful examination can be performed.

Altered Relationships in the Presence of Rotational Drawer

The following discussions are based on a scheme of Castaing et al. (1972) and Bousquet (1972) and its refinement by Müller (1982) based on new discoveries in physiopathology. A knowledge of the functional synergisms of the ligaments forms the basis for the evaluation. This means that not one, but two or more ligaments are responsible for a given function in the knee. The structure chiefly responsible for that function is called the primary restraint (primary stabilizer), and the others are called secondary restraints (secondary stabilizers). This principle is illustrated by the synergism that exists between the ACL, the posterior oblique ligament of Hughston (1976) and the posterior horn of the meniscus. These structures must act in concert so that full stability can be achieved. In 30° of flexion, the collateral ligaments are chiefly responsible for stabilizing the knee in the frontal plane, so they are the primary restraints. The examiner should bear in mind that there is always a mild degree of varus laxity in the normal knee. The lateral collateral ligament does not become tense until a mild varus stress is applied; this is easily confirmed by palpation. In 60° and 90° of flexion, external rotation of the tibia is associated with an anterior displacement of the medial tibial plateau and a posterior displacement of the lateral plateau. This causes an immediate tightening of the medial collateral ligament (Fig. 6). Because the medial collateral ligament inserts at a relatively low level on the tibial metaphysis, about 11 cm distal to the articular surface, the adjacent tibial plateau is free to move over a somewhat greater range until it is finally restrained by the semimembranosus corner. The posterior displacement of the lateral tibial plateau during external rotation, more pronounced than the anterior displacement of the medial plateau, is checked by the lateral collateral ligament and to a degree by the popliteus tendon. The greatest freedom of external rotation, then, resides in the lateral compartment, where rotation is definitively restrained by lateral ligaments and tendons. External rotation decreases tension in the ACL. Anterior drawer testing, then, simultaneously tests the integrity of the medial and lateral capsuloligamentous structures, which function as secondary restraints to anterior tibial motion depending on the rotational position of the joint (Fig. 7). If the secondary restraints are intact, the clinical drawer test, which uses a relatively low tensile force, will demonstrate little or no anterior laxity. This implies that an isolated rupture of the ACL cannot be definitively diagnosed by

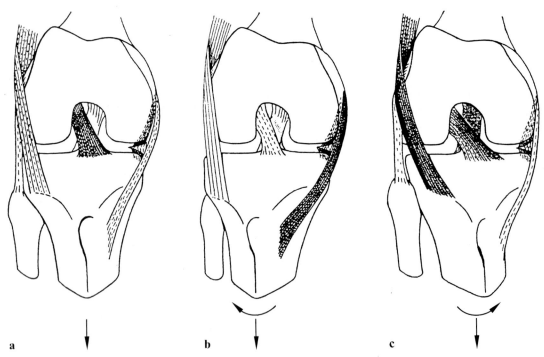

Fig. 6a–c. Ligamentous stability during anterior drawer testing in the flexed knee. **a** Neutral rotation: The ACL, lax in flexion, is made taut by pulling the tibia forward. This ligament is the primary restraint to anterior tibial motion. Slight tension is placed on the secondary restraints: the semimembranosus corner and anterolateral femorotibial ligament. **b** External tibial rotation: The medial collateral liagment, semimembranosus corner, and lateral collateral ligament come under greatest tension; they are the primary restraints. Both cruciate ligaments are lax in the externally rotated knee. **c** Internal tibial rotation: As a primary restraint, the ACL becomes tight when the tibia is pulled forward. Both internal rotation and anterior traction on the tibia make the ACL tense. Internal rotation places the greatest tension on the semimembranosus corner and iliotibial tract. (From drawings by Müller)

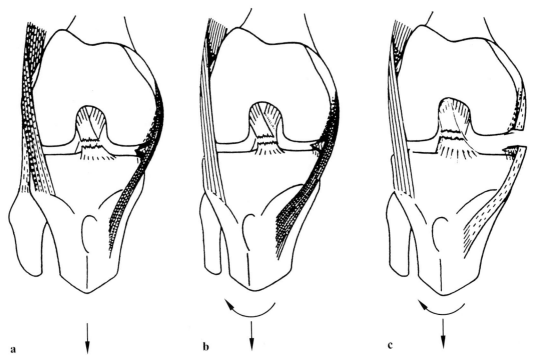

Fig. 7 a–c. Anterior drawer associated with rupture of the ACL. **a** With isolated division of the ACL, the secondary restraints permit very little drawer motion in neutral rotation compared with the uninjured knee. **b** When testing is performed in external rotation, there is no change relative to the unaffected side. The primary restraints are the medial collateral ligament, semimembranosus corner, and lateral collateral ligament. **c** Concomitant rupture of the the medial secondary restraints permits a massive anterior drawer that is checked only by the tertiary restraints

drawer testing. If the secondary restraints are lax, whether due to concomitant injury or gradual elongation in chronic instability, a more obvious drawer sign will be obtained.

Anterior drawer testing should be performed from a position of neutral rotation, located by allowing the tibia to rotate freely in the direction where anterior motion is most easily elicited. In this way the greatest extent of the displacement can be ascertained. Drawer testing in 15° of external or internal rotation, as we formerly suggested, forces the tibia to assume a position in which twisting of the peripheral capsule and ligaments creates an increased tension that restricts anterior mobility. No drawer motion is elicited in positions of extreme internal or external rotation. Rotational stability testing, together with lateral stability testing in flexion and extension, provides information on the complexity of the ligament damage and the stability of the secondary restraints. Drawer testing in the slightly flexed knee (Lachman) and testing for subluxation due to anterolateral instability are simpler studies that offer a higher predictive value in the diagnosis of acute or chronic injury to the ACL.

Lachman Test

As early as 1971, Trillat noted the importance of drawer testing in a position of slight flexion. At the time, we underrated this truly useful examination. In 1976 Torg et al. published their first description of the simple, reliable test taught to them by Lachman. The test is performed with the knee slightly flexed to about 15°. The examiner holds the femur with one hand and pulls the tibia forward with the other. A positive test is one in which there is demonstrable tibial motion with respect to the femur, terminating in a soft or "mushy" end point. A hard end point signifies some stablity of the ACL. If a hard end point is reached within 3 mm, the ligament is completely stable. A hard end point reached at 5 mm or more indicates a relative stability, perhaps associated with prior stretching of the ACL. At our department (Bertschmann et al. 1981) we tested the predictive value of the Lachman test in 36 fresh ligamentous knee injuries. We performed the test under general anesthesia, simultaneously testing posterior tibial displacement so that we could differentiate the anterior and posterior components more precisely. The setup involves placing a roll about 8 cm in diameter beneath the proximal tibia or distal femur (see Fig. 3). Anterior displacement is elicited by pressing down on the femur and ipsilateral foot while the roll is beneath the upper tibia. The radiographic values correlate well with the lesions identified at operation. We had no false-positive results in either of 2 separate comparative studies in our patients (Bertschmann et al. 1981; Stäubli et al. 1983a). Torg and we obtained false-negative tests in ACL ruptures that were accompanied by an incarcerated bucket-handle fragment of meniscus. A radiographic mobility of $10.8 +/- 4.0$ mm in 4 joints with interposed menisci increased to $16.0 +/- 2.0$ mm following reduction of the meniscal fragment. All patients with a ruptured ACL (n = 27) exhibited anterior drawer mobility in the extended knee. All patients with a ruptured PCL (n = 7) showed significant posterior tibial displacement in extension.

The obvious advantages of the Lachman test are its high predictive accuracy and the lack of need for general anesthesia. The relatively flat contact surface of the femoral condyles near extension causes much less interference to anterior motion of the tibia and menisci. Moreover, a hamstring spasm does little to restrict anterior tibial motion due to the unfavorable lever arm created by the extended joint position. A positive Lachman test is significant because a small amount of drawer motion near extension can be more disabling than greater drawer motion in 90° flexion, which is remarkably well tolerated by many patients.

Anterolateral Instability

Anterolateral instability is a type of rotatory instability. It differs from a simple one-plane instability like that associated with laxity of the medial collateral ligament. Rotatory instability is a complex form involving a rotational motion about an imaginary axis with concomitant translation. There are 3 axes of translation – medial-lateral, compression-distraction, and anterior-posterior, the latter forming the salient component of anterolateral instability. In anterolateral rotational instability (ALRI), the most common rotatory instability, the lateral tibial plateau rotates and slips forward beneath the lateral femoral condyle. If the tibia is held in place, the lateral femoral condyles slips backward while moving on a curved path about a medially displaced rotational axis. This type of motion in ALRI is opposite to the screw-home mechanism of the knee in terminal extension.

If the screw-home mechanism augments stability as the knee approaches extension, clearly the loss of this mechanism will cause instability to be most pronounced near extension, i. e., in the range between 0° and 30° of flexion. The structure that, when intact, guarantees maintenance of the screw-home mechanism, and thus of stability in the extended knee, but permits ALRI when defective is the ACL. The clinical severity of ALRI is demonstrated by drawer testing in approximately 25° of flexion. During activities of daily living such as turning the knee while standing on one leg, ALRI causes a subluxation that the patient may describe as a "giving way," "going out," or "catching" of the knee. This is even more common during athletics, especially competitive sports such as soccer, handball, and basketball, or when the patient lands on the leg with the foot turned slightly inward. Muscular effort cannot compensate for ALRI, because the subluxation is of sudden onset, and neither the powerful quadriceps nor the hamstrings can check the rotation.

The clinically significant ALRI with subluxation near extension should be distinguished from ALRI in flexion. ALRI in flexion may be viewed as the lateral counterpart of a mild anteromedial rotatory instability. It usually results from a stretch or occasionally a fresh tear of the lateral capsule, arcuate ligament, and iliotibial tract. There are no symptoms aside from a mildly positive anterior drawer sign in medial rotation, and the anterior instability is not pronounced.

Pathomechanics of the Subluxation Test

A "central" knee ligament in every sense of the term, the ACL is responsible for the rolling-gliding mechanism of femorotibial articulation. If the ligament is absent or defective, the rolling phase becomes prolonged under weight bearing, permitting anterior subluxation of the lateral tibial plateau. At about 25° of flexion the iliotibial tract moves from the extensor to the flexor side of the joint and, through its action as a flexor, effects a sudden reduction of the subluxation. Anterior subluxation in the lateral compartment is favored by the slight anatomic convexity of the lateral tibial plateau. This convexity results in a "misfit" between the femorotibial articular surfaces in the lateral compartment, which therefore lacks the stability that congruity would provide. In the past there has been some confusion about the exact causative lesions of ALRI. Today it is agreed that the key to this instability is a deficient ACL. The main credit for this discovery belongs to Jakob (1981), who ex-

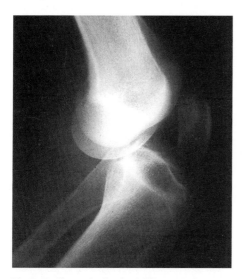

Fig. 8. Radiograph of a pivot shift test under general anesthesia. Marked anterior subluxation of the tibia on the lateral and medial sides results from ruptures of the ACL, semimembranosus corner, the anterior third of the lateral capsule, and a partial rupture of the medial collateral ligament. This case illustrates how a recurrent pivot shift can separate the menisci from the posterior capsule

perimented with cadaveric knees. An anterolateral instability develops, notes Jakob, when the ACL is torn and there is concomitant stretching or tearing of the lateral capsule and ligaments. Isolated division of the ACL is sufficient to produce a positive pivot shift experimentally, but the sign is less positive than when the peripheral capsule and ligaments are also damaged. When the ACL is intact, a pivot shift sign cannot be elicited. A lesion of the lateral capsular ligaments alone cannot incite a true pivot shift and can cause only an inconstant snap due to entrapment or surmounting of the lateral meniscus. In our own studies of 15 stable cadaver knees with no history of pathology in which the ACL was selectively sectioned through a small arthrotomy, we were able to confirm that an isolated lesion of the ACL is sufficient to produce a pivot shift. Patients with an isolated lesion of the ACL exhibit a mildly positive pivot shift that cannot be elicited by muscular tension. The peripheral capsular structures become stretched over time, increasing the amount of anterolateral rotational instability and the degree of pivot shift. In a young soccer player (Fig. 8) who underwent a preoperative examination under anesthesia, we X-rayed the knee during the subluxation phase of the pivot shift. On viewing the film, we were amazed at the degree of subluxation, which approached an anterior dislocation. Of course a very strongly positive drawer sign could be elicited in the neutral position. At sub-

sequent operation we confirmed that the ACL rupture was accompanied by ruptures of the anterior third of the lateral capsule, the semimembranosus corner, and a two-thirds tear of the medial collateral ligament.

The lesions on the medial side were just extensive enough to permit marked anterior translation of the medial tibial plateau. A complete rupture of the medial capsule and ligaments makes it impossible to apply the valgus stress needed in the pivot shift to press the articular surfaces in the lateral compartment together so that they can roll upon each other. Division of the iliotibial tract increases the degree of anterolateral subluxation, but it significantly weakens the clinically relevant phase of painful reduction.

Subluxation Tests in Patients with Anterolateral Instability

The diagnosis is established by a maneuver that attempts to reproduce the subluxation that occurs in ALRI. Although several subluxation tests have been described by different authors, there is only one form of ALRI, so there is only one subluxation that can be elicited, regardless of the method used. The basic motion in a positive test is an internal rotation of the tibia and a flexion-extension movement in which the iliotibial tract glides from the extensor side to the flexor side of the joint or vice-versa. Some tests start in the extended subluxated position and go to the flexed reduced position, while others proceed in the opposite direction.

Pivot Shift Test of Galway et al. (1972)

The examiner picks up the foot of the extended leg with one hand, and with the other he pushes the knee into flexion while applying a mild valgus stress. The tibia rotates and translates anterolaterally into the subluxated position. At 25° of flexion the iliotibial tract moves behind the flexion axis and, acting as a flexor, abruptly pulls the tibia back into the normal starting position (Fig. 9).

Jerk Test of Hughston et al. (1976)

From a position of about 60° flexion, the knee is extended while the tibia is in slight internal rotation. When about 20° of flexion is reached, the lateral ti-

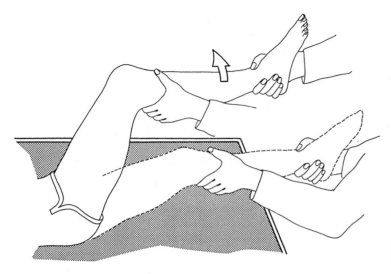

Fig. 9. Schematic drawing of the jerk test. While the pivot shift is tested by moving the knee from extension to flexion, the jerk test is performed by moving the joint from flexion to extension. (From Jakob et al. 1981)

bial plateau slips forward with a sudden jerk. To the eye, this motion appears more like an abrupt posterior subluxation of the lateral femoral condyle (see Fig. 9).

Anterior Subluxation Test of Losee et al. (1979)

The left foot is picked up in the examiner's left hand and is held in slight external rotation with the knee flexed 30°. The right hand grasps the knee, placing the thumb behind the head of the fibula. While exerting a valgus stress (by pulling the foot laterally and pushing the knee medially with the abdomen), the examiner slowly extends the knee, allowing the foot to rotate internally. In a positive test the tibia will subluxate anterolaterally just before extension is reached.

Anterolateral Rotatory Instability Test of Slocum et al. (1976)

This test is useful in apprehensive patients with hamstring guarding that would make other types of examination difficult. The patient lies on the uninvolved side and holds the upper, injured leg in extension with the foot turned slightly inward. In this position the weight of the leg exerts a slight valgus stress on the injured knee. One hand holds the distal femur while the other hand grasps the tibial plateau with the thumb behind the fibular head. As the extended knee is flexed, the examiner palpates for subluxation and subsequent reduction. This test allows for complete relaxation of the quadriceps, which can be advantageous.

Subluxation Test of Jakob et al. (1977)

The patient leans with his sound side against a wall, his weight distributed evenly on both legs. From there the procedure is the same as for the Slocum test.

Flexion-Rotation Drawer Test of Noyes (1980)

The author of this test claims that it combines the features of the pivot shift test and Lachman test. The knee is held in 20° of flexion and neutral rotation. If the ACL is lax, the weight of the thigh will cause the femur to sag backward and rotate externally relative to the stationary tibia. This is the rotational component of the anterolateral subluxation. The examiner then flexes the knee about an additional 10° while pushing backward on the tibia, causing the femur to rotate internally (reduction). Alternate subluxation and reduction can be elicited by gentle flexion and extension of the limb. This test is most useful in knees with mild (grade I) anterolateral laxity, which is not plainly demonstrated by the reduction maneuver of the pivot shift (Fig. 10).

Posterolateral Involvement

The PCL is much more commonly involved in acute complex injuries than is generally assumed. These concomitant, often mild posterior instabilities are not obvious on clinical inspection or laxity testing. A stress radiograph of anterior drawer displacement near extension (Lachman) and of posterior displace-

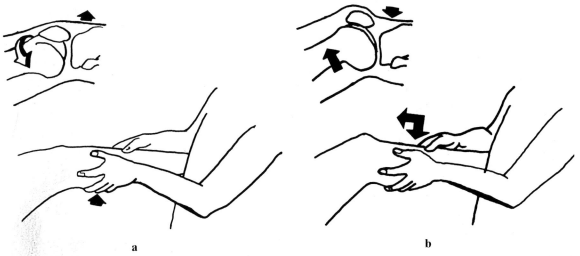

a   **b**

Fig. 10 a, b. Flexion-rotation drawer test of Noyes (1980a). **a** Subluxated position with the tibia in neutral rotation. With the examiner supporting the knee in slight flexion, the femur drops backward and rotates externally when the ACL is deficient.

b As the knee is flexed with a downward push on the leg, the joint will reduce. This tests the function of the ACL in the control of both translation and rotation

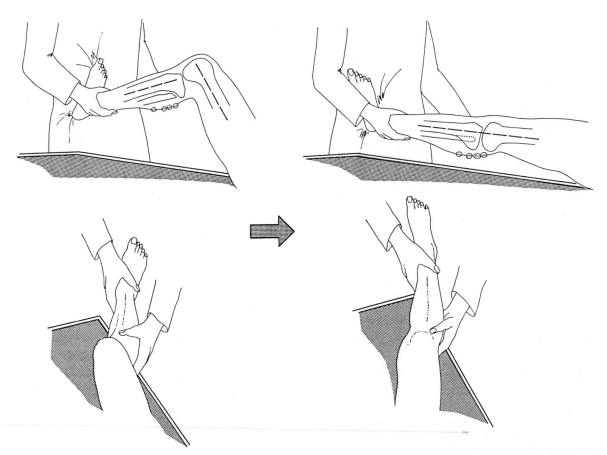

Fig. 11. Reversed pivot shift test for posterolateral rotatory instability. The examiner picks up the right foot with the right hand, bracing the foot against the iliac spine. The left hand supports the lateral aspect of the lower leg. The knee is flexed 70°–80°, and the foot is externally rotated to elicit posterior subluxa-tion of the lateral tibial plateau. The knee is then extended while a mild valgus stress is applied, and the tibial plateau reduces forward abruptly when the knee reaches 20°. (From Jakob et al. 1981)

ment as described yields accurate information on the degree of the instability. In cases where an anterior instability is managed by an extraarticular "lateral repair," careless dissection in the region of the arcuate ligament can predispose to subsequent posterolateral laxity. The arcuate complex, responsible for supporting the central pivot of the cruciate ligaments posterolaterally by coapting the articular surfaces and restricting external rotation, can be attenuated. The result is hypermobility of the lateral compartment in the direction of external rotation.

The anterolateral subluxation in ALRI involves increased anterior rotation on the lateral side. This exerts a permanent stress on the scarred tissues, especially in genu varum, and often gives rise to a second-

ary laxity. The varus stretches the ACL and popliteus tendon. The flexing action and posterior drawer stresses imposed on the knee by the kinetic forces associated with walking and deceleration are an additional factor that can stretch the structures that control external rotation. In every knee with chronic anterolateral instability, the examiner should look for evidence of posterolateral stretching with lateral hypermobility. Jakob and Stäubli (1981) were the first to describe the pivot shift-imitating phenomenon of posterolateral instability, referring to it as the "reversed pivot shift" (Fig. 11).

The patient is positioned supine. To test the right knee, the examiner stands at the foot of the table, picks up the right foot with his right hand, and braces

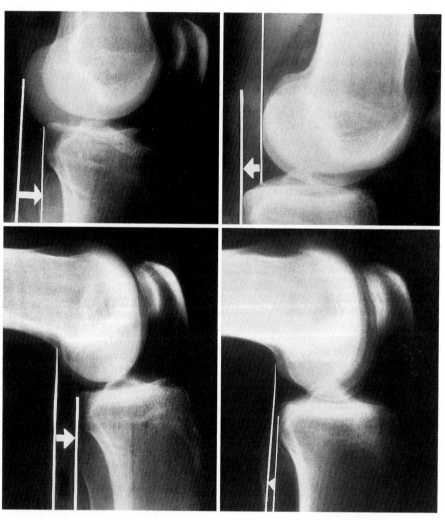

Fig. 12. Man 20 years of age with clinically diagnosed anterior instability. Stress radiographs taken under anesthesia confirmed the clinically apparent pattern of instability. *Above:* positive anterior and posterior drawer signs near extension. *Below:* anterior drawer positive in 90° flexion, posterior drawer negative. This peculiar posterior instability that is apparent near extension but disappears in flexion has been noted in several patients

the foot against his right iliac spine. The left hand supports the posterolateral side of the lower leg at the level of the proximal fibula. The knee is now flexed to 70°–80°. In that position, external rotation of the foot will cause the lateral tibial plateau to subluxate posteriorly. The examiner then slowly extends the knee while exerting a gentle valgus stress. When the knee reaches about 20° of flexion, it will reduce abruptly with a visible and palpable anterior motion of the tibial plateau. The sign can also be tested in the reverse direction, so alternate subluxation and reduction can be elicited.

In joints with combined anterolateral and posterolateral laxity, the rotational position of the foot is useful for differentiating between them. An obvious jerky motion elicited in internal rotation indicates a true pivot shift, while a motion that is more apparent with the foot externally rotated signifies the reversed pivot shift of posterolateral instability. From cadaveric studies on the pathomechanics of the reversed pivot shift, Jakob et al. concluded that the sign is prevented by the intact function of the popliteus tendon, arcuate ligament, and lateral collateral ligament. By far the most important structures are the popliteus muscle and popliteus tendon with its expansions to the arcuate ligament. These studies indicate that the reversed pivot shift is paralleled by a posterior drawer motion in flexion and external rotation. With every lesion that produces a marked reversed pivot shift, the posterior drawer in external rotation is always more pronounced.

In detailed comparative studies of freshly operated and previously operated patients, we have made some interesting findings with regard to the amounts of drawer mobility present near extension and in 90° flexion. There are patients who have a markedly positive posterior drawer sign in extension but show no evidence of posterior instability in the flexed knee and have a firm end point on posterior drawer testing (Fig. 12). Posterior subluxation can be elicited in these patients near extension, but the posterior drawer sign is negative in flexion. Arthroscopy and subsequent operation in these cases disclosed only an old rupture of the ACL and a longitudinal tear of the medial meniscus in the posteromedial corner. It must be assumed that different structures act as restraints to posterior displacement in flexion and extension. This cannot be the posterior capsule, which is taut in extension but lax in flexion. So far we have been unable to account for this phenomenon. This shows that, even with stress radiographic measurements of drawer displacement in flexion and extension under anesthesia, there are knee joints that we still cannot fully analyze or comprehend in terms of their stability.

Now and in the future, we must examine knee joints with our senses alert and our eyes open, and we must continue to perform studies in cadaveric knees so that we can comprehend more fully the pathomechanics of this fascinating joint. The diagnosis of instability relating to a defective ACL is a basic prerequisite for effective therapy, and it continues to be a challenge for the physician.

References

Abbott LC, Saunders JB, Bost FC, Anderson CE (1944) Injuries to the ligaments of the knee joint. J Bone Joint Surg [Am] 26: 503–521

Benedetto KP, Glotzer W, Sperner G (1984) Die Bedeutung des Akutarthroskopie für die Verifizierung der frischen Kreuzbandrupturen. Acta Traumatol 14: 227–231

Bertschmann W, Stäubli HU, Noesberger B (1981) Stellenwert einfacher diagnostischer Tests bei frischer Kniegelenksläsion. Helv Chir Acta 48: 685–691

Bousquet G (1972) Le diagnostic des laxités chroniques du genou. Rev Chir Orthop 58: 71–77

Butler DL, Noyes FR, Grood ES (1980) Ligamentous restraints to anterior-posterior drawer in the human knee. J Bone Joint Surg [Am] 62: 259–270

Castaing J, Burding P, Mougin M (1972) Les conditions de la stabilité passive du genou. Rev Chir Orthop 58: 34–48

Daniel D, Malcolm L, Stone ML, Barnett P, Biden E (1983) The active drawer test Syllabus. The measurement of knee instability. Syllabus Kaiser Permanente Medical Center, San Diego

Ellison AE (1980) The pathogenesis and treatment for anterolateral rotatory instability. Clin Orthop 147: 51–55

Figueras JM, Escalas F, Vidal A, Morgenstern R, Buló JM, Merino JA, Espadaler-Gamisans JM (1987) The anterior cruciate ligament injuri in skiers skiing trauma and safety. Sixth International Symposium ASTM STP 938. American Society for Testing and Materials, Philadelphia, pp 55–60

Galway RD, Beaupré A, McIntosh DL (1972) Pivot-shift: A clinical sign of symptomatic anterior cruciate insufficiency. J Bone Joint Surg [Br] 54: 763–764

Gillquist J, Hagberg G, Oretorp N (1977) Arthroscopy in acute injuries of the knee joint. Acta Orthop Scand 48: 190

Grood ES, Noyes FR, Butler DL, Suntay WJ (1981) Ligamentous and capsular restraints preventing straight medial and lateral laxity in intact human cadaver knees. J Bone Joint Surg [Am] 63: 1257

Hackenbruch W, Henche HR (1981) Diagnostik und Therapie von Kapselbandläsionen am Kniegelenk. Eular, Basel

Hughston JC, Andrews JR, Cross JM, Moschi A (1976) Classification of knee ligament instabilities. Part I: The medial compartment and cruciate ligaments. Part II: The lateral compartment. J Bone Joint Surg [Am] 65: 145–179

Jacobsen K (1976) Stress radiographical measurement of the anteroposterior, medial and lateral stability of the knee joint. Acta Orthop Scand 47: 335–344

Jacobsen K (1977) Stress radiographical measurement of post traumatic knee instability. Acta Orthop Scand 48: 301–310

Jakob RP, Noesberger B, (1976) Das Pivot shift Phänomen, ein neues Zeichen der Ruptur des vorderen Kreuzbandes und die spezifische laterale Rekonstruktion. Helv Chir Acta 43: 451–456

156   B. Noesberger

Jakob RP, Stäubli H-U (1981) Das umgekehrte Pivot shift Phänomen (reversed pivot shift) - ein neues Zeichen der postero-lateralen Knieinstabilität. In: Jäger M, Hackenbroch MH, Refior JH (Hrsg) Kapselbandläsionen des Kniegelenkes. Thieme, Stuttgart New York, S 135-140

Jakob RP, Noesberger B, Saxer U (1977) Der Wert des Pivot shift Phänomens und der lateralen Rekonstruktion; zur Diagnose und Therapie der vorderen Kreuzbandruptur. Schweiz Z Sportmed 2: 69-84

Jakob RP, Hassler H, Stäubli H-U (1981) Observations on rotatory instability of the lateral compartment of the knee. Acta Orthop Scand [Suppl 191] 52: 1-32

Kennedy JC, Weinberg MW, Wilson AS (1974) The anatomy and function of the anterior cruciate ligament. As determined by clinical and morphological studies. J Bone Joint Surg [Am] 56: 223-235

Losee RE, Johnson TR, Southwick WO (1978) Anterior subluxation of the lateral tibial plateau. A diagnostic test and operative repair. J Bone Joint Surg [Am] 60: 1015-1030

Müller We (1983) The knee. Form, function and ligament reconstruction. Springer, Berlin Heidelberg New York Tokyo

Nielson S, Ovesen J, Rasmussen O (1984) The anterior cruciate ligament in the knee. An experimental study of its importance in rotatory knee instability. Arch Orthop Trauma Surg 103: 170-174

Noyes FR, Grood ES, Butler DL, Paulos LE (1980a) Clinical biomechanics of the knee - Ligament restraints and functional stability. In: Funk FJ jr (ed) The American Academy of Orthopedic Surgeons: Symposium of the Athlete's Knee. Mosby, St. Louis, pp 1-35

Noyes FR, Basset RW, Grood ES, Butler DL (1980b) Arthroscopy in acute traumatic hemarthrosis of the knee. Incidence of anterior cruciate tears and other injuries. J Bone Joint Surg [Am] 62: 687-695

Noyes FR, Mooar PA, Matthews DS, Butler DL (1983) The symptomatic anterior cruciate-deficient knee. Part I. The long-term functional disability in athletically active individuals. J Bone Joint Surg [Am] 65: 154-162

Odensten M (1984) Treatment of the torn anterior cruciate ligament. Linköping University Medical Dissertations No 177. Linköping, Sweden

Palmer I (1938) On the injuries of the ligaments of the knee joint: A clinical study. Acta Chir Scand [Suppl 81] 53: 1-282

Segond P (1979) Recherches cliniques et experimentables sur les epauchements sanguins du genou par entorse. Prog Med 7: 297-299, 319-321, 340-341, 379-381, 400-401, 419-421

Simonsen D, Jensen J, Mouritsen P, Lauritzen J (1984) The accuracy of clinical examination of injury of the knee joint. Injury 16: 96-101

Slocum DB, Larson RL, (1968) Rotatory instability of the knee. Its pathogenesis and a clinical test to demonstrate its presence. J Bone Joint Surg [Am] 50: 211-225

Slocum DB, James SL, Larson RL, Singer KM (1976) Clinical test for antero-lateral rotatory instability of the knee. Clin Orthop 118: 63-69

Stäubli H-U, Noesberger B (1985) Anterior-posterior knee instability and stress radiography. A prospective biomechanical analysis with the knee in extension. in: Perren SM, Schneider E (eds) Biomechanics: Current interdisciplinary research. Nijhoff, The Hague, pp 397-402

Stäubli H-U, Jakob RP, Noesberger B (1981a) Experimentelle Grundlagen zur Diagnostik der postero-lateralen Knierotationsinstabilität. In: Jäger M, Hackenbroch MH, Refior JH (Hrsg) Kapselbandläsionen des Kniegelenks. Thieme, Stuttgart New York, S 109-116

Stäubli H-U, Jakob RP, Noesberger B, (1981b) Die posterolaterale Knierotationsinstabilität. Experimentelle Grundlagen zur Diagnostik und Therapie. Helv Chir Acta 48: 693-696

Stäubli H-U, Noesberger B, Jakob RP (1983a) Radiologische Messtechnik der extensionsnahen Schubladenverschieblichkeit des Kniegelenkes. Unfallheilkunde 165: 28

Stäubli H-U, Noesberger B, Jakob RP (1983b) The drawer sign of the knee in extension. A prospective study. J Bone Joint Surg [Am] 7: 585

Torg JS, Conrad W, Kalen V (1976) Clinical diagnosis of anterior cruciate ligament instability in the athlete. Am J Sports Med 4: 84-93

Trillat A (1971) Chirurgie du genou. Journées Lyonnaises. Simép, Villeurbanne

Woods GW, Chapman DR (1984) Repairable posterior menisco-capsular disruption in anterior cruciate ligament injuries. Am J Sports Med 12: 381-385

Pathomechanical and Clinical Concepts of the Pivot Shift Phenomenon

R. P. Jakob and H.-U. Stäubli

With recent advances in our understanding of the diagnosis, pathoanatomy, and pathomechanics of ligamentous knee injuries, the pivot shift sign continues to be an important clinical and conceptual entity. Though it was observed some 50 years ago, the sign is most commonly associated with the names of MacIntosh and Galway and their excellent description published in 1972 (Galway et al. 1972). The pivot shift was a source of controversy in the early 1970s, and 4 years passed before the sign and its importance became generally acknowledged. This was a time in which our knowledge of the biomechanics of the knee was expanded through the work of O'Donoghue, Slocum, Hughston, Kennedy, Trillat, and others. In the present chapter we shall explore the history, clinical presentation, and pathology of the pivot shift phenomenon, and we shall propose recommendations for treatment.

Historical Aspects of the Pivot Shift Phenomenon

In reviewing the literature on the pivot shift, one is faced with a bewildering array of descriptions and interpretations. The phenomenon was probably first described in 1913 by Jones and Smith, who reported the "rocking knee" as the main symptom of the stretched anterior cruciate ligament (ACL). They described a testing method (quoted in Arnold et al. 1979) in which "placing the hands on the joint, the femur seemed to be suddenly displaced inward just before extension was completed, constituting the slipping of which the patient complained."

Hey Groves in 1920 described the symptoms of injury to the ACL as follows:

On passive manipulation, the head of the tibia can be moved forwards on the femur. In active exercise, when the foot is put forward and the weight of the body pressed on the leg, the tibia slips forward. Sometimes this forward-slipping of the tibia occurs abruptly with a jerk: often it is under the patient's control, but if he hurries or forgets to control his knee, the subluxation will suddenly occur, giving him a sense of insecurity, or actually "throwing him down" (Hey Groves 1920, p. 508).

The simplicity and accuracy of this description are remarkable and represent only a sample of the wealth of information contained in this classic article.

In 1934 Felsenreich became the first German author to describe the pivot shift:

In a slow demonstration of the sign, it can be shown how the lateral femoral condyle glides over the lateral tibial condyle with internal rotation and increasing flexion, snapping past the lateral meniscus (Felsenreich 1934, p. 381).

Lemaire published the first French account of the phenomenon in 1967:

A sign that is seen inconsistently appears to be pathognomonic for lesions of the ACL: an antero-internal subluxation of the knee that can be elicited in terminal extension. The foot is placed in internal rotation, the knee in extension. When the muscles are completely relaxed, small movements of flexion and extension, and anterior and internal subluxation can be elicited by pushing slightly on the fibular head. By working very gently, the examiner can produce a spring-like phenomenon at the start of flexion, recreating the mechanism of the injury in a manner that the patient can recognize. The sign is difficult to elicit due to the difficulty of attaining muscular relaxation. When the examination is performed under anesthesia, the sign can be frequently found, thus confirming a rupture of the ACL (Lemaire 1967).

From this description, Lemaire subsequently developed his extraarticular (lateral) repairs, which are still widely practiced in Europe today.

Also in the late 1960s, MacIntosh was working with the pivot shift sign on the North American continent, and in 1972 he published the following vivid description with his co-authors Galway and Beaupré:

The pivot shift is characterized by forward subluxation of the lateral tibial plateau on the femoral condyle in extension and spontaneous reduction in flexion. It occurs at the time of sudden directional change. This sign can be reproduced on physical examination. The majority of patients with this type of instability do not have medial collateral laxity, but all have demonstrable anterior instability. This subluxation is responsible for other entities, including flattening of the femoral condyle, cartilage, and the lateral meniscal tears seen in the majority of instances. The anterior drawer sign is not a good indicator of ACL insufficiency, the pivot shift "being present" when the drawer sign is equivocal (Galway et al. 1972, p. 763).

Galway, who had worked with MacIntosh in the cadaver experiments, was largely responsible for some of the stimulating encounters between Mac-Intosh and Kennedy.

Meanwhile, Losee (1983; Losee et al. 1978), working independently, had recognized the phenomenon in 1969 and had corresponded with Kennedy on the subject in the early 1970s. He did not formally report his findings until 1978, however.

Other tests, which were basically variations on the same theme, were described later by Hughston et al. (1976) (jerk test), Slocum et al. (1976) (anterior lateral rotatory instability test), Losee (1983; Losee et al. 1978), and Noyes et al. (1980) (flexion-rotation drawer). All of these signs have the same pathomechanical cause.

Stimulated by MacIntosh in 1973 and 1974, we brought the sign back to Switzerland and analyzed its pathology with regard to the function of the iliotibial tract (Hassler and Jakob 1981; Jakob 1987 a,b; Jakob et al. 1976, 1977, 1981, 1987, 1988).

Clinical Presentation and Pathomechanics of the Pivot Shift Sign

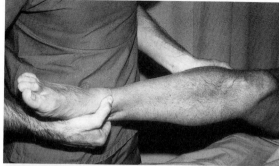
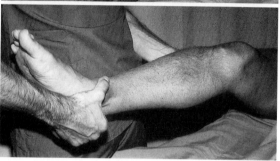

Fig. 1. Position for eliciting the pivot shift sign starting from full extension (see text)

As Galway et al. noted in 1972, the pivot shift is both a subjective symptom that is perceived by the athlete on the playing field and a physical sign that can be demonstrated on the examining table. On the playing field, the anterior subluxation occurs close to full extension when the foot is forcefully planted to make a sudden stop or to change direction by turning the upper torso away from the involved leg. Thus, when the right foot is planted, the upper body turns away at a right angle toward the left, and the body weight pivoting on the lateral tibial plateau imposes a valgus stress on the right knee. The strong quadriceps contraction required to keep the knee extended pulls the tibia forward beneath the femoral condyles. This process is significant in isolated cruciate ligament ruptures in skiers who perform a very powerful quadriceps contraction aimed at maintaining an upright posture in response to a backward shift of the body weight.

With the tibia in anterior subluxation, the athlete feels a sensation of "going out" or "coming apart," accompanied by severe pain as the supporting secondary capsular structures are stretched. Reduction occurs with a jerky or springlike motion as the knee is flexed further, probably accompanied by a reflex inhibition of the quadriceps. This is reinforced by the tense iliotibial tract, which at about 30°–40° of flexion moves from an extensor position anterior to the lateral epicondyle to a flexor position behind the flexion axis.

The description of the history is often so typical that a classic pivot shift test can be predicted. The classic history is that of an athlete who sustains a knee injury followed by recurrent episodes of giving way and locking consistent with a torn meniscus. After undergoing meniscectomy and resuming athletics, he notices that his knee suddenly and periodically gives way. This, together with recurrent bouts of symptomatic knee effusions, finally suggests the strong presumptive diagnosis of an ACL insufficiency.

The pivot shift test is performed with the patient supine and relaxed. The examiner holds the limb in extension, cradling the heel in one hand and placing the other behind the proximal tibia and fibula (Fig. 1). In this position the tibia will begin to subluxate anteriorly when a valgus pressure is applied to the lateral side of the knee. The excursion in anterior subluxation depends on the amount of valgus stress applied. We find that it is easier to elicit the sign when the patient's leg is held against the examiner's hip to transmit axial pressure. When the knee reaches 20°–40° of flexion, reduction occurs. The degree of flexion depends on the degree to which the tibia has subluxated. With a small amount of anterior translation, reduction will occur earlier. The diagnosis is supported by the patient's observation that the test reproduces the typical giving-way episodes experienced during athletics.

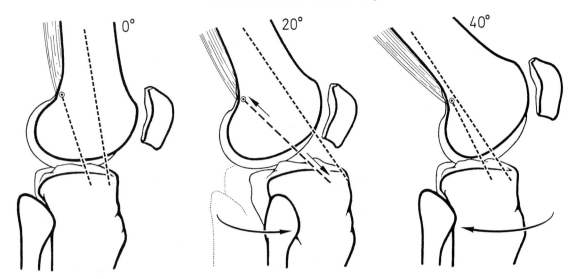

Fig. 2. Pathomechanics of the pivot shift phenomenon (see text). (From Jakob 1987a)

Later tests involved modifications of the MacIntosh maneuver. Hughston et al. (1976) described the "jerk test" in which the knee is flexed 90° and then gradually extended to elicit an anterior subluxation. Slocum et al. (1976) placed the patient in a lateral decubitus position with the affected side up, allowing the knee to fall into a valgus position. Losee (1983) and Losee et al. (1978) modified the test by holding the patient's knee with the thumb on the fibular head to control rotation. Noyes et al. (1980) stabilized the leg by grasping the upper tibia with a hand on each side and clamping the patient's foot between the examiner's arm and chest.

We do not feel that the particular method used is as important as the examiner's proficiency in performing at least one test correctly. We would, however, recommend the Noyes modification for apprehensive patients who have difficulty relaxing their hamstrings.

The *pathomechanics* of the pivot shift sign has been investigated by numerous authors. Galway and MacIntosh (1980) gave an excellent description highlighting the importance of the topographic anatomy of the lateral compartment (Fig. 2). The lateral tibial plateau is relatively short and convex, with the tibial articular cartilage forming a sharp drop-off posteriorly. This contrasts with the longer and inherently more stable medial plateau. When the ACL is deficient, the lateral femoral condyle glides farther posteriorly than normal and slips off the back of the plateau. As an expression of the pathologic rolling-gliding mechanism (Wirth and Artmann 1974), the knee remains in that position until it is reduced by flexion. The depth and contour of the lateral femoral condyle and the "limiting groove" probably also play a role.

In the mild and moderate forms of the pivot shift phenomenon, the medial compartment forms the kinematic center and rotational axis of the knee. Motion in that compartment is stabilized by the tension of the medial collateral structures and is largely rotational due to the congruity of the medial articular surfaces.

Subluxation of the lateral femoral condyle with respect to the anterior and posterior contours of the tibial plateau occurs only when those surfaces are pressed together by a valgus stress. The initial subluxating force is generated by quadriceps contraction aimed at stabilizing the knee during athletic activities in which the body weight is multiplied by landing from a jump or changing direction abruptly (cutting). As the tibia subluxates forward, the femorotibial fibers of the iliotibial tract become increasingly tense until a critical point is reached, at about 20°–40° flexion, where fiber tension is sufficient to reduce the tibia posteriorly (see Fig. 2).

The distracting forces during the subluxations progressively stretch the peripheral structures, leading to the development of a global anterior instability. As the posteromedial and posterolateral corners become lax, a secondary posterolateral instability also may develop.

The described pressure increase in the lateral compartment is produced by a valgus stress. This stress can augment the pivot shift phenomenon only as long as the medial collateral ligament retains some functional integrity. With complete rupture of that ligament, the pivot shift may disappear (Fig. 3a) (Jakob et al. 1976, 1977, 1981). The iliotibial tract plays a sig-

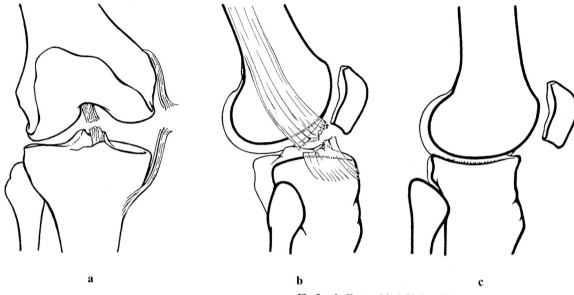

a   b   c

Fig. 3 a–d. Even with ACL insufficiency, a true pivot shift may not occur due to **a** a complete rupture of the medial collateral ligament, **b** rupture of the iliotibial tract, **c** a bucket-handle meniscus tear, or **d** progressive osteoarthritis of the lateral compartment. (From Jakob 1987 a)

d

nificant role in controlling the degree of the phenomenon. In cadaver experiments, we showed that division of the iliotibial tract increases the degree of anterior subluxation caused by severing the ACL, underscoring the importance of the tract as a secondary restraint to anterior translation. When the iliotibial tract is divided, the total reducing force is diminished, and the degree of pivot shift is markedly reduced. The tibia remains in anterior subluxation until the knee is flexed to 70°–80° (Fig. 3 b). A bucket handle tear of the meniscus also may dampen the subluxation and reduction maneuver (Fig. 3 c).

The impact of the phenomenon on the menisci, cartilage, and ligaments was vividly described by Galway

et al. (1972) and Galway and MacIntosh (1980) in their description of the "ACL syndrome" (Fig. 4). Although most of the anterior subluxation takes place in the lateral compartment, secondary damage is more apt to occur in the medial compartment. This is because there is a greater amount of stress transfer in the medial compartment, where loads are further compounded by progressive laxity of the lateral collateral structures and the development of a secondary progressive varus angulation. This damages the posterior horns of the menisci and leads to erosive changes in the cartilage on the femoral condyles. The forces acting on the lateral compartment tend to round off the convexity of the tibial plateau, molding it to the shape of the femoral condyle, with a consequent loss of mobility. The lateral condyle becomes flattened, while the tibial plateau develops anterior and posterior osteophytes which account for the self-stabilizing effect of the osteoarthritis and the disappearance of the pivot shift sign with increasing joint stiffness (see Fig. 3 d). The femoropatellar joint undergoes pathologic changes due to the increased medial and lateral pressure that develop in accordance with the limb morphotype and preexisting constitutional laxity.

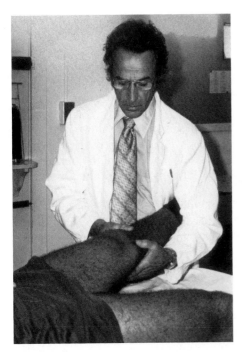

Fig. 4. The pivot shift test as performed by Dr. D. MacIntosh (photographed in 1973). Note how Dr. MacIntosh grasps the knee with both hands while immobilizing the foot between the elbow and torso

Grading the Pivot Shift

The pivot shift phenomenon demonstrates anterior instability in a Lachman position, i. e., near extension. The degree of anterior subluxation measured on Lachman stress radiographs reflects the anterior translation of the medial and lateral tibial plateaus. In most cases of global anterior laxity, translation is somewhat more pronounced on the lateral side than on the medial side. The degree of pivot shift subluxation is closely related to the instability of the medial compartment. The greater the amount of anterior subluxation on the medial side, the more pronounced the translation on the lateral side, and the greater the magnitude of the subluxation and subsequent reduction. MacIntosh himself stressed the importance of the anterior subluxation of the medial tibial condyle, which can be accurately assessed while observing the phenomenon in the patient's knee.

Grading the pivot shift poses certain difficulties. For example, the examiner must analyze both components of the elicited motion, i. e., translation and rotation of the tibia on the femur. Existing classifications are based on the simple impression of the intensity of the reduction maneuver and depend greatly on the technique of the examiner and the ability of the patient to relax his muscles.

Knee motions are characterized by the interplay and coupling of translations and rotations. The pivot shift phenomenon is an example of a coupled motion. The amount of translation observed depends on the degree of tibial rotation, with full translation requiring a particular rotational position. The principle of our classification is based on the attempt to intervene in the dynamic, coupled motion pattern and "uncouple" it by constraining tibial rotation.

In defining the position of rotation, it must be considered that both the hip and knee joints are involved, i. e., internal rotation of the knee joint is paralleled by internal rotation at the hip. This biarticular rotation can affect the tension of the iliotibial tract. Internal rotation at the hip and knee lengthens and tightens the tensor fasciae latae, causing a rise of pressure in the lateral compartment. External rotation relaxes the iliotibial tract and lowers the compartmental pressure. Maximum internal rotation will check anterior translation of the lateral plateau by imparting tension to the iliotibial tract. While this tension lessens the degree of the subluxation, reduction will occur with a more perceptible jerk in patients with a mildly positive pivot shift. A grade I pivot shift often cannot be elicited unless the limb is internally rotated; external rotation may abolish it. For a grade III pivot shift, though, slight external rotation during the test can increase the anterior translation of the upper tibia owing to the pronounced loosening effect on the posteromedial corner and anteromedial subluxation. This also lengthens the path of tibial reduction.

Conversely, maximum external rotation at the hip and knee in a forced terminal position can make it impossible to elicit a pivot shift sign, because this locks the tibia in an externally rotated position.

Abduction and adduction of the hip also influence the tension of the iliotibial tract. It has been shown, for example, that hip abduction produces a greater degree of pivot shift than adduction (Bach et al. 1988). Other factors such as hip flexion may also play a role.

In the classification proposed by us (Jakob et al. 1984), the following grades of pivot shift are recognized by degree of intensity:

– Grade I (1 +) pivot shift: Abnormal tibial translation occurs only when the tibia is held in maximum internal rotation; it is absent in neutral or external rotation (Fig. 5a). This shift can be perceived as a slight slip, is accompanied by pain in awake patients, and is somewhat easier to palpate in the

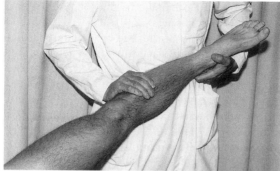

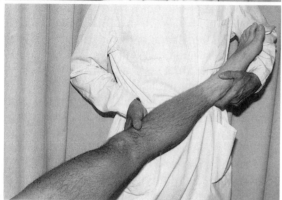

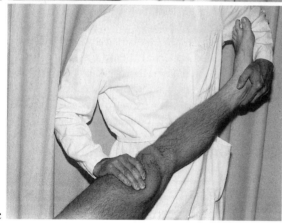

Fig. 5 a–c. Various rotational positions are used to grade the intensity of the pivot shift: **a** forced internal rotation (grade I pivot shift), **b** neutral rotation (grade II pivot shift), **c** external rotation. The right hand rotates the femur internally, the left hand rotates the tibia externally (grade III). The position in **c** makes it difficult to elicit a grade I pivot shift because the external tibial rotation reduces the anterior subluxation. (From Jakob 1987 b)

anesthetized joint. This grade corresponds to the American "trace" pivot shift and the French "ressaut en bâtard."

– Grade II (2 +) pivot shift: The test is positive in neutral and internal rotation but negative when the tibia is held in definite external rotation (Fig. 5 b). Translation on the lateral side is easily perceived visually and by palpation. A less obvious anterior shift of the medial tibial plateau can be detected by noting a change in the medial step-off between the femoral condyle and tibial plateau with the palpating finger. A distinct "clunk" is perceived when the tibia is in the internally rotated position.

Examination with this technique allows a clear distinction between a grade I and grade II pivot shift, both by the rotational position of the tibia and by the qualitative difference in the intensity of the subluxation.

– Grade III (3 +) pivot shift: Abnormal translation with a pronounced "clunk" can be elicited when the tibia is held in neutral or external rotation (Fig. 5 c). The sign is less obvious in internal rotation. A grade III shift is seen in acute injuries with moderate damage to posteromedial and posterolateral structures and a complete rupture of the ACL. It is also seen in knees with severe chronic instability and associated stretching of the secondary posterior restraints.

These three grades of pivot shift represent a progression from mild anterolateral laxity in grade I to increasing anterior translation of both compartments in grade III. The successive use of three positions of tibial rotation selects the most clinically significant points from this continuum.

This grading system was developed on the basis of a parallel study in which the degree of anterior translation on Lachman stress radiographs was determined for the medial and lateral tibial plateaus (Fig. 6 a = grade II pivot shift, Fig. 6 b = grade III pivot shift). In knees with a grade I pivot shift, the medial tibial plateau showed an average anterior displacement of 5 mm, the lateral plateau 12 mm (Fig. 6 c); the Lachman test showed an average shift of 9 mm measured at the level of the tibial tuberosity.

The grade II pivot shift was associated with an average of 10 mm medial and 18 mm lateral plateau displacement, the Lachman test indicating 10–15 mm of motion. This instability is common after an isolated rupture of the ACL, both in acute and chronic cases. The grade III pivot shift gave an average subluxation of 15 mm medially and 22 mm laterally, with a 15-mm displacement in the Lachman test (Fig. 6 c).

One difficulty in the pivot shift test lies in distinguishing the true pivot shift from the reversed pivot shift, a dynamic sign that reflects posterolateral rotatory instability, increases with external tibial rotation, and decreases with internal rotation (Fig. 7). The differentiation between these signs and the grading of the pivot shift provide the basis for a better under-

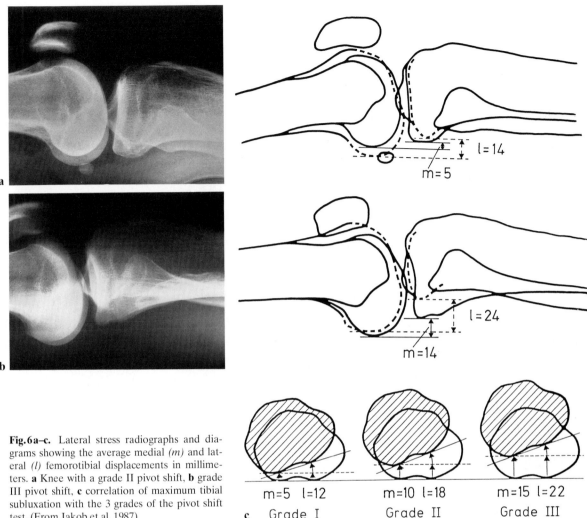

Fig. 6a–c. Lateral stress radiographs and diagrams showing the average medial *(m)* and lateral *(l)* femorotibial displacements in millimeters. **a** Knee with a grade II pivot shift, **b** grade III pivot shift, **c** correlation of maximum tibial subluxation with the 3 grades of the pivot shift test. (From Jakob et al. 1987)

standing of the pathomorphology and management of anterior instability.

Therapeutic Aspects of the Pivot Shift

The pivot shift phenomenon has been called a "lateral compartment event" for the following reasons: (1) As noted above, the lateral compartment displaces somewhat more than the medial compartment. (2) The pivot shift phenomenon is possible only when there is greater stress transfer in the lateral compartment, i.e., when a varus stress is applied. (3) The pivoting is made possible by the biconvexity of the lateral articular surfaces. Since the inception of the pivot shift concept, surgical attention has focused on the treatment of the lateral side. The value or benefit of a grading system depends ultimately on its useful-

ness as an aid to therapeutic planning. During the past 6 years we have used this grading system as a decision-making criterion in the evaluation, treatment, and follow-up of patients with a positive pivot shift.

Several authors have independently developed surgical procedures that attempt to duplicate the function of the ACL with an extraarticular substitute. These extraarticular reconstructions are designed so that the redirected fibers of the substitute run parallel to the ACL, forming a lateral femorotibial ligament. Lemaire (1967), Galway et al. (1972), Galway and MacIntosh (1980), Losee (1983), Losee et al. (1978), Arnold et al. (1979), and Jakob et al. (1988) have used distally based strips of fascia lata routed beneath the lateral collateral ligament or passed through an osseous tunnel to construct a femorotibial ligament. Galway et al. (1972) and Galway and MacIntosh (1980) demonstrated the effect of this technique by inserting a Kirschner wire through the iliotibial tract

Internal rotation   Neutral rotation   External rotation

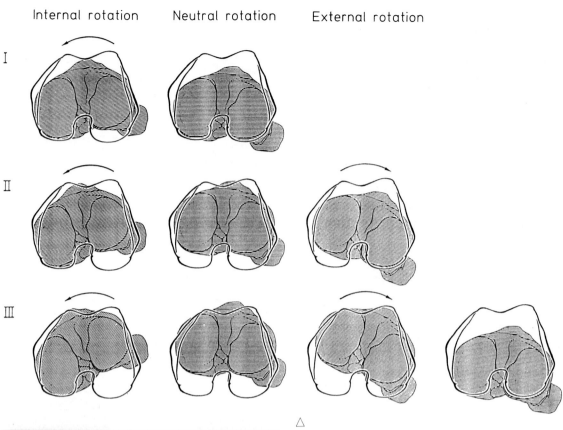

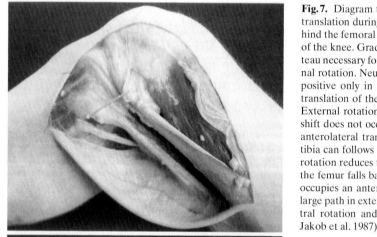

△

Fig. 7. Diagram to illustrate how the amount of anterior tibial translation during pivot shift, represented by the clear area behind the femoral condyles, is affected by the rotational position of the knee. Grade I: The anterior translation of the lateral plateau necessary for a grade I pivot shift occurs in maximum internal rotation. Neutral or external rotation reduces it. The test is positive only in internal rotation. Grade II: Marked anterior translation of the tibia occurs in internal and neutral rotation. External rotation reduces the lateral compartment, so a pivot shift does not occur. Grade III: Pronounced anteromedial and anterolateral translation. In neutral and external rotation the tibia can follows the path to maximum anterior laxity. Internal rotation reduces the posteromedial corner. In external rotation the femur falls backward due to gravity while the tibia initially occupies an anteriorly displaced position, then reduces over a large path in external rotation. Pivot shift is pronounced in neutral rotation and is accentuated by external rotation. (From Jakob et al. 1987)

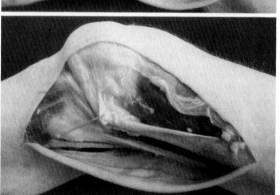

◁

Fig. 8. Demonstration of the effect of fixation of the iliotibial tract with a Kirschner wire inserted anteriorly at the level of the lateral epicondyle in the flexed knee. By redirecting the course of the tract fibers, the wire restraints anterior tibial displacement as the knee extends. This classic experiment of MacIntosh demonstrates the effect of lateral extraarticular reconstructions of the ACL

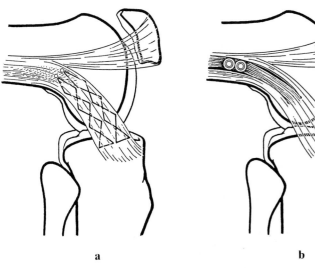

a   b   c

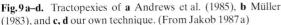

Fig. 9 a–d. Tractopexies of **a** Andrews et al. (1985), **b** Müller (1983), and **c, d** our own technique. (From Jakob 1987 a)

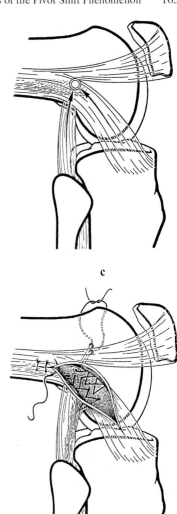

d

at the level of the femoral epicondyle with the knee flexed (Fig. 8). This abolished the pivot shift phenomenon at once, because the intact fibers of the iliotibial tract were now rerouted behind the wire and became tense as the flexed knee was extended. Running parallel to the ACL, these fibers held the knee in a reduced position.

Experience has shown that these techniques can eliminate the dynamic pivot shift phenomenon in patients with mild or moderate instabilities. Because these procedures do not involve entry into the joint space itself, the risk of postoperative scarring is decreased. It is known, however, that in joints with progressive anterior instability where there is marked translation of the medial tibial plateau, a lateral repair is inadequate and is prone to secondary loosening. Even if the procedure eliminates the pivot shift initially, it will culminate in a recurrence approximately equal in severity to the original instability. We feel that these procedures also carry a risk of secondary varus instability since they compromise the integrity of the iliotibial tract. It is our experience, moreover, that the excessive removal of tract material leads to a secondary posterolateral instability that frequently is manifested by a slight reversed pivot shift.

Andrews et al. (1985) developed a technique in which the whole iliotibial tract is fixed to the lateral femoral condyle with transosseous sutures to create a lateral femorotibial ligament (Fig. 9 a). Müller (1983) proposed using a strip of iliotibial tract isolated by anterior and posterior longitudinal incisions, leaving the strip attached proximally and distally (Fig. 9 b).

This isolated fascia lata strip was then fastened to the lateral aspect of the femur directly anterior to the lateral intermuscular septum. For some time we used a technique in which a distally based fascia lata strip was routed beneath the common femoral attachment of the lateral collateral ligament and popliteus tendon and then sutured to itself, but mild degrees of ensuing secondary posterolateral instability led us to adopt a simple tractopexy in which a small-fragment screw with plastic washer is inserted through all layers of the iliotibial tract at an isometric site (Fig. 9 c). Unfortunately this tractopexy has led to instances of painful bursitis and restricted motion, demonstrating the importance of free gliding of the iliotibial tract over the lateral epicondyle.

We are now convinced that sacrificing or refixing portions of the iliotibial tract may be harmful for several

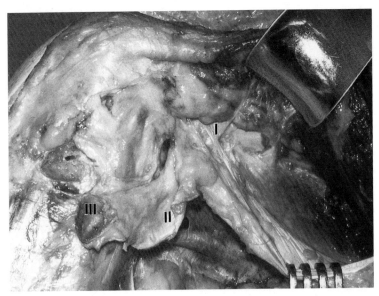

Fig. 10. Anatomy of the iliotibial tract (lateral aspect of the left knee). *I* Attachment of the Kaplan fibers to the intermuscular septum on the femur. Tract fibers arise 1 cm distal to that point and pass distally *(II)* to the tubercle of Gerdy *(III)*, here detached. This structure forms a lateral femorotibial ligament that functions as a lateral tension band to withstand varus loading. It correlates with the retrograde fiber tract of Lobenhoffer and is also mentioned by Müller (1985). Over the lateral epicondyle, these fibers connect with deeper structures by areolar tissue. Terry et al. (1986) described a relation to the aponeurosis of the lateral gastrocnemius and plantaris muscles

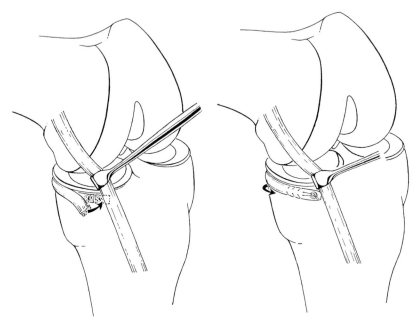

Fig. 11. The horizontal arm of the semimembranosus tendon is detached on a bone fragment and advanced beneath the medial collateral ligament to reinforce the posteromedial capsule in patients with marked anteromedial instability. (From Jakob 1987b)

reasons: Terry et al. (1986) have identified connections between the deep capsulo-osseous layer of the iliotibial tract and the aponeurosis of the lateral gastrocnemius and plantaris muscles, which perform a restraining function. When substantial portions of the iliotibial tract are removed and reattached elsewhere, this posterolateral protective function is lost to the knee.

The iliotibial tract is an important reinforcing structure for the weak lateral collateral ligament and counteracts the extrinsic varus-producing effect of the medial body-weight axis in the one-legged stance phase (Bousquet and Rhenter 1982). As noted with reference to the pathomechanics of medial cartilage degeneration, a loss of lateral coaptation in the knee due to weakness of the iliotibial tract could account for the varus tendency and thus for the mechanical overload on the medial side. It is our current belief that the iliotibial tract with its femorotibial connections is basically an anisometric structure, a belief supported by the fact that the tract is controlled by a muscle, the tensor fasciae latae, at its proximal end. To a degree, however, the iliotibial tract may also be regarded as isometric. For the past 3 years, therefore, we have used a lateral repair designed to reinforce the lateral femorotibial ligament and restrain anterolateral displacement. This technique reinforces the "retrograde fiber tract" described by Lobenhoffer et al. (1987), which we illustrated in a somewhat different form in 1981 (Fig. 10) (Jakob et al. 1981).

Drawing on the techniques of Andrews et al. (1985) and Müller (1983), we incise the superficial layer of the iliotibial tract at its anterior border and sharply dissect it from the deep layer. We then pass heavy nonabsorbable sutures through the deep layer and fix it to an isometric site on the femur using transosseous threads brought out on the medial side or pullout threads from a cruciate ligament-bone block anchored to the femur. The isometric site corresponds to the prolongation of the supracondylar contour of the femoral condyle where the condyle tapers to unite with the shaft at the insertion of the Kaplan fibers (Fig. 9 c). Following fixation of the deep tract layer, the superficial layer is closed with a row of absorbable sutures that encompass part of the deep layer. The repair also reinforces the posterolateral corner through the deep capsulo-osseous attachments with the arcuate complex. This lateral reinforcement technique supplements our cruciate ligament reconstruction with the patellar ligament, and our experience in the past 2 years has been favorable.

While we treat moderately severe anterior instabilities with a grade II pivot shift by reconstruction with the central one-third of the patellar ligament attached with 2 bone blocks and reinforced by the extraarticular tractopexy described above, we feel that an extra measure is needed for more severe forms. A grade III pivot shift with massive subluxation in external rotation is invariably associated with significant medial or posteromedial attenuation. In these cases we add a medial reconstruction in which the horizontal arm of the semimembranosus tendon is advanced beneath the medial collateral ligament to tighten the posteromedial capsule (Fig. 11). This demonstrates the potentially great value of a precise description of the pivot shift phenomenon based on a specific classification in directing therapeutic planning.

We thank Mr. W. R. Hess, Department of Instructional Medicine, University of Bern and Inselspital Bern, for providing the illustrations (Figs. 2, 3, 7, 9).

References

Andrews JR, Sanders RA, Morin B (1985) Surgical treatment of anterolateral rotatory instability. Am J Sports Med 73: 112–119

Arnold JA, Coker TP, Heaton LM et al. (1979) Natural history of anterior cruciate tears. Am J Sports Med 7: 305–313

Bach BR, Warren RF, Wickiewicz TL (1988) The pivot shift phenomenon: results and description of a modified test for anterior crucial ligament in sufficiency. Am J Sports Med 16/6: 571–576

Bousquet G, Rhenter JL (1982) Illustré du genou. Mure, Le Coteau

Felsenreich F (1934) Klinik der Kreuzbandverletzungen. Arch Klin Chir 179: 375–408

Galway HR, MacIntosh DL (1980) The lateral pivot shift. A symptom and sign of anterior cruciate ligament instability. Clin Orthop 147: 45

Galway HR, Beaupré A, MacIntosh DL (1972) Pivot shift. A clinical sign of anterior cruciate ligament instability. J Bone Joint Surg [Br] 54: 763

Hassler H, Jakob RP (1981) Ein Beitrag zur Ursache der anterolateralen Instabilität des Kniegelenkes. Eine Studie an 20 Leichenknien unter besonderer Berücksichtigung des Tractus iliotibialis. Arch Orthop Trauma Surg 98: 45–50

Hey Groves EW (1920) The crucial ligaments of the knee joint: Their function, rupture, and the operative treatment of the same. Br J Surg 7: 505–515

Hughston JD, Andrews JR, Cross MJ et al (1976) Classification of knee ligament instabilities. Part I. The medial compartment and cruciate ligaments. J Bone Joint Surg [Am] 58: 159

Jakob RP (1987 a) Pathomechanical and clinical concepts of the pivot shift sign. Semin Orthop 2: 9–17

Jakob RP (1987 b) Indikation, Behandlung und Evaluation bei chronischer vorderer Kreuzband-Instabilität. Orthopade 16: 130–139

Jakob RP, Noesberger B, Saxer U (1976) Der Wert des Pivot-shift-Phänomens und der lateralen Rekonstruktion; zur Diagnose und Therapie der vorderen Kreuzbandruptur. Annual Meeting of the Schweiz Gesellschaft für Sportmedizin, Fribourg, October 21. Haupt, Bern, S 69-84

Jakob RP, Noesberger B, Müller ME (1977) The diagnostic value of the pivot shift sign in anterior instability of the knee and specific lateral repair. In: Chapchal G (ed) Injuries of the ligaments and their repair. Hand - knee - foot. Seventh International Symposium on Topical Problems in Orthopaedic Surgery Lucerne. Thieme, Stuttgart, pp 95-102

Jakob RP, Hassler H, Stäubli H-U (1981) Observations on rotatory instability of the lateral compartment of the knee. Acta Orthop Scand 52 [Suppl 191]

Jakob RP, Stäubli H-U, Deland JT (1987) Grading the pivot shift. Objective tests with implications for treatment. J Bone Joint Surg [Br] 69: 294-299

Jakob RP, Kipfer W, Klaue K, Stäubli H-U, Gerber C (1988) Étude critique de la reconstruction du ligament croisé antérieur du genou par la plastie pédiculée sur le Hoffa à partir du tiers médian du tendon rotulien, 50 genoux opérés avec recul de 2 à 4 ans. Rev Chir Orthop 74: 44-51

Jones R, Smith A (1913) On rupture of the crucial ligaments of the knee and on fractures of the spine of the tibia. Br J Surg 1: 70-89

Lemaire M (1967) Ruptures anciennes du ligament croisé antérieur du genou. J Chir (Paris) 93: 311-320

Lobenhoffer P, Posel P, Witt S, Piehler J, Wirth CJ (1987) Distal femoral fixation of the iliotibial tract. Arch Orthop Trauma Surg 106: 285-290

Losee RE (1983) Concepts of the pivot shift. Clin Orthop 172: 45-51

Losee RE, Johnson TR, Southwick WO (1978) Anterior subluxation of the lateral tibial plateau. A diagnostic text and operative repair. J Bone Joint Surg [Am] 60: 1015

Müller We (1983) The knee. Form, function and ligament reconstruction. Springer, Berlin Heidelberg New York Tokyo

Noyes FR, Basset RW, Grood ES et al. (1980) Arthroscopy in acute traumatic hemarthrosis of the knee. J Bone Joint Surg [Am] 62: 687-695

Slocum DB, James SL, Larson RL et al. (1976) Clinical test for anterolateral rotatory instability of the knee. Clin Orthop 118: 63

Terry GC, Hughston JC, Norwood LA (1986) The anatomy of the iliotibial tract. Am J Sports Med 14: 39-45

Wirth CJ, Artmann M (1974) Verhalten der Roll-Gleit-Bewegung des belasteten Kniegelenkes bei Verlust und Ersatz des vorderen Kreuzbandes. Arch Orthop Unfallchir 78: 356

Anterior Subluxation in Knees with Chronic Anterior Cruciate Ligament Insufficiency: A Comparison of Arthrometry and Stressradiography

H.-U. Stäubli, R. P. Jakob, and B. Noesberger

It is generally acknowledged that the severity of a knee injury can be assessed by the clinical testing of knee stability. Although a number of objective test procedures have been devised (Kennedy and Fowler 1971; Markolf et al. 1978; Jacobsen 1981; Stedtfeld and Strobel 1988; Shino et al. 1984; Daniel et al. 1985; Edixhoven 1986; Edixhoven et al. 1987; Kärrholm et al. 1988), the diagnosis of a knee instability is based largely on the systematic evaluation of the primary and secondary restraints of the knee joint. Although some instability tests are widely used, there are significant examiner-dependent variations in terms of the starting position for varus-valgus testing and the resting position prior to anteroposterior drawer testing. Systematic preoperative stability testing of the cruciate and collateral ligaments can be hampered by various factors such as pain, effusion, and muscle spasm. Thus, systematic instability testing under anesthesia, as recommended by the Swiss OAK knee group (Müller et al. 1988), is preferred over clinical testing without anesthesia for the documentation of comparable, reproducible physical findings.

An established clinical test for diagnosing anterior cruciate ligament (ACL) insufficiency is the Lachman test, popularized by Torg et al. (1976). Anteroposterior drawer testing near extension (20°–25° flexion) has been advocated by Torg et al. (1976), Trillat et al. (1978), Stäubli et al. (1985), and Müller et al. (1988) as an important clinical sign for the evaluation of ACL deficiency. In this test attention is given to the direction and amount of anteroposterior translation and to the resilience of the anterior or posterior end point in order to assess the restraining action of the ACL or PCL. The resulting anterior-posterior displacements of the medial and lateral tibial plateaus with respect to the medial and lateral femoral condyles are estimated separately for each compartment and are stated in millimeters. When this test is performed in the supine patient with distal thigh support, the force of gravity causes a slight posterior sag of the tibia relative to the femur. This resting position is affected by quadriceps and hamstring tone in the sense that a slight tensing or contraction of the quadriceps generates an *anterior* force vector (Daniel et al. 1985) while hamstring contraction creates a *posterior* force vector acting on the upper tibia. These effects alter the resting position of the joint, i.e., the position of the tibia in relation to the femur. Performing the Lachman test in the prone patient, as recommended by Feagin, permits painless anterior drawer testing with relaxation of the quadriceps and hamstrings, even in acute trauma cases with hemarthrosis (Feagin 1988). Anterior displacement of the tibia with respect to the femur in the slightly flexed knee accompanied by an altered end-point resilience is diagnostic of ACL insufficiency (Torg et al. 1976). Posterior displacement of the tibia near extension signifies a lesion of the PCL (Stäubli and Jakob 1990) and/or associated lesions of the posterolateral corner of the capsule (Stäubli and Birrer 1990). Definition of the starting position, resting position, neutral position, state of quadriceps tension, constitutional ligament quality, morphotype, and the direction, nature, and magnitude of applied forces and torques with respect to a given knee position enable us to make an accurate clinical assessment of the integrity, partial deficiency, or complete incompetence of the primary and secondary restraints of the knee joint. Large discrepancies in the stability test results reported by different examiners (Daniel 1989; Noyes et al. 1989) and the difficulty of defining the neutral position have led to the development of objective methods for the measurement of femorotibial displacement. In this chapter we shall examine several types of knee testing apparatus and their principles of operation. Generally these test devices measure the relative mobility of the femorotibial joint at a designated flexion angle while defined forces and moments are applied.

These devices provide output data in the form of continuously recorded force-displacement curves or displacements measured at a point, i.e., positions measured at the end point and representing the limits of pathologic motion between the femur and tibia. The test conditions in these studies can be precisely defined, and the applied forces and torques can be accurately measured. Femorotibial displacement depends on the angle of knee flexion, the three planes

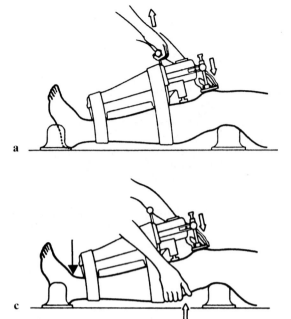

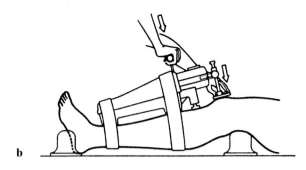

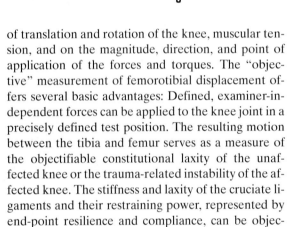

Fig. 1a–c. The KT 1000 arthrometer of Daniel et al. (1985). **a** Anterior drawer stress of 10 kp. **b** Measurement of posterior drawer motion after applying a posterior force of 10 kp. **c** Maximum manual anterior drawer stress. Care is taken that the heel is not lifted from the foot rest *(arrow)*

of translation and rotation of the knee, muscular tension, and on the magnitude, direction, and point of application of the forces and torques. The "objective" measurement of femorotibial displacement offers several basic advantages: Defined, examiner-independent forces can be applied to the knee joint in a precisely defined test position. The resulting motion between the tibia and femur serves as a measure of the objectifiable constitutional laxity of the unaffected knee or the trauma-related instability of the affected knee. The stiffness and laxity of the cruciate ligaments and their restraining power, represented by end-point resilience and compliance, can be objectively measured and compared with a normal population (Edixhoven 1986).

Clinical Testing Devices

The KT 1000 or KT 2000 Arthrometer of Daniel

This knee testing apparatus (Fig. 1 a–c) developed by Daniel, Stone, and Sachs uses patellar and tibial-tuberosity sensor pads to measure the relative patellotibial displacement of the knee under various applied loads. Right-left differences and compliance values, i.e., data on the distensibility of the ACL, can be measured and compared for anterior applied forces of 89 N (10 kp) and 67 N (7.5 kp). These measurements, together with the maximum manual anterior displacement, permit an accurate assessment of

the functional competence of the ACL in 90% of subjects tested (Daniel et al. 1985).

The numerical data output is plotted continuously during the test. Daniel claims that the readouts are sufficient to differentiate between a cruciate ligament-intact and cruciate ligament-deficient population.

The KT 1000 arthrometer includes a thigh rest that is placed beneath the distal femur to give proximal support to the knee. A foot rest is used to control tibial rotation. With the knee positioned at 20°–30° flexion, an anteriorly directed force of 67 or 89 N is administered through a force-sensing handle without anesthesia. The measurements taken for the two loads are supplemented by a determination of the maximum manual anterior displacement, which proved to be diagnostic in more than 90% of patients with a disruption of the ACL (Daniel et al. 1985). Care must be taken, however, that application of a maximum posteroanterior force does not lift the heel from the foot rest and that the knee flexion angle and relative positions of the patellar and tuberosity sensor pads are not disturbed. Another critical point is the definition of the resting position, since the tibia sags several millimeters under its own weight when the distal femur is supported. The calibration of the neutral, resting or starting position, then, is not identical with the anatomically defined neutral position of bony contour tangents (to the femoral condyles or tibial plateaus) in the sagittal plane (Stäubli 1990).

Similar testing devices such as the Stryker Laxity Tester, Knee Signature System (KSS), and the portable

UCLA knee tester of Markolf are based on similar principles of measuring patellotibial displacement.

The Portable UCLA Knee Tester

The portable knee testing apparatus developed by Markolf at the University of California in Los Angeles in 1976 (Fig. 2) uses a spring-scale principle to give a continuous force-displacement readout of femorotibial motion during the application of an anteroposterior force with the knee flexed 15°. The distal femur is clamped in place during the test by a framework containing three sand-filled pads. A force of 200 N is applied manually through a spring-loaded plunger strapped to the proximal lower leg. The displacement picked up by the calibrated measuring unit is continuously recorded on an X-Y plotter. Laxity, represented by the degree of displacement in relation to the applied force, and stiffness, represented by the slope of the force-displacement curves, can be read directly on the X-Y plotter.

Using the UCLA tester on knees positioned in 20° of flexion, Markolf et al. (1978) showed that a significant preoperative anterior displacement averaging 12.2 mm in ACL-deficient knees could be reduced to a residual value of 5.7 mm 3 years after anterior cruciate reconstruction. This portable knee tester can provide objective, examiner-independent information on laxity and stiffness without anesthesia in normal and cruciate ligament-deficient knees. Markolf notes that this biomechanical testing of anterior cruciate parameters provides a means of comparing populations with ACL insufficiency that have been treated by different methods. Markolf et al. (1978) note the possibility of making an objective, subject-independent, reproducible, noninvasive evaluation of knee stability and residual laxity, with a side-to-side comparison, before and after ACL reconstruction. Sherman et al. (1987) compared a new model of the portable UCLA tester with the KT 1000 arthrometer for measuring anterior laxity in normal and ACL-deficient knees. Normal ranges for both devices were established for a control group of 48 subjects with intact cruciate ligaments. With the UCLA device at 200 N of applied anterior force, 95% of the normal knees had a physiologic anterior laxity less than 8 mm and a right-left difference less than 2 mm. The corresponding values for the KT 1000 at 89 N were 9 mm and 2 mm, respectively. Thus, despite the application of more than twice the force, measurements taken with the UCLA device were smaller than with the KT 1000 arthrometer.

When anterior laxity was measured in 19 ACL-defi-

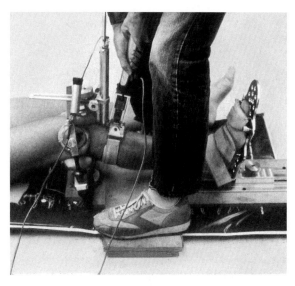

Fig. 2. UCLA knee tester of Markolf (1984 version). The distal femur and anterior patellar surface are clamped against a rest, fixing the knee in a position of 25° flexion. A spring scale equipped with a load cell measures anteroposterior patello-femoral displacement while the tibia is held in neutral rotation by a foot plate. This system measures femorotibial displacement with constrained rotation

cient knees, both devices showed that the anterior displacement was approximately twice that on the normal side. A 1:1 correlation was not found for the two devices. Both demonstrated an objectifiable anterior laxity in 90%–95% of ACL-deficient knees, whose degree of laxity was outside the normal range. A direct comparison of mean laxities at 89 N showed that the UCLA measurements were markedly smaller than the KT 1000 in both normal and cruciate ligament-deficient knees. Sherman (1987) attributes this discrepancy to the fact that the UCLA device clamps the femur in place while the KT 1000 does not, the femur simply resting on a thigh support. Another possible cause, Sherman suggests, is that clamping the distal thigh in the UCLA device may cause spasm or increased tension of the quadriceps and hamstrings, which could affect the resting position of the knee joint.

Drawer Tester of Edixhoven

Edixhoven et al. reported in 1987 on the accuracy and reproducibility of drawer measurements with their instrumented knee testing apparatus. The apparatus used by these authors (Fig. 3) consists of a comfortable seat that places the patient's hip in approximately 90° of flexion. The distal femur is se-

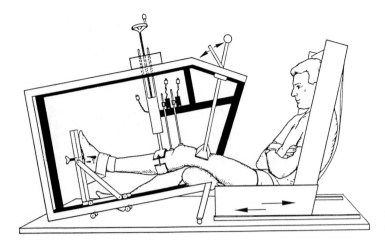

Fig. 3. AP drawer tester of Edixhoven et al. (1987)

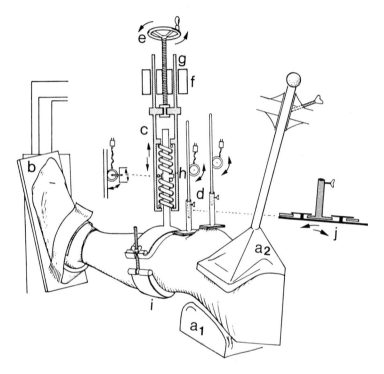

Fig. 4. Schematic diagram of the AP drawer tester of Edixhoven et al. (1987). *a1*, *a2*, Thigh holder; *b*, foot holder to control tibial rotation; *c*, cross section of the spring used to administer AP force; *d*, electropotentiometers for measuring relative motion between the anterior surfaces of the patella and tibial tuberosity; *e*, spindle; *gf*, load cell. (From Edixhoven et al. 1989)

cured with a thigh holder that compresses the quadriceps anteriorly and the hamstrings posteriorly. The tibia is held in a stable rotational position by a footplate, and anteroposterior forces are applied to the proximal tibia with a spindle. Displacement transducers are positioned on the tibial tuberosity and the anterior surface of the patella to measure relative displacement in the anteroposterior direction. The schematic view of the apparatus in Fig. 4 shows the components of the thigh holder, the fixation of tibial rotation by an adjustable footplate, and the strap encircling the ankle. The anteroposterior forces administered by the spindle and spring-scale principle and

the potentiometers for measuring relative patellotibial motion in units of electrical potential are also graphically shown.

Comparing the findings in 29 ACL-deficient knees with a normal population of 64 knees with intact cruciate ligaments, the authors found that both a significant anterior and posterior displacement could be demonstrated with their apparatus (see Fig. 4). Instrumented measurements in 28 patients with PCL insufficiency showed that, compared with the normal population (Fig. 5a), the starting position of the knee joint prior to application of an anteroposterior force was shifted 3.5 mm posteriorly (Fig. 5b). The effect of

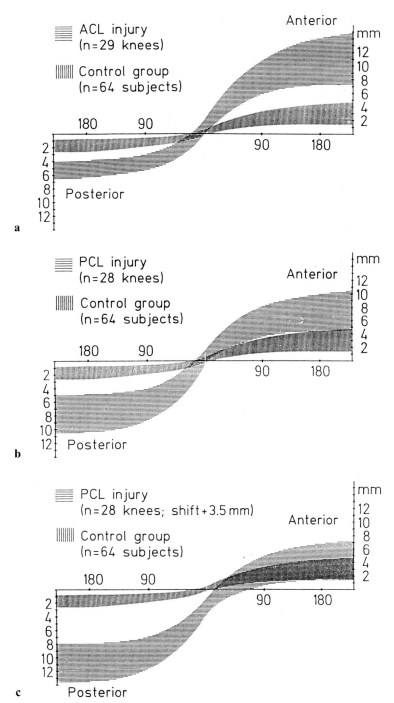

Fig. 5. a Anteroposterior displacement measured by the AP drawer tester of Edixhoven (1986) in a group of patients with chronic anterior cruciate insufficiency (n = 29) compared with a normal population with an intact ACL (n = 64). The chronic group shows a markedly increased anterior instability combined with a slight posterior instability. (After Edixhoven 1986.) **b** A group of 28 patients with chronic posterior cruciate insufficiency compared with a normal population of 64 cruciate ligament-intact subjects. The somewhat more posterior (3.5 mm), non-gravity-corrected starting position of the tibia results in a significant posterior displacement and a marked associated anterior laxity. **c** With + 3.5 mm gravity correction for the posterior sag, the posterior laxity is more clearly appreciated. The scatter and extent of the accompanying anterior laxity in this PCL-deficient population are greater than the physiologic anterior joint play in normal subjects with an intact ACL. (From Edixhoven et al. 1989)

gravity compard with a normal population is shown graphically in Fig. 5 c, which demonstrates a significantly more pronounced posterior subluxation of the tibia.

Problems with Clinical Knee Testing Devices

The designers of the various testing systems claim that their devices can objectively record anteroposterior femorotibial displacement as an index of cruciate ligament insufficiency. Indeed, sensor plates are positioned on the patella and tibial tuberosity in a designated angle of knee flexion, a defined force is applied, and the resulting displacement is measured. As this occurs, the patella is pressed against the femoral trochlea. It is assumed that motion of the patella is representative of femorotibial displacement. Pathomechanics tells us, however, that an anterior drawer stress applied to a knee joint near extension always elicits a coupled motion. This consists of anterior translation and internal rotation of the tibia in both normal and ACL-deficient knees (Stäubli 1990). Conventional test devices represent these coupled motions as pure translation on the force-displacement curve, although in a knee with an "isolated" anterior cruciate deficiency, for example, one can demonstrate an almost exclusive anterolateral unicompartmental motion, which is much more pronounced than the anteromedial motion. Objective test devices record combined motions like coupled anterior translation and internal rotation as pure translational motions. Thus, effective compartmental motions that occur physiologically with an intact cruciate ligament or following loss of the primary restraint are replaced by central anteroposterior motion patterns. Another problem with knee testers is the difficulty of measuring and defining the neutral point or neutral position and the resting or starting position of the joint (Edixhoven 1986). One way to determine the neutral starting position is proposed by Daniel (1985), who defines the "quadriceps neutral" angle at 70° of knee flexion, where the patella and thus the patellar ligament are directly above the insertion of the patellar tendon over the tibial tuberosity. In this position, according to Daniel (1989), extensor contraction produces no anterior or posterior displacement of the tibia with respect to the femur. At the quadriceps neutral angle neither a spontaneous *posterior sag* nor an *actively induced anterior drawer* can be demonstrated in awake subjects (Daniel 1989).

The state of tension of the quadriceps and hamstrings is a very important factor when near-extension drawer testing is performed with an instrumented device. In 20° of flexion the patella and patellar ligament are anterior to the tibial tuberosity. When the femur is supported distally in this position, the tibia normally sags 2–3 mm posteriorly due to gravity, even when the PCL is intact. Quadriceps contraction will produce a relative anterior shift of the tibia from this initial position. This raises the problem of differentiating between an effective, active, quadriceps-induced anterior tibial shift in the anterior cruciate-deficient knee and a reduction of the tibia from posterior subluxation into the neutral position in a knee with a deficient PCL (Stäubli and Jakob 1990).

New concepts in the clinical evaluation of knee instability stress the importance of analyzing the limits of compartmental motion in the knee. This involves the clinical measurement of the anterior displacements of the medial and lateral compartments of the joint (International Knee Documentation Committee of the AOSSM/ESKA 1988/1989). The extent, direction, and nature of the displacements and the anterior and posterior end-point resiliencies are carefully recorded. Test devices that use sensors placed against the outer contours of the knee "lump together" abnormal coupled motions (such as coupled translation and internal rotation of the tibia with respect to the femur) into a global, centralized motion; at present these devices are unable to analyze the separate motions of the individual compartments. Edixhoven et al. developed an instrumented drawer tester for the in vivo measurement of anteroposterior displacement (Edixhoven 1986; Edixhoven et al. 1987). Because the neutral position cannot be measured objectively, the extent of the anterior and posterior motion segment does not agree with the recorded motion segments in the determination of total anteroposterior displacement.

Clinical Importance of Arthrometry

Arthrometry, denoting the measurement of anterior-posterior subluxation or medial-lateral joint space opening between the femur and tibia, is generally performed with the patient awake and unanesthetized. Clamping the distal femur in a leg holder, as in the UCLA and Edixhoven devices, can be quite uncomfortable, as we know from personal testing of both devices. Pain due to compression of the quadriceps and hamstrings against the femur may cause tension in these muscle groups, which in turn can affect the outcome of passive drawer testing when a large force is used. The advantage of these methods is that, correctly performed, they provide an examiner-independent measurement of global tibial displacement with respect to the femur. Another advantage is that they permit defined, measurable forces to be administered to the knee in a designated test position. The devices can record continuous force-displacement curves, measure the compliance of the intact ACL and PCL, and identify motion limits in cruciate ligament-deficient knees.

The disadvantage of these test devices lies the inevitability of soft-tissue interference in the measurement of femorotibial displacement. Basically the devices measure the motion of the patella, stabilized in the femoral trochlea, in relation to the tibial tuberosity; this is why coupled motions such as combined translation and internal rotation cannot be separately evaluated. A disadvantage of these indirect, outer-contour-oriented methods is that the neutral point, or the normal relationship of the medial and lateral femorotibial compartments on the sagittal plane and the femorotibial relation in the resting or starting position, cannot be precisely defined. As a result, patients with constitutional posterolateral laxity, posterior laxity coexisting with ACL insufficiency, or a predominantly posterior instability are not adequately evaluated.

If the patient lies supine while the distal femur is supported by a rest or clamped in a holder, gravity causes a slight posterior sag of the tibia when the extensors are relaxed (Edixhoven 1986). If now a posteroanterior force is applied for testing anterior displacement in 20° of knee flexion, the deflection of sensors positioned on the outer limb contours will indicate the total anteroposterior excursion from the resting position to the limit of anterior motion. The whole anteroposterior laxity pattern cannot be resolved into an anterior and posterior motion segment. Only the total sagittal displacement between the femur and tibia is determined. Consequently, the values measured with a testing apparatus are somewhat greater than the displacements recorded simultaneously by stress radiography, which indicates pure anterior displacement with respect to the anatomic neutral position (Stäubli and Jakob 1990).

Discussion

The results of manual clinical stability testing are highly variable from one examiner to the next. As a rule, unknown forces and moments are applied to the knee joint, and the test position of the knee, muscular

tension, gravitational effects, and the control of the resulting pathologic mobility cannot be precisely defined. Thus, a true rationale appears to exist for the use of simple, objective, noninvasive test devices for measuring femorotibial displacement. The problems with instrumented arthrometric devices relate to the fact that they basically record displacements between the patella and tibial tuberosity. Because soft-tissue structures of variable thickness and prominence occur between the external reference points and the underlying bony skeleton, the potential effect of soft-tissue interference on the arthrometric data must be taken into account. To control the test position, most arthrometric devices are equipped with a distal thigh holder and a footplate to define the position of tibial rotation. In interpreting the test data, therefore, the principle of constrained motion testing applies. In arthrometric measurements of a knee joint with chronic ACL insufficiency, which generally produces a combined anterior translation and internal rotation of the tibia with respect to the femur, we feel that the measurement error is rather negligible since the translational component of both compartments exceeds the internal rotational component. In knees with an "isolated" anterior cruciate insufficiency, characterized by a slight anterior translation and a pronounced degree of internal rotation (grade I pivot shift), the effective amount of anterior displacement of the lateral tibial plateau cannot be determined by the constrained arthrometric method, i.e., the arthrometric data associated with this type of cruciate ligament insufficiency are below the anterolateral subluxation values as determined by anterior compartmental drawer stressradiography.

References

Butler DL, Noyes FR, Grood ES (1980) Ligamentous restraints to anterior-posterior drawer in the human knee. A biomechanical study. J Bone Joint Surg [Am] 62: 259–270

Daniel DM (1989) Assessing the limits of knee motion. 6th Congress of the International Society of the Knee, 8th–12th May, Rome

Daniel DM, Malcom LL, Losse G, Stone ML, Sachs R, Burks R (1985) Instrumented measurement of anterior laxity of the knee. J Bone Joint Surg [Am] 67: 720–726

Edixhoven P (1986) De geinstrumenteerde schuifladestest van de knie in vivo. On-line Vormvervaardiging, Nijmegen

Edixhoven P, Huiskes R, deGraaf R, van Rens TJG, Sloof TJ (1987) Accuracy and reproducibility of an instrumented knee-drawer tests. J Orthop Res 5: 378–387

Edixhoven P, Huiskes R, de Graaf R (1989) Anteriorposterior drawer measurements in the knee using an instrumented test device. Clin Orthops 247: 232–242

Feagin JF (1988) The prone Lachman test. In: Feagin JA jr

(ed) The crucial ligaments. Churchill Livingstone, New York Edinburgh London Melbourne, p 55

Fukubayashi T, Torzilli PA, Sherman MF, Warren RF (1982) An in vitro biomechanical evaluation of anterior-posterior motion of the knee. Tibial displacement, rotation, and torque. J Bone Joint Surg [Am] 64: 258-264

Heigaard N, Sandberg H, Jacobsen K (1983) Prospective stressradiography in 38 old injuries of the ligaments of the knee joint. Acta Orthop Scand 54: 119-125

Jacobsen K (1981) Gonylaxometry. Stress radiographic measurement of passive stability in the knee joints of normal subjects and patients with ligament injuries. Accuracy and range of application. Acta Orthop Scand 52 [Suppl 194]

Kennedy JC, Fowler PJ (1971) Medial and anterior instability of the knee. An anatomical and clinical study using stress machines. J Bone Joint Surg [Am] 53/7: 1257-1270

Kärrholm J, Selvik G, Elmquist LG, Hansson L, Jonsson H (1988) Three-dimensional instability of the anterior cruciate deficient knee. J Bone Joint Surg [Br] 70: 777-783

Markolf KL, Graff-Radford A, Amstutz HC (1978) In vivo knee stability. A quantitative assessment using an instrumented testing apparatus. J Bone Joint Surg [Am] 60: 664-674

Müller We, Biedert R, Hefti F, Jakob RP, Munzinger U, Stäubli H-U (1988) OAK knee evaluation. A new way to assess knee ligament injuries. Clin Orthop 232: 37-50

Sherman OH, Markolf KL, Ferkel RD (1987) Measurements of anterior laxity in normal and anterior cruciate absent knees with two instrumented test devices. Clin Orthop 215: 156-161

Shino K, Ohta N, Horibe S, Ono K (1984) In vivo measurement of A-P instability in the ACL-disrupted knees and in postoperative knees. Trans Orthop Res Soc 9: 394

Stäubli H-U, (1990) Limits of compartmental knee motion: Acta Orthop Scand [Suppl] (submitted for publication)

Stäubli H-U, Birrer ST (1990) The popliteus tendon and its fascicles at the hiatus popliteus. Functional arthroscopic evaluation in ACL deficient knees. Arthroscopy 6, 3: 209-220

Stäubli H-U, Jakob RP (1990) Assessment of posterior instability of the knee near extension. J Bone Joint Surg [Br] 72: 225-230

Stäubli H-U, Jakob RP, Noesberger B (1985) Anterior-posterior knee instability and stressradiography. A prospective biomechanical analysis with the knee in extension. In: Perren SM, Schneider E (eds) Biomechanics. Current interdisciplinary research. Nijhoff, Dordrecht Boston Lancaster, pp 397-402

Stedtfeld M, Strobel HW (1988) Diagnostik des verletzten Kniegelenkes. Marseille, München

Torg JS, Conrad W, Kalen V (1976) Clinical diagnosis of anterior cruciate ligament instability in the athlete. Am J Sports Med 4: 84-92

Torzilli PA, Greenberg RL, Insall J (1981) An in vivo biomechanical evaluation of anterior-posterior motion of the knee. Roentgenographic measurement technique, stress machine and stable population. J Bone Joint Surg [Am] 63: 960-968

Trillat A, Dejour H, Bousquet G (1978) Chirurgie du genou. 3èmes Journées (Lyon), Septembre 1977. Simep Villeurbanne

Our Current Technique of Stressradiography Near Extension

H.-U. Stäubli and R. P. Jakob

Various authors (Nyga 1970; Leven 1977; Kennedy and Fowler 1971; Jacobsen 1976, 1981; Torzilli et al. 1981) have discussed the radiographic documentation of relative femorotibial motion in 90° of knee flexion. Fukubayashi et al. (1982) noted the distinction between measuring translation with and without constraint of tibial rotation, finding that values were 30% higher when rotation was unconstrained. Gollehon et al. (1987) determined the physiologic increase of rotation that accompanies increasing flexion of the knee. The next logical step, it seemed, was to measure translation in the position of near extension, since it is reasonable to expect that the degrees of freedom of coupled rotation will be less near extension than in 90° of flexion. To document the clinically determined amounts and limits of sagittal translation at small angles of knee flexion, Stäubli et al. (1985) developed a new technique for the radiographic measurement of drawer signs near extension: Standardized stressradiographs taken under anesthesia are used to analyze the relative displacement of the medial and lateral femorotibial joint compartments in the anterior and posterior directions. This technique can be used to document subluxation phenomena as well as to grade the pivot shift (Jakob et al. 1987). Also, the direction of the displacement with respect to the neutral position can be determined radiometrically; anterior translation can be differentiated from posterior translation. The physiologic limits of anteroposterior motion, or the limits of motion in the cruciate-ligament-intact knee, can be distinguished radiographically from the increased anterior, posterior, or combined anteroposterior limits of subluxation. This enables the physician to identify coupled motions, such as combined translations or rotations, during radiographic anterior and posterior drawer stress testing. This can be done separately for both the medial and lateral compartments. The quantifiable subluxations yield objective data on the direction, type, and degree of the subluxation, guiding the physician in selecting patients for primary repair, evaluating residual laxities, and performing disability assessments.

Definition of the Neutral Position

The neutral position of the knee is defined as the position in which lines drawn tangent to the posterior borders of the medial and lateral tibial plateaus, running parallel to the posterior tibial cortex at the middle third of the tibial shaft, coincide with tangents to the posterior borders of the medial and lateral condyles of the femur. The neutral position in stressradiography provides a baseline for determining the anterior and posterior components of medial and lateral compartmental motions in the knee (Fig. 1).

Posterior Displacement of the Tibia

The tibia is posteriorly displaced when the tangents to the posterior borders of the tibial plateaus are located behind the posterior femoral tangents, either spontaneously due to gravity or in response to an applied posteroanterior force. The distance between the tibial and femoral tangents is a measure of the relative posterior displacement of the medial and lateral compartments with respect to the neutral position on the sagittal plane. Three basic patterns of posterior compartmental subluxation are recognized:

– *Posterior subluxation* involves a "pure" posterior translation in which both tibial plateaus move an equal distance posteriorly.
– *Posterolateral subluxation* is present when the posterior subluxation is coupled with external rotation, i.e., both tibial plateaus move backward, the lateral plateau moving a greater distance posteriorly than the medial plateau.
– *Posteromedial subluxation* is one in which the posterior displacement of the medial plateau exceeds that of the lateral plateau.

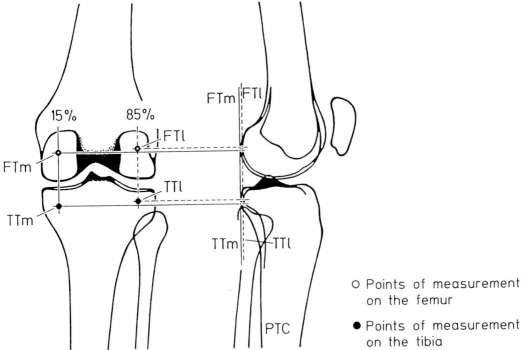

Fig. 1. Neutral position of the joint compartments on the sagittal plane. The neutral position is defined as that in which the posterior compartmental tangents drawn parallel to the posterior tibial shaft cortex (PTC at mid-third level) coincide. *FTm*, Medial femoral tangent; *FTl*, lateral femoral tangent; *TTm*, medial tibial tangent; *TTl*, lateral tibial tangent; *PTC*, posterior tibial cortex (reference line); *PFC*, posterior femoral cortex (reference line)

Anterior Displacement of the Tibia

The tibia is anteriorly displaced with respect to the femur when lines parallel to the posterior tibial shaft cortex and tangent to the posterior borders of the tibial plateaus pass in front of the posterior femoral tangents. The distance between the tibial and femoral tangents is a measure of the anterior displacement of the medial and lateral compartments with respect to the neutral position on the sagittal plane. Three basic patterns of anterior compartmental displacement or anterior tibial subluxation are recognized:

– *Anterior subluxation* involves a "pure" anterior translation in which both tibial plateaus travel an equal distance forward.
– *Anterolateral subluxation* is present when the anterior translation is associated with increased anterior displacement of the lateral tibial plateau. This coupled motion is defined as anterior translation plus internal rotation of the tibia.
– *Anteromedial subluxation* is present when the anterior translation is associated with a demonstrable increase in the anterior displacement of the medial tibial plateau. This coupled motion is

defined as anterior translation plus external rotation of the tibia.

Technique of Stressradiography on the Sagittal Plane Under Anesthesia

Indications

In a patient presenting with a history of significant knee trauma, with an initial sensation of tearing or giving way, followed by effusion and subjective instability, we recommend the following procedure:

1. Systematic examination of the knee without anesthesia, *active drawer testing*, and exclusion of a spontaneous gravity-induced *posterior subluxation* of the tibia. A sag can be objectively demonstrated by measuring the level of the tibial tuberosity in millimeters with the thigh supported distally and the knee flexed 20° and comparing the measurement with the uninjured side. The following active tests have proven useful for distinguishing between an anterior and posterior drawer in the slightly flexed knee:

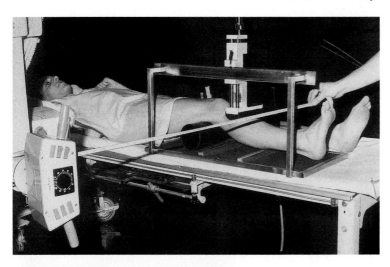

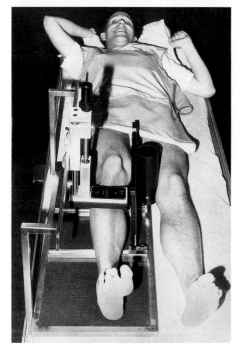

Fig. 2. Knee positioning device with Telos unit; setup for posterior stressradiography. The X-ray cassette is placed against the medial side of the knee, and the film-focus distance is 120 cm. The cross-table beam is angled 5°–8° distally

◁ **Fig. 3.** Positioning device set up for posterior stressradiography, axial view

2. Supplementation of the systematic knee exam by stability testing under peridural anesthesia according to the guidelines of the OAK group (Müller et al. 1988) and according to the recommendations of the IKDC (International Knee Documentation Committee)
3. Stress radiographs on the sagittal and frontal planes during the application of defined forces and torques, with documentation of the terminal positions
4. Functional knee arthroscopy with probing to define structural anatomic lesions

Radiographic Technique

– The "active Lachman test" for anterior cruciate ligament (ACL) insufficiency (quadriceps contraction pulls the involved tibia from the starting position to a position of anterior subluxation)
– Reduction of a spontaneous posterior subluxation: In the knee with a deficient posterior cruciate ligament (PCL) and a gravity-induced posterior sag, quadriceps contraction reduces the spontaneous posterior subluxation to the neutral position (Stäubli and Jakob 1990). This provides a way to distinguish an active anterior subluxation ("positive active Lachman test") from the reduction of a gravity-induced posterior subluxation to the neutral position (sign of PCL deficiency).

The patient is positioned supine. Following the induction of anesthesia and full muscular relaxation, a special positioning device with a load arm (Telos, Germany) is used to apply the desired stress to the immobilized knee while radiographs are taken (Fig. 2). The device incorporates a hard base on which, for posterior drawer stressradiography, a bolster 11.5 cm in diameter is placed beneath the distal femur 10 cm proximal to the joint line of the knee. This places the knee in a position of 10°–20° flexion depending on the limb length and constitution of the patient. For anterior drawer stressradiography, a 7.5-cm bolster is placed beneath the center of the lower leg. A 20 × 40-cm cassette is positioned vertically against the medial side of the knee in a special holder. The film-focus distance is 120 cm, and a lateral-to-medial cross-table projection is used with the central beam angled 5°–8° distally to superimpose the posterior knee contours and provide an orthograde view of the femoral condyles on the sagittal plane.

Technique of Posterior Stressradiography (Fig. 3)

The patient is positioned supine with the distal femur supported on an 11.5-cm bolster placed 10 cm proximal to the lateral joint space of the knee. The Telos load arm is positioned 10 cm distal to the knee joint, below the tibial tuberosity. The electronic measuring unit of the Telos arm is adjusted for a net anterior-to-posterior force of 20 kp. The tibia is not immobilized, so tibial motion is unconstrained. Before taking an exposure, the examiner moves the knee through two complete cycles of anteroposterior motion while applying maximum manual force. After a constant posterior force of 20 kp has been applied for 10 s with the Telos unit, an exposure is taken in the posteriorly subluxated position. This film documents the terminal position at the posterior limit of motion.

Technique of Anterior Stressradiography

A medium-size bolster 7.5 cm in diameter is placed beneath the center of the lower leg, and the thigh support is removed. The Telos unit is positioned above the knee so that the load arm is 3 fingerwidths proximal to the base of the patella. At that site a posteriorly directly force of 20 kp is applied to the unconstrained femur from the anterior side. While the force is applied, the foot is held against the base with a strap or manually by the examiner. This causes an anteriorly directed force vector to act upon the proximal tibia. The resulting anterior displacement of the tibia or posterior displacement of the femur relative to the fixed tibia is documented with respect to the neutral position.

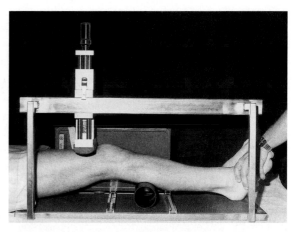

Fig. 4. Positioning device set up for anterior stressradiography, lateral view

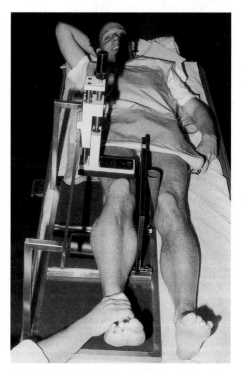

Fig. 5. Positioning device set up for anterior stressradiography, axial view

Analysis of the Stressradiographs

Tangents are drawn to the posterior borders of the medial and lateral femoral condyles and the medial and lateral tibial plateaus, parallel to the posterior tibial cortex at the mid-shaft level. The degree of compartmental displacement can now be measured as the distance in millimeters between the posterior tangents of the corresponding compartments. These data on compartmental displacement are based on an area defined by points located at approximately 15% and 85% of the total coronal width of the knee (see Fig. 1).

The magnification factor of 1.1 (10%) is disregarded during the measurements. Generally a coupled anterior translation and internal rotation are found on the

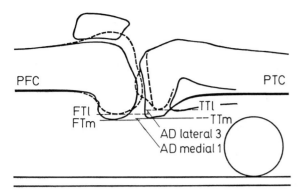

Fig.6. Taking measurements from AP stressradiographs (*dashed line*, lateral compartment; *solid line*, medial compartment). *FTl*, Lateral femoral tangent; *FTm*, medial femoral tangent; *TTl*, lateral tibial tangent; *TTm*, medial tibial tangent; *PFC*, posterior femoral cortex; *PTC*, posterior tibial cortex (reference line); *AD*, anterior displacement

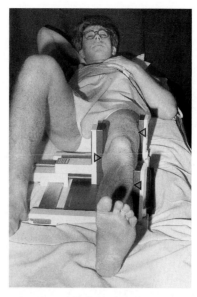

Fig.7. Stressradiography on the frontal plane: varus stress (left knee). Positioned medially at the supracondylar level, the Telos arm exerts a force of 20 kp against the padded proximal and distal posts on the lateral side, producing a combination of medial compression, lateral distraction, medial translation, and axial rotation

radiographs of intact knees subjected to an anterior stress of 20 kg. This pattern is present if the anterior displacement of the lateral tibial plateau exceeds that of the medial plateau. If both tibial plateaus undergo equal anterior motion, we describe the result as equidistant bicompartmental unidirectional anterior displacement, which corresponds to a pure anterior translation. A greater relative anterior displacement of the medial tibial plateau indicates that anterior translation is coupled with external tibial rotation. We can define an anterior and a posterior motion segment as well as the limits of anterior and posterior motion on the sagittal plane with respect to the neutral position.

Stressradiography in the Frontal Plane

If there is interest in documenting the pre- or postoperative varus-valgus stability of the knee, the Telos apparatus can be used to perform stressradiography under a defined varus or valgus stress of 20 kp in extension. When a varus stress is applied, the condition of the articular cartilage in the compressed medial femorotibial compartment can be evaluated along with the integrity of the primary and secondary lateral restraints. When a valgus stress is applied, the cartilage thickness in the lateral femorotibial compartment and the laxity of the medial capsule and ligaments can be documented.

Anteroposterior stressradiography under standard conditions provides a means of differentiating anterior and posterior motion components with respect to the neutral position and distinguishing physiologic

from abnormal limits of anterior motion. The anterior displacements of the lateral and medial compartments can be separately determined. In healthy knees the study demonstrates physiologic patterns and limits of motion, documenting the integrity of the primary restraints to anteroposterior displacement. In knees with combined anteroposterior instabilities, in knees with anterior instability combined with a preexisting posterolateral, constitutional laxity factor, or in knees with posterior instabilities, three main physiologic and pathologic motion patterns can be identified:

– If the ACL is intact, the anterior drawer stress will generally elicit anterior translation combined with a slight internal rotation.
– If the ACL is deficient, the stress will elicit a significantly greater anterior translation with equal motion of both tibial plateaus. Greater anterior displacement of the lateral compartment represents a coupled anterior translation and medial rotation, a typical finding with chronic ACL deficiency (see Fig.9 *top*). The physiologic posterior mobility associated with an intact PCL generally consists of a slight posterior translation combined with external tibial rotation with respect to the femur. A tear of the PCL generally leads to a significant posterior translation of the tibia relative to the femur (see

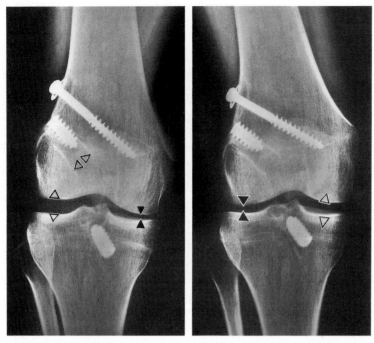

Fig. 8. Stressradiographs of the right knee on the frontal plane. **a** Varus stress, **b** valgus stress. The varus stress film, taken 1 year after intraarticular reconstruction of the ACL, documents compression of the medial compartment with loss of normal cartilage thickness and lateral joint distention with residual varus laxity (Stäubli 1990 a, b)

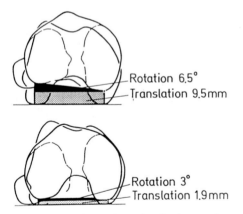

Fig. 9. Translation and rotation in the anterior cruciate ligament-deficient knee. The anterior compartmental displacements measured by stressradiography in the presence of a deficient *(top)* and intact *(bottom)* anterior cruciate ligament are graphically shown

Fig. 9 *bottom*). A PCL tear combined with damage to posterolateral structures leads to posterolateral subluxation, while a posterior cruciate tear combined with damage to posteromedial structures leads to significant posteromedial subluxation (Stäubli and Jakob 1990).

Comparison of Instrumented Arthrometry and Stressradiography

When we contrast the two major clinical measuring systems, we note the following differences: Arthrometry generally employs anterior sensor elements that detect relative motion of the anterior patellar surface stabilized in the femoral trochlea with respect to the tibial tuberosity. In stressradiography, posterior tangents serve as reference lines for measuring compartmental displacements and their limits separately for the medial and lateral compartments. Defining the neutral position as the alignment of the posterior tibial and femoral tangents makes it possible to differentiate between anterior and posterior components of motion. The problem with arthrometric devices is that the resting position, i.e., the initial femorotibial relation, cannot be precisely defined on the basis of external contours. As Edixhoven et al. (1987) have shown, a deficient PCL permits a spontaneous posterior subluxation averaging 3.5 mm when the knee is flexed 25°. This sag in the PCL-deficient knee must be taken into account when measuring the deflection produced by a posterior drawer force in order to obtain data that are comparable to values measured by stressradiography. In a comparative study of the UCLA testing apparatus and the KT 1000 arthrometer, Sherman et al. (1987) found that the results depended on the device used, the KT 1000 yielding consistently higher measurements. Stäubli and Jakob (1991) noted the same trend in a prospective comparison of the KT 1000 and simultaneous stressradiography.

Given the current trend toward the clinical measurement of compartmental motion limits in the knee, we predict an increasing reliance on the use of objective, reproducible, noninvasive, portable measuring systems for the objective analysis of relative compartmental motions between the femur and tibia.

References

Edixhoven PF, Huiskes R, Graaf de R, Rens van TJG, Sloof TJ (1987) Accuracy and reproducibility of instrumented knee-drawer tests. J Orthop Res 5: 378–387

Fukubayashi T, Torzilli PA, Sherman MF, Warren RF (1982) An in vitro biomechanical evaluation of anterior-posterior motion of the knee. Tibial displacement, rotation and torque. J Bone Joint Surg [Am] 64: 258–264

Gollehon DL, Torzilli PA, Warren RF (1987) The role of the posterolateral and cruciate ligaments in the stability of the human knee. J Bone Joint Surg [Am] 69: 233–242

Jacobsen K (1976) Stress radiographical measurement of the anteroposterior, medial and lateral stability of the knee joint. Acta Orthop Scand 3: 335

Jacobsen K (1981) Gonylaxometry. Stress radiographic measurement of passive stability in the knee joints of normal subjects and patients with ligament injuries. Accuracy and range of application. Acta Orthop Scand 52 [Suppl 194]: 1–263

Jakob RP, Stäubli H-U, Deland JT (1987) Grading the pivot shift. J Bone Joint Surg [Br] 69: 294–299

Kennedy JD, Fowler PJ (1971) Medial and anterior instability of the knee. J Bone Joint Surg [Am] 53: 1257–1270

Levén H (1977) Determination of sagittal instability of the knee joint. Acta Radiol 18: 689–697

Müller We, Biedert R, Hefti F, Jakob RP, Munzinger U, Stäubli H-U (1988) OAK Knee Evaluation. A new way to assess knee ligament injuries. Clin Orthop 232: 37–50

Nyga W (1970) Röntgenologische Darstellung von Kreuzbandverletzungen des Kniegelenkes. Z Orthop 107: 340–344

Sherman OH, Markolf KL, Ferkel RD (1987) Measurements of anterior laxity in normal and anterior cruciate absent knees with two instrumented test devices. Clin Orthop 215: 156–161

Stäubli H-U (1990a) Stressradiography: Measurements of knee motion limits. In: Daniel D, Akeson W, O'Connor J (eds) Knee ligaments: Structure, function, injury and repair. Raven Press, New York, pp. 449–459

Stäubli H-U (1990b) Limits of compartmental knee motion. Acta Orthop Scand [Suppl] (submitted for publication)

Stäubli H-U, Jakob RP (1990) Assessment of posterior instability of the knee near extension. J Bone Joint Surg [Br] 72: 225–230

Stäubli H-U, Jakob RP (in press) Anterior knee motion analysis with KT-1000. Tibial position in ACC-intact and ACC-deficient knees at arthrometry and simultaneous radiography. Am J Sports Med

Stäubli H-U, Jakob RP, Noesberger B (1985) Anterior-posterior knee instability and stress-radiography. A prospective biomechanical analysis with the knee in extension. In: Perren SM, Schneider E (eds) Biomechanics: Current interdisciplinary research. Nijhoff, Dordrecht Boston Lancaster, pp 397–402

Torzilli PA, Greenberg RL, Insall JN (1981) An in vivo biomechanical evaluation of anterior posterior motion of the knee. Roentgenographic measurement technique, stress machine and stable population. J Bone Joint Surg [Am] 63: 960–968

Anterior Subluxation in the Chronically Anterior Cruciate Ligament-Deficient Knee: Comparison of Simultaneous Arthrometry and Stressradiography Using the KT 1000

H.-U. Stäubli and R. P. Jakob

Anterior drawer testing of the knee in 20° of flexion is widely acknowledged as a reliable clinical procedure for diagnosing chronic anterior cruciate ligament (ACL) deficiency (Torg et al. 1976; Trillat et al. 1978; Stäubli et al. 1985; Daniel et al. 1985; Müller et al. 1988). The direction, type, degree, and end point or limit of anterior tibial displacement are tested in patients with suspected ACL deficiency. Examiners have used a variety of methods for the objective testing of anteroposterior knee stability in vivo (Daniel et al. 1985; Jacobsen 1981; Markolf et al. 1978; Shino et al. 1984; Torzilli et al. 1981; Sherman et al. 1987). Daniel (personal communication, 1988), Markolf et al. (1978), and Edixhoven (1986) measured the central displacement of external bony landmarks by placing one sensor of a test device on the patella and another on the tibial tuberosity. Stäubli et al. (1985) discussed stressradiographic drawer testing in the slightly flexed knee, which involves measuring the displacement of radiographic reference points on the posterior bony contours to document the limits of anteroposterior knee motion.

Our goal in the present article is to evaluate the accuracy of measurements of anterior tibial subluxation in 20° of knee flexion on the basis of a prospective study (Stäubli and Jakob 1990). Readings taken with the KT 1000 arthrometer (MEDmetric Corp., San Diego, CA) were compared with values measured on simultaneous stressradiographs. Anterior tibial displacement in a group of patients with chronic ACL deficiency was measured and compared with measurements in healthy knees. Then the mean anterior displacements determined by both methods and the differences of the means in ACL-deficient knees were compared with those of control knees with an intact ACL. Both arthrometry and stressradiography, which were performed simultaneously under anesthesia with adherence to standard conditions, were diagnostic. We suggest that both methods be regarded as mutually complementary for the objective measurement and documentation of anterior knee instability or anterior subluxation in knees with chronic ACL deficiency.

Materials and Methods

Sixteen patients (9 women, 7 men) with documented, symptomatic, chronic ACL deficiency in one knee were enrolled in the study. Their average age was 28.4 +/− 10 years, with a range from 16 to 53 years. The opposite knee (with an intact ACL) was examined under identical conditions to serve as a control.

Use of the KT 1000 arthrometer for documenting the limits of anterior knee motion followed the guidelines specified by Daniel et al. (1985). The KT 1000 is a manual test device with an integrated foot rest for controlling tibial rotation (Fig. 1). A dial indicator displays the relative motion (in millimeters) between sensor pads in contact with the patella and the tibial tuberosity. Force is applied to the tibia through a handle. In our study two anteroposterior force cycles were applied before measurements were begun. The patients were examined under anesthesia prior to open or arthroscopic knee surgery.

The prescribed motion tests were performed in accordance with the recommendations of Daniel et al. (1985) and the personal instructions of Marie Lou Stone (Fig. 1). We obtained simultaneous stressradiographs using the technique described in a previous publication (Stäubli et al. 1985).

Resting Position = Starting Position

Daniel et al. (1985) state that, after strapping the arthrometer to the lower leg with the knee flexed 20°, the examiner must apply a maximum manual force to the limits of anteroposterior displacement in two complete load cycles before measuring anterior displacement. The resting position is defined as the position that is assumed spontaneously after a posterior force of 10 kp (89 N) has been applied and released.

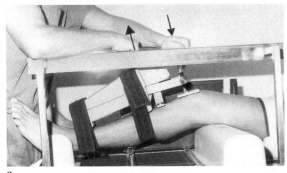

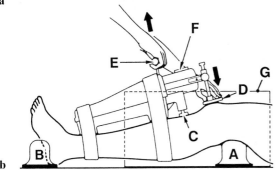

Fig. 1a, b. For testing with the KT 1000 arthrometer, the knee is flexed 20°. A 10-kp (89-N) anterior force *(left arrow)* is applied to the proximal tibia through a handle. Posterior pressure *(right arrow)* on the patellar sensor pad *(D)* stabilizes the patella in the femoral trochlea. *A,* Thigh support; *B,* foot rest; *C,* tibial sensor pad; *D,* patellar sensor pad; *E,* handle; *F,* displacement dial indicator; *G,* 20 × 40-cm X-ray cassette at medial side of knee

Anterior Subluxation Test
with a 10-kp Anterior Drawer Stress

The knee was flexed over the thigh support, generally resulting in a 20° flexion angle, and an anterior force of 10 kp (89 N) was applied manually through the handle. When an audible signal confirmed that the 10-kp load had been reached, an anterior drawer stress lateral-projection radiograph was taken; this was always done by the same examiner and the same radiology assistant (Fig. 1). The compliance of the ACL, defined as the anterior displacement elicited by an anterior force of 7.5–10 kp, was determined without taking an additional stressradiograph.

Stressradiographic Technique

The stressradiographs taken during the arthrometry document the direction and degree of the compartmental displacement of posterior reference points, located by drawing tangents to the posterior borders of the femorotibial compartments. The anterior drawer stress film demonstrates the knee in the anteriorly subluxated position, the X-ray tube being angled 6°–8° distally across the knee to center the beam on the superimposed posterior condyles (Fig. 2).

The film-focus distance is 120 cm. The 20 × 40-cm X-ray cassette is held vertically against the medial side of the knee in a holder. The posterior reference lines consist of tangents to the posterior borders of the medial and lateral tibial plateaus and to the femoral condyles. These are drawn parallel to the posterior cortex of the middle third of the tibial shaft. When viewed from behind the knee, the medial and lateral lines pass through points located at 15% and 85% of the total knee width. The posterior reference tangents are used to determine the anteroposterior displacement of the corresponding knee compartments. The arithmetic mean of the anterior displacement of the medial and lateral compartments is defined as the central anterior displacement.

Evaluation and Results

In each patient the 10-kp anterior drawer test with the KT 1000 arthrometer was performed on both knees, and simultaneous stressradiographs were obtained. The anterior displacement values were determined, and the mean values obtained by arthrometry and by stressradiography were calculated. The compliance index was determined by arthrometry only. The results were statistically evaluated by the comparison of paired values. Correlation coefficients and probabilities were statistically computed.

In our analysis of anterior drawer displacements determined by arthrometry and simultaneous stressradiography, the arthrometric values were analyzed in relation to the resting position and the radiographic values in relation to the anatomic compartmental neutral position on the sagittal plane (Fig. 3).

The KT 1000 arthrometer indicated a mean anterior displacement of 11.9 +/− 3.1 mm in the ACL-deficient group versus 6.2 +/− 2.5 mm in the ACL-intact group (Fig. 4).

Simultaneous stressradiography showed a mean cen-

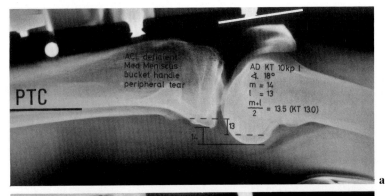

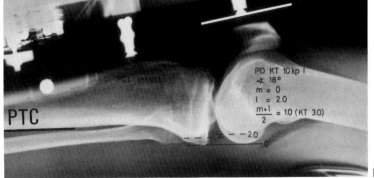

Fig. 2a, b. Stressradiographs of the knee joint in the anteriorly subluxated position **(a)** and in the posteriorly stressed position **(b)** during KT 1000 arthrometry. The central beam is angled 6°–8° distally across the joint to center it on the superimposed posterior femoral condyles. Patellar-trochlear contact and the parallel alignment of the sensor pad and anterior patellar surface *(white line)* are documented on both films. In this patient with chronic ACL deficiency and a reduced peripheral bucket-handle tear, the KT 1000 arthrometer measured an anterior displacement of 13.0 mm while the simultaneous stressradiograph showed a central displacement of 13.5 mm **(a)**. The arthrometry indicated a posterior displacement of 3.0 mm, versus a central posterior displacement of 1.0 mm measured by simultaneous stressradiography **(b)**

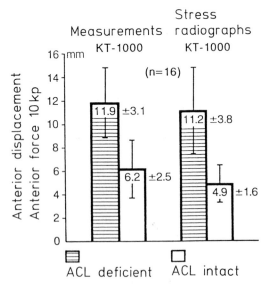

Fig. 3. Anterior tibial displacement with respect to the femur produced by an anterior drawer stress of 10 kp, as determined by the KT 1000 arthrometer *(left columns)* and simultaneous stressradiography *(right columns)* for cruciate ligament-deficient and cruciate ligament-intact knee groups (mean values in millimeters +/− 1 SD)

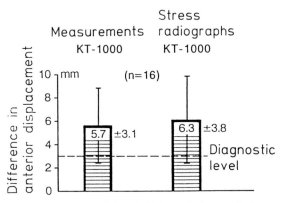

Fig. 4. Mean ACL deficient-ACL intact differences in the anterior displacements measured by arthrometry with the KT 1000 *(left)* and by simultaneous stressradiography *(right)* in millimeters +/− 1 SD. On average, both methods yielded values surpassing the diagnostic level of 3 mm

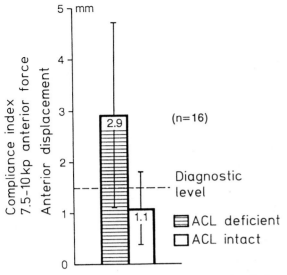

Fig.5. Compliance index measured over the anterior displacement produced by an anterior force of 7.5–10 kp. The diagnostic level of 1.5 mm was exceeded on average in the ACL-deficient group

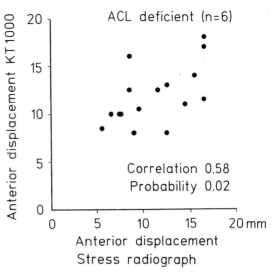

Fig.6. Scattergram to illustrate the anterior displacements measured by arthrometry *(vertical)* and simultaneous stress-radiography *(horizontal)*. The correlation coefficient in the ACL-deficient group was 0.58 with a significance of 0.02

tral anterior displacement of $11.2 +/- 3.8$ mm in the deficient group versus $4.9 +/- 1.6$ mm in the intact group (see Fig.4).

Both methods showed a significant ($p < 0.01$) anterior displacement in the 10-kp anterior drawer test when an ACL-deficient group was compared with an intact group (see Fig.4). Both methods showed a significant increase of anterior displacement by a 10-kp anterior drawer stress when the mean values in the deficient knees were compared with those in the controls. Both methods yielded mean difference values above the diagnostic level of 3-mm anterior displacement (arthrometric mean 5.7 mm, radiographic mean 6.2 mm) when ACL-deficient knees were compared with intact knees (Fig.5).

The mean compliance index on arthrometry was 2.9 for the ACL-deficient group and 1.1 for the intact group (Fig.6). A mean value of 1.5 is considered diagnostic of ACL insufficiency (Daniel et al. 1985).

On comparing the paired measurements yielded by both methods, we found a slight correlation in the ACL-deficient group (correlation = 0.58, probability = 0.02). We found no correlation between the arthrometric and radiographic values in the intact control group. These results are presented in the scattergrams in Figs.6 and 7. We found no correlation when we compared the paired difference values in the ACL-deficient group with those in the intact population (Table 1).

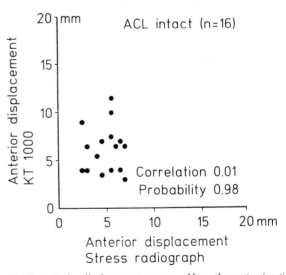

Fig.7. Anterior displacements measured by arthrometry *(vertical)* and simultaneous stressradiography *(horizontal)* in the ACL-intact group. The correlation coefficient was 0.01 with a significance of 0.98

Table 1. Anterior displacement in an ACL-deficient group and ACL-intact control group measured by KT 1000 arthrometry and simultaneous stressradiography

	KT 1000 (mm)	Stress-radiographs (mm)	Correlation	Probability
ACL deficient	11.9 +/− 3.1	11.2 +/− 3.8	0.58[a]	0.02
ACL intact	6.2 +/− 2.5	4.9 +/− 1.6	0.01[b]	0.98
Difference	5.7 +/− 3.1	6.2 +/− 3.8	0.38[b]	0.14

[a] Statistically slight correlation between the two methods.
[b] No statistical correlation of measured values.

Discussion

In a prospective study, we analyzed the anterior displacement of the knee joint with the KT 1000 arthrometer and simultaneous stressradiographs in 16 knees with documented chronic ACL deficiency. The intact contralateral knee of each patient served as a control. The ACL-intact and ACL-deficient knees of each patient were tested under anesthesia by the same examiner using the same technique.

Both arthrometry and stressradiography with an anterior drawer stress of 10 kp yielded values diagnostic for ACL deficiency. The increase of mean anterior displacement in the ACL-deficient knees was significant in relation to the controls ($p < 0.01$). The simultaneous stressradiographs yielded greater mean difference values than arthrometry. These discrepancies may relate to various factors: differences in the definition of the resting and neutral position, soft-tissue interference with arthrometry, different measuring techniques (anterior sensor pads in arthrometry, posterior tangents in stressradiography), and the magnification factor of 1.1 (10%) on the stressradiographs.

For arthrometry with the KT 1000, one sensor pad is placed on the tibial tuberosity and a second on the anterior patellar surface. This arrangement measures central patellotibial displacement. For measurements on stressradiographs, posterior reference tangents are defined which determine the degree of osseous femorotibial displacement for each compartment. The arithmetic mean of the compartmental femorotibial displacements on the stressradiographs was defined as the measure of central knee displacement. In the present study, then, we were comparing an anterior and a posterior measuring system applied under identical conditions in the same individual under anesthesia. The arthrometric measurements

for a 10-kp anterior drawer stress and the difference between the chronically ACL-deficient and intact populations are comparable to the anterior displacements measured by Daniel et al. (1985) in 129 knees with chronic ACL deficiency. Our data showed a mean difference of 5.7 mm in the anterior displacements measured in a small group of 16 patients with chronic ACL deficiency. Daniel et al. (personal communication, 1988) found a mean difference of 5.8 mm in the anterior displacements measured under a drawer stress of 10 kp. The stressradiographs in our study indicated a mean difference of 6.2 mm based on measurements of osseous femorotibial displacement using reference lines. Both arthrometry and stressradiography yielded values significantly above the 3-mm diagnostic level. According to Daniel et al. (1985), these values are diagnostic of ACL deficiency.

Comparing our study with investigations by other authors (Daniel et al. 1985; Edixhoven 1986; Edixhoven et al. 1987; Jacobsen 1981; Heigaard et al. 1983; Shino et al. 1984; Sherman et al. 1987), we may draw the following conclusions: Both arthrometry and simultaneous stressradiography were diagnostic in patients with chronic ACL deficiency (tested under anesthesia with a 10-kp anterior drawer stress and 20° flexion). The mean difference in anterior displacements between the ACL-deficient and ACL-intact groups as determined by stressradiography was 0.5 mm greater on average than that determined by simultaneous arthrometry (6.2 mm for stressradiography vs. 5.7 mm for arthrometry).

We feel that the slight difference in anterior displacements determined by arthrometry and stressradiography relate to different definitions of the resting or neutral position and the different measuring techniques employed. Both methods showed a significant side-to-side difference in anterior displacements in chronically ACL-deficient knees selected for surgical repair. Both methods objectively documented a significant increase of anterior central displacement in symptomatic ACL-deficient knees.

These results agree with the results of biomechanical studies on the restraining function of the ligaments, as reported by Butler et al. (1980). Our in vivo data correlate well with the in vitro data of authors such as Fukubayashi et al. (1982), who studied anteroposterior motion in cadaver knees under similar conditions.

On comparing the two methods of measurement, we found a slight correlation in the differences measured in the ACL-deficient group, but no correlation in the ACL-intact group. Our results suggest that instrumented arthrometry tends to measure higher values than those determined by simultaneous stress-radiography. Previous studies and our own results indicate that both arthrometry with the KT 1000 and simultaneous stressradiography using a 10-kp anterior drawer stress and anesthesia are reliable procedures for documenting anterior subluxation of the tibia in chronically ACL-deficient knees.

References

Butler DL, Noyes FR, Grood ES (1980) Ligamentous restraints to anterior-posterior drawer in the human knee. A biomechanical study. J Bone Joint Surg [Am] 62: 259–270

Daniel DM, Malcom LL, Losse G, Stone ML, Sachs R, Burks R (1985) Instrumented measurement of anterior laxity of the knee. J Bone Joint Surg [Am] 67: 720–726

Edixhoven P (1988) De geinstrumenteerde schuifladestest van de knie in vivo. On-line vormvervaardiging, Nijmegen

Edixhoven P, Huiskes R, deGraaf R, van Rens TJG, Sloof TJ (1987) Accuracy and reproducibility of an instrumented knee-drawer tests. J Orthop Res 5: 378–387

Edixhoven P, Huiskes R, de Graaf R (1989) Anteroposterior drawer measurements in the knee using an instrumented test device. Clin Orthop 248: 232–242

Forster IW, Warren-Smith CD, Tew M (1989) Is the KT 1000 Knee Ligament Arthrometer reliable? J Bone Joint Surg [Br] 71: 843–847

Fukubayashi T, Torzilli PA, Sherman MF, Warren RF (1982) An in vitro biomechanical evaluation of anterior-posterior motion of the knee. Tibial displacement, rotation, and torque. J Bone Joint Surg [Am] 64: 258–264

Heigaard N, Sandberg H, Jacobsen K (1983) Prospective stressradiography in 38 old injuries of the ligaments of the knee joint. Acta Orthop Scand 54: 119–125

Jacobsen K (1981) Gonylaxometry. Stress radiographic measurement of passive stability in the knee joints of normal subjects and patients with ligament injuries. Accuracy and range of application. Acta Orthop Scand 52 [Suppl 194]

Markolf KL, Graff-Radford A, Amstutz HC (1978) In vivo knee stability. A quantitative assessment using an instrumented testing apparatus. J Bone Joint Surg [Am] 60: 664–674

Müller We, Biedert R, Hefti F, Jakob RP, Munzinger U, Stäubli H-U (1988) OAK knee evaluation. A new way to assess knee ligament injuries. Clin Orthop 232: 37–50

Sherman OH, Markolf KL, Ferkel RD (1987) Measurements of anterior laxity in normal and anterior cruciate absent knees with two instrumented test devices. Clin Orthop 215: 156–161

Shino K, Ohta N, Horibe S, Ono K (1984) In vivo measurement of A-P instability in the ACL-disrupted knees and in postoperative knees. Trans Orthop Res Soc 9: 394

Stäubli H-U, Jakob RP (1990) Anterior knee motion analysis with KT-1000. Tibial position in ACC-intact and ACC-deficient knees at arthrometry and simultaneous radiography. Am I Sports Med (in press)

Stäubli H-U, Jakob RP, Noesberger B (1985) Anterior-posterior knee instability and stressradiography. A prospective biomechanical analysis with the knee in extension. In: Perren SM, Schneider E (eds) Biomechanics. Current interdisciplinary research. Nijhoff, Dordrecht Boston Lancaster, pp 397–402

Torg JS, Conrad W, Kalen V (1976) Clinical diagnosis of anterior cruciate ligament instability in the athlete. Am J Sports Med 4: 84–92

Torzilli PA, Greenberg RL, Insall J (1981) An in vivo biomechanical evaluation of anterior-posterior motion of the knee. Roentgenographic measurement technique, stress machine and stable population. J Bone Joint Surg [Am] 63: 960–968

Trillat A, Dejour H, Bousquet G (1978) Chirurgie du genou. 3èmes Journées Lyon, Septembre 1977. Simep, Villeurbanne

The Various Faces of Anterior Cruciate Ligament Tears During Arthroscopic Examination

A. Gächter

Arthroscopy is unique among diagnostic modalities in its ability to provide a clear picture of anterior cruciate ligament (ACL) tears. The examiner can not only assess the damage to the anterior cruciate ligament but very often can identify associated injuries of the semimembranosus corner, menisci, or cartilage. This clarity can greatly aid the physician in devising a treatment plan and selecting an appropriate operative procedure. Faster rehabilitation and an improved therapeutic outcome are achieved as a result of the minimal surgical exploration.

Diagnosis of Acute Tears

With an acute rupture of the ACL, the patient very often hears or feels a pop in the knee "like a rope snapping." In most cases hemarthrosis ensues within minutes, although absence of this hemorrhage does not exclude a ligament rupture. In examining the hemarthrotic knee, the arthroscopist should watch for floating fat globules, which usually signify leakage of fat marrow secondary to an osteochondral fracture. When arthroscopy is performed in gas, these shimmering fat globules are very easy to identify (caution: air embolism).

The clinical examination of an acutely torn ACL is often difficult because of pain. The most rewarding clinical test is undoubtedly the Lachman drawer test, which can be performed without eliciting much pain.

Diagnostic arthroscopy can easily be performed under local anesthesia. Severe pain about the medial collateral ligament can be managed by adding a local block of the infrapatellar branch of the saphenous nerve. An existing hemarthrosis must be aspirated, and if need be the joint irrigated, before intraarticular anesthetic is injected.

A major purpose of the arthroscopic examination, besides diagnosing an ACL tear, is to detect and identify associated injuries. Generally an acute lesion can be distinguished from an older injury, although this can pose major difficulties in rare cases. A probe with an embossed scale can be used during arthroscopy to measure the degree of tibial translation. With the arthroscope in an anterolateral portal, a graduated probe is passed into the intercondylar notch from the anterior side and hooked over the tibial plateau. As the upper tibia is pulled forward, the probe will move with it, and the scale can be read as it emerges from behind the lateral femoral condyle (Fig. 1).

There are associated injuries that are easily missed by careless arthroscopic technique, such as a coexisting incomplete tear of the posterior cruciate ligament (PCL). Close inspection of knees with a torn ACL will generally reveal bloody suffusions about the PCL as well, and it can be difficult to appreciate the precise extent of the associated laxity. A peripheral posterior horn tear of the medial meniscus is also apt to be missed, so probing should be an essential part of the examination. Tears of the lateral meniscus are

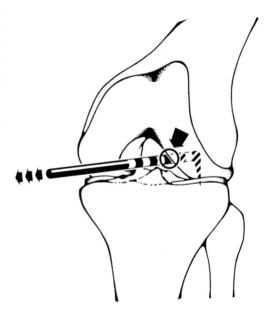

Fig. 1. Arthroscopic quantitation of anterior drawer displacement: The test can be performed near extension or in 60° or 90° flexion. Color markers on the probe shank are easily read at the anterior border of the lateral femoral condyle (with the scope in an anterolateral portal)

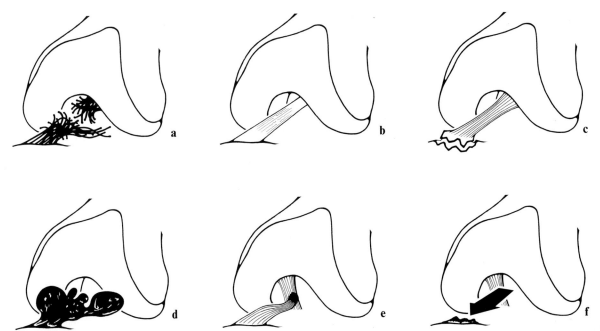

Fig. 2a–f. Classification of complete tears of the anterior cruciate ligament. **a** Type I (mop-end type). The torn ends of the ACL appear frayed and moplike, the individual fiber bundles lying in disarray. Some bundles may be caught between the medial or, more commonly, the lateral joint surfaces, causing a block to extension. Rupture sites are usually visible over a large portion of the ligament (especially in histologic sections), and individual fibers are elongated. If the fiber ends are clumped together and show a clublike distention, the rupture is at least several weeks old. **b** Type II is an intrasynovial rupture in which the investing synovium is completely intact, or at least appears to be. In many acute cases the upper end of the synovial sleeve can be hooked with the arthroscopic probe and pulled down to expose the underlying torn bundles. In older tears the cruciate ligament may be scarred and elongated within an intact synovial sleeve, or it may be complete resorbed leaving only an incompetent synovial tube. Probing will usually clarify the situation. Hemarthrosis can recur with each episode of "shifting," signifying recurrent tearing of the synovial sleeve. **c** Type III is a bony avulsion of the ACL from the tibia; on occasion the avulsion may also involve the PCL, which inserts far more distally. Because of the bony lesion, fat globules are usually present in the hemarthrosis. Proximal bony avulsions of the ACL are very rare. Equally rare are true periosteal avulsions, which usually occur only in children and adolescents and are relatively easy to repair. **d** Type IV. The ends of the torn ACL have retracted, show clubhead distention, and assume a rounded or oval shape. Viewed arthroscopically, they may resemble loose bodies. A tear with this appearance is at least a month old and perhaps much older. **e** Type V. The ACL has been torn or avulsed proximally and has fallen upon the PCL, to which it has become attached. Its distal attachment is normal, but fibers no longer pass to the lateral femoral condyle. The proximal attachment is vacant. **f** Type VI. The ruptured ACL has been completely resorbed, and only the tibial attachment can still be recognized. A period of weeks to years may be required for the resorption to occur

considerably easier to detect by arthroscopy than by an open arthrotomy. Finally, lesions of the femoropatellar joint are apt to be missed or misinterpreted during arthroscopic examination; rupture of the ACL is associated with a concomitant patellar dislocation in approximately 3%–5% of cases. Evidence may include a bloody suffusion in the region of the retinaculum and associated cartilage damage.

A rupture of the PCL should always be considered in the differential diagnosis of a lax ACL. This injury may allow the tibial plateau to slip into a posterior drawer position, causing a laxness of the ACL that may be misinterpreted. Doubts are resolved by performing an anterior drawer maneuver that restores tension to the intact ACL.

Older Tears

The main indication for arthroscopy in chronic ACL injuries is to evaluate for associated lesions. When there is advanced pathology in the medial compartment, for example, consideration should be given to performing a tibial valgus osteotomy in addition to the ACL reconstruction. Frequently there are associated meniscal tears that have progressed since the acute trauma, eventually causing mechanical interference with joint motion. The older cruciate ligament tear can present in various "guises," the most important of which are reviewed in Fig. 2. An older anterior cruciate tear can easily be misinterpreted as an "intact cruciate ligament," an error just as apt to be made at open arthrotomy. This is particularly true when the ligament retains an intact synovial sleeve or the distal stump has fallen upon the PCL and gained attachment there (types II and V). Fiber bundles that show "clubhead" distention at their torn ends may be mistaken for loose bodies (type IV).

An older, associated rupture of the PCL is difficult to detect precisely by arthroscopic examination. It is our experience that most older ACL tears are accompanied by an instability component involving damage to the PCL.

New Imaging Techniques

A. Gächter

Of the new imaging modalities, magnetic resonance imaging (MRI) seems to have acquired a particularly favorable track record in examinations of the knee. In addition to MRI, we shall also briefly discuss the diagnostic applications of sonography and computed tomography in this region.

Sonography

Sonography in the knee is used mainly for the diagnosis of cystic abnormalities (Baker's cysts, meniscal cysts, etc.). Its use for diagnosing meniscal injuries remains controversial. Methods have been described for quantitative interpretation of the Lachman test using ultrasound, but their accuracy does not appear to surpass that of other instrumented techniques (e.g., the KT 1000 arthrometer). Also, more costly and complex equipment is required. We see no other potential applications of ultrasound for the evaluation of anterior cruciate ligament (ACL) abnormalities.

Computed Tomography

Computed tomography (CT) is best suited for evaluating the bony structures of the knee. The patellofemoral joint surfaces, for example, are well delineated on axial scans. The cruciate ligaments are very poorly demonstrated by CT, due partly to the fact that the scan planes do not follow the course of the ligaments. The best application of CT is for checking the placement and condition of drill channels following cruciate ligament reconstructions.

Today MRI has almost completely superseded CT for evaluating the ligaments and menisci of the knee.

Magnetic Resonance Imaging (MRI)

Within a short time, MRI has earned an established place in the evaluation of knee disorders, including lesions of the articular cartilage and subchondral structural changes. MRI is also very well suited for examining the menisci, since imaging can be done on virtually any plane desired.

MRI is impressive in its ability to delineate the cruciate ligaments. Especially the posterior cruciate ligament (PCL), which is difficult to see and evaluate by arthroscopy, can easily be surveyed over its entire course. Indeed, MRI can provide excellent images of all the soft-tissue structures about the knee (e.g., the popliteal fossa region) (Figs. 1 and 2). Since scanning can even be performed on oblique planes, the entire course of the ACL can be visualized, although it is not always easy to assess the quality or competence of

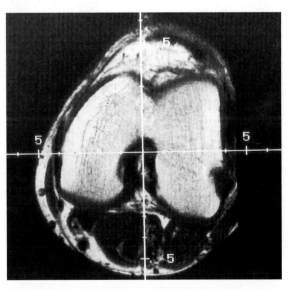

Fig. 1. MR image. The bony structure of the femoral condyles is plainly demonstrated on this tunnel-like view. The course of the PCL is delineated within the intercondylar notch. The groove for the popliteus tendon is visible on the lateral *(right)* side. The periarticular structures, most notably the muscles, blood vessels, and nerves, are seen in cross section

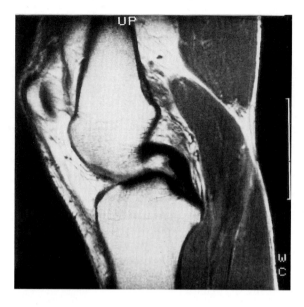

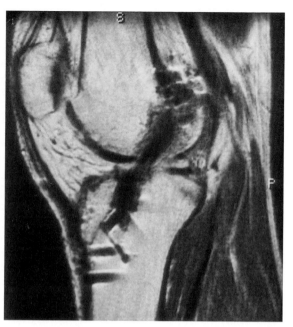

Fig. 2. Longitudinal MR scan through the knee. The PCL is seen passing far downward and backward from its femoral attachment to its tibial insertion. The gastrocnemius muscle mass is visible posteriorly. The patellar ligament with its merging Sharpey fibers is clearly shown anteriorly

Fig. 3. Sagittal MR scan through the knee following reconstruction of the ACL with a patellar tendon graft. The proximal attachment was routed through drill channels using the "through the top" technique (see article by Gächter, p. 384 ff.). The distal bone block was inlaid into a slot and the previously detached bone wedge "stacked" over it. Cartilage lesions are visible within the femoropatellar compartment

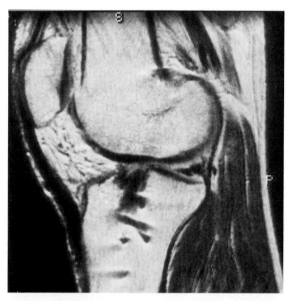

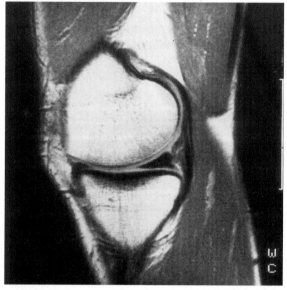

Fig. 4. Lateral parasagittal MR scan following ACL reconstruction, showing a bucket-handle tear in the posterior segment of the lateral meniscus. The tibial plateau is convex superiorly. The scan clearly shows the variable cartilage thickness on the patella and femoral condyle

Fig. 5. Parasagittal MR scan shows the slightly concave medial tibial plateau with increased subchondral bone density. The meniscus appears as an intact wedge anteriorly and posteriorly, much as on an arthrogram. The posterior capsular structures appear as a thick layer of low signal intensity

the ligament. We feel that MRI can also be very useful in evaluating the status of a reconstructed ACL following surgery (Fig. 3). The course of the graft and its points of attachment are well demonstrated. Image distortion is negligible when small, nonmagnetic implants (e. g., titanium clips) are used for attaching the graft (Figs. 3 and 4). "Graft hyperplasia" (see article by Stäubli and Jakob, p. 589 ff.) also can be readily detected by MRI. Prosthetic cruciate ligaments made of polymeric materials are poorly demonstrated, however, as they do not generate an adequate MR signal.

MRI is a noninvasive examination technique that permits a very good assessment of the anterior and posterior cruciate ligaments. It can demonstrate associated injuries of cartilage and bone (Figs. 3 and 4), and any meniscal lesions can be discerned (Figs. 4 and 5). MRI has proven to be fully competitive with arthroscopy, especially in postoperative evaluations, although it can be difficult to obtain a high-quality image of the cruciate ligament. Misinterpretations are also possible in evaluations of the menisci.

Arthroscopy retains the advantage of providing *color* images while permitting a *functional* evaluation. Also, diagnostic arthroscopy can be immediately followed by a surgical arthroscopic procedure. A major disadvantage of both modalities is that they are highly "examiner specific."

References

Braunstein EM (1982) Anterior cruciate ligament injuries: a comparison of arthrographic and physical diagnosis. AJR 138: 423–425

Federle MP, Brant-Zawadzki M (eds) (1982) Computed tomography in the evaluation of trauma. Williams & Wilkins, Baltimore

Kean DM, Worthington BS, Preston BJ et al. (1983) MR imaging of the knee: example of normal anatomy and pathology. Br J Radiol 56: 355–364

Li KC, Henkelmann M, Poon PY, Robenstein J (1984) MR imaging of the normal knee. J Comput Assist Tomogr 8: 1147–1154

Moon KL, Genant HK, Helms CA, Chafetz NI, Crooks LE, Kaufman L (1983) Muscoloskeletal applications of NMR. Radiology 147: 161–171

Schmid A, Schmid F, Tiling T (1988) Stellenwert der Arthrosonographie beim Lachman-Test. In: Beck E (Hrsg) Arthroskopie bei Instabilität des Kniegelenkes. Enke, Stuttgart, S 27–37

Turner DA, Prodomos CC, Clark JW (1984) MRI in detecting acute injury of ligaments of the knee. Vortrag, Annual Meeting of the Radiological Society of North America, Washington/DC, November 1984

The Drawer Simulator: A Practice-Oriented Training Device for Anteroposterior Stability Testing in the Knee

M. H. Oswald, S. Christen, and R. P. Jakob

The accurate diagnosis of a knee injury is often difficult, and it is frequently impossible to identify the precise underlying structural lesions. Yet the functional incompetence of anatomic structures and the subsequent biomechanical effects can and must be ascertained prior to operative treatment.

Every ligamentous lesion of the knee permits an abnormal displacement of the tibia relative to the femur. This may amount to several millimeters, depending on the severity of the injury. The degree of joint instability is a key factor determining the course of action following examination of the injured knee. This is particularly true with lesions of the anterior and posterior cruciate ligaments, for they are of central importance to the stability of the knee. Tears of the cruciate ligaments are manifested clinically by "drawer signs," or anteroposterior translations of the tibia with respect to the femur.

We know from experience that cruciate ligament injuries are often missed because the degree of anteroposterior displacement is incorrectly assessed. There are several reasons for this, including joint effusion, restriction of knee motion by hamstring or other muscle spasm, a physician with small hands attempting to examine a large knee, and the extreme difficulty of quantitating an observed translation and expressing it in units. The latter is a particular problem for beginners, many of whom are unsure about the examination technique and the correct assessment of the pathologic motion that is found.

At our hospital in Bern, we have for some time stated the findings of clinical instability tests in millimeters to avoid the inaccuracies inherent in the traditional classification (0–2 mm of displacement = normal, 3–5 mm = 1 +, 6–10 mm = 2 +, more than 10 mm = 3 +).

Our goal in the present study was to answer the following questions:

– Is it possible to develop a simple testing and training device on which the novice can practice the examination of anteroposterior knee instabilities, i.e., anterior and posterior drawer testing, in a realistic way?
– Can repeated practice on such a device improve the results of the examination?
– Can such a device affect the quality of the examination?

Given the central importance of the cruciate ligaments, we have confined our attention to a device that permits just two simple tests providing direct information on the status of the cruciate ligaments: the traditional drawer test in 90° flexion, and the Lachman drawer test in the minimally flexed knee.

Both tests are advantageous over the pivot shift test in that they are simpler to learn and perform, and they can be more easily quantified.

The Model[1]

The main problem in developing a knee simulator was to abstract complex physiologic processes and translate them into a simple mechanical model. This problem was greatly simplified by confining motion to flexion-extension and eliminating rotational and varus-valgus mobility.

The drawer simulator is a steel and plastic model of a right leg that has full mobility in flexion-extension and a variable degree of anterior and/or posterior drawer motion that is adjustable over a range of 40 mm.

The femur and tibia are represented by two steel tubes 42 and 40 cm in length. The knee joint is constructed as follows: A square metal base rigidly mounted on top of the tibia carries two vertical end plates interconnected by two anteroposterior bearing spindles. A metal yoke slides forward and backward on the spindles, assisted by ball bearings. The yoke has two vertical jaws that support an additional, transverse spindle. While the two lower spindles define the gliding plane of the knee in the anteroposterior direction, the upper transverse spindle bears

[1] We again express thanks to Mr. A. Keller, precision mechanic and engineer in Vico-Soprano, Greece, for his outstanding work in the manufacture of the steel joint.

the femoral shaft and defines the flexion axis of the joint (Fig.1).

This design permits flexion-extension over a range of about 0° to 110° while allowing 40 mm of anteroposterior motion. Rotational and varus-valgus motion are prevented.

Anteroposterior (drawer) displacement is controlled by two screw stops that travel on guide rods; each can permit up to 20 mm of anterior or posterior motion. The guide rods enter the joint from the popliteal side and are mounted in the rear end plate of the base. The screw stops can be adjusted to define any desired range of AP travel of the yoke on the bearing spindles. A millimeter scale between the guide rods allows for an accurate, reproducible setting of the anterior and posterior drawer values. With this system, simulator adjustments can be made quickly and easily. The screw stops are easily accessible in the popliteal fossa and do not interfere with the examination.

Variations of end-point resilience – changes in the perceived firmness of the end point during stability testing – are simulated by foam rubber pads of varying hardness.

The metal parts about the joint are overlaid with molded plastic "bones" to reproduce the anatomic contours of the knee. The soft tissues of the thigh and lower leg are modeled from fine-grained Styropor, and the whole limb is encased in two elastic stockings of different hardness.

The drawer simulator can be clamped to a table or desk with a special holding fixture with a movable arm that can be locked in any position desired (Fig.2).

The steel construction imparts the necessary stability to mechanically stressed parts while giving the simulator the approximate weight of a normal lower limb. The clarity of the bony structures and the firmness of the soft tissues provide a realistic context for performing the various drawer tests (Figs.3, 4). The textured outer sleeve affords the examiner a positive grip, although it may be slightly irritating since it is rougher than normal skin.

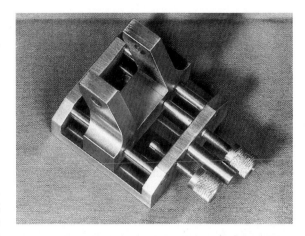

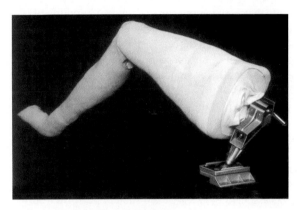

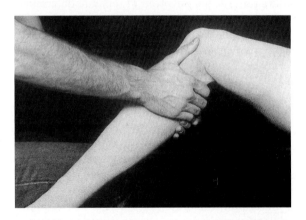

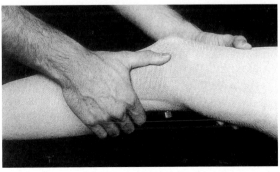

Fig.1. The metal construction of the knee joint, viewed obliquely from above

Fig.2. The assembled drawer simulator with holding fixture

Fig.3. Performing a drawer test on the simulator

Fig.4. The Lachman test performed on the simulator. A palpable "step-off" between the femoral condyles and tibial plateau aids the examiner in performing either the classic or Lachman form of the test

Evaluation

In the first phase of the evaluation, we wished to have experienced surgeons rate the drawer simulator with regard to its realism, handling, and clinical relevance. For this purpose the simulator was introduced to a total of 48 participants at a knee workshop organized by the Swiss OAK group in September of 1985. At least 90% of all those queried welcomed this kind of training device enthusiastically, confirming its clinical relevance in terms of usefulness and demand.

Approximately three-fourths of the experienced knee examiners polled (examiners with more than 5 years' experience) gave the drawer simulator an overall "good" rating. Although some reservations were expressed about the realism and handling of the device, it was found that the model simulates a human leg so well that essentially the same visual and tactile effect is produced on the examiner as with a real limb, and the same results can be achieved.

The results of this initial phase confirmed one of our working hypotheses, since the results of three different test series correlated very highly on average with the level of examiner experience (Fig. 5).

The second phase of the evaluation dealt with determining the efficacy of the drawer simulator as a teaching tool. A possible short-term learning effect was assessed by having each subject perform a series of drawer tests that involved 14 separate determinations. An openly displayed control series of 5 values was interjected into the subject's test series, giving the subject the opportunity to check his results by direct feedback. The values reported by the subject immediately before and after the control series were compared.

A long-term learning effect was tested by having each subject perform 3 test series at intervals of 2–4 days, which were then compared.

The subjects consisted of several senior staff physicians and a larger number of residents in various surgical specialities (n = 24).

With regard to a short-term learning effect, we found no significant difference between the values reported before and after the control series. It was obvious that experience from a control series could not be productively applied to a subsequent test series in the short term. Indeed, most subjects with initially good results were only confused by the control series, as indicated by their subsequently poorer results. This implies that brief practice on the simulator shortly before a clinical examination would not improve the results of the examination.

We define a long-term learning effect as an improvement that is noted from one test series to the next

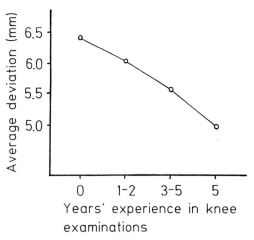

Fig. 5. Average deviation of estimated from true (set) values, correlated with the experience of the examiner

Table 1. Results of two subjects on the drawer simulator (average deviation in mm)

	Subject A	Subject B
Series 1	2.76	1.89
Intervening period	2 days	3 days
Series 2	0.56	1.50
Intervening period	10 days	3 days
Series 3	1.11	1.10

average deviation of the reported values from the true (set) values decreases by 20% to a final value of 1.13 mm. The scatter of the results also declines from 0.65 mm in series 1 to 0.22 mm in series 3. If we exclude the initially good results (no more than 1 mm deviation of reported from true value) from the review, we find that the average deviation improves by 50% to a final value of only 1.10 mm (n = 8; Fig. 6). Viewed individually, the results varied substantially among different subjects. We found that prolonged interruptions had a marked adverse effect on the accuracy of the drawer determinations, whereas regular practice led to a steady improvement of results. This is illustrated by the examples in Table 1.

The drawer simulator provides the trainee with a tool that, with regular practice, can improve his accuracy in performing and interpreting the classic drawer and Lachman tests. The purpose of the device is two-fold: to improve the examiner's proprioceptive sensation while also training him in examination techniques. It cannot help the trainee become more proficient in differential diagnosis, which must be acquired by experience with live patients.

Finally we compiled all the determinations (n = 1151 values) and broke them down by the magnitude of

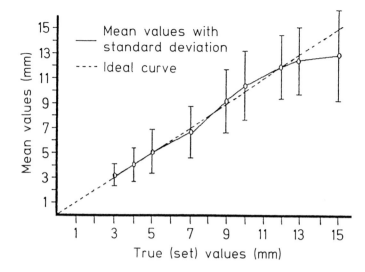

Fig.6. Mean values of all anterior drawers versus the true (set) values

when the series are repeated at intervals of 2–4 days (regular participants n = 11).

Reviewing the results of all subjects, we observe a marked improvement from series 1 to series 3. The the drawer sign. We wished to learn whether there were any general trends in the drawer determinations.

Figure 7 shows the mean values and standard deviations of the reported drawer values with respect to the true (set) values. It can be seen that, up to 12 mm, the average deviations of the reported from the true values are quite small. The highest deviation of 0.42 mm occurs at 10 mm, while the mean reported values decline markedly at displacements of 13 and 15 mm.

Looking now at the standard deviations, we find that those at 9 and 10 mm are markedly higher than those at 12 and 13 mm. Apparently this is the range of greatest uncertainty, as it is the range where large upward and downward deviations can occur.

From a clinical standpoint, it should be noted that the marked decline of reported mean values at 13 and 15 mm is of little clinical relevance. The large standard deviations at 9 and 10 mm are of greater importance, because that range has a greater practical bearing on clinical diagnosis and treatment planning. Selective training on the drawer simulator in this range would be of definite benefit in improving diagnostic proficiency.

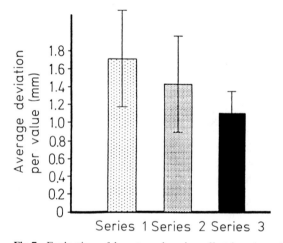

Fig.7. Evaluation of long-term learning effect based on the average deviation of reported values from true values. Initially good results (average deviation 1 mm or less) are disregarded. The test series were performed at intervals of 2–4 days

Conclusions

We can now answer the questions posed initially as follows:

– The drawer simulator is a valid model for simulating pathologic anteroposterior displacements in knees with ligamentous injury. The imitation of natural anatomic forms closely approximates the experience of examining a real limb. Our simulator confirms the feasibility of using a model to practice clinical methods of direct anteroposterior stability testing in the knee.

– Our findings show that practice on the simulator does not produce a short-term learning effect, i.e.,

there is no demonstrable improvement in results after a single use of the drawer simulator. However, a significant learning effect is seen following repeated, regular practice on the model. It is reasonable to assume that regular use of the device as an adjunct to daily practice can lead to a permanent improvement in diagnostic proficiency.
– The quality of the examination is influenced to the degree that the individual examination technique is strengthened by increasing practice and improved results. This presupposes that the learner already knows the correct manipulations or is trained in them initially by a tutor using the model.

The results of our inquiry show that there is a significant demand among physicians for a training device on which clinical examination techniques can be practiced. From this standpoint our drawer simulator satisfies a definite need.

A common suggestion expressed during our evaluation was to expand the simulator into a complete knee model useful for learning and practicing various examination techniques, most notably the pivot shift test. Interest was also expressed in a complex device that would pose problems of differential diagnosis by presenting the learner with various types of instability. It is clear, however, that a device able to simulate these complex motions would have a highly complicated design more consistent with the requirements of a mechanically perfect prosthetic knee than a training device.

It has been suggested that our drawer simulator can be improved by incorporating electronic control elements into the device. While this might make the simulator somewhat easier to handle, it must be emphasized that our purely mechanical model satisfies all essential requirements and performs all assigned tasks.

References

Abbott LC, Saunders M (1944) Injuries to the ligaments of the knee joint. J Bone Joint Surg 26: 503–521

Brantigan OC, Voshell AF (1941) The mechanics of the ligaments and menisci of the knee joint. J Bone Joint Surg 23: 44–66

Furman W, Marshall JL, Girgis FG (1976) The anterior cruciate ligament. J Bone Joint Surg [Am] 58: 179–185

Jakob RP, Noesberger B (1976) Das Pivot-Shift-Phänomen, ein neues Zeichen der Ruptur des vorderen Kreuzbandes und die spezifische laterale Rekonstruktion. Helv Chir Acta 43: 451–456

Marshall JL, Wang JB, Furman W, Girgis FW, Warren R (1975) The anterior drawer sign: What is it? Am J Sports Med 3: 152–158

Müller We (1982) Das Knie. Form, Funktion und ligamentäre Wiederherstellungschirurgie. Springer, Berlin Heidelberg New York

Torg JS, Conrad W, Kalen V (1976) Clinical diagnosis of anterior cruciate instability in the athlete. Am J Sports Med 4: 84–93

Morphology and Function of the Cruciate Ligaments in a Computer Simulation Model

B. Schneider, P. Wirz, and R. P. Jakob

In this article we present a computer model of the knee that was developed to address the following specific questions:

- Question 1: Is there a direct relationship among the shape of the femoral condyles, the knee ligaments, and the shape and position of the tibial plateau, i.e., can the femoral contours be reconstructed from radiographic or MR images using a mathematical geometric model?
- Question 2: Can the different shapes of the lateral and medial tibial plateaus account for the different shapes of the lateral and medial femoral condyles?
- Question 3: How do changes in ligament parameters affect the shape of the condyles?
- Question 4: How do changes in the shape and position of the tibial plateau affect the shape of the condyles?
- Question 5: How do ligamentous changes affect the strain behavior of the ligaments during motion?
- Question 6: Can the model offer an explanation for clinical findings such as a flexion or extension deficit or instabilities?
- Question 7: What is the significance of the Burmester curve?

Assumptions

We employ a two-dimensional model in which the knee is represented as a projection onto the sagittal plane. The longitudinal axis of the femur runs vertically, and the femur remains stationary while the tibia moves in flexion-extension. The right knee is viewed from the medial to lateral aspect in our model, or the left knee from lateral to medial. The tibial plateau is represented schematically as a linear or circular arc segment. When the tibial plateau moves, the cruciate ligaments determine the path of the motion. There are isometric points on the femur and tibial plateau that always maintain a constant distance from each other during motion (see chapter by Friederich and O'Brien, p. 78 ff.). The sites of attachment of the cru-

ciate ligaments correspond to these points in our model. The tibial plateau contacts the femoral articular surface at one point in each position of motion. In every position, then, the portion of the tibial surface in contact with the femur represents a tangent (linear or circular arc segment) to the condylar surface. The complete set of contact points defines the shape of the femoral condyle.

Method

The cruciate ligaments are modeled as lines connecting 2 points on the sagittal plane (Fig. 1). The lengths of the ligaments and their points of attachment can be arbitrarily selected in the model.

The cruciate ligaments are motion-controlling elements. They do not alter their length during joint motion, i.e., the points of tibial attachment move on circular paths about the points of femoral attachment.

The tibial plateau is alternatively represented as a convex or concave circular arc or as a linear segment. When it is represented as a circular arc segment, the radius and associated center of the circle can be varied. When it is represented as a linear segment, the distance from the plateau to the tibial attachment points and the slope of the plateau relative to the femoral axis can be varied.

Two different plateaus can be selected, leading to the computation of two different femoral condyles, although each is based on the same ligament parameters (Fig. 1).

Collateral ligaments can be added to the model if desired. While these ligaments do not perform a controlling function in the model, it is nevertheless interesting to calculate the strain behavior of the ligaments during articular motion. The points of attachment of the collateral ligaments can be sited on the "Burmester curve." This curve is determined exclusively by the cruciate ligaments (for more details, see below or Menschik 1987) (see Fig. 1).

The following parameters, then, provide a complete description of the modeled knee:

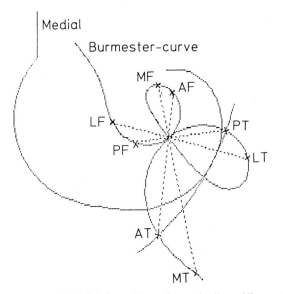
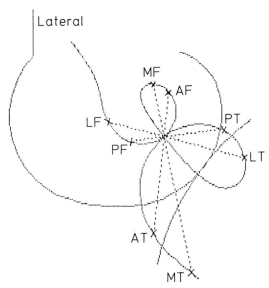

Fig. 1. Model simulations with cruciate and collateral ligaments for a concave medial and convex lateral tibial plateau. The collateral ligaments insert on the Burmester curve. *AF*, Femoral attachment of ACL; *AT*, tibial attachment of ACL; *PF*, femoral attachment of PCL; *PT*, tibial attachment of PCL; *LF*, femoral attachment of LCL; *LT*, tibial attachment of LCL; *MF*, femoral attachment of MCL; *MT*, tibial attachment of MCL

– The length of the cruciate ligaments
– The distances between the femoral and tibial attachments of the cruciate ligaments
– The shape and position of both tibial plateaus
– If needed, a definition of the cruciate ligaments (see Fig. 1)

The condylar shape is calculated as follows:

– The points of attachment of the cruciate ligaments remain equidistant from each another during motion, i.e., the tibial attachments move in circular paths about the femoral attachments, which remain stationary.
– The tibial attachment of the anterior cruciate ligament (ACL) moves on a small circular arc about the femoral attachment. Because the tibial attachment of the posterior cruciate ligament (PCL) also moves on a circular path about the femoral attachment of the ligament, and the distance between the tibial attachment sites remains unchanged, their new position is uniquely defined. Both attachment points determine the new position of the tibial plateau, and thus the distal attachment points of the cruciate ligaments as well. The position of the cruciate ligaments and tibial plateau, moreover, determine the point of femorotibial contact. It is constructed by finding the point of intersection of the tibial plateau with a line perpendicular to the tibial plateau through the instant center of rotation, the instant center coinciding with the crossing point of

the cruciate ligaments. The sum of these contact points defines the shape of the femoral condyle.

Use of the Model

The following steps are followed in using the model:

1. First the parametric values of the knee are determined from an X-ray or MR image or from empirical data (length of the cruciate ligaments, distances between the femoral and tibial points of attachment, shape and position of the tibial plateau, points of attachment of the collateral ligaments if desired).
2. The cruciate ligament parameters (lengths and attachments) are entered on the computer screen either by moving the points of attachment or by typing in numerical values.
3. The cruciate ligament parameters can be used to plot the Burmester curve (see below). If collateral ligaments are desired, their points of attachment can be defined.
4. Both tibial plateaus are defined.
5. From these data (ligament apparatus and tibial plateaus), the outlines of the femoral condyles are computed.
6. The calculated curves can be graphically displayed and compared with the radiographs.

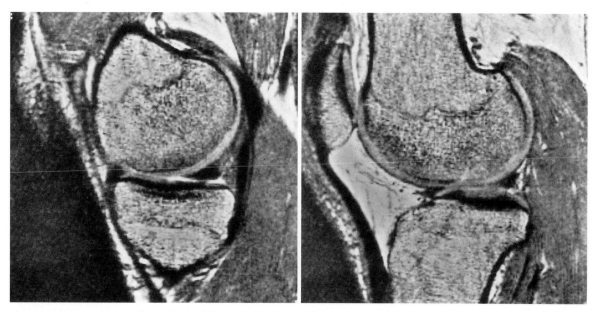

Fig. 2. MR images of the medial and lateral joint compartments. Presumed sections through the planes of motion

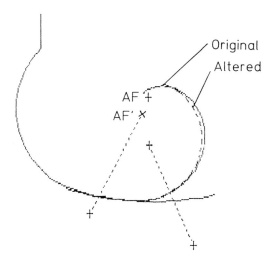

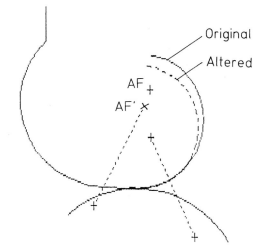

Fig. 3. The femoral attachment of the anterior cruciate ligament *(AF)* was placed too far anteriorly (approx. 6 mm) in the extended position. This results in about a 6-mm shortening of the ligament, which becomes stretched as the knee is flexed.

This stretching effect is manifested by the marked discrepancy in the old and new condyle shapes. Because the new condyles lie inside the old ones, stretching occurs. The effects on the lateral and medial sides of the joint are different

7. Next, the ligament parameters and the shape and position of the tibial plateau can be manipulated as desired (e.g., by moving the points of cruciate ligament attachment or moving the tibial plateau to a designated position of flexion).

8. The altered values define a new situation, for which the corresponding condyle shapes can be recomputed.

9. The recomputed condylar shapes can now be compared with the old shapes (Fig. 3).

10. A movement can be simulated by having the tibial plateau move while guided by the old ligament apparatus. During this motion a record can be generated of the strain (length change) experienced by the new ligaments.

Results

Relationship Between Femoral Condyle Shapes, Ligament Parameters, and Shape and Position of the Tibial Plateaus (Questions 1, 2, and 4)

The ligament lengths, distances between attachments, and the shapes and position of the tibial plateaus were determined from the MR images of a volunteer (see Fig. 2). These data were then fed into the model to compute the condylar shapes (see Fig. 4). The calculated shapes of the condyles and the shapes from the MR images show good agreement up to about 100° of flexion (see Figs. 2, 4). Past 100° flexion,

the medial condyle deviates sharply from the MR image. We therefore attempted to use a strongly convex tibial plateau past 100° of flexion. This change improved the computed femoral shape. The two different condyles are shown in Fig. 5. Presumably the approximation of the tibial plateau as a purely convex or concave circular arc is not accurate enough for very large flexion angles. Because the contact point moves backward on the tibial plateau with increasing flexion (Fig. 6) and the medial plateau becomes somewhat convex posteriorly (see Fig. 2), the computed condyle deviates from the original shape in extreme flexion.

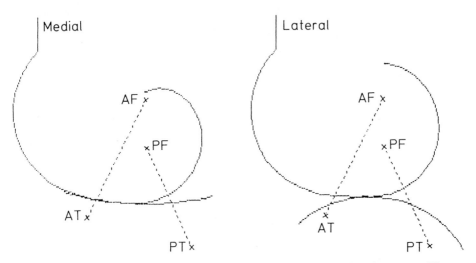

Fig. 4. Reconstruction of the condylar shapes by the computer model based on the presumed ligament lengths and distances between attachment points taken from Fig. 2. Abbreviations as in Fig. 1

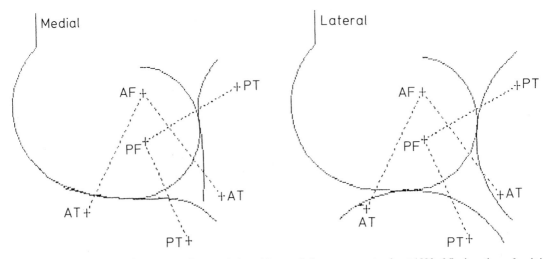

Fig. 5. The medial plateau is represented as consisting of 2 parts. It is concave up to about 100° of flexion, thereafter it is strongly convex. Abbreviations as in Fig. 1

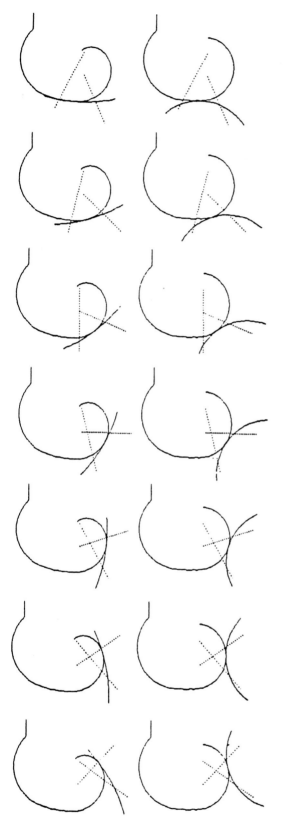

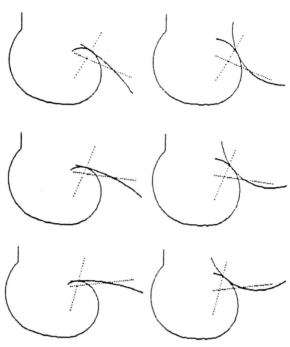

Fig. 6. Ten phases of a computer-generated motion from extension to full flexion. The *left* image in each pair represents the medial side of the joint, the *right* image the lateral side. The points of femorotibial contact move posteriorly during the motion

Even this initial example clearly demonstrates a functional relationship between the ligament apparatus, the shape of the tibial plateau, and the shape of the femoral condyle. Although our model is a gross simplification (only 2 dimensions, only 1 ligament fiber, a linear or circular arc segment for the tibial plateau), its relation to reality is quite good. In particular, it can account for the varying shapes of the lateral and medial condyles associated with changes in the tibial plateaus. The importance of the shape of the tibial plateau can be appreciated in Figs. 4 and 5. A concave plateau leads to greater curvature of the femoral condyle with increasing flexion.

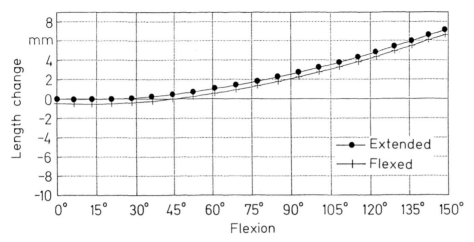

Fig. 7. The change from Fig. 6 was made in extension and in approximately 45° of flexion. When the change is made in flexion, the ACL is slightly lax in extension and is stretched less in flexion

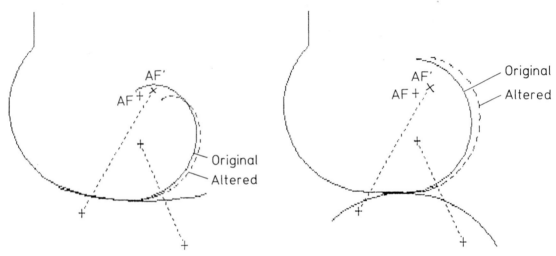

Fig. 8. The femoral attachment of the anterior cruciate ligament *(AF)* was transposed about 6 mm posteriorly in the extended position. This results in an approximately 4-mm lengthening of the ligament, which becomes lax with increasing flexion. This effect is manifested by the marked discrepancy in the old and new condyle shapes. Because the new condyles lie outside the old ones, laxness occurs. The effects on the lateral and medial sides of the joint are different

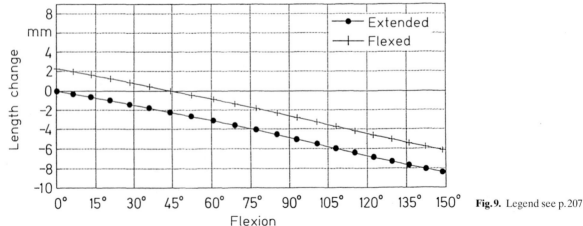

Fig. 9. Legend see p. 207

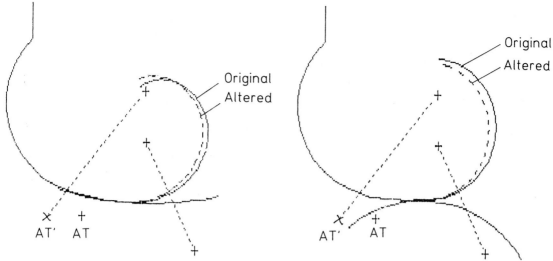

Fig. 10. The tibial attachment of the ACL *(AT)* was advanced about 12 mm anteriorly in the extended position. This results in an approximately 6.5-mm lengthening of the ligament, which becomes stretched with increasing flexion. This effect is mani- fested by the marked discrepancy in the old and new condyle shapes. Because the new condyles lie inside the old ones, stretching occurs. The effects on the lateral and medial sides of the joint are different

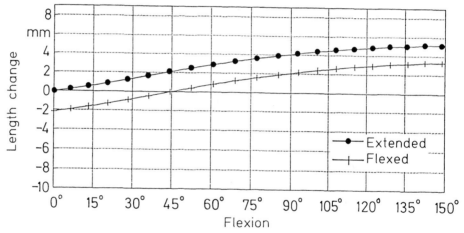

Fig. 11. The change from Fig. 10 was made in extension and in approximately 45° of flexion. When the change is made in flex- ion, the ACL is slightly lax in extension and is stretched less in flexion

Effects of Changing Ligament Parameters on Condyle Shape and Ligament Strain (Questions 3 and 5)

The following changes were made in the subject-defined parameters used in Fig. 4:

- The femoral attachment of the ACL was moved approximately 6.5 mm anteriorly. This change was

◁ **Fig. 9.** The change from Fig. 8 was made in extension and in ap-proximately 45° of flexion. When the change is made in flexion, the anterior cruciate ligament is slightly overstretched in exten-sion and is stretched less in flexion

made both in extension (see Fig. 3) and in about 45° of flexion. The strain behavior of the ligament is shown in Fig. 7.
- The femoral attachment of the ACL was moved approximately 6 mm posteriorly. This change was made both in extension (Fig. 8) and in about 45° of flexion. The strain behavior of the ligament is shown in Fig. 9.
- The tibial attachment of the ACL was moved ap-proximately 12 mm anteriorly. This change was made both in extension (Fig. 10) and in about 45° of flexion. The strain behavior of the ligament is shown in Fig. 11.

– The tibial attachment of the ACL was moved approximately 12 mm posteriorly. This change was made both in extension (Fig. 12) and in about 45° of flexion. The strain behavior of the ligament is shown in Fig. 13.

During motion the tibial plateau was guided by the original ligament apparatus, i.e., the tibial plateau enveloped the original condyle during the course of the movement. The length change in the ligament (strain) was computed at each point of the motion.

If the new computer-generated condyle shape is inside the outline of the original shape, then for motion to occur, either the ligaments must be stretched or a portion of the articular cartilage must be removed. If the new condyle shape is outside the original shape, the ligaments must become lax during joint motion, i.e., they will cease to function as restraints, and the joint will become unstable.

In our model, moving the femoral attachment of the ACL anteriorly leads to a shortening of the ligament, which consequently becomes stretched with increasing flexion. This effect is manifested in Fig. 6 by the marked deviation of the new condyle shapes from the original shapes. If the change is introduced in the

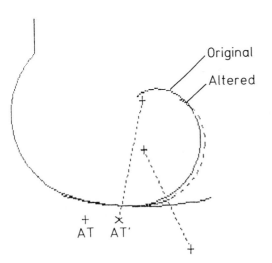 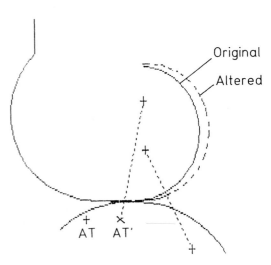

Fig. 12. The tibial attachment of the ACL *(AT)* was transposed about 12 mm posteriorly in the extended position. This results in an approximately 4-mm shortening of the ligament, which becomes lax with increasing flexion. This effect is manifested by

the marked discrepancy in the old and new condyle shapes. Because the new condyles lie outside the old ones, laxness occurs. The effects on the lateral and medial sides of the joint are different

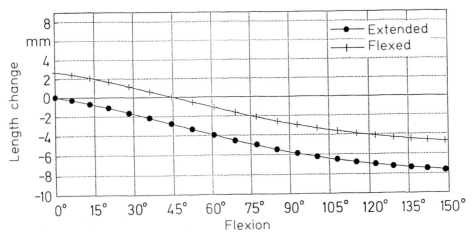

Fig. 13. The change from Fig. 12 was made in extension and in approximately 45° of flexion. When the change is made in flex-

ion, the ACL is slightly stretched in extension and is less lax in flexion

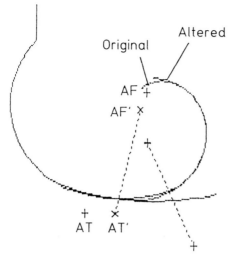
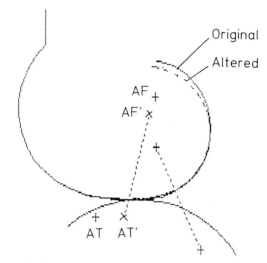

Fig. 14. The tibial attachment of the ACL *(AT)* was transposed about 10 mm posteriorly and its femoral attachment *(AF)* about 6 mm anteriorly. Made at about 45° of flexion, these changes result in about 12-mm shortening of the ligament, which is slightly stretched in both flexion and extension, although the deviations are relatively small. Moving the tibial attachment posteriorly compensates to a degree for the anterior advancement of the femoral attachment

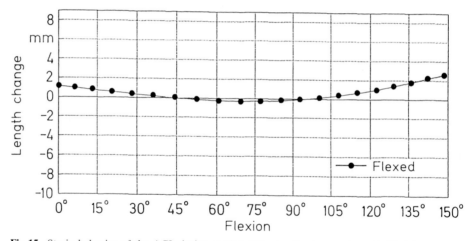

Fig. 15. Strain behavior of the ACL during motion following the changes shown in Fig. 14

flexed position, ligament stretching is reduced in flexion, but the ACL becomes slightly lax in extension.

Moving the femoral attachment of the ACL posteriorly causes the ACL to become lax in flexion. If the change is made in the flexed position, the ligament becomes overstretched in extension (see Figs. 8, 9).

Moving the tibial attachment of the ACL anteriorly leads to stretching of the ligament in flexion (see Figs. 10 and 11). Moving the tibial attachment posteriorly causes the ligament to become lax in flexion (see Figs. 12, 13).

These findings suggested that ligament stretching caused by placing the femoral attachment of the ACL too far anteriorly (see Figs. 6, 7) could be partially corrected by moving the tibial attachment posteriorly (see Figs. 12, 13). This change was simulated, and the results are shown in Figs. 14 and 15. Although the two sets of ligament parameters are quite different (see Figs. 4, 14), in both cases the tibial plateaus trace out almost identical condyle shapes.

Explanation of Clinical Findings (Question 6)

The expected results were compared with the results generated by the computer model, and reasonably good agreement was found. The model can furnish explanations for certain clinical findings. It can identify situations in which ligament stretching will occur (see Fig.3). For motion to proceed normally in these cases, either several millimeters of cartilage material must be removed from the old condyles, or the ligament must stretch accordingly.

The effects on the lateral and medial joint compartments are not necessarily the same (see Fig.8). This is illustrated by the change in Fig.8, which has a greater effect medially than laterally. This could be one cause of the varus limb morphotype.

On the Burmester Curve (Question 7)

The computer model also aids us in understanding the significance of the Burmester curve.

As noted earlier, the Burmester curve is determined entirely by the cruciate ligaments. At a given flexion angle, the curve passes through all points that are at the vertex of their path in that position of motion, i.e., the radius of curvature of the paths of these points is maximal in that position. Menschik (1987) states that the collateral ligaments insert on the Burmester curve for the position in which lines connecting the tibial and femoral attachments of the cruciate ligaments are almost parallel, or more precisely, where the tibial plateau is inclined about 4° posteriorly from the parallel position (see Fig.1).

In working with the model, we made the following discoveries:

- When the collateral ligaments insert on the Burmester curve as described, the distances between their points of attachment remain virtually unchanged throughout joint motion (Fig.16).

- The collateral ligaments are slightly lax in full extension and flexion; they attain their maximum length in intermediate flexion.
- If the attachments of the collateral ligaments are moved off the Burmester curve (Fig.17), the ligaments are alternately lax and stretched during motion (Fig.18), and the length changes are generally greater.

Comparison with Other Studies

To see how our results compared with the current state of research in this area, we selected two representative studies and compared them with our computer knee model (Hoogland and Hillen 1984; chapter by Friederich and O'Brien, p.78 ff.).

Hoogland and Hillen used cadaver knees to investigate motion-related length changes in ACLs attached at various sites. They tested 3 attachment sites on the femur and 4 on the tibia (Fig.19). Each of the femoral sites was connected to each of the tibial sites, and the length changes were graphically recorded for 4 different knees. The results of this study are shown in Fig.20.

These same changes (Fig.19) were simulated by our computer model. The results are shown in Figs.21–23. In contrast to the Hoogland-Hillen study, our results were obtained mathematically rather than mechanically. As we have seen, moving the femoral attachment of the ACL posteriorly (position C in Fig.19) causes the ligament to become lax in flexion and stretched in extension. Moving the femoral at-

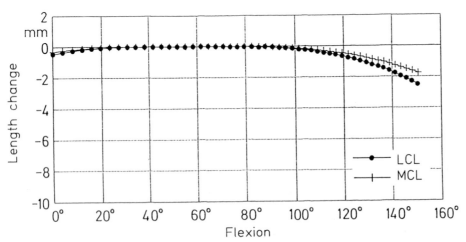

Fig.16. Strain behavior of collateral ligaments inserting on the Burmester curve (see Fig.1). There is no point at which the collateral ligaments become stretched during joint motion. The length changes are relatively small. *LCL* Lateral collateral ligament, *MCL* medial collateral ligament

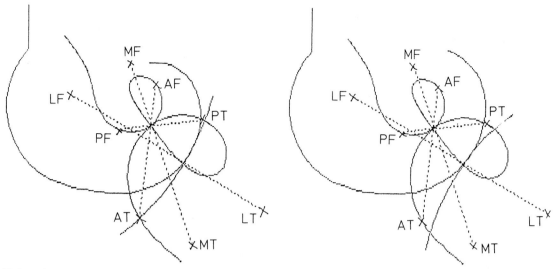

Fig. 17. Insertion of the collateral ligaments adjacent to the Burmester curve. Abbreviations as in Fig. 1

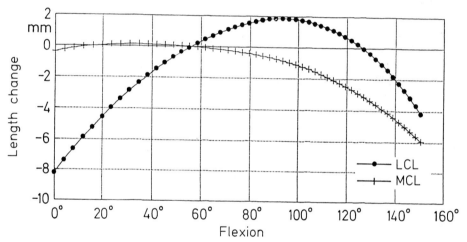

Fig. 18. Strain behavior of collateral ligaments that insert off the Burmester curve (see Fig. 17). The collateral ligaments are alternately lax and stretched during flexion. The length changes are relatively large

tachment anteriorly (position A) produces the opposite effect. Moving the tibial attachment of the ACL anteriorly or posteriorly either compensates for these effects or compounds them. In Fig. 21, for example, shifting the tibial attachment to position 3 (posteriorly) partly compensates for the advanced position of the femoral attachment. However, moving the tibial attachment to position 3 in Fig. 23 (posteriorly) causes even greater stretching of the ligament in extension.

Although the results of our model basically agree with the results of Hoogland and Hillen, the absolute values of their measurements are not exactly comparable to our results.

In the chapter by Friederich and O'Brien (p. 78 ff.), the sites of attachment of the cruciate ligament are studied in greater detail, and the existence of a "transition line" is demonstrated experimentally. Ligaments that insert on the transition line do not become lax or stretched in extension or in about 140° of flexion. It was shown experimentally that the farther the ligaments are attached from the isometric point and from the transition line, the greater the length change experienced by the ligaments during joint motion. Moving the attachment site along the transition line produces the smallest changes; moving it perpendicular to the transition line produces the greatest changes.

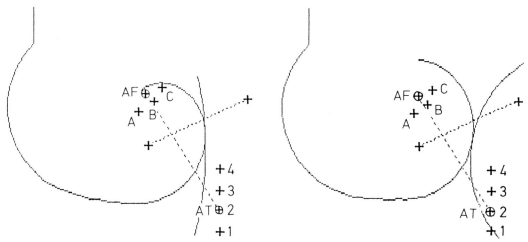

Fig. 19. Experimental arrangement like that used by Hoogland and Hillen (1984). Three femoral attachment points *(A, B, C)* and 4 tibial attachments *(1, 2, 3, 4)* are selected. In the study, each of the femoral points *(AF)* was connected to each of the tibial points *(AT)* (Hoogland and Hillen used cadaver material; we used our computer model)

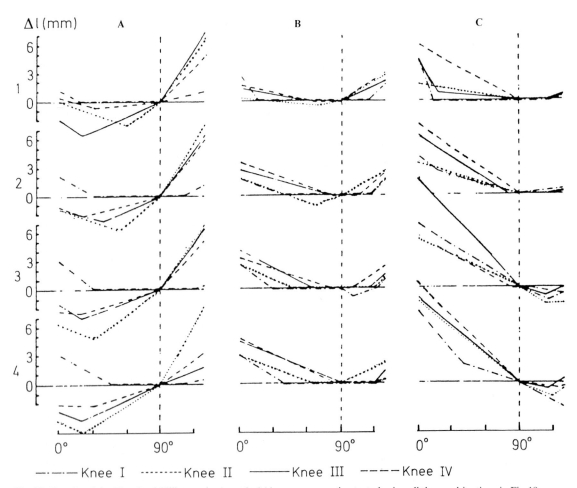

Fig. 20. Results of the Hoogland-Hillen study. A total of 4 knees were motion tested using all the combinations in Fig. 19

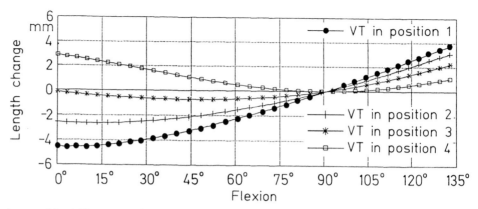

Fig. 21. The femoral attachment of the ACL was moved to position A (too far anterior). Placing the tibial attachment in position 3 (too far posterior) partly corrects the femoral deviation. Placing it in position 4 leads to stretching of the ACL in extension, while positions 2 and 1 lead to ACL slackness in extension. In each case the ACL is lax beyond 90° flexion (see Fig. 19)

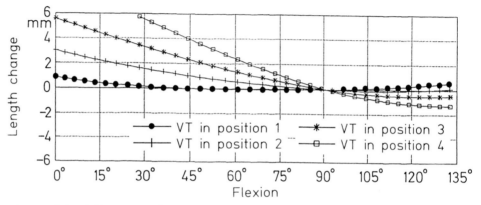

Fig. 22. The femoral attachment of the ACL was moved to position B (too far posterior). Placing the tibial attachment in position 1 (too far anterior) partly corrects the femoral deviation. Placing it farther posteriorly (positions 2, 3, and 4) leads to stretching of the ACL in extension (see Fig. 19)

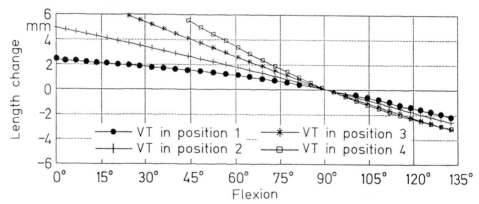

Fig. 23. The femoral attachment was moved to position C (too far posterior). Placing the tibial attachment *(AT)* in position 1 (too far anterior) partly corrects the femoral deviation. Placing it farther posteriorly (positions 2, 3, and 4) leads to stretching of the ACL in extension. However, the degree of stretch is greater than in Fig. 22. The ACL is slightly lax in flexion (see Fig. 19)

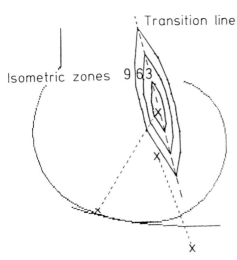

Fig. 24. The transition line and zones of isometry were calculating using the computer model

We used our model to calculate the femoral transition line of the ACL and lines with equivalent ligament length changes for a concrete situation. The femoral attachment of the ACL was repositioned at several points, and the length changes of the ligament during motion were calculated. Linear extrapolation then was used to construct the lines with 3, 6 and 9 mm of length change. The result is shown in Fig. 24 (see Fig. 6a in the chapter by Friederich and O'Brien, p. 84). Once again, our model confirmed the experimental results, including the existence of the transition line. When we placed the femoral attachment of the ACL on this line, the length of the ligament showed absolutely no change at 0° and 140° of flexion.

This finding validates the basic assumptions underlying our model, while also confirming the experimental results of other authors.

Potential Applications

We can envision several potential applications for this model:

- Surgeons in training could use the model to study visually the effects of altering ligament positions and the consequences of faulty insertion sites without the need for costly cadaver studies. Changes are easy to reverse or modify, and all experiments are reproducible.
- Students could use the model to learn more about the function of the knee joint, and teachers could use it to demonstrate certain types of clinical finding.

- The model could aid physiotherapists in determining whether a given motion can be safely performed or whether a forced movement would cause irreparable ligamentous injury. It could also be used to inform patients about the effects of surgical procedures.
- Another area of application is in prosthetics. What shape must a partial joint replacement have in order to protect ligament integrity? The model has already been used to calculate the condylar shapes for two mechanical knee models (see chapter by Wirz et al., p. 215 ff.).
- The model is also useful for research purposes, as it can provide the mathematical background for certain types of experiment. The results are fully reproducible.

Concluding Remarks

Our model, which is based on a somewhat modified form of the crossed four-bar linkage, can demonstrate graphically the relationships between the ligaments, tibial plateau, and femoral condyles and the effects of ligament transpositions and thus can furnish an explanation for certain findings. Computer simulation provides a new source of information that can supplement the traditional mode of data acquisition through physical experiment. Simulator experiments are less costly and fully reproducible. Still, it is well to keep in mind the distinction between a model and reality. A model can simulate reality only within a limited realm. Our model, for example, lacks the third dimension and does not include elements of the muscular system. Nevertheless, it is surprising how capably our model can reproduce experimental results, explain clinical findings, and reconstruct the shapes of the femoral condyles.[1]

References

Menschik A (1987) Biometrie. Konstruktionsprinzip des Kniegelenks, des Hüftgelenks, der Beinlänge und Körpergröße. Springer, Berlin Heidelberg New York Tokyo

Müller We (1982) Das Knie. Form, Funktion und ligamentäre Wiederherstellungschirurgie. Springer, Berlin Heidelberg New York Tokyo

Hoogland T, Hillen B (1984) Intra articular reconstruction of the anterior cruciate ligament. Clin Orthop 185: 197–202

[1] The computer model can be run on any IBM-compatible PC with at least 256K RAM and a graphics card. The software is available from the senior author.
The study was funded by a generous research grant from the Maurice E. Müller Foundation in Bern.

Production of Mechanical Knee Models for Training

P. Wirz, B. Schneider, and R. P. Jakob

Background

Students, physiotherapists, and even physicians often find it difficult to comprehend the complex functional mechanisms of the knee joint.

Because the accurate diagnosis of potential instabilities is crucial to effective treatment planning, major importance is attached to the correct conduct and interpretation of knee examinations. Persons suffering from a knee disorder do not make appropriate "training objects."

Statement of Problem

There is need for a sophisticated teaching model that permits a comprehensive demonstration of the functional, physiologic, and pathologic motions of the knee. The dynamic stability tests are of special concern, for they are technically demanding and cause significant patient discomfort. Thus, as a supplement to the Lachman simulator (see chapter by Oswald et al., p. 196 ff.), there is interest in developing a model knee that can reproduce not just drawer displacements but also rotational motions and the more complex motions that are associated with dynamic testing.

One of our goals in developing a new model was to replicate the anatomy of the articular surfaces as accurately as possible. A second, parallel goal was to analyze geometrically the ligament system and motion characteristics of the knee so that an optimum articular shape could be computed. The synthesis of anatomy and mathematics should yield a knee model that possesses sufficient but not excessive ligamentous restraint and is a faithful reproduction of the knee in terms of its anatomy and function (especially with regard to motion characteristics).

Design of Models that Allow Motion on the Sagittal Plane

We approached the complex mechanics of the knee joint in stages, beginning with the design of two initial models that permit only the principal knee motion of flexion-extension. The kinematic core of each model is a crossed four-bar linkage with rigid steel connectors that have ball bearings at their hinge points. Regarding the articular surfaces, a special computer program was used to calculate the shapes of the femoral condyles from the defined parameters of the cruciate ligaments and tibial plateau, and also to illustrate the effects of ligament manipulations (see chapter by Schneider et al., p. 201 ff.).

Below we shall describe and illustrate the steps followed in the production of the demonstration model and its didactic use.

A series of magnetic resonance images of the left knee of the senior author (P. W.) were obtained in 1:1 scale. Figure 1 shows a sagittal scan through the intercondylar notch.

We recognize the ACL (1) with its tibial and femoral attachments.

We determined the isometric points of the cruciate ligament attachments, drawing on the experiments of Friederich et al.: femoral attachment of the ACL (2), tibial attachment of the ACL (3) (see also chapter by Friederich and O'Brien, p. 78 ff.).

The following structures are also easily identified: patella (7), patellar ligament (8), quadriceps tendon (9).

The location of the isometric points and the shape and position of the tibial plateau provided the input data for calculating the shape of the femoral condyle using the computer model (Fig. 2).

The computer program offers the option of printing out the coordinates of the condylar points. For a previously selected number of points, this option provides the x value, y value, local radius of curvature for milling, and sequential point numbering.

The patellar surface was configured so that it conformed closely to anatomy. Starting from the point of

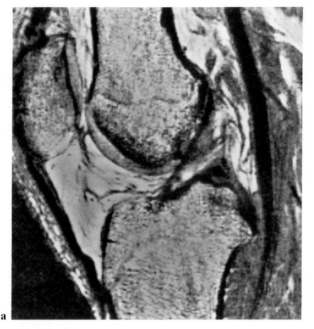

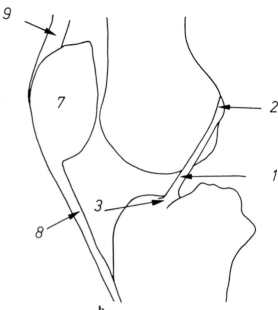

Fig. 1 a, b. MR image with explanatory drawing

Lengths stated in mm
Condyles: Peter Wirz standard
Ligament lengths:
    Anterior cruciate ligament: 47.000
    Posterior cruciate ligament: 38.005
Distance between cruciate ligament attachment points:
    Femur = 18.000
    Tibia = 40.000
Coordinates of ligament attachment points:
Anterior cruciate ligament: AF (0.000,   0.000),
                             AT (−25.598, −39.418)
Posterior cruciate ligament: PF (−1.256, −17.956),
                             PT (11.783, -53.654)

Medial tibial plateau:
    Plateau is straight:
    RTP = 0.000, δ = 80.000
Condyles:
    Medial condyle:

	Point 1 = (− 42.156, 12.805)
Radius = 31.000 →	Point 2 = (− 45.367, 8.459)
Radius = 31.000 →	Point 3 = (− 47.775, 3.621)
Radius = 31.000 →	Point 4 = (− 49.306, − 1.561)
Radius = 31.000 →	Point 5 = (− 49.914, − 6.930)
Radius = 31.000 →	Point 6 = (− 49.580, −12.323)
Radius = 31.000 →	Point 7 = (− 48.315, −17.577)

Fig. 2. Listing of coordinates: Peter Wirz standard

femorotibial contact in extension, the values were precisely calculated according to the dimensions of the cruciate ligaments and the shape of the tibial plateau. The calculated data were loaded into the memory of a computer-controlled milling machine, which cut into preformed steel blanks of the femur and tibia the condylar shape conforming to the ligament and tibial parameters, as well as the tibial platform itself (Fig. 3). A fixed reference system was created by mounting the workpieces on positioning pins set into a base plate (*1* = steel femur workpiece, *3* = milling spindle with bit, *4* = positioning pins for tibial workpiece).

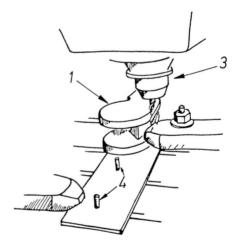

Fig. 3. Milling the femoral condyle

Further details on the manufacture of the model would exceed the scope of this article. The finished components are shown in Fig. 4.

An aperture in the femoral condyle permits an observer to view the arrangement and interplay of the cruciate ligaments. Figure 5a,b shows the model, with its straight tibial plateau, in the extended position; Fig. 5c,d shows the model positioned in approximately 90° flexion.

It can be seen how flexion is associated with a descent of the ACL (4) onto the tibial plateau, and with a recession of the patella. This recession demonstrates that an "olecranization" of the knee joint (immobilizing the patella in a fixed position with respect to the tibia) would prohibit normal motion in a joint with intact cruciate ligaments. The model further illustrates how the quadriceps muscle becomes stretched during flexion. The cruciate ligaments, true to their name, form an almost equilateral cross.

Following the same basic principle, we constructed a second model in which the flat tibial plateau was replaced by a plateau that was concave medially and convex laterally (Fig. 6). For this purpose we had to determine the radii and corresponding centers of curvature of the plateaus from the MR images. MR demonstrated a concave medial tibial plateau articulating with a somewhat squat medial condyle. The lateral plateau was strongly convex, and the lateral condyle displayed a fuller shape. Measurements indicated a radius of curvature of 167 mm on the medial side (concave plateau) and 43 mm on the lateral side (convex plateau). In accordance with the different medial and lateral radii of curvature on the tibia, the computer calculations generated different shapes for the medial and lateral femoral condyles.

Figure 6 shows a lateral view of the model flexed to about 160°. To better demonstrate the rolling-gliding motion of the joint, fine markings are placed along the borders of the femur and tibia to indicate the points of femorotibial contact (a). The tibial markings are spaced at regular intervals. With increasing flexion, the corresponding femoral contact points are spaced closer and closer together. This shows that gliding predominates at the start of flexion, while a greater degree of rolling occurs as flexion proceeds, shifting the contact point posteriorly (b).

A front view of the model (Fig. 7) shows how the ACL (4) impinges against the roof of the intercondylar notch (a) in the extended knee, preventing hyperextension. A rear view into the workings of the joint (Fig. 8) shows how the different-shaped tibial plateaus are matched with different condylar shapes. It can be seen how the lateral condyle (a) terminates at a higher level than the medial condyle.

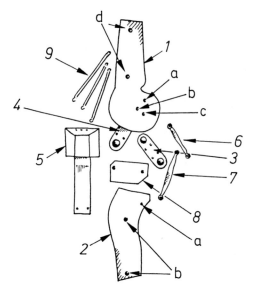

Fig. 4. The disassembled model

1 Femur with:
   a Drill hole for ACL
   b Drill hole for PCL
   c Drill hole for medial collateral ligament
   d Drill holes to position the workpiece for milling
2 Tibia with:
   a Drill hole for medial collateral ligament
   b Drill holes to position the workpiece for milling
3 Posterior cruciate ligament with ball bearing seats
4 Anterior cruciate ligament
5 Patella with patellar ligament
6 Medial collateral ligament
7 Lateral collateral ligament
8 Tibial insert for attaching the cruciate ligaments with:
   a Drill hole for ACL
   b Drill hole for PCL
9 Springs representing the quadriceps muscle bellies

The models are swivel-mounted on a flat stand, on the underside of which is printed:

Two-Dimensional Knee Joint Model (Left Knee).

Features

1. The cruciate ligaments are designed as a four-bar linkage with rigid attachments (flat bars with ball bearings at the hinge points).
2. The collateral ligaments consist of a flexible copper wire mesh. They change their length during motion: lateral length change 3.2 mm = 6.4%, medial length change 1.5 mm = 2.3%. They are stretched at 100° of flexion.
3. The quadriceps femoris muscle group is represented by 3 springs.
4. For simplicity, the tibial plateau is flat on its medial and lateral sides and has a 10° slope.

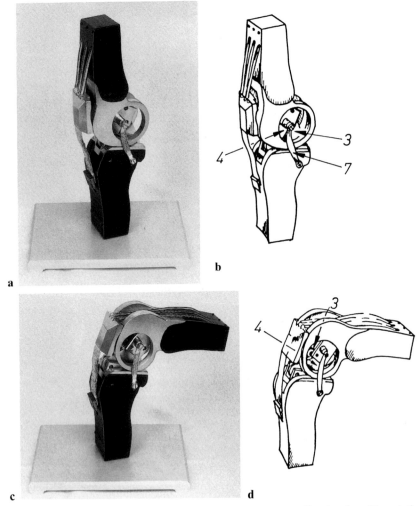

Fig. 5 a–d. First model in extension and flexion, with corresponding drawings. The relationships in the assembled model are the same as in the disassembled state

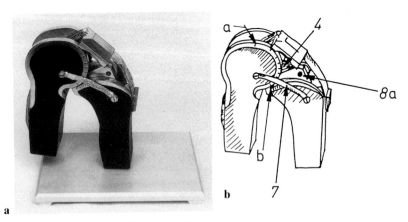

Fig. 6 a, b. Second model viewed from the side

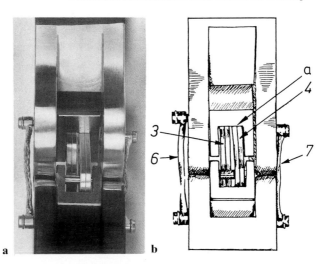

Fig. 7 a, b. Anterior view   **a**   **b**

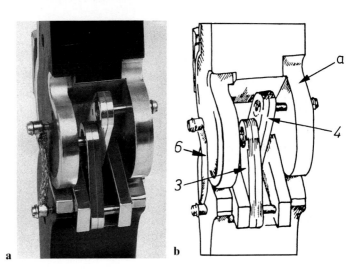

Fig. 8 a, b. Posterior view   **a**   **b**

5. The femoral condyle shape is computer-calculated from the following data: length of ACL 47 mm, length of PCL 38 mm, distance between cruciate ligament attachments 18 mm on the femur, 40 mm on the tibia.

Two-Dimensional Knee Joint Model (Right Knee).

Features

1. The cruciate ligaments are designed as a four-bar linkage with rigid attachments.
2. The collateral ligaments are flexible. They change their length during motion: lateral length change 3.2 mm = 6.4%, medial length change 1.5 mm = 2.3%. They are stretched at 100° of flexion.
3. The femoral condyle shape is computer-calculated from the following data: length of ACL 47 mm, length of PCL 38 mm, distance between cruciate ligament attachments 18 mm on the femur, 40 mm

on the tibia; lateral tibial plateau convex, R = 43 mm; medial plateau is concave, R = 167 mm. (Note the resulting change in the femoral contours.)

4. The lateral borders of the femur and tibia are *marked to indicate the corresponding contact points* and *demonstrate the rolling-gliding mechanism.*

Models with Three-Dimensional Motion and Adjustable Ligament Lengths

The design of these models was based on a series of sagittal MR images taken at 1.8-mm intervals through the knee of the senior author.

A computer program was used to convert the MRI-defined joint contours into digitized instructions for cutting out identically contoured metal plates on a

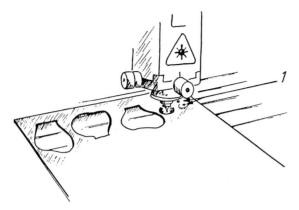

Fig. 9. Laser cutter. Three contours have already been cut from the plate stock

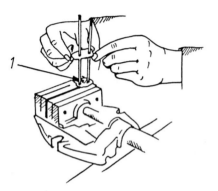

Fig. 10. Assembly of the plate cutouts

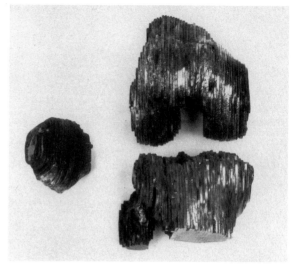

Fig. 11. Raw model

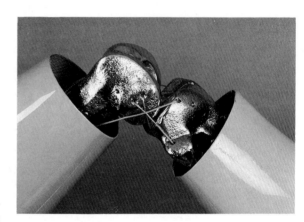

Fig. 12. Lateral view

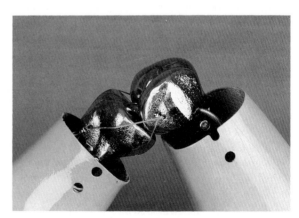

Fig. 13. Medial view

laser cutting bench (Fig. 9). The program also positioned reference holes on the plates *(1)* that, when laser drilled, served as guides for accurately assembling the contoured plates over long positioning pins (Fig. 10). Before each new plate is added, soft solder *(1)* and flux are placed on the underlying plate. When all the plates have been stacked, the assembly is heated to bond the pieces together. This relief model of the femur and tibia is ground smooth and used to make a mold, which is then used to cast the finished joint components from hardenable steel (Fig. 11). Finally the cast components are drilled for insertion of the wire ligaments and the screw threads for attaching the joint to the thigh and lower leg.

A lateral view of the fully assembled model (Fig. 12) demonstrates the complexity of a mechanical knee: The cable forming the lateral collateral ligament emerges from the proximal drill hole in the femur. To the right of it is the origin of the popliteus tendon. The tendon of the iliotibial tract passes over both structures to the tubercle of Gerdy. Two ligaments are visible from the medial aspect: the medial collat-

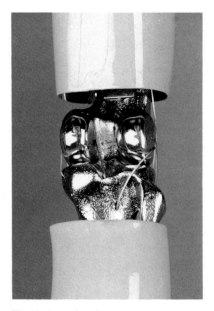

Fig. 14. Posterior view

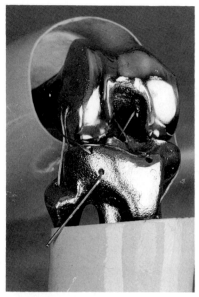

Fig. 15. Anterior view

eral ligament and the posterior oblique ligament. From the posterior side, the PCL and ACL are seen within the joint. Figure 15 shows the knee from the anterior aspect. The hollow wrench is used to adjust the ligaments to the correct length.

General View of the Knee Simulator (Fig. 16)

The following subunits are visible in a general view of the simulator: the mechanism for adjusting the lengths and elasticities of the ligaments, the wires with cable guides that pass through the thigh to the femur, the hip joint with table clamp, and the model joint with thigh and lower leg attached.

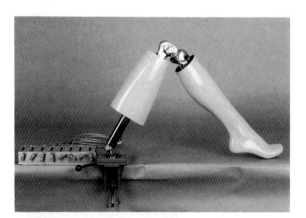

Fig. 16. Overall view of the third model

Both the lengths and the elasticities of the ligaments are adjusted with a control mechanism specially developed for the knee simulator. The front plate on the mechanism can be slid over to hide the ligament settings from the examiner.

The adjustable components are, from medial to lateral, the posterior oblique ligament, the medial collateral ligament, the anterior cruciate ligament, the lateral collateral ligament, the iliotibial tract, and the popliteus tendon.

Drawer testing (Figs. 18, 19) is performed in the neutral position with no external or internal rotation of the tibia:

1. Holding the simulator in the starting position, the examiner immobilizes the foot with his thigh.
2. A positive anterior drawer (Fig. 18) on the simulator, as in clinical testing, signifies slackness of the

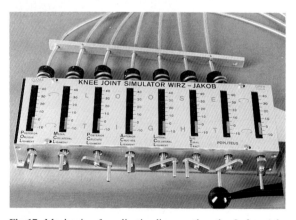

Fig. 17. Mechanism for adjusting ligament lengths. *Left to right:* controls for the iliotibial tract, popliteus tendon, lateral collateral ligament, anterior cruciate ligament, posterior cruciate ligament, and medial collateral ligament

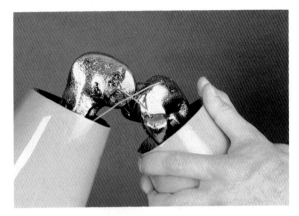

Fig. 18. Anterior drawer test

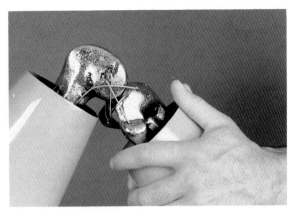

Fig. 19. Posterior drawer test

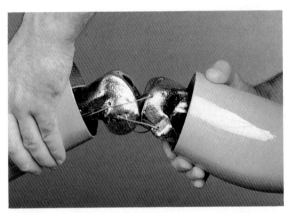

Fig. 20. Anterior subluxation in the Lachman test

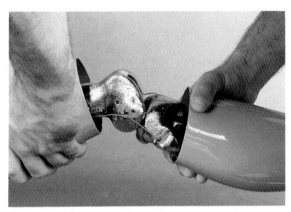

Fig. 21. Posterior subluxation in the Lachman test

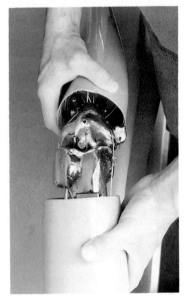

Fig. 22. Lachman test (overhead view)

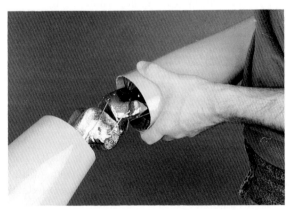

Fig. 23. Lateral pivot shift test near extension

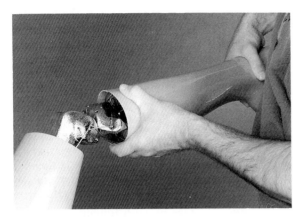

Fig. 24. Lateral pivot shift test in flexion

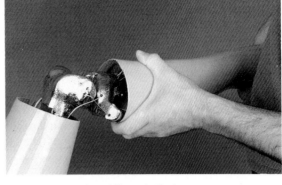

Fig. 25. Reverse pivot shift test in flexion

ACL and iliotibial tract. (Note the restraining action of the Kaplan fibers against further subluxation in the anterior cruciate-deficient joint.)
3. Pushing the tibia posteriorly (Fig. 19) elicits a posterior drawer sign (relative posterior subluxation) when the PCL and lateral collateral ligament are lax. The popliteus muscle also can function as a restraint to posterior drawer.

For anterior and posterior drawer testing in the Lachman position (Figs. 20–23) the knee is flexed to only about 25°:

1. In the *anterior Lachman test* (Fig. 20) the iliotibial tract is almost perpendicular to the knee joint line, so it is a less efficient restraint to anterior tibial translation, which is restrained chiefly by the ACL and medial collateral ligament.
2. *Posterior displacement of the tibia* (Fig. 21) is restrained by the PCL, the popliteus tendon (both of which pass over the posterior aspect of the tibia), and the lateral collateral ligament.
3. Overhead view (Fig. 22).

A positive pivot shift test signifies laxness of the ACL. The test involves holding the tibia in internal rotation and, while applying a valgus stress and axial pressure, slowing moving the knee joint from extension to flexion. The deficient ACL will permit excessive internal rotation and anterior translation. Resistance increases due to blockage of the lateral condyle. With further flexion (past about 30°) the tibia abruptly reduces backward from an anteriorly subluxated position (Figs. 23, 24). This jerky motion is produced by the muscular tension of the iliotibial tract in the presence of a torn ACL.

The reverse pivot shift test is positive with laxness or rupture of the PCL and popliteus muscle. We con-

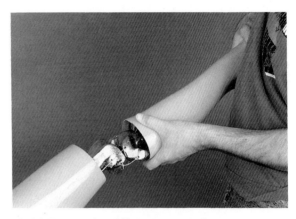

Fig. 26. Reverse pivot shift test near extension

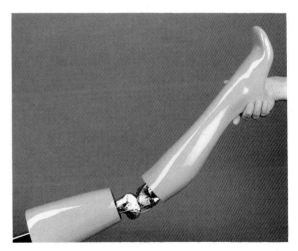

Fig. 27. Hyperextension

firmed this on our knee simulator by loosening both structures before performing the test.

The test is performed with the knee flexed 60°–90°, the tibia externally rotated, and the application of valgus pressure. The lax PCL and popliteus muscle permit a high degree of external rotation, placing the lateral tibial condyle in a position of posterior subluxation (Fig. 25). As the leg is extended, a jerk will be felt as the force vector of the iliotibial tract crosses over the femorotibial contact point, causing the tibia to jump from posterior subluxation to a neutral position (Fig. 26).

With concomitant laxness of the ACL and PCL and their associated secondary posterolateral restraints, the knee will sag into hyperextension under its own weight (Fig. 27).

Conclusion

The first two models provide valuable insight into the mechanics of the knee joint. The third model is a more general-purpose simulator that can train examiners in the practice and interpretation of commonly used knee tests. It is also excellent for demonstrating the course and stabilizing action of ligaments and tendons. We plan soon to add a digital indicator that will give a numerical readout of translation and rotation. Combined with a stocking drape, this device will help train the examiner in the quantification of translation and rotation. At present, such training models are being successfully used at a number of centers in Europe and the USA.

Femoropatellar Problems Associated with Anterior Cruciate Ligament Insufficiency

C. Gerber

The essential clinical manifestation of anterior cruciate ligament (ACL) insufficiency is femorotibial instability. If recurring episodes of subluxation have caused damage to the menisci, meniscal symptoms may become predominant. Animal studies have shown that experimental transection of the ACL gives rise to a functional instability that is followed within a short time by the formation of marginal osteophytes, remodeling of the articular surface, meniscal deterioration, and osteoarthritis of the knee (Marshall and Olson 1971; Paatsama and Sittnikow 1972). These experimental findings have since been confirmed by clinical studies showing that 10 years after rupture of the ACL, a progressive, radiographically apparent osteoarthritis will develop in approximately 25% of patients who received conservative or unsuccessful operative treatment for their injury (Aubriot and Rivat 1983; Dejour et al. 1987; Feagin et al. 1982; Gerber and Matter 1983; Jacobsen 1977; Kannus and Järvinen 1987). The degenerative changes in these cases follow a characteristic pattern (Feagin et al. 1982): Within 6–12 months after the rupture, X-rays show peaking of the intercondylar eminence, followed by hypertrophy and osteophytosis in that region. By 12–18 months osteophytes appear at the inferior pole of the patella, followed by osteophytic stenosis of the intercondylar notch. Joint-space narrowing becomes apparent at about 5–6 years, usually commencing in the medial femorotibial compartment. Some authors (Casscells 1985; Funk 1983; McDaniel and Dameron 1980) found that significant degenerative disease was rather uncommon in knees with chronic ACL insufficiency and rightly pointed out that less than 10% of severe osteoarthritis cases requiring treatment are caused by cruciate ligament instability. These data are based on advanced osteoarthritis cases from the early 1980s. Dejour et al. (1987) have shown that the clinical tolerance for instability-related osteoarthritis is high. In their series of 64 patients, those with an isolated cruciate ligament defect required treatment for osteoarthritis an average of 35 years (10–50 years) after their injury, whereas patients with accompanying meniscal lesions required treatment after an average of 25 years. On the other hand, patients who had unsuccessful or inadequate surgical treatment of their ligament injury required osteoarthritis surgery after a much shorter time (11 years). Because the incidence of cruciate ligament injuries has been rising in recent years due to greater athletic participation by the population as a whole, we may expect to see a significant increase in degenerative knee disease due to ACL insufficiency in the near future.

The wealth of clinical data on degenerative disease of the femorotibial joint, which clearly is accelerated by meniscal pathology, contrasts with the relative paucity of data on femoropatellar joint problems. Experiments in dogs have shown osteophytic changes in the intercondylar notch region and decreased distal patellar radiopacity developing within 3 weeks after section of the ACL, and significant osteophytosis involving the intercondylar notch and lower pole of the patella within 4–6 weeks (Paatsama and Sittnikow 1972). This is consistent with the reports by Dejour et al. (1987) and Feagin et al. (1982) on early osteophytic stenosis of the intercondylar notch, and it helps explain why Segal et al. (1980) described patellar chondromalacia in 34% of their 110 knees treated for anteromedial instability. The incidence of clinically overt femoropatellar problems may be quite low (16.7% according to Mansat et al. 1977) or extremely high depending on the series and perhaps on the method of history taking. In the prospective series of Kannus and Järvinen (1987), 78% of patients reported patellar complaints.

Femoropatellar problems must be sought not just in the literature but also during history taking and clinical evaluation. Even when present, they may be eclipsed by the more dramatic giving way episodes and feelings of instability. On occasion, however, femoropatellar problems may directly warrant treatment and must be recognized preoperatively so that they will not mar the outcome of a successful stabilizing procedure.

Below we shall describe the most salient femoropatellar problems that we have encountered in association with treated and untreated acute and chronic ruptures of the ACL.

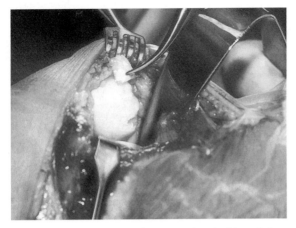

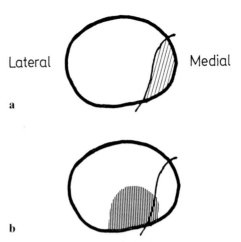

Fig. 1. Acute rupture of the ACL associated with an infero-medial flake fracture of the patellar cartilage

Femoropatellar Chondropathy and Osteoarthritis

Acute lesions of the ACL are occasionally associated with damage to the posterior patellar surface in the form of an impacted chondral fracture or flake fracture (Fig. 1). Occasionally they result from violent knee trauma producing multiple lesions (ACL, medial collateral ligament, meniscus), possibly accompanied by subluxation or dislocation of the patella. The incidence of such lesions is unknown, because many of these fresh ligament ruptures are operatively treated under emergent conditions and are not thoroughly documented. For actuarial and other reasons, it would be desirable if the condition of the posterior patellar surface and trochlea were consistently documented for every case.

In our own consecutive, prospective series of 38 ACL reconstructions performed for *chronic* insufficiency, 12% of the patients complained spontaneously of significant, disabling femoropatellar pain after surgery. When we specifically questioned our postoperative patients about this, a total of 42% reported femoropatellar joint symptoms (Gerber and Jakob 1983). At operation 76.6% exhibited femoropatellar cartilage lesions, with 58% showing fissuring and ulceration corresponding to grade II or grade III disease by the Ficat classification. As expected, however, the correlation between visible cartilage pathology and femoropatellar pain was poor. Of the 29 patients with patellar cartilage lesions, 15 had no pain, and 14 reported pain. Of the 9 patients with normal-appearing cartilage, 7 had no femoropatellar pain, and 2 were symptomatic. This is not surprising when we compare these findings with the results of arthroscopy

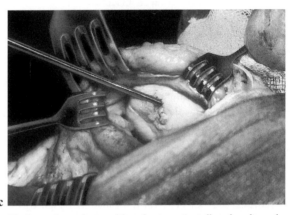

Fig. 2 a–c. In patients with refractory "patellar chondromalacia," cartilage degeneration is usually limited to the odd facet and is often considered physiologic **(a)**. With chronic lesions of the ACL, the patellar cartilage damage usually involves the contact area at about 20° of flexion **(b)**. Clinical example of chondropathy secondary to a chronic lesion of the ACL **(c)**

copy in 50 cases of refractory "patellar chondromalacia" (DeHaven et al. 1979), where cartilage lesions were noted in only 40% of the patients.

The cartilage lesions of patellar chondromalacia are confined to the medial "odd facet" of the patella (Fig. 2) and thus to the area of patellofemoral contact at approximately 130° of flexion. In this area grade I surface degeneration of the patellar cartilage is considered a normal finding (Goodfellow et al. 1976). In our patients with cruciate ligament tears, by contrast, the patellar cartilage lesions were not only more severe but were located more distally and centrally. Figure 2 shows that the affected area on the patellar surface corresponds to the patellofemoral contact area at about 20° of flexion – precisely the angle at which the pivot shift phenomenon occurs. It is quite possible that the pivoting traumatizes the cartilage at that site, whether in a violent initial event (see Fig. 1) or in repeated, smaller traumas associated with episodes of recurrent instability (Gerber and Matter 1983; Johnson 1959).

Two years after a successful ACL repair or reconstruction, approximately half of patients still experience femoropatellar symptoms. The frequency of complaints or objective pathologic findings was not influenced in our prospective study by postoperative immobilization in a long leg cast as compared with early mobilization in a hinged cast.

In summary, we find that cartilage lesions are present on the posterior patellar surface in three-fourths of our patients with chronic instabilities of the ACL. The lesions are located distally and medially, involving the patellofemoral contact area at 20° of flexion (Goodfellow et al. 1976). Only 42% of the patients have femoropatellar complaints, with about every 10th patient spontaneously reporting patellar problems. These complaints were not relieved by effective postoperative stabilization or by early mobilization of the operated limb.

Stenosis of the Intercondylar Notch

In contrast to the patella, the femoral trochlea is an uncommon site for true cartilaginous injuries. Consistent with the changes found by Paatsama and Sittnikow (1972) in animal studies, typical narrowing of the intercondylar notch develops within a short time following rupture of the ACL (Fig. 3). This change is distinguished from the patellar lesion not only by its pathogenesis, which is more reactive than traumatic, but also in its clinical significance. The patellar damage leads to a disturbance of femoropatellar tracking with consequent abrasion of the articular cartilage surface. Intercondylar notch stenosis, though located topographically within the femoropatellar joint, does not produce a clinically relevant change in femoropatellar mechanics. Its clinical significance lies, rather, in its constraining effect on the motion of the ACL. The stenosing osteophyte must be removed at the time of ACL reconstruction to ensure that the reactive anterior roof of the intercondylar notch will not act like a guillotine on the substitute ligament during knee extension. Given the common practice of attaching the graft in the extended knee, an omitted or inadequate notch plasty (widening of the intercondylar notch) can sometimes account for persistence of anteroposterior laxity in flexion despite an isometric graft placement and good stability in extension.

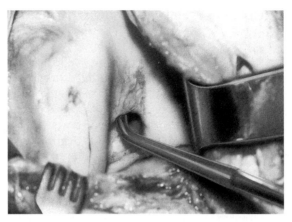

Fig. 3. Stenosis of the intercondylar notch following a tear of the ACL. A "notch plasty" is required at the time of reconstruction

The notch should not be widened past the anatomic limits. The plasty must not damage the attachment of the posterior cruciate ligament on the medial femoral condyle, nor should cartilage-bearing portions of the femorotibial joint be resected.

Postoperative Patella Baja

Centering of the patella may be altered in various ways following surgery for lesions of the ACL. The former practice of transferring the central one-third of the patellar tendon occasionally led to an excessive lateral pressure syndrome with increasing pain.

There are two mechanisms by which patella baja can develop following removal of the central third of the patellar tendon: First, sewing the remaining medial and lateral portions of the tendon together tends to shorten the tendon, causing distalization of the patella. Because of this problem we no longer suture the remaining limbs of the patellar tendon together before closing. Second, contracture of the infrapatellar fat pad can distalize the patella, leading to a painful excessive pressure syndrome that is most pronounced in flexion. The main cause of this condition is trauma to the infrapatellar fat pad caused, for example, by the use of a patellar tendon graft. In our experience (Jakob et al. 1988) there is no advantage to using a graft based on the infrapatellar fat pad, and there is the disadvantage of occasional patellar descent, so we have abandoned that technique. If the surgeon uses a free patellar tendon graft, he should be careful to avoid trauma to the fat pad.

Extension Loss Following Patellar Tendon Transfer

In a broad sense, femoropatellar problems include the loss of extension that may occur following a vascularized patellar tendon transfer based on the infrapatellar fat pad (Jakob et al. 1988). The apparent cause is a relative compromise of blood flow to the infrapatellar fat pad, which undergoes scarring and hypertrophy. This firm mass in the anterior part of the knee then creates a block to extension, which must be removed by excision. At resection the former fat pad appears as a firm mass that is difficult to separate from the anterior horns of the menisci. It presents histologically as a densely bundled, vascularized scar tissue devoid of fat. We have found that resection of the hypertrophied infrapatellar fat pad significantly improves the active and passive extension deficit. This complication can also be avoided by using a free patellar tendon graft. This again underscores the risk of basing the graft on the infrapatellar fat pad for an ACL reconstruction.

Extensor Apparatus

Combined injuries of the medial collateral ligament and ACL may rarely be associated with a patellar dislocation, resulting in a weakened medial retinaculum. This is accompanied by an atrophy of the vastus medialis during postoperative care, necessitating passive mobilization to keep the patella mobile and prevent lateralization. In addition to this pathology, we have noted significant quadriceps atrophy in patients with ACL lesions as well as a selective atrophy of the vastus medialis resulting from chronic instability (Gerber et al. 1985). These changes in the active extensor muscles are probably caused not by femoropatellar pain but by the general functional derangement in the complex knee joint. They may even represent an active, compensatory stabilizing mechanism in which the hamstrings undergo significantly less atrophy than the quadriceps. We do not believe that quadriceps atrophy, which is commonly observed and is not specific for ACL injuries, is an indication for quadriceps training in patients with existing lesions and subjective instability, as this will exacerbate the ligamentous instability and cannot replace the function of the ACL. However, once the knee joint is optimally stabilized and the reconstructed ligament has healed and remodeled, there is no question that complete quadriceps rehabilitation will improve the function of the lower extremity (Gerber et al. 1980).

Femoropatellar problems are frequently neglected in the treatment of ACL tears. However, many of these lesions occur in athletes who must be rehabilitated to complete recovery. This is feasible only if proper attention is given to the full spectrum of knee pathology, including femoropatellar problems.

References

Aubriot JH, Rivat P (1983) Arthrose femoro-tibiale et laxité du genou avec atteinte du ligament croisé antérieur. Rev Chir Orthop 69: 291–294

Casscells SW (1985) The torn meniscus, the torn anterior cruciate ligament, and their relationship to degenerative joint disease. Arthroscopy 1/1: 28–32

DeHaven KE, Dolan WA, Mayer PJ (1979) Chondromalacia patellae in athletes. Am J Sports Med 7: 5–11

Dejour H, Walch G, Deschamps G, Chambat P (1987) Arthrose du genou sur laxité chronique antérieure. Rev Chir Orthop 73: 157–170

Feagin JA, Cabaud HE, Curl WW (1982) The anterior cruciate ligament: Radiographic and clinical signs of successful and unsuccessful repairs. Clin Orthop 164: 54–58

Funk FJ (1983) Osteoarthritis of the knee following ligamentous injury. Clin Orthop 172: 154–157

Gerber C, Matter P, Chrismas OD, Langhans M (1980) Funktionelle Rehabilitation nach komplexen Knieverletzungen. Wissenschaftliche Grundlagen und Praxis. Schweiz Z Sportmed 28: 37–56

Gerber C, Jakob RP (1983) Das Femoro-Patellargelenk bei vorderer Kreuzbandinsuffizienz. Hefte Unfallheilkd 165: 231–233

Gerber C, Matter P (1983) Biomechanical analysis of the knee after rupture of the anterior cruciate ligament and its primary repair. J Bone Joint Surg [Br] 65: 341–399

Gerber C, Hoppeler H, Claassen H, Robotti G, Zehnder R, Jakob RP (1985) The lower-extremity musculature in chronic symptomatic instability of the anterior cruciate ligament. J Bone Joint Surg [Am] 67: 1034–1043

Goodfellow J Hungerford DS, Zindel M (1976) Patello-femoral joint mechanics and pathology, part 1 and 2. J Bone Joint Surg [Br] 58: 287–290, 291–299

Jacobsen K (1977) Osteoarthrosis following insufficiency of the cruciate ligaments in man. Acta Orthop Scand 48: 520–526

Jakob RP, Kipfer W, Klaue K, Stäubli H-U, Gerber C (1988) Étude critique de la reconstruction du ligament croisé antérieur du genou par la plastie pédiculée sur le Hoffa a partir du tiers médian du tendon rotulien. Rev Chir Orthop 74: 44–51

Johnson LC (1959) Kinetics of osteoarthritis. Lab Invest 8: 1223–1241

Kannus P, Järvinen M (1987) Conservatively treated tears of the anterior cruciate ligament. J Bone Joint Surg [Am] 69: 1007–1012

Mansat C, Duboureau L, Cha P, Dorbes R (1977) Déséquilibre rotulien et instabilité rotatoire externe du genou. Rev Rhum Mal Osteoartic 44/21: 115–123

Marshall JL, Olsson SE (1971) Instability of the knee. J Bone Joint Surg [Am] 53: 1561–1570

McDaniel WJ, Dameron TB (1980) Untreated ruptures of the anterior cruciate ligament. J Bone Joint Surg [Am] 62: 696-704

Paatsama S, Sittnikow K (1972) Early changes in the knee joint due to instability induced by cutting of the anterior cruciate ligament. Acta Radiol [Suppl] 319: 169-173

Segal Ph, Lallement JJ, Raguet M et al. (1980) Les lésions ostéo-cartilagineuses de la laxité antéro-interne du genou. Rev Chir Orthop 66: 357-366

Classification of Meniscal Tears Associated with Lesions of the Anterior Cruciate Ligament

We. Müller

Although meniscal tears are highly diverse in their morphology, they have certain internal characteristics in common. The anatomic structure and design principle of the meniscus, together with its pattern of loading during function, account for the development of various types of tear that, far from being random, are more or less inevitable.

These tears are more frequent and severe in the knee with a deficient anterior cruciate ligament (ACL), where the menisci must function more rigorously as secondary restraints or "brakes" to anteroposterior tibial motion. This subjects the menisci to increased wear and tear, as described in the chapter by Dupont and Scellier in this volume (p. 246 ff.).

Ontogenic and Functional Aspects

The menisci and cruciate ligaments are already present in the embryo with a CRL of 29 mm, before the the joint space of the knee has formed. The menisci are still fused to the tibia at this time and do not partially separate from it until the joint becomes mobile

and a joint space appears. However, the menisci retain their firm attachments with the cruciate ligaments and the capsular ligament system. The menisci and cruciate ligaments have been described as a functional composite system having the configuration of a deformable figure-of-8 loop (Fig. 1).

The functional relationship between the menisci and cruciate ligaments is underscored by the increased concentration of neuroproprioceptive elements located in the posterior horns of the menisci at their junction with the cruciate ligaments (Cerulli, personal communication). Not infrequently, an almost characteristic residual painful zone remains at that location following arthroscopic surgery under local anesthesia.

The attachments of the menisci to the ligamentous capsule, specifically to the posterior oblique ligament medially in the semimembranosus corner and to the arcuate complex laterally, contribute significantly to the mechanical stability of both articular compartments (Fig. 2). Without its attachment to the posterior oblique ligament and the meniscotibial coronary ligament, the meniscus cannot function as a restraint to anterior tibial motion.

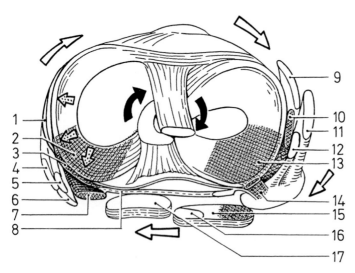

1 Medial collateral ligament
2 Posterior horn of medial meniscus
3 Posterior oblique ligament
4 Sartorius muscle
5 Gracilis muscle
6 Semitendinosus muscle
7 Semimembranosus muscle
8 Oblique popliteal ligament
9 Iliotibial tract
10 Popliteus tendon
11 Biceps muscle
12 Lateral collateral ligament
13 Posterior horn of lateral meniscus
14 Arcuate ligament
15 Lateral gastrocnemius
16 Plantaris muscle
17 Medial gastrocnemius

Fig. 1. Semischematic representation of the menisci and their attachment to the cruciate ligaments in the form of a figure-of-8 loop

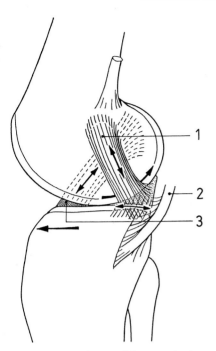

Fig.2. The attachment of the posterior horn of the medial meniscus to the posterior oblique ligament and its synergism with the ACL
1 Posterior oblique ligament
2 Semimembranosus muscle
3 ACL

Classification of Meniscal Tears

Peripheral Detachments of the Meniscus

With an apparent isolated rupture of the ACL with no initial evidence of damage to the meniscus or to the medial collateral ligament-posterior oblique ligament system, there may be an occult posteromedial rupture of the coronary ligament behind the medial collateral ligament, hidden beneath the meniscus (Fig.3).

In other cases the whole meniscal cartilage may be peripherally detached from the capsule (Fig.4a). The gap between the meniscus and capsule may become spontaneously bridged by loose synovial and granulation tissue (Fig.4b). With or without a loose tissue bridge, the joint is predisposed to the "signo del salto" (jump sign) instability described by Finocchietto (1930). The entire body of the meniscus subluxates and then reduces with a palpable and audible jumping-snapping action (Fig.5).

Tears in the Substance of the Meniscus

There are several other, atypical types of meniscal tear that are located more centrally than the peripheral detachments described above. The shapes of these tears are so diverse that they may appear random to the casual observer.

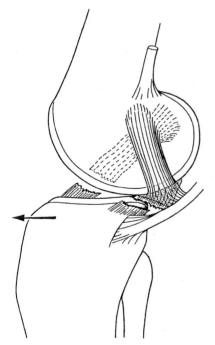

Fig.3. Rupture of the ACL combined with an occult, predominantly ligamentous meniscotibial avulsion

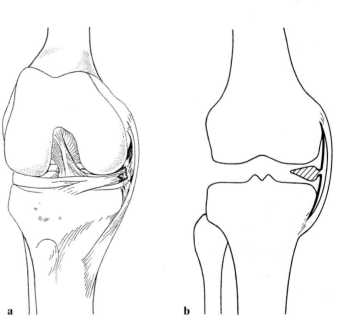

Fig.4. a Peripheral separation of the meniscus. **b** Healing of the injury by bridging synovial tissue

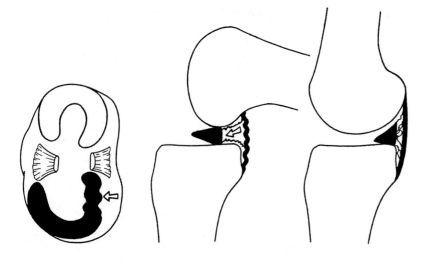

Fig. 5. "Jump sign" due to incarceration of a hypermobile meniscus

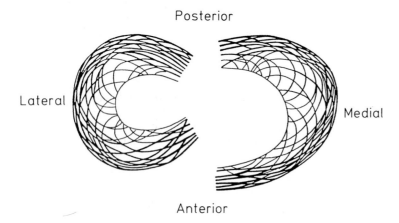

Posterior

Lateral

Medial

Anterior

Fig. 6. Fiber architecture of the menisci according to Wagner

The architecture of the meniscus, in which the cartilage matrix is reinforced by collagenous fibers arranged in a systematic pattern (Fig. 6), conveys an immediate sense of how meniscal tears follow lines of predilection defined by the fiber architecture. Years ago, Trillat (1962, 1971 a, b) classified these tears into basic groups (Fig. 7); his classification will be expanded here.

Transverse or Radial Tears

Viewing the fiber pattern of the menisci as described by Wagner (1976) (see Fig. 6), we notice at once that the dense, parallel fiber arrangement in the outer third of the meniscus gives way to a less dense, more radially oriented pattern in the inner third. Consequently, the inner border of the meniscus is relatively prone to tearing by a longitudinally directed force. Normally this is not a problem because the meniscus is naturally protected from this type of stress. But if

an individual falls, say, onto the internally rotated tibia while the knee is flexed, the main effect is a posterior displacement of the tibia relative to the femur in the lateral joint compartment, exerting longitudinal traction on the inner border of the lateral meniscus that can cause radial tearing (Fig. 8). A wide meniscus is predisposed to this type of injury.

In the various forms of discoid meniscus, a sudden axial compressive load can deform the meniscus and generate stresses at its inner edge sufficient to cause a transverse tear.

Primary Posterior Horn Flap Tear

This tear, commonly known as a "parrot beak tear," is classically located in the posterior segment of the meniscus, where, in contrast to the middle third, the fibers are less radially oriented and follow a more arched path to the inner border of the meniscus (Fig. 9). As with transverse tears, anteroposterior

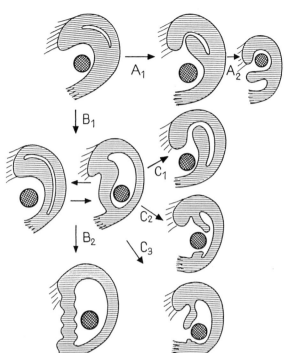

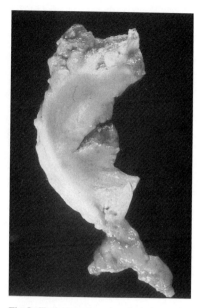

Fig. 8. Transverse tear in a broad, nearly discoid meniscus

Fig. 7. Classification of meniscal tears according to the Trillat scheme. A classic longitudinal tear of the posterior horn of the medial meniscus *(upper left)* may progress along line *A* to produce a parrot-beak tear A_2 or along line *B* to form a complete longitudinal tear that becomes a bucket handle tear B_1 with consequent locking. The bucket handle fragment may remain incarcerated, in which case the tear will enlarge as in B_2, perhaps to the point where it no longer blocks extension. If the bucket handle continually slips in and out of the intercondylar notch, it may tear secondarily through its posterior (C_1), central (C_2), or anterior portion (C_3). The *dark circle* represents the area of femorotibial contact

translation, perhaps combined with rotation, is a major causal mechanism. This translation tends to be greater in knees with inherently large "joint play" or with acquired pathologic laxity due, say, to a partial insufficiency of the ACL or, more rarely, the posterior cruciate ligament.

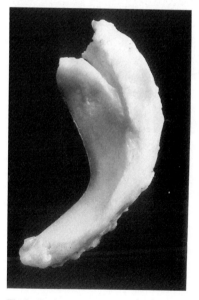

Fig. 9. Typical posterior flap tear with a parrot-beak configuration

Longitudinal Tears

These tears, too, can be understood in terms of the meniscal fiber architecture. They occur at sites in the meniscal substance where the peripheral longitudinal fiber pattern, which provides ideal tensile strength along the circumference of the disc, abruptly gives way to a less tear-resistant structure (see Figs. 6, 10). The site of predilection for longitudinal tears, then, is the transition zone from a circumferential to a more radial fiber orientation.

Longitudinal tears can range from a few millimeters in length to very extensive bucket-handle lesions. Well-defined longitudinal tears are a good indication for suture repair. Repair is particularly appropriate for short tears and tears located close to the periphery.

Posterior
oblique ligament

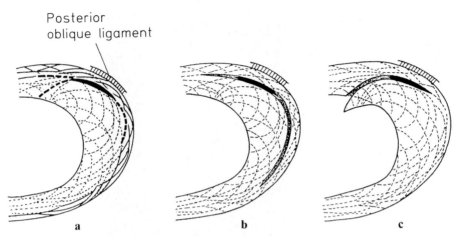

Fig. 10 a–c. Tears at sites of predilection defined by the fiber architecture of the meniscus (see Fig. 6)

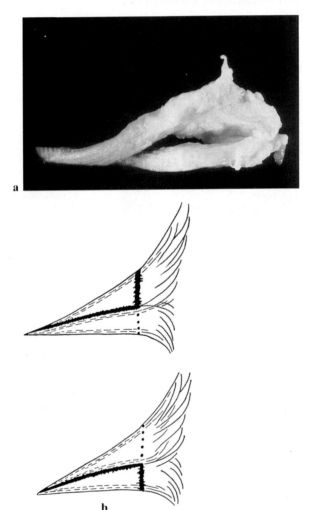

Fig. 11. a Typical large cleavage tear (still) without flap formation. **b** Cross-sectional view of the meniscal fiber structure, showing the site of predilection for horizontal cleavage

Secondary Flap Tears

A chronically subluxating bucket-handle fragment may become detached posteriorly, centrally, or anteriorly to form various types of flap tear (see Fig. 7), e. g., an anteriorly based flap, a posteriorly based flap, or a pair of flaps based anteriorly and posteriorly.

Horizontal Tears

The alternate term for horizontal tears, cleavage tears, aptly describes how this lesion occurs. A cross-sectional view of the fiber architecture of the meniscus (Fig. 11) demonstrates how a central fiber layer approximately bisects the meniscal wedge and forms a plane of predilection on which the upper half of the meniscus may separate from the lower (Fig. 12). Each half, in turn, can undergo further disintegration along the lines of a primary flap tear. The end result of this process is highly variable, although, with experience, it is possible to recognize the lesion as having originated from a cleavage tear.

Crush Lesion (Fig. 13)

A meniscus may undergo a gradual chronic disintegration, similar to the horizontal cleavage process, in which the meniscus is grossly deformed but preserves its internal continuity. The affected segment appears thinned and widened, as if "rolled out" by extreme pressure. The accompanying mucoid degeneration (Fig. 14) in turn promotes the mechanical process causing the deformation shown in Fig. 13.

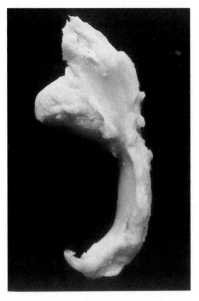

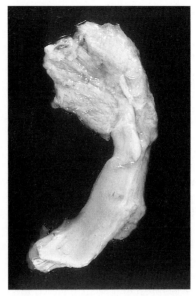

Fig. 12. Example of a flap tear caused mainly by horizontal cleavage of the meniscus

Fig. 13. Crush lesion. A meniscal segment has been crushed and flattened by chronic pressure from the femoral condyle, somewhat similar to the flap tear in Fig. 12. Unlike a cleavage or flap tear, however, meniscal continuity is preserved. The affected segment appears abnormally glossy and exhibits mucoid degeneration and swelling

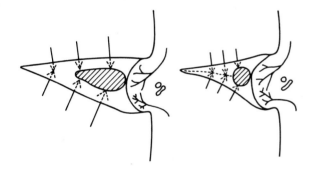

◁

Fig. 14. The meniscus derives its nutrition from peripheral capillaries and by diffusion from the joint cavity through its upper and lower surfaces. The nutritionally critical central zone is a site of predilection for mucoid degeneration and cyst formation. The size of the zone is proportional to the volume of the meniscus

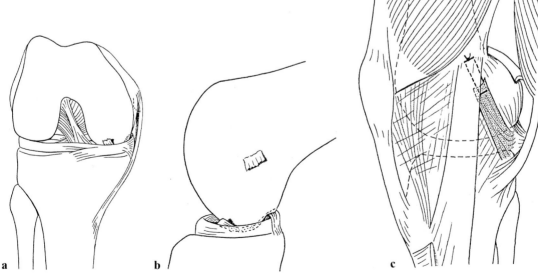

Fig. 15 a–c. "Meniscal tear" in the semimembranosus corner. This type of injury can produce the symptoms of a torn meniscus. Outwardly similar, the different forms of injury can be quite diverse in their anatomic details

Meniscal Tears and Cysts

The central portion of the meniscus is more poorly nourished than the periphery, which receives nutrition from the peripheral capillaries and by diffusion from the meniscal surface. Mucoid degeneration can be an early result of mechanical disruption associated with a catabolic state (Fig. 15). Its focus at the center of the meniscus lies close to preformed rupture lines, which can cause cysts and tears to have a common appearance. This has led some authors (e.g., Jackson) to suggest an inverse pathogenesis for meniscal cysts: A unidirectional pump mechanism injects synovial fluid into the body of the meniscus through a tear. This fluid then inspissates and drives the walls of the meniscus apart at the center (Jackson, personal communication; Jaffres 1975).

Years ago these cases were managed by total excision of the tear and cyst to forestall a recurrence. Today, owing to greater interest in preserving the mechanically important meniscus, a partial arthroscopic resection is preferred in which the cyst is opened and drained internally. Additional time and follow-up are needed to determine whether this can prevent the once-common recurrences, which may extend well outside the joint.

"Meniscal Tear" in the Semimembranosus Corner

This type of injury is uncommon. It may present clinically as a constant pain on motion or weight bearing in a patient with an old knee injury. Its symptoms resemble those of a torn meniscus, but palpation elicits the greatest tenderness proximal to the joint line.

In some cases the lesion presents as a capsular flap on arthroscopy. In other cases arthroscopy shows only a scarred synovium, with subsequent arthrotomy, if required, revealing a continuity disruption with an unstable scar in the region of the posterior oblique ligament and capsule (Biedert and Müller 1986).

Residual complaints may be so disabling in competitive athletes, especially soccer players and martial artists, that a meticulous open repair is warranted. Extreme care should be taken to spare the nerve branches that are encountered at operation.

Note: The figures showing the meniscectomy specimens in this article are 18–25 years old. These total excisions are wholly inconsistent with contemporary concepts favoring partial resections that spare a maximum amount of functional meniscal tissue.

References

Biedert R, Müller We (1986) Spezielle Verletzungen des Semimembranosuseckes. Schweiz Z Sportmed 2: 87–91

Finocchietto (1930) El signo del salto. Press Med Argent

Jaffres R (1975) Les kystes méniscaux. Considérations thérapeutiques et pathogéniques. Rev Rhum Mal Osteoartic 42: 519–526

Trillat A (1962) Lésions traumatiques du ménisque interne du genou. Rev Chir Orthop 48: 551–560

Trillat A (1971a) Les lésions méniscales internes. Rev Chir Orthop 57: 318

Trillat A (1971b) Les lésions méniscales externes. Rev Chir Orthop 57: 318

Wagner HJ (1976) Die Kollagenfaserarchitektur der Menisken des menschlichen Kniegelenkes. Z Mikrosk Anat Forsch 90: 302–324

Natural History of Untreated Tears of the Anterior Cruciate Ligament

H.-U. Stäubli and R. P. Jakob

The natural history of acute tears of the anterior cruciate ligament (ACL) is controversial (Balkfors 1982; Beaver et al. 1982; Chambat 1985; Clancy et al. 1982; Fetto and Marshall 1980; Giove et al. 1983; Hejgaard et al. 1984; Hey Groves 1920; Hughston 1983; Larson 1983; McDaniel and Dameron 1980; Noyes et al. 1980a, 1983a; Odensten and Gillquist 1985; Rowere and Adain 1983; Satku et al. 1986).

Various authors state that the predictable course of a conservatively treated ACL insufficiency is characterized by a progressive deterioration of knee function, with the incidence of secondary meniscal tears and severity of articular cartilage lesions increasing over time in proportion to the severity of the instability (Feagin 1979; Marshall and Rubin 1977). Late sequelae include instability-related degenerative arthritis (Balkfors 1982; Chambat 1985; Fairbank 1948; Feagin et al. 1982; Jacobsen 1977).

Satku et al. (1986) reviewed 97 untreated complete ruptures of the ACL. Despite objective evidence of instability in all cases, the degree of functional disability varied significantly: 6% of the patients had to restrict their daily activities, 31% returned to normal activities but gave up sports, and 63% resumed their preinjury level of sports activity following the initial phase of treatment. Functional deterioration was noted at 6-year follow-up; only 46% of the patients were able to maintain the same level of sports activity (Satku et al. 1986).

Kennedy et al. (1974) compared a group of conservatively treated ACL ruptures with a group treated by primary surgical repair. The follow-up examinations were performed at 44 and 88 months postinjury. While there was no significant difference between the two groups at 44 months, the results in the conservatively treated group were markedly poorer at 88 months than in the group managed by primary repair.

McDaniel and Dameron (1980) compared the natural history of untreated ACL ruptures at 10 and 14 years. In evaluating 52 knees 14 years after injury, they noted a decline in the frequency of giving-way episodes while the clinical signs of anterior and rotatory instability remained constant relative to the 10-year finding. Three-fourths of the patients remained athletically active, although 86% required a unilateral or bilateral meniscectomy, and 33% showed radiographic signs of early osteoarthritis in the form of joint-space narrowing and increased subchondral sclerosis.

Table 1. Factors affecting the course of an untreated ACL rupture

1. Mechanism of injury and severity of ligament insufficiency	Chambat (1985) Montmollin and Le Coeur (1980) Norwood and Cross (1979)
2. Type of tear and degree of incompetence	Cabaud et al. (1974) Cabaud (1983) Chick and Jackson (1978) Kennedy et al. (1974) Kennedy et al. (1976) Lipscomb and Anderson (1986) Müller (1982)
3. Pathomechanics in the ACL-deficient knee	Butler et al. (1980) Cabaud (1983) Fukubayashi et al. (1982) Furman et al. (1976) Hejgaard et al. (1984) Jacobsen (1981) Lipke et al. (1981) Losee et al. (1978) Noyes et al. (1980b) Stäubli et al. (1985)
4. Rupture and associated lesions	Hamberg et al. (1983) Shoemaker and Markolf (1986)
5. Insufficiency, constitutional ligament laxity and morphotype	Bousquet et al. (1980)
6. Insufficiency, age, and level of sports activity	Giove et al. (1983) Noyes et al. (1983a) Satku et al. (1986)
7. Insufficiency and osteoarthritis	Chambat (1985) Fairbanks (1948) Feagin et al. (1982) Jacobsen (1977) Lemaire (1975)

In several follow-up studies, knee function deterio-
rated in the years following an acute rupture in proportion to the frequency of giving-way episodes
(Fairbank 1948; Feagin et al. 1982; Feagin 1979;
Satku et al. 1986). The symptomatic meniscal and
cartilage lesions associated with these episodes
eventually progressed to the syndrome of the chronic
ACL-deficient knee (Feagin 1979).

The factors that influence the natural history of an
untreated ACL rupture are listed in Table 1.

Mechanisms and Severity
of ACL Insufficiency

Partial Rupture

Various authors have disputed the existence of a partial rupture of the ACL (Hughston and Barrett 1983;
O'Donoghue 1959). Johnson et al. (1984), however,
verified a large number of partial ACL ruptures in
arthroscopic examinations of knees with posttraumatic hemarthrosis (Dandy et al. 1982; DeHaven
1980, 1983; Johnson et al. 1983).

When the knee is internally rotated while weight
bearing, the anteromedial bundle of the ACL comes
under the greatest stress and is apt to rupture first
(Chambat 1985). If the internal rotation forces are
not checked, the tear can extend to involve the remaining bundles. This mechanism can produce
various grades of severity of partial ACL rupture
(Norwood and Cross 1979) (see Fig. 1 b).

Complete ("Isolated") Rupture

Two mechanisms can cause an "isolated" rupture of
the ACL: rotation and hyperextension. According to
DeMontmollin and le Coeur (1980), maximal quadriceps contraction while the tibia is internally rotated
can produce an isolated tear through the substance of
the ligament. The hyperextension mechanism first
stretches the posterolateral bundle of the ACL
(Fig. 2a). Unchecked, the hyperextension forces can
cause a complete rupture as the anteromedial and intermediate bundles are stretched and torn against the
anterior edge of the intercondylar shelf (Feagin and
Curl 1976; McMaster et al. 1974; Müller 1982; Norwood and Cross 1979) (Fig. 2 b).

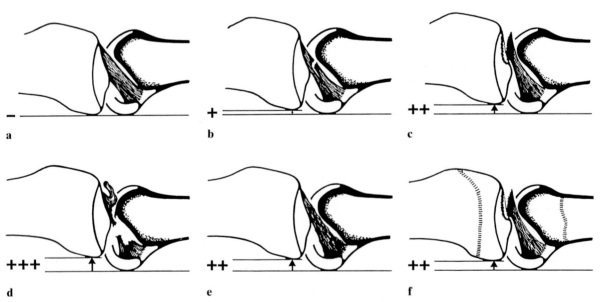

Fig. 1a–f. ACL tears and associated grades of functional incompetence. Right knee, medial aspect, with medial femoral
condyle removed. **a** Normal ligament. Tibial attachment: anterior intercondylar area and anterior border of intercondylar
eminence. Femoral attachment: lateral femoral condyle at posterolateral border of intercondylar notch. **b** Incomplete rupture
with partial incompetence: 1 + anterior subluxation near extension with an intact anterior end point. **c** Bony avulsion from the
anterior intercondylar area with complete incompetence:
2 + anterior subluxation near extension with an altered or absent anterior end point. **d** Complete midsubstance tear with
complete incompetence: 3 + anterior subluxation near extension with loss of the anterior end point. **e** Interstitial stretching
with partial incompetence: 2 + anterior subluxation near extension with an altered anterior end point. **f** Bony avulsion in an
adolescent with complete incompetence: 2 + anterior subluxation near extension with an altered or absent anterior end point

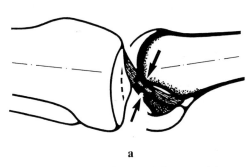 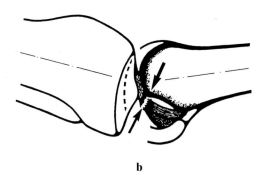

a   b

Fig. 2 a, b. Hyperextension mechanism producing a partial or complete ACL rupture. **a** Partial rupture with insufficiency of the posterolateral bundle and incipient interstitial stretching.

b Unchecked hyperextension can produce a complete midsubstance tear by the shearing action of the anterior edge of the intercondylar shelf

Associated Medial Injuries

Medial capsuloligamentous injuries can accompany an ACL rupture when combined valgus-external rotation moments act upon the slightly flexed knee. Tearing of the medial collateral ligament, the suspensory (meniscofemoral and meniscotibial) ligaments of the medial meniscus, the posterior oblique ligament, and the ACL was described by Pallmer in 1938 and termed the "unhappy triad" by O'Donoghue in 1950. The resulting instability consists of valgus instability and a combined anteromedial/ anterolateral subluxation of the tibia (Lipke et al. 1981), which can be demonstrated by various clinical tests (Galway et al. 1972; Hughston 1983; Kennedy and Fowler 1971; Lemaire and Miremed 1983; Losee et al. 1978; Stäubli et al. 1985; Torg 1976).

Associated Lateral Injuries

Varus-internal rotation forces acting on the slightly flexed knee can lead to combined injuries of the ACL and lateral ligaments (Chambat 1985; Müller 1982), i.e., tearing of the ACL and the middle third of the lateral capsular ligament or meniscal suspensory ligament, concomitant injury of the iliotibial tract fibers attaching to the anterolateral tubercle ("anterolateral femorotibial ligament" of Müller 1982), and variable lesions of the arcuate complex (Müller 1982). The resulting instability consists of varus laxity combined with a predominantly anterolateral subluxation of the tibia and signs of posterolateral rotatory subluxation (Bousquet et al. 1980; Chambat 1985; Jakob et al. 1981; Müller 1982).

Associated Posterior Injuries

Besides a complete ACL rupture, unchecked hyperextension forces can cause a partial rupture of the posterior cruciate ligament, frequently combined with posterior capsuloligamentous disruption. This aggravates the already increased hyperextensibility of the knee that is typically noted after a complete rupture of the ACL.

Types of Tear and Grades of Incompetence

Interstitial Stretching (Fig. 1 e)

A variety of physical forces acting upon the knee joint lead to varying degrees of ACL disruption (DeMontmollin and le Coeur 1980; Müller 1982; Norwood and Cross 1979). Relatively small, secondarily checked physical forces can cause a partial rupture, while more severe forces can produce a bony avulsion. Unchecked forces can lead to complete interstitial failure of the primary restraint (the ACL) with varying degrees of associated insufficiency of the secondary restraints (Butler et al. 1980; Müller 1982; Noyes et al. 1980 a, 1984).

Partial incompetence of the ACL can result from stretching of the ligament alone. The partial insufficiency is manifested clinically by a demonstrable increase in anterior tibial displacement with an altered anterior end point. Arthroscopic inspection and probing reveal only sites of subsynovial hemorrhage (Johnson et al. 1984). If the synovial covering of the ACL is still intact, a partial ligament rupture can occasionally be demonstrated by opening the synovial sleeve (Müller 1982) (Fig. 1 e).

Complete Midsubstance Tear (Fig. 1 d)

A complete midsubstance tear of the ACL is manifested clinically by increased anterior tibial displacement near extension with no palpable anterior end point. The clinical tests used to detect complete ACL insufficiency are the Lachman test (Torg et al. 1976), the pivot shift test (Galway et al. 1972), the Losee test (Losee et al. 1979), and the jerk test of Hughston (1983). Noyes noted the importance of the flexion-rotation drawer test for diagnosing complete ACL insufficiency (Noyes 1983 a, b).

These clinical tests demonstrate a combined anteromedial/ anterolateral subluxation of the tibia with respect to the femur (Lipke et al. 1981).

Bony Avulsion (Fig. 1 c)

Noyes et al. (1984) showed experimentally that forces applied gradually to the knee can produce avulsion fractures of the ACL, their experiments demonstrating combinations of bony avulsions with interstitial stretching of the ligament. When there is a displaced bone fragment avulsed from the anterior intercondylar area, generally there is coexisting injury to the area of attachment of the anterior horn of the lateral meniscus. This associated anterior horn injury is produced by tension on the fibers passing from the anteromedial bundle of the ACL to the anterior horn attachment area of the lateral meniscus.

Pathomechanics of the ACL-Deficient Knee

Stressradiographs have provided objective evidence of the femorotibial displacement in the sagittal plane that occurs near extension in the ACL-deficient knee (Chambat 1985; Hooper 1986; Stäubli et al. 1985).

Translation and Rotation in the ACL-Intact Knee

When the ACL is intact, normal constitutional ligamentous laxity permits an anterior tibial displacement of 2.8–4.0 mm relative to the femur in the slightly flexed knee (Stäubli et al. 1985). Clinical testing of physiologic anterior joint play near extension in the ACL-intact knee generally demonstrates a firm anterior end point, indicating that the physiologic restraining force of the primary restraint is preserved (Butler et al. 1980). Stressradiographs show only a slight translation and internal rotation, with a 2.8-mm

displacement of the medial compartment and 4.0-mm displacement of the lateral compartment (Stäubli et al. 1985).

Translation and Rotation with a Partial and Isolated Complete ACL Rupture

As the severity of the insufficiency increases, the restraining force of the ACL is progressively lost (Lipke et al. 1981). Stressradiographs of the knee near extension (Stäubli et al. 1985; Hooper 1986) demonstrate a predominantly anterolateral subluxation of the tibia, meaning that the internal rotation component, and thus the anterior displacement of the lateral tibial plateau, exceeds the anterior displacement of the medial plateau (Stäubli et al. 1985). This accounts for the simultaneous anterior translation of both plateaus coupled with internal rotation (Fig. 3 a).

Translation and Rotation with ACL Rupture and Medial Capsuloligamentous Injury (Fig. 4 b)

As noted above, the loss of the primary restraint occasioned by a complete rupture of the ACL leads to a small amount of translation combined with a marked anterolateral subluxation component (see Fig. 3 a). The degree of insufficiency of the secondary medial restraints depends on the extent and severity of associated posteromedial injuries. Pathomechanically, there is a combined anteromedial/anterolateral forward subluxation of the tibia distinguished by an increased simultaneous anterior translation of both plateaus (Lipke et al. 1981; Stäubli et al. 1985). The instability includes a predominantly anterolateral rotatory component, but this is of minor significance in clinical and stressradiographic testing (Fig. 3 b).

Anterior subluxation testing demonstrates a marked anterior displacement of the medial tibial plateau and an even greater anterior displacement of the lateral plateau (Stäubli et al. 1985; Galway et al. 1972).

Translation and Rotation with ACL Rupture and Lateral Capsuloligamentous Injury

The pathomechanical outcome of a flexion-varus-internal rotation injury that ruptures the ACL and damages the arcuate complex is a combined anteromedial/anterolateral subluxation of the tibia with respect to the femur. A more or less marked posterolateral rotatory component can be demonstrated, de-

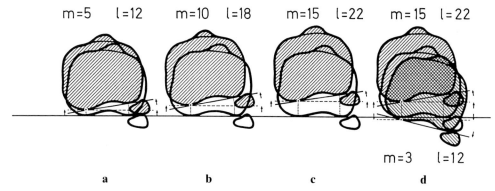

Fig. 3 a–d. Tibial subluxation and grades of pivot shift. **a** Isolated rupture: slight increase in both medial and lateral translation with an anterolateral rotatory component. Pivot shift 1 + in IR, – in NR, – in ER. **b** Rupture with insufficiency of the semimembranosus corner: marked increase in both medial and lateral translation with an anterolateral rotatory component. Pivot shift 2 + in IR, 1 + in NR, – in ER. **c** Complete rupture with insufficiency of the semimembranosus corner and anterolateral secondary complex: pivot shift 3 + in IR, 2 + in NR, 1 + in ER. **d** Complete rupture with insufficiency of the semimembranosus corner and the anterolateral and posterolateral complex (arcuate complex): pivot shift 3 + in IR, 2 + in NR, 1 + in ER. Reversed pivot shift 1 + . *m*, Anterior displacement of medial tibial plateau in mm; *l*, anterior displacement of lateral tibial plateau in mm

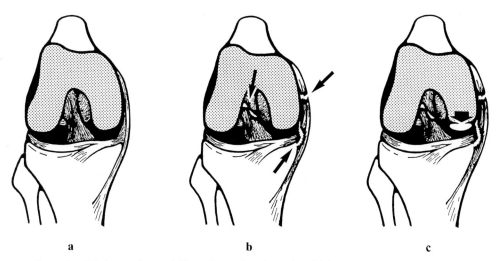

Fig. 4 a–c. Insufficiency and associated lesions. **a** Intact ACL. **b** Complete midsubstance tear with insufficiency of the semimembranosus corner (medial collateral ligament, meniscofemoral and meniscotibial coronary ligaments, posterior oblique ligament). **c** As in **b** but also with an osteochondral fracture of the medial femoral condyle

pending on the severity of the injury to the arcuate complex (Jakob et al. 1981).

Translation and Rotation with Chronic ACL Insufficiency

Chronic insufficiency is generally characterized by a marked anterior subluxation of the tibia (Stäubli et al. 1985). In patients with a genu varum morphotype and loss of secondary restraints to anterolateral subluxation, associated pathology will develop in the posterolateral corner, either primarily or secondarily due to distention. The pathomechanical consequence is a marked, global anterior translation of both tibial plateaus with an accompanying anterolateral rotatory component and posterolateral subluxation (Jakob et al. 1981). Clinical tests demonstrate anterior subluxation of the tibia with signs of posterolateral rotatory subluxation and varying degrees of varus laxity (Bousquet et al. 1980; Jakob et al. 1981; Müller 1982) (Fig. 3 d).

In a prospective study of the popliteal hiatus in knees with acute and chronic ACL insufficiency, coexisting lesions of the superior and inferior fascicles of the popliteomeniscal attachments were consistently detected (see chapter by Stäubli and Birrer, p. 495 ff.).

Lesions Associated with ACL Rupture

Meniscal Lesions

The cruciate ligaments are the primary stabilizers of the knee. Butler et al. (1980) state that the ACL provides 86% of the total restraining force to anterior drawer. As a result, any elongation or disruption of the ACL will permit varying degrees of anterior tibial subluxation (Stäubli et al. 1985). During the first episode of anterior subluxation, both menisci initially remain intact in 50% of cases. Peripheral posterior meniscocapsular injuries treatable by primary repair are sustained in 27.7% of cases. In chronic ACL insufficiency with persistent anterior tibial subluxation, only 12.3% of both menisci remain intact, and 29.5% sustain reparable tears (Woods and Chapman 1984).

Clancy et al. (1982) found meniscal lesions in 86% of patients examined 2 years following an unrepaired ACL rupture, significant cartilage pathology involving at least one femorotibial compartment in 54%, and marked retropatellar cartilage lesions in 28%. The increased episodes of anterior tibial subluxation place a greater strain on the taut suspensory ligaments of the menisci (Shoemaker and Markolf 1986). This subjects both the medial and lateral menisci to increased shearing forces in the posterior compartment, typically leading to posteromedial and posterolateral meniscal tears. Most of these lesions are still reparable initially, but as the degree of instability progresses, irreparable types of meniscal tear become more prevalent (Woods and Chapman 1984) (see Fig. 4 b).

Cartilage Lesions

Depending on the degree of instability, the morphotype, and constitutional laxity, the recurrent episodes of subluxation subject the cartilage to excessive shearing forces that incite degenerative changes in the corresponding medial or lateral compartment of the knee (Clancy et al. 1982). In the medial femorotibial compartment, these forces cause superficial flaking or a characteristic rippling of the articular cartilage on the weight-bearing portion of the femoral condyle as this area impinges on the posterior edge of the menisci (Fig. 5). Cartilage lesions on the posterior portion of the tibial plateau are seen with increasing frequency as a sequel to posterior horn meniscectomy (Fig. 5). The lateral femorotibial compartment, which is physiologically "hypermobile" (Bousquet et al. 1980), is prone to developing secondary de-

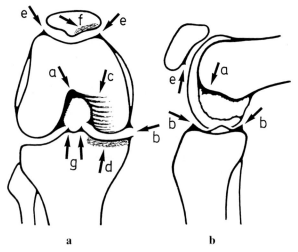

Fig. 5a, b. Radiographic signs of osteoarthritis in the chronic ACL-deficient knee. **a** Frontal plane, **b** sagittal plane. *a*, Superolateral narrowing of the intercondylar notch by marginal osteophytosis *b*, "guillotine osteophyte" at the anterior edge of the intercondylar roof; marginal osteophytes expanding the articular surface; *c*, rippling of the articular cartilage on the medial femoral condyle (detectable by arthroscopy); *d*, increased subchondral sclerosis, pronounced in genu varum following medial meniscectomy; *e*, marginal osteophytes in the femoropatellar joint; *f*, increased subchondral sclerosis in the lateral patellar region; *g*, peaking of the intercondylar tubercles

generative changes, especially if a partial or complete lateral meniscectomy has been performed. Cartilage damage is also observed on the femoropatellar articular surfaces (Clancy et al. 1982). Magnetic resonance imaging reveals various forms of cartilage lesion and subchondral bone damage in knees with acute ACL tears.

ACL Insufficiency, Constitutional Ligamentous Laxity, and Morphotype

Various types of constitutional, physiologic ligamentous laxity are encountered ranging from lax knee ligaments that allow a high degree of constitutional anteroposterior and rotatory joint play and hyperextension to relatively tight ligaments that reduce joint play and hyperextensibility. Radiographs of knees with lax ligaments show a relative hypoplasia of the intercondylar tubercles of the tibia, a narrow intercondylar notch, and occasionally a relative patella alta with lateral subluxation of the patella. In individuals with tight ligaments, the intercondylar tubercles appear well developed, the intercondylar notch is relatively wide, the patella is normally positioned, and a fabella is generally present. A relatively minor trauma in individuals with constitutionally lax ligaments can cause severe disruption of the ACL, while a similar trauma in individuals with tight ligaments may cause only a partial tear. At the same time, this type of knee may occasionally sustain chondral or osteochondral fractures during a weight-bearing rotational injury due to the high coaptation pressure between the articular surfaces (Fig. 4 c). By contrast, the relatively low coaptation pressure in the lax knee appears to protect the articular surfaces from osteochondral fracture.

ACL Insufficiency, Age, and Level of Sports Activity

In their analysis of 103 patients with symptomatic ACL insufficiency, Noyes et al. (1983 a,b) noted a significant increase of functional knee instability in patients who continued to participate in sports at the preinjury level. Reinjury rates rise when a high level of sports activity is maintained. Secondary meniscal damage, secondary lesions of the articular cartilage surfaces, and increasing instability during daily activities are the result (Noyes et al. 1983 a,b) (see Fig. 3 d).

Chronic ACL Insufficiency and Secondary Osteoarthritis

If painful subluxation episodes persist in the presence of chronic ACL insufficiency despite activity modification, the syndrome of the chronic ACL-deficient knee will develop (Feagin 1979). Radiographic signs of degenerative joint disease are few initially but gradually become more prominent (Balkfors 1982; Chambat 1985; Jacobsen 1977). Osteoarthritis of the knee associated with ACL instability following partial bilateral meniscectomy is characterized radiographically by a flattening of the femoral condyles on the frontal and sagittal planes, changes in the intercondylar eminence, and marginal osteophyte formation in the intercondylar notch (Fairbank 1948; Feagin 1979; Jacobsen 1977) (see Fig. 5).

The superolateral portion of the intercondylar fossa ("Grant's notch") is markedly narrowed by osteophytosis (Fig. 5). In the late stage of chronic ACL deficiency, marginal "guillotine osteophytes" may appear at the anterior rim of the intercondylar shelf (Fig. 5). These excrescences may be large enough to fill Grant's notch, which should be adequately widened (notch plasty) during secondary reconstruction of the ACL.

The natural history of nonoperatively treated chronic ACL insufficiency is determined by the type of primary injury, the level of sports activity, primary and secondary irreparable meniscal and cartilage lesions, and by constitutional ligamentous laxity and morphotype. Patients with pronounced genu varum show twice the incidence of degenerative arthritis as individuals with a normal limb axis (Chambat 1985).

These findings were confirmed by McDaniel and Dameron (1980), who identified excessive body weight, sports activity level, genu varum, and prior medial meniscectomy as predisposing factors in the early development of osteoarthritis in the chronically ACL-deficient knee.

A protocol for studying the natural history of an acute rupture or chronic insufficiency of the ACL should take into account the following factors on a prospective basis:

- Age, occupation, and level of sports activity at the time of injury
- Mechanism of injury, pattern of injury, degree of subjective instability
- Type of tear and degree of incompetence of the ACL (clinical tests, arthroscopy, stress radiography)
- Identification of associated lesions: cartilage surfaces, meniscal lesions, capsuloligamentous injuries (MRI, arthroscopy)
- Constitutional ligamentous laxity (degree of laxity on sagittal and frontal planes)
- Morphotype (genu varum, valgum, recurvatum, antecurvatum)
- Prior knee surgery (transarthroscopic, open)

We thank Mr. C. Langenegger, Department of Instructional Media, University of Bern and Inselspital Bern, for the excellent illustrations.

References

Balkfors B (1982) The course of knee-ligament injuries. Acta Orthop Scand 53 [Suppl]: 198

Beaver PF, Frank CB, Rademaker AW, Becker K (1982) A computerised study of anterior cruciate injuries: Repaired versus removed. J Bone Joint Surg [Br] 64: 261

Bousquet G, Millon J, Bascoulergue G, Rhenter JL (1980) La réfection du ligament croisé antérieur par plastie activo-passive du pivot central et des points d'angle. Rev Chir Orthop [Suppl] 2: 66

Butler DL, Noyes FR, Grood ES (1980) Ligamentous restraints to anterior-posterior drawer in the human knee. A biomechanical study. J Bone Joint Surg [Am] 62: 259

Cabaud HE (1983) Biomechanics of the anterior cruciate ligament. Clin Orthop 172: 26

Cabaud HE, Rodkey WG, Feagin JA (1974) Experimental studies of acute anterior cruciate ligament injury and repair. Am J Sports Med 7: 18

Chambat (1985) Le ligament croisé antérieur. Cahiers d'enseignement de la SOFCOT, pp 79–101

Chick RR, Jackson DW (1978) Tears of the anterior cruciate ligament in young athletes. J Bone Joint Surg [Am] 60: 970

Clancy WG jr, Nelson DA, Reider B, Narechania RG (1982) Anterior cruciate ligament reconstruction using one-third of the patellar ligament. Augmented by extra-articular tendon transfers. J Bone Joint Surg [Am] 64: 352–359

Dandy DJ, Flanagan JP, Steenmeyer V (1982) Arthroscopy and the management of the ruptured anterior cruciate ligament. Clin Orthop 167: 43

DeHaven KE (1980) Diagnosis of acute knee injuries with hemarthrosis. Am J Sports Med 8: 9–14

DeHaven KE (1983) Arthroscopy in the diagnosis and management of the anterior cruciate ligament deficient knee. Clin Orthop 172: 52–56

Fairbank TJ (1948) Knee joint changes after meniscectomy. J Bone Joint Surg [Br] 30: 664–670

Feagin JA jr (1979) The syndrome of the torn anterior cruciate ligament. Orthop Clin North Am 10: 81

Feagin JA, Curl WW (1976) Isolated tear of the anterior cruciate ligament. 5 year follow-up study. Am J Sports Med 4: 95

Feagin JA jr, Cabaud HE, Curl WW (1982) The anterior cruciate ligament: radiographic and clinical signs of successful and unsuccessful repairs. Clin Orthop 164: 54–58

Fetto JF, Marshall JL (1980) The natural history and diagnosis of anterior cruciate ligament insufficiency. Clin Orthop 147: 29–38

Fukubayashi T, Torzilli PA, Sherman MF, Warren RF (1982) An in vitro biomechanical evaluation of anterior-posterior motion of the knee. J Bone Joint Surg [Am] 64: 258

Furman W, Marshall JL, Girgis FG (1976) The anterior cruciate ligament. J Bone Joint Surg [Am] 56: 179

Galway RD, Beaupré A, MacIntosh DL (1972) Pivot shift: a clinical sign of symptomatic anterior cruciate insufficiency. J Bone Joint Surg [Br] 54: 763

Giove TP, Miller SJ III, Kent BE, Sanford TL, Garrick JG (1983) Non-operative treatment of the torn anterior cruciate ligament. J Bone Joint Surg [Am] 65: 184–192

Hamberg P, Gillquist J, Lysholm J (1983) Suture of new and old peripheral meniscus tears. J Bone Joint Surg [Am] 65: 193

Hejgaard N, Sandberg H, Hede A, Skive L, Jacobsen K (1982) Prospective stress radiographic study of knee liga-ment injuries in 62 patients treated by acute repair. Acta Orthop Scand 53: 285

Hejgaard N, Sandberg H, Hede A, Jacobsen K (1984) The course of differently treated isolated ruptures of the anterior cruciate ligament as observed by prospective stress radiography. Clin Orthop 182: 236

Hey Groves WE (1920) The crucial ligaments of the knee joint: Their function, rupture, and the operative treatment of the same. J Surg 7: 505–515

Hooper GJ (1986) Radiological assessment of anterior cruciate ligament deficiency. J Bone Joint Surg [Br] 68: 292–296

Hughston JC (1983) Anterior cruciate deficient knee. Editorial. Am J Sports Med 11: 1–2

Hughston JC, Barret GR (1983) Acute anteromedial rotatory instability: long-term results of surgical repair. J Bone Joint Surg [Am] 65: 145–153

Jacobsen K (1977) Osteoarthrosis following insufficiency of the cruciate ligaments in man: a clinical study. Acta Orthop Scand 48: 520–526

Jacobsen K (1982) Gonylaxometry. Stress radiographic measurements of the passive instability in the knee joint of normal subjects and patients with ligaments injuries. Accuracy and range of application. Acta Orthop Scand 52 [Suppl 194]: 1–263

Jacobsen K, Rosenkilde P (1977) A clinical and stress radiographical follow-up investigation after Jones' operation for replacing the anterior cruciate ligament. Injury 8: 221

Jakob RP, Hassler H, Stäubli H-U (1981) Observations on rotatory instability of the lateral compartment of the knee. Acta Orthop Scand 52 [Suppl 191]

Johnson RJ, Eriksson E, Haggmark T, Pope MH (1984) Five-to-ten-year follow-up evaluation after reconstruction of the anterior cruciate ligament. Clin Orthop 183: 122–140

Kennedy JC, Fowler PJ (1971) Medial and anterior instability of the knee. An anatomical and clinical study using stress machines. J Bone Joint Surg [Am] 53: 1257

Kennedy JC, Weinberg HW, Wilson AS (1974) The anatomy and function of the anterior cruciate ligament: as determined by clinical and morphological studies. J Bone Joint Surg [Am] 56: 223–235

Kennedy JC, Hawkins RJ, Willis RB, Danylchuk KD (1976) Tension studies of human knee ligaments. Yield point, ultimate failure and disruption of the cruciate and tibial collateral ligaments. J Bone Joint Surg [Am] 58: 350

Larson RL (1983) The knee – the physiological joint. Editorial. J Bone Joint Surg [Am] 65: 143–144

Lemaire M (1967) Ruptures anciennes du ligament croisé antérieur du genou. J Chir (Paris) 93: 311–320

Lemaire M, Mimerad C (1983) Les instabilités chroniques antérieures et internes du genou. Etude théorique, diagnostic clinique et radiologique. Rev Chir Orthop 69: 16

Lipke JM, Janecki CJ, Nelson CL, McLeod P, Thompson C, Thompson J, Haynes DW (1981) The role of incompetence of the anterior cruciate and lateral ligaments in anterolateral and anteromedial instability. J Bone Joint Surg [Am] 63: 954–960

Lipscomb AB, Andersen AF (1986) Tears of the anterior cruciate ligament in adolescents. J Bone Joint Surg [Am] 68: 19–28

Losee RE, Johnson TR, Southwick WO (1978) Anterior subluxation of the lateral tibial plateau. A diagnostic test and operative repair. J Bone Joint Surg [Am] 60: 1015–1030

McDaniel WJ jr, Dameron TB jr (1980) Untreated ruptures of the anterior cruciate ligament: a follow-up study. J Bone Joint Surg [Am] 62: 696–705

McMaster JH, Weinert CR jr, Scranton P (1974) Diagnosis and management of isolated anterior cruciate ligament tears. J Trauma 14: 230

Marshall JL, Rubin RM (1977) Knee ligament injuries – a diagnostic and therapeutic approach. Orthop Clin North Am 8: 641–668

Montmollin B, le Coeur P (1980) La rupture isolée fraîche du ligament croisé antérieur du genou. Rev Chir Orthop 66: 48

Müller We (1982) Das Knie. Form, Funktion und ligamentäre Wiederherstellungschirurgie. Springer, Berlin Heidelberg New York

Norwood LA, Cross MJ (1979) Anterior cruciate ligament: functional anatomy of its bundles in rotatory instabilities. Am J Sports Med 7: 23

Noyes FR, Bassett RW, Grood ES, Butler DL (1980a) Arthroscopy in acute traumatic hemarthrosis of the knee: incidence of anterior cruciate tears and other injuries. J Bone Joint Surg [Am] 62: 187–195

Noyes FR, Grood ES, Butler DL, Malek M (1980b) Clinical laxity tests and functional stability of the knee: biomechanical concepts. Clin Orthop 146: 84–89

Noyes FR, Mooar PA, Matthews DS, Butler DL (1983a) The symptomatic anterior cruciate-deficient knee. Part I: The long-term functional disability in athletically active individuals. J Bone Joint Surg [Am] 65: 154–162

Noyes FR, Matthews DS, Mooar PA, Grood ES (1983b) The symptomatic anterior cruciate-deficient knee. Part II: the results of rehabilitation, activity modification, and counseling on functional disability. J Bone Joint Surg [Am] 65: 163

Noyes FR, Butler DL, Grood ES, Zernicke RF, Hefzy MS (1984) Biomechanical analysis of human ligament grafts used in knee ligament repairs and reconstructions. J Bone Joint Surg [Am] 83: 344–352

Odensten M, Gillquist J (1985) Functional anatomy of the anterior cruciate ligament and a rationale for reconstruction. J Bone Joint Surg [Am] 67: 257–262

O'Donoghue DH (1959) Injuries of the knee. Am J Surg 98: 463

Rowere GD, Adain DM (1983) Anterior cruciate deficient knees: a review of the literatur. Am J Sports Med 11

Satku K, Kumar VP, Ngoi SS (1986) Anterior cruciate ligament injuries. J Bone Joint Surg [Br] 68: 458–461

Shoemaker SC, Markolf KL (1986) The role of the meniscus in the anterior-posterior stability of the loaded anterior cruciate-deficient knee. J Bone Joint Surg [Am] 68: 71–78

Stäubli H-U, Jakob RP, Noesberger B (1985) Anterior-posterior knee instability and stress radiography. A prospective biomechanical analysis with the knee in extension. In: Perren SM, Schneider E (eds) Biomechanics: Current interdisciplinary research. Nijhoff, Dordrecht Boston Lancaster, pp 397–402

Torg JS, Conrad W, Kalen V (1976) Clinical diagnosis of anterior cruciate ligament instability in the athlete. Am J Sports Med 4: 84–93

Woods GW, Chapman DR (1984) Repairable posterior, meniscoscapular disruption in ACL injuries. Am J Sports Med 12: 381–385

Natural History of Associated Intraarticular Pathology in the Chronic Anterior Cruciate Ligament-Deficient Knee

J. Y. Dupont and C. Scellier

The natural history of injuries of the anterior cruciate ligament (ACL) has been the focus of numerous studies (Dejour et al. 1983; Fetto and Marshall 1980; McDaniel and Dameron 1983; Noyes et al. 1983). These studies have consistently shown that osteoarthritis of the knee can develop within 10 years after rupture of the ACL. This instability-induced arthrosis may remain asymptomatic for some time. The methodology of these retrospective studies is open to question, however, because the need for arthrotomy constitutes a negative selection criterion as it selects only those patients who are most troubled by the instability.

Method

Arthroscopy, a relatively noninvasive procedure, is well tolerated by patients and permits a thorough examination of intraarticular structures (cruciate ligaments, menisci, cartilage surfaces).
Functional complaints, degree of knee laxity, and the type and extent of meniscal and articular cartilage lesions were evaluated in a series of 375 patients with varying degrees of arthroscopically confirmed ACL insufficiency in relation to the interval between the initial injury and arthroscopy.
Due to the potential for statistical error in this type of approach, our findings should be viewed as tendencies rather than hard conclusions.

Case Analysis

Knee arthroscopy was performed in 375 patients with ACL injuries (250 men, 125 women). Eighty-nine percent of the patients sustained their initial knee injury while playing sports. The age at initial injury ranged from 10 to 59 years, with an average of 26 years (only patients with a typical mechanism of injury were included in the study). We excluded patients with an acutely torn ACL with hemarthrosis.

The average interval from injury to arthroscopy was 4 years, with a range from 1 month (21 cases) to more than 20 years (12 cases). All patients who had undergone a knee reconstruction prior to arthroscopy were excluded from the study, but those who had only had a meniscectomy were included. To compare these highly diverse cases, we devised a functional instability score based on the frequency and precipitating mechanisms of subjective complaints (total of 20 points) and an anatomic laxity scheme (23 points) based on the Lachman test, anterior drawer in neutral and external rotation, dynamic subluxation phenomena in internal and external rotation, and varus laxity in flexion (all tests performed under anesthesia). A score was also assigned to chondropathy or chondral changes (20 points based on the location, depth, and extent of cartilage lesions). Only one surgeon performed the clinical and arthroscopic examinations.

Results

Functional complaints occurring outside episodes of instability (pain, crepitation, swelling, locking) were not significantly influenced by passage of time. Pain bore no apparent relation to the development of chondral changes. Instability, however, showed a progressive development over time (Fig. 1). The average instability score increased in the period from 1 month to 2 years, stabilized at about 10 years, then began to decline. During the first 2 years, 30% of the patients had no complaints relating to functional instability. After 5 years, all the patients were more or less unstable. Measurable knee laxity increased over time, the laxity curve showing good agreement with the instability curve (Fig. 2). Without anesthesia, 20% of the knee joints showed no objectively demonstrable laxity. Under general anesthesia the Lachman sign (anterior drawer near extension with absence of an anterior end point) seemed to be a more reliable test, especially during the initial months, than the classic anterior drawer sign, which was mainly elicited an

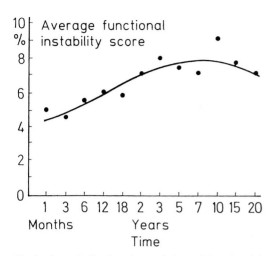

Fig. 1. Score indicating the evolution of functional instability over time. *0* = No instability, *2–8* = moderate instability, *>10* = severe instability

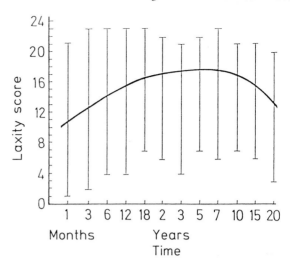

Fig. 2. Increase in knee laxity tested under anesthesia (general instability score and patient distribution pattern). Patients are included with a minimum and maximum laxity score in each time interval. Note the very wide distribution

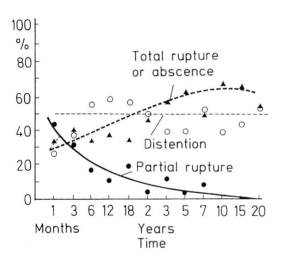

Fig. 3. Types of ACL injury in patients with chronic knee laxity

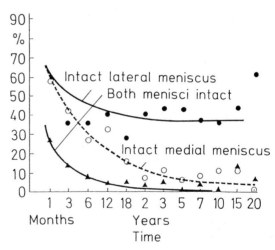

Fig. 4. Number of intact menisci

average of 2 years after the onset of instability and signified progressive stretching of the peripheral capsule and ligaments. The pivot shift test in internal rotation (an important sign) was positive in 30% of cases immediately after the initial injury and in 80% of cases at 2 years postinjury. Associated injuries of the medial structures (in 20% of cases) showed no laxity change over time compared with initial findings. The higher the patient's level of sports activity, the earlier he sought medical help, and the more pronounced the initial laxity. The development of secondary osteoarthritis reduced the degree of anterior knee laxity after 10 years or more.

The types of ACL injury varied over time (Fig. 3). Partial ruptures and partial functional incompetence decreased with passage of time; they disappeared after approximately 3 years. Complete absence of the ACL, which generally was noted 6–12 years postinjury, was demonstrable in 3 of 5 cases after 1 year. There was a close correlation between the instability or laxity score and the presence or absence of an ACL that was still partly functional.

Associated lesions of the menisci progressed over time in both prevalence (Fig. 4) and type (Fig. 5). Some 78% of the medial menisci and 62% of the lateral menisci developed tears, with lesions of both

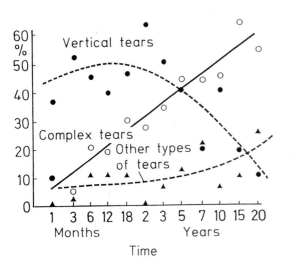

Fig. 5. Types and progression of medial meniscal lesions associated with chronic anterior knee laxity

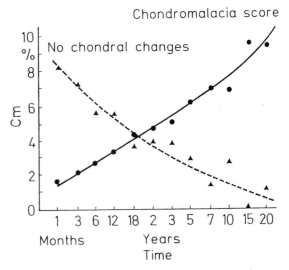

Fig. 6. Follow-up study of chondral changes score and percentage of patients without changes

menisci demonstrable in 1 of 2 patients (178 cases). Only 7% of non-meniscectomized patients retained intact menisci (27 cases), and only within 1 year post-injury. The number of medial meniscus lesions increased rapidly over time, while the number of lateral meniscus lesions remained constant after 2 years (40% remained intact). The more time had passed since the initial injury, the more severe the meniscal lesions.

Articular cartilage lesions increased over time (Fig. 6) and were consistently present after 10 years, with 1 in 3 cases displaying global osteoarthritis at 10 years. Osteoarthritic changes generally began in the medial femorotibial compartment, then spread to the femoropatellar compartment before finally involving the lateral femorotibial compartment as well. Of the 45 patients who underwent meniscectomy prior to arthroscopy, 42 had demonstrable osteoarthritis of the involved compartment. Meniscectomy significantly worsened the spontaneous course, but it did not appear to affect the progression of laxity (perhaps due to the swift secondary development of osteoarthritis).

Conclusions

Our prospective studies conducted over a 4-year period permit the following conclusions to be drawn.

Pathophysiology

Our study confirms the concepts of the various restraints to anterior tibial subluxation developed by Noyes et al. (1983): Functional incompetence of the primary restraint (the ACL) leads to a progressive stretching out of the secondary restraints, leading in turn to anterior drawer laxity and a pivot shift in internal and external rotation. The patient may experience no functional disability for the first 2 years, but functional instability eventually ensues and becomes worse with passage of time. As expected, continued athletic activity has a deleterious effect on the knee.

Methods of Surgical Reconstruction

The preferred reconstructive techniques are those in which the defective ACL is replaced by an intra-articular substitute. We believe that techniques which purport to correct the functional instability without correcting the anatomic lesion at the center of the joint (e. g., extraarticular ligament transfers to block the pivot shift and active techniques) are, by their very concept, doomed to failure.

Indications for Knee Reconstruction

We do not believe that primary conservative treatment, with its lengthy rehabilitation period, can be seriously regarded as the therapy of first choice. As a matter of principle, isolated or total meniscectomies should be withheld whenever possible, though occasionally they are unavoidable. Avoidance of athletic activities can be incorporated into the treatment plan of patients who experience instability only during sports. If reconstructive surgery is planned, it should be done at a time when knee laxity has not yet stretched out the peripheral structures, the meniscal tears are still reparable, and the cartilage lesions can still be stabilized within the first 2 years after the initial injury. Reconstructive knee surgery should correct any anatomically determined laxity whenever possible.

References

Butler DL, Noyes FR, Grood ES (1980) Ligamentous restraints to anterior drawer posterior drawer. A biomechanical study. J Bone Joint Surg [Am] 62: 259–270

Dejour H et al. (1983) Les résultats du traitement des laxités antérieures du genou. Symposium. Rev Chir Orthop 64: 255–301

Fetto JF, Marshall JL (1980) The natural history and diagnosis of anterior cruciate ligament insufficiency. Clin Orthop 147

Jacobsen K (1977) Osteoarthrosis following insufficiency of the cruciate ligaments in man. Acta Orthop Scand 48: 520–526

McDaniel WJ, Dameron TB (1983) Untreated ruptures of the anterior cruciate ligament. A follow-up study. J Bone Joint Surg [Am] 62: 696–705

Noyes FR, Mooar PA, Metthews DS, Butler DL (1983) The symptomatic anterior cruciate-deficient knee. J Bone Joint Surg [Am] 65: 154–174

Scellier (1985) Les symptomes et les lésions des laxités chroniques du genou par atteinte du ligament croisé antérieur. Thèse médecine, Amiens

Aplasia of the Cruciate Ligaments

H.-U. Stäubli, R. P. Jakob, P. Witschger, and R. Ganz

Aplasia of the cruciate ligaments is rare (DeLee and Curtis 1983; Giorgi 1956; Johansson and Aparisi 1983; Torode and Gillespie 1983). Giorgi (1956), in a retrospective analysis of 2500 radiographs of the knee, found one instance in which complete absence of the intercondylar tubercles was present as a morphologic correlate of cruciate ligament aplasia (Fig. 1 a–c). Besides flattening of the intercondylar eminence, Johansson and Aparisi (1983) noted hypoplasia of the intercondylar notch as a morphologic correlate of congenital absence of the cruciate ligaments (Fig. 1 c). Two variants of intercondylar eminence dysplasia may be seen on radiographs: *hypoplasia* and *aplasia*. Hypoplasia (Fig. 1 b) is characterized by a flattening of the intercondylar eminence, which projects only slightly above the articular surface of the tibial plateaus compared with the normal joint (Fig. 1 a). Aplasia (Fig. 1 c) of the intercondylar eminence (and thus of the cruciate ligaments) is characterized by the complete absence of an elevation in the intercondylar region (DeLee and Curtis 1983; Giorgi 1956).

Kaelin et al. (1986) pointed to the relationship between congenital aplasia of the cruciate ligaments and hypoplasia of the lateral femoral condyle. Souryal et al. (1988) found significant hypoplasia of the intercondylar notch in a group of 45 patients with consecutive bilateral insufficiency of the anterior cruciate ligament (ACL) (Fig. 1 b).

In functional tests Johansson and Aparisi (1983) and Torode and Gillespie (1983) demonstrated a sagittal laxity in the flexed knee (Fig. 2). Jones and Moseley (1985) noted the danger of posterior subluxation of the knee during femoral lengthening (Fig. 3). Torode and Gillespie (1983) documented subluxation of the flexed knee both clinically and radiographically (on stress films) in patients with femoral, tibial and fibular hypoplasia and with varying degrees of proximal femoral focal dysplasia (PFFD) or deficiency.

In this article we are concerned with identifying the morphologic and radiographic features of hypoplasia or aplasia of the cruciate ligaments. The direction, type, and amount of sagittal knee laxity near extension were documented preoperatively on stress-radiographs taken while an anterior and posterior drawer stress was applied (Fig. 4) (Stäubli et al. 1985). The congenital knee laxities were classified by clinical and stressradiographic criteria as isolated anterior laxity, isolated posterior laxity, or combined anteroposterior laxity.

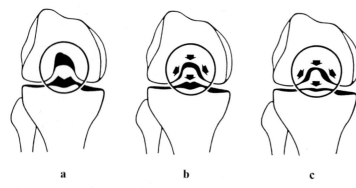

a   b   c

Fig. 1 a–c. Morphology of the intercondylar tubercles. **a** Normal-appearing intercondylar eminence with normal height of the medial and lateral tubercles and normal widths of the anterior intercondylar area and intercondylar notch. **b** Hypoplasia of the intercondylar tubercles and intercondylar notch. **c** Aplasia with complete absence of the intercondylar eminence, flattening of both tibial plateaus, and marked dysplasia of the intercondylar notch

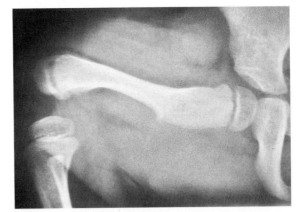

Fig. 2. Posterior subluxation of the tibia in flexion associated with hypoplasia of the posterior cruciate ligament and of the femur

Fig. 3. Posterior subluxation of the tibia near extension following femoral shaft lengthening in a patient with congenital aplasia of the posterior cruciate ligament

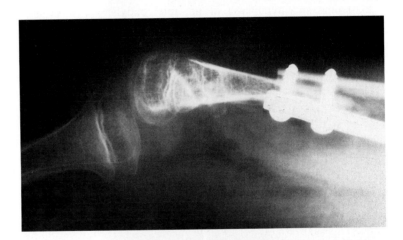

Fig. 4. Stressradiographs documenting a combined anterior *(above)* and posterior *(below)* knee laxity in extension with femoral hypoplasia. Arthroscopy showed a functionally incompetent synovial band in place of the anterior cruciate ligament and a hypoplastic posterior cruciate ligament

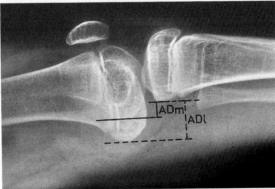

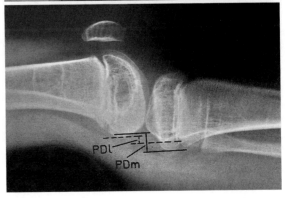

Material and Method

Of 23 patients treated operatively for congenital leg-length discrepancy between 1972 and 1984, 13 showed morphologic signs of intercondylar eminence dysplasia on X-rays. These 13 patients with congenital limb deficiencies were examined clinically for sagittal knee laxity near extension and near flexion. The sagittal knee instabilities and laxities were classified clinically and by stressradiography (see Fig. 4) into *anterior*, *posterior*, and *combined anterior and posterior knee laxities* near extension.

Results

Tables 1 and 2 shows the results of clinical and stress radiographic knee laxity testing near extension in 10 patients with femoral hypoplasia and 3 patients with tibial hypoplasia.

Anterior laxity was demonstrated clinically and by stressradiography in 3 cases, posterior laxity in 7, and a combined anterior-posterior laxity in 3 (see Table 2).

We observed the following morphologic signs of cruciate ligament dysplasia on radiographs of our patients:

– Flattening and hypoplasia of the intercondylar tubercles.

Table 1. Hypoplasias and leg-length discrepancy

Type of hypoplasia	Femoral hypoplasia	Tibial hypoplasia
Number of patients	10	3
Average age	10.6 years	8.6 years
Mean leg-length discrepancy	− 7.2 cm	− 3.5 cm

– Narrowing of the anterior intercondylar area.
– Hypoplasia of the intercondylar notch (Fig. 5)
– Hypoplasia of the lateral femoral condyle (Fig. 6)
– Flattening of the tibial plateau

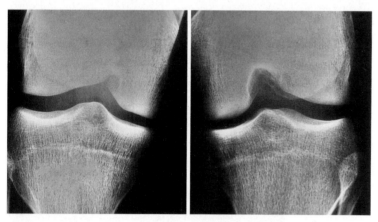

Fig. 5. Hypoplasia *(right)* and dysplasia *(left)* of the intercondylar notch

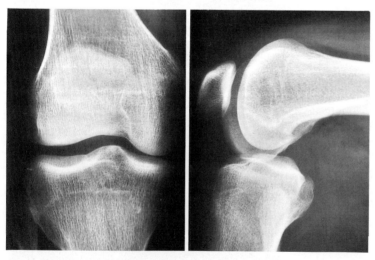

Fig. 6. Hypoplasia of the right intercondylar eminence and lateral femoral condyle in a knee with cruciate ligament hypoplasia

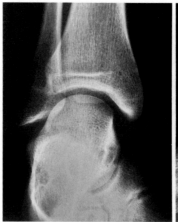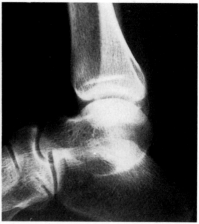

Fig. 7. Incidental finding of talocalcaneal coalition ("ball and socket joint") in a patient with documented ipsilateral cruciate ligament aplasia

Table 2. Type and direction of knee laxity

	Femoral hypoplasia	Tibial hypoplasia
Knee laxity near extension (n)		
Anterior knee laxity	1	2
Posterior knee laxity	6	1
Combined knee laxity	3	0
Total	10	3

Dysmelias or dysplasias in the same extremity are common, as illustrated by the incidental finding of a "ball and socket joint" in a patient with cruciate ligament aplasia.

Discussion

Johansson and Aparisi (1983) described the combination of congenital femoral hypoplasia and cruciate ligament aplasia. Clinical drawer testing in flexion was supplemented in 3 cases by arthroscopy, which in each case showed complete absence of the cruciate ligaments.

Kaelin et al. (1986), on arthroscopy of 6 patients with congenital aplasia of the cruciate ligaments, found absence of the ACL in 4 cases and a nonfunctional synovial band in 2 cases with radiographic signs of hypoplasia of the lateral femoral condyle. They additionally described hypoplasia or aplasia of the intercondylar notch and flattening of the intercondylar eminence.

Torode and Gillespie (1983) stressed the importance of sagittal knee testing in flexion for providing early evidence of congenital limb deficiency (see Fig. 3). X-ray morphologic signs of hypoplasia or aplasia of the intercondylar eminence generally cannot be confidently interpreted as signifying cruciate ligament aplasia until adolescence, when there is sufficient skeletal maturation of the knee (DeLee and Curtis 1983; Giorgi 1956). To avoid posterior subluxation of the knee complicating a planned lengthening of the femur (see Fig. 3), we feel it is important to clinically test sagittal knee laxity in flexion and near extension and document the laxity preoperatively by drawer stress radiographs in 10° of flexion (Stäubli et al. 1985) (see Fig. 4). If knee laxity is pronounced, knee-stabilizing measures should be discussed prior to the limb-lengthening procedure as a means of avoiding progressive posterior subluxation of the tibia during femoral lengthening (Torode and Gillespie 1983).

In patients who develop consecutive bilateral cruciate ligament insufficiency and in patients who experience significant laxity following a trivial knee injury, clinical testing and stressradiography should be used to evaluate constitutional laxity and look for morphologic evidence of cruciate ligament dysplasia.

We thank Mr. C. Langenegger, Department of Instructional Media, University of Bern and Inselspital Bern, for the excellent illustrations.

References

DeLee JC, Curtis R (1983) Anterior cruciate ligament insufficiency in children. Clin Orthop 172: 112

Giorgi B (1956) Morphologic variations of the intercondylar eminence of the knee. Clin Orthop 8: 209

Johansson E, Aparisi T (1983) Missing cruciate ligament in congenital short femur. J Bone Jt Surg [Am] 65: 1109

Jones DC, Moseley CF (1985) Subluxation of the knee as a complication of femoral lengthening by the Wagner technique. J Bone Jt Surg [Br] 67: 33

Kaelin A, Hulin PH, Carlioz H (1986) Congenital aplasia of the cruciate ligaments: A report of six cases. J Bone Jt Surg [Br] 68: 827-828

Souryal TO, Moore HA, Evans JP (1988) Bilaterality in anterior cruciate ligament injuries: Associated intercondylar notch stenosis. Am J Sports Med 16: 449-454

Stäubli H-U, Jakob RP, Noesberger B (1985) Anterior-posterior knee instability and stress radiography: A prospective biomechanical analysis with the knee in extension. In: Perren SM, Schneider E (eds) Biomechanics: current interdisciplinary research. Nijhoff, The Hague pp 397-402

Torode IP, Gillespie R (1983) Anteroposterior instability of the knee: A sign of congenital limb deficiency. J Pediatr Orthop 3: 467

Concepts and Experience
in the Treatment
of Anterior Cruciate Ligament
Disorders

Healing Processes

F. Hefti

Several authors have published experimental studies on the healing processes in ligaments. Nearly all have made their observations in the medial or lateral collateral ligament of the knee (e.g., Miltner and Hu 1933; Jack 1950; Clayton and Weir 1959; O'Donoghue et al. 1961). While the authors disagree in some of their conclusions, all observed more or less complete healing of the medial collateral ligament in 6–8 weeks. Frank et al. (1983) published basic but elegant studies on spontaneous healing of the medial collateral ligament. They ruptured the medial collateral ligament in 64 male New Zealand rabbits with a wire, leaving the ends of the ligaments unapproximated. The contralateral knees were sham-operated. All ligaments "healed" within 14 days by scar-tissue filling of the defects. The ligaments appeared grossly normal at that time, but histologic examination revealed a vascularized inflammatory infiltrate within the rupture zone. By 14 weeks the ligaments showed improved remodeling; there were many longitudinally oriented fibroblasts, and the tissue was less cellular. Even by 40 weeks, however, differences were still apparent between the scar tissue and normal ligamentous tissue. Rupture strength testing of the ligaments showed increased compliance and decreased load even after 40 weeks.

The only previous study on spontaneous healing of the anterior cruciate ligament (ACL) was published by O'Donoghue et al. (1966). In this experimental study in dogs, the ACL was completely transected at its tibial attachment in 24 animals and partially severed in 12. All the animals were immobilized. Pairs of animals were then examined at 1, 2, 4, 6, 8, and 10 weeks. Finally a histologic evaluation was performed. Mechanical testing of the ligaments was originally intended but was omitted because the authors were unable to fix the bones to the testing apparatus so that the bone would not break during the testing of intact ligaments. At 10 weeks they found no evidence of regeneration in the completely transected ligaments, but there was some degree of scar-tissue replacement in the partially sectioned ligaments. Because mechanical tests were not performed and the number of animals was small, this study yields little

meaningful data. Ligaments were also sutured in the same study. When the torn ends were well approximated, the authors observed good scar formation, and the ACL regained its functional competency. Cabaud et al. (1980) published another study on healing processes in the repaired ACL. These authors compared simple suture repair of the ligament with augmentation of the ligament by a strip of patellar tendon. They found better mechanical properties in the augmented ligaments than in the repaired, non-augmented ligaments.

We know that the regeneration of a ligament or tendon proceeds essentially from its surroundings; the "soft tissue envelope" plays a critical role. Owing in large part to the studies of Frank et al. (1983), we have learned much about healing processes in the medial collateral ligament. The ACL presents quite a different situation, however. This ligament is not surrounded by other soft tissues, and its regeneration cannot proceed from its environment. We still know little about the spontaneous healing processes in the ACL. This prompted us to conduct experimental studies designed to answer the following questions:

- How does spontaneous healing of the ACL proceed in the long term following *partial* sectioning of the ligament?
- Can the ACL heal spontaneously following *complete* transection?
- Is there a difference in spontaneous healing between *mature* and *immature* animals?
- How is healing affected by cast *immobilization*?
- How is healing affected by *mobilization*?

Experimental Studies

Materials and Methods

We performed our experimental studies on 404 knees in 202 rabbits. In each case the ACL was completely or partially sectioned in the right knee, and the left knee was sham-operated. Thirty-nine rabbits were killed immediately after the operation; in the other rabbits, ACL regeneration was tested at 2 and 6 weeks and at 3 and 12 months. *Male* rabbits were used for the experiment itself, and several females formed a subgroup of controls. The ligaments from 2 animals per group were *histologically* examined, and the others were mechanically tested. A few cases in each group were unsuitable for evaluation.

The study included *young* rabbits with an average age of 3.25 months at operation (3.1–3.7 months) as well as older, *fully grown* rabbits with an average age of 8.53 months at operation (8.17–8.96). The young rabbits had an average body weight of 2375 g, the adult rabbits 4083 g.

Young and adult rabbits with a partially sectioned ACL were examined in groups of 13–15 specimens after the prescribed intervals. Because no regeneration was observed initially after complete division of the ACL, we used smaller groups of only 6 animals that were examined at 6 weeks and at 3 and 12 months. Additional control groups consisted of animals that were not just mobilized in their cages but were also free to exercise outdoors for 1 h twice daily. In another group the hind limb was immobilized in a plaster cast after surgery. Both these groups were examined after 6 weeks. Two other control groups consisted of female rabbits that were examined immediately after surgery and at 6 weeks. Finally we examined a control group in which the intact ACL was ruptured at a slower rate than in the other cases.

The *operation* was performed under halothane anesthesia. The ACL in the right knee was partially or completely transected with a knife, leaving 1 mm of the approximately 4- to 5-mm width of the ligament intact. The anteromedial bundle was always severed, and in partial cases only a portion of the posterolateral bundle was left intact. The opposite side was sham-operated by opening the knee joint and doing nothing to the ACL. After the designated observation period, the animals were killed with an overdose of Pentothal administered under halothane anesthesia.

Two ligaments from each group were examined histologically. The specimens, which included the femoral condyles and proximal tibia, were embedded in paraffin, and serial longitudinal sections were cut with a microtome. The sections were then alternately stained with PAS, H&E, Pasini, and van Gieson-eosin.

The mechanical properties of the specimens were tested with a tensile test apparatus (Sadamel) in which the distal femur and proximal tibia were held by 2 clamps. Interconnected only by the ACL, the femur and tibia were mechanically distracted. The clamp mechanism on the femoral side was connected to a spring bar with a known elastic constant. The ligament strain and rupture force were measured simultaneously using displacement pickups and measuring amplifiers. The curves were plotted on an x-y recorder, fed directly into a computer, and statistically analyzed.

Results

The *immediate postoperative* maximum load on the partially sectioned side was reduced to 1/3 that on the sham-operated side in young animals and to 1/4 in adult animals.

At *2 weeks* postoperatively all ligaments showed a significant reduction of maximum load and decreased stiffness on both the partially sectioned and sham-operated sides. Histology revealed massive tissue infiltration by leukocytes, lymphocytes, and mast cells.

At *6 weeks* postoperatively no regeneration was apparent in the completely transected ligaments. Twenty percent of the partially sectioned ligaments went on secondarily to complete rupture. In the rest, the maximum load of the ligaments in young and adult animals was approximately equal to the immediate postoperative state on both the partially sectioned and sham-operated sides. Stiffness was still markedly reduced. Histologically, the defect was filled with disordered scar tissue. Fibroblasts and collagen fibers were abundant and arranged in whorls. Animals that were actively mobilized after partial sectioning showed similar ACL stiffness and rupture strength values. In animals whose limb had been immobilized in a long cast, the rupture strength of the partially sectioned ACL was significantly reduced, and its compliance was increased.

At *3 months* postoperatively there was still no evidence of regeneration in the completely transected ligaments. About 25% of the partially sectioned ligaments underwent complete secondary rupture. In the rest, the maximum load of the ACL on the operated side was approximately 2/3 that on the sham-operated side, indicating that the ligament had become significantly stronger. Its stiffness was comparable to that on the opposite side. In adult animals the rupture strength on the partially sectioned side was about half that on the sham-operated opposite side, but again the stiffness was within normal limits. Histologically, the replacement tissue was still clearly distinguishable from normal surrounding ligamentous tissue. It was more cellular, but most of the fibroblasts already showed a largely parallel arrangement, and the collagen fibers also showed a very regular, parallel structure.

By *1 year* postoperatively the transected ligaments still showed no evidence of regeneration. In most cases the stumps of the ACL were resorbed, and sometimes they were adherent to the posterior cruciate ligament. Severe osteoarthritic changes were invariably present. In the partially sectioned group, approximately 20% of the ligaments had undergone secondary complete rupture by this time – the same percentage noted at 3 months. In the rest the maximum load on the partially sectioned side was 2/3 that on the sham-operated side in young animals and 3/4 in adult animals. The stiffness of the ligaments was equal on both sides. Length measurements showed that the ligaments on the partially sectioned side were longer than on the sham-operated side. This was a marked tendency in the young animals, and the difference was statistically significant in the adults. Histologically, the appearance of the replacement tissue was almost indistinguishable from that of normal ligamentous tissue. The replacement tissue was still slightly more cellular and somewhat more compact but showed a regular structure with a parallel arrangement of fibrocytes and collagen fibers.

In summary, no regeneration was observed in the completely transected ACLs, and severe osteoarthritic changes ensued. Partially sectioned ligaments went on to complete secondary rupture in 1/5–1/4 of cases. In the rest, (incomplete) regeneration and strengthening were observed following an initial weakening of all the ligaments at 2 weeks, an apparent result of the surgical trauma. In young animals the maximum load on the partially sectioned side increased from 1/3 that on the sham-operated side to 2/3 by 3 months, with no further significant strengthening thereafter. In the adults the maximum load strength increased from an initial 1/4 to 3/4 at 1 year. Stiffness normalized in only 3 months. While active exercise had no measurable effect on regeneration, cast immobilization had a deleterious effect. We observed no differences between males and females. At 1 year the partially sectioned ligaments were slightly longer than on the sham-operated opposite side; this difference was significant in adult animals but not in young animals.

Discussion

An issue in every animal experiment is whether the results are applicable to humans. In a *biomechanical* sense, the animal knee is vastly different from the human knee: It is habitually flexed and cannot be fully extended; knee motions are always coupled with motion at the ankle joint because the extensor digitorum tendon attaches to the lateral femoral condyle and bridges both joints; also, animal knees have less freedom of rotation than the human knee. Our inquiry, however, is less biomechanical than *biological*. The biologic situation of the ACL is very similar in animals and humans, especially with regard to blood supply. The surrounding structures and the course of the ligament within the joint cavity are also comparable to those in humans. Thus, our study provides useful analogies with the human condition, even though we must be somewhat careful in interpreting the results.

Another basic question is whether the surgical incision of a ligament is comparable to a traumatic rupture. Obviously there are fundamental differences. In a partial rupture, individual fiber bundles have been torn apart longitudinally, creating a very irregular disruption. Our attempts to partially rupture the ACL mechanically with a wire were unsuccessful due to the highly variable extent of the resulting tear. In order to obtain meaningful results, we had to adopt a standardized technique. We therefore sectioned the ligaments with a knife, in partial cases leaving 1 mm of the ligament width intact. Given the thinness of the ACL in young animals, this left a somewhat greater percentage of the ligament intact in the adult animals.

In cases with complete transection of the ACL, we saw absolutely no evidence of subsequent regeneration. All the animals showed severe osteoarthritic changes at 3 months. At 1 year we observed very severe deformities of the knee joint along with secondary damage to the menisci and posterior cruciate ligament. These observations are consistent with those of O'Donoghue et al. (1966), who likewise saw no regeneration 10 weeks after transection of the ACL in dogs. We know from clinical experience that a completely ruptured ACL frequently undergoes subsequent resorption. We have seen several human cases in which the ruptured ACL gained attachment to the posterior cruciate ligament. Nevertheless, the biomechanical effects of an isolated ACL rupture are not entirely comparable in animals and man. For example, severe osteoarthritic changes never develop as swiftly in humans with an isolated ACL tear as in animals, where the ACL apparently plays a more dominant role. This is due largely to the habitually flexed knee position, which deemphasizes the role of secondary restraints. We know that rupture of the ACL in dogs causes a profound functional disability that usually necessitates operative treatment.

We observed significant regeneration of the partially sectioned ACL in both young and adult animals. The regeneration was not complete, however, as the partially sectioned ligament attained only about 3/4 the maximum load of the opposite ligament. It was slightly elongated but showed normal stiffness. These facts were not previously known, and there has been no prior study demonstrating the basic regenerative capacity of the ACL. It appears possible, then, for a partially torn ACL to "recover" as long as an intact guide structure is present (i.e., the unruptured portion of the ligament) and the residual ligament retains an adequate blood supply. The onset of regeneration was somewhat more rapid in young animals than in adults, although at 1 year postoperatively it was no more complete. In 20%–25% of cases the partial section progressed to a complete rupture, apparently during the first 3 months. This occurred even in limbs immobilized in plaster, and it was not significantly more frequent in animals allowed to roam freely than in animals given "functional" therapy in their cages. This suggests that secondary ruptures of this kind do not always have a "traumatic" etiology but may also relate to a proteolytic process that is most apt to occur when there is significant compromise of local blood flow. When examined, most of the secondarily ruptured ligaments had been completely resorbed through proteolysis.

Despite all reservations about the applicability of animal findings to man, our study suggests very strongly that operative treatment can be withheld for most isolated incomplete tears of the ACL (with intact secondary restraints), as there is an excellent prospect for significant regeneration. It must be clearly established, however, that the ligament is not completely torn, and at present this requires the use of arthroscopy with a probing hook. If the rupture is complete, there is no reasonable prospect of regeneration. The decision to operate will depend on the age of the patient, the intergrity of the secondary restraints, and the patient's desire to participate in sports. In every case functional mobilization of the limb appears to be more favorable than cast immobilization.

Therapeutic Implications

Our experimental study confirms the clinical experience that a completely divided ACL does not regenerate. We frequently observe complete absence of the ACL in knees with chronic anterior instability. In other cases the ACL is still present and has gained attachment to the posterior cruciate ligament. Apparently this can occur with proximal ligament avulsions, for example. We saw several cases of this in our animal experiments. In cases where the ACL was absent, we invariably noted extensive degenerative joint disease at 1 year. We know that in human patients with an isolated ACL rupture and intact secondary restraints, the ACL insufficiency does not necessarily produce clinically overt instability and does not always incite a severe osteoarthritis. Associated primary or secondary damage to the secondary restraints must be present in order for decompensation to occur. Apparently the secondary restraints are less effective in the rabbit knee due to the habitually flexed joint position.

Our experimental study has also shown that a partially torn ACL can regenerate (though incompletely) in cases where secondary complete rupture does not supervene. Barring secondary rupture, regeneration appears to require no more than a residual guide structure with adequate blood flow, even though the ACL is surrounded by very few soft tissues. In humans as well, arthroscopic examination often gives the impression that the ACL is indeed present as a complete band, but that "something must have happened at some time" even though the patient does not recall an injury. These are probably cases where the ACL has regenerated from a previous partial tear. We are concerned by our finding that the ACL did not exhibit a normal length after regeneration but was somewhat elongated, especially in adult animals. This means that isometry is not ensured in every case. Nevertheless, we believe we may conclude from our study that, barring injury to the secondary restraints, nonoperative treatment should be adequate in most cases for an isolated incomplete rupture of the ACL. Of course the diagnosis should first be established by arthroscopy with probing, since it is not uncommon for a complete ACL rupture to be mistaken for an incomplete tear. We feel that this recommendation is especially important in view of the disappointing results of cruciate ligament repairs, which have caused most centers to adopt primary reconstruction as the first-line treatment even for acute tears.

With an isolated tear, there is ample justification for managing the patient nonoperatively and waiting for clinically overt instability to appear. The operative procedure is still the same as if primary surgical treatment had been elected.

References

Cabaud HE, Feagin JA, Rodkey WG (1980) Acute anterior ligament injury and augmented repair. Experimental studies. Am J Sports Med 8: 395–401

Clayton ML, Weir GJ (1959) Experimental investigations of ligamentous healing. Am J Surg 98: 373–378

Frank C, Schachar N, Dittrich D (1983) Natural history of healing in the repaired medial collateral ligament. J Orthop Res 1: 179–188

Jack EA (1950) Experimental rupture of the medial collateral ligament of the knee. J Bone Joint Surg [Br] 32: 396–402

Miltner LJ, Hu CH (1933) Experimental reproduction of joint sprains. Proc Soc Exp Biol Med 30: 883–884

O'Donoghue DH, Rockwood CA, Zaricznyj B, Kenyon R (1961) Repair of knee ligaments in dogs. I. The lateral collateral ligament. J Bone Joint Surg [Am] 43: 1167–1178

O'Donoghue DH, Rockwood CA, Frank GR, Jack SC, Kenyon R (1966) Repair of the anterior cruciate ligament in dogs. J Bone Joint Surg [Am] 48: 503–519

Morphologic Ultrastructure of Repaired and Reconstructed Ligaments

W. Hackenbruch and H. Arnold-Schmiebusch

We have combined arthroscopic and electron microscopic studies in an effort to identify objective criteria governing the fate of the repaired or reconstructed anterior cruciate ligament (ACL). Other objective methods (e.g., mechanical rupture tests or the complete histologic workup of a whole cruciate ligament) are inappropriate for use in human subjects on ethical grounds.

A major advantage of electron microscopy is that it can be performed on minute tissue samples that do not affect the stability of the knee. A biopsy specimen no larger than 1×1 mm is sufficient.

Although the examination of large numbers of patients is not feasible or justifiable, to date we have been able to analyze 52 electron microscopic specimens: 41 obtained after repair or reconstruction of the ACL and 11 control specimens (Table 1).

In the patients with ACL repair or reconstruction, 9 specimens were obtained in reoperations and 32 during arthroscopy. Most reoperations were performed for significant residual instability, and arthroscopy for severe residual complaints (meniscal and cartilage lesions). The biopsy was documented photographically or on video tape using a standardized technique. An effort was made to take the biopsy specimen at a consistent site located 1 cm anterolateral to the tibial attachment of the ligament.

The biopsy specimen was fixed at once in buffered glutaraldehyde solution and stored at a constant temperature of $4°C$ until processed for electron microscopy using the classic technique.

Our population was too small and heterogeneous for a meaningful statistical evaluation. It is likely, moreover, that the results are nonrepresentative and tend to be poorer than average, since the series consisted almost entirely of patients with poor outcomes (residual instability, meniscal or cartilage lesions).

From the wealth of documented material, we have selected several characteristic electron micrographs for presentation in this chapter (Figs. 1–5).

Ultrastructural analysis of the repaired or reconstructed ligaments indicated the following:

- The autologous ACL substitute survives within the knee.
- With an isometric reconstruction, the collagen fibers become oriented along lines of tensile stress.
- In agreement with clinical and macroscopic findings, the patellar tendon makes the most suitable autologous substitute for the ACL.
- Dysplastic collagen structures and irregular fibril patterns were mostly observed in the repaired ACL and in other autologous grafts (iliotibial tract). With passage of time, the ultrastructure of the graft approaches that of the ACL through remodeling. This is consistent with clinical experience that good intermediate-term results (1–2 years) portend good late results (5–8 years).

Despite the confidence of our findings, additional questions remain. For example, it would be of great interest to document in detail the progression of ligamentous healing on electron micrographs. The biopsies in the present study were taken from 3 to 72 months postoperatively. It would also be interesting to learn whether proprioceptive nerve structures can be detected in the ACL. To date we have been unable to find any recognizable tactile corpuscles in our specimens.

Table 1. Biopsies of repaired and reconstructed ACLs

Replacement with a free patellar tendon graft	21
Replacement with a patellar tendon strip based on the infrapatellar fat pad	13
Repair with pull-through sutures	3
Reattachment of a distal bony avulsion	1
Replacement with a vascularized strip of iliotibial tract	1
Repair by a nonspecific operative procedure	2
Total	41
Control specimens:	
Anterior cruciate ligament	6
Posterior cruciate ligament	1
Patellar tendon	2
Patellar tendon reconstruction of the ACL in experimental animals (see article by Drobny et al., p.)	
Total	11

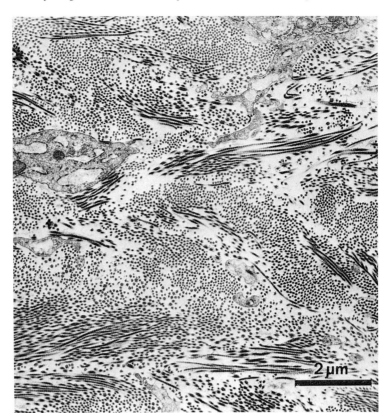

Fig. 1. Electron micrograph of a grossly intact ACL biopsied during open meniscectomy in a 63-year-old man. Note the regular fibril arrangement and homogeneous ultrastructure

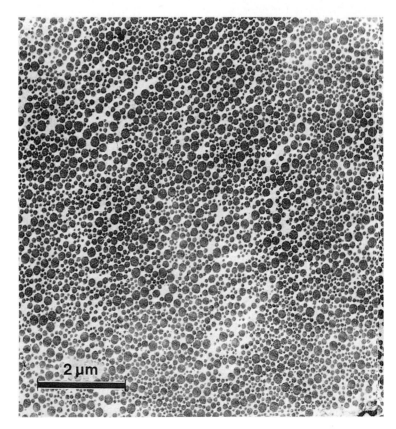

Fig. 2. Electron micrograph of the patellar tendon of a 20-year-old woman shows a completely homogeneous ultrastructure with a symmetrical arrangement of the collagen fibrils

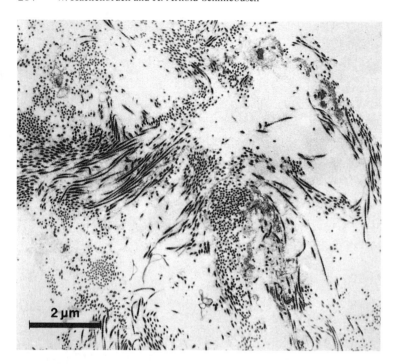

Fig. 3. Electron micrograph 1 year after ACL reconstruction with a vascularized iliotibial tract transfer. The patient, a 19-year-old male, shows significant residual instability with an unsatisfactory clinical result. There is marked collagen dysplasia with irregular fibril patterns and cellular ingrowths

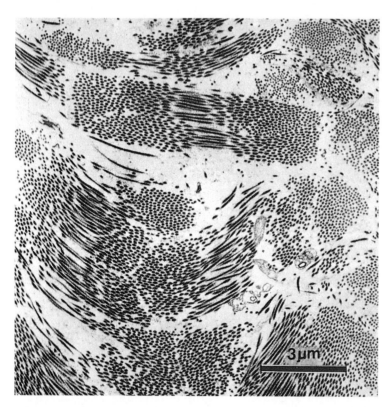

Fig. 4. Electron micrograph 1 year after ACL replacement with a free patellar tendon graft. The fibrils show a relatively uniform arrangement with symmetrical calibers. The clinical and arthroscopic results in this 36-year-old man are good

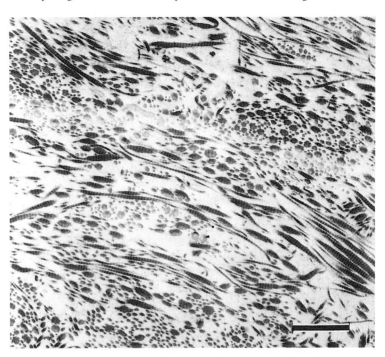

Fig.5. Electron micrograph 2 years after patellar tendon reconstruction of the ACL. Clinically the patient, a 31-year-old woman, had minimal residual instability near extension and residual complaints due to retropatellar chondropathy. The electron microscopic image (enlarged) shows a regular, homogeneous arrangement of the collagen fibrils with no dysplasia or cellular ingrowths

The answers to these and many other questions will require continued research. It would be of significant help to clinical and surgical practitioners if these questions could be more fully explored.

References

Alm A, Gillquist J, Strömberg B (1974) The medial third of the patellar ligament in reconstruction of the anterior cruciate ligament. Acta Chir Scand [Suppl] 445: 5

Arnoczky S, Rubin R, Marshall J (1979) Microvasculature of the cruciate ligament and its response to injury. J Bone Joint Surg [Am] 61: 1221

Hackenbruch W, Henche HR, Kentsch A (1981) Arthroskopische Nachuntersuchungen bei primärer Kreuzbandnaht und Kreuzbandplastik. In: Jäger M, Hackenbroch M, Refior H (Hrsg) Kapselbandläsionen des Kniegelenkes. Thieme, Stuttgart, S 194–202

Hackenbruch W, Schmiebusch H, Müller W, Staubesand J (1986) Arthroscopy and electron microscopy following anterior cruciate reconstruction: In: Trickey, EL, Hertel P (eds) Surgery and Arthroscopy of the Knee. Springer, Berlin Heidelberg New York Tokyo, pp 192–200

Müller We (1982) Das Knie. Springer, Berlin Heidelberg New York

Salamon A, Mayer F, Temes G (1970) Der experimentelle Ersatz des vorderen Kreuzbandes im Kniegelenk durch Transplantate verschiedenen Typs. Bruns Beitr Klin Chir 218: 182

Indications for the Operative and Conservative Treatment of Cruciate Ligament Injuries

C.J. Wirth

The decision whether to manage cruciate ligament injuries operatively or conservatively is controversial. The insistence in former years on the necessity of surgical repair for a torn cruciate ligament was based on the experience that the anterior cruciate ligament (ACL) in particular would not heal with conservative therapy. Nonoperative treatment was thought to result in resorption of the torn ends, leaving the knee permanently unstable. However, since the results of stabilizing procedures on the knee have been evaluated and scored by functional outcomes (Lysholm score), there is a growing sense that even untreated cruciate ligament injuries, especially when "isolated," do not seriously compromise knee function.

The advocates of a nonsurgical approach base their position largely on retrospective studies of untreated "isolated" cruciate ligament injuries. In patients with isolated ACL tears, these studies have shown good to excellent functional outcomes, often with no restriction of sports activities, in 47%–83% of cases (Arnold et al. 1979; Chick and Jackson 1978; Fowler and Regan 1987; Gudde and Wagenknecht 1973; Joke et al. 1984; McDaniel and Dameron 1980, 1983; Paterson and Trickey 1983; Puddu et al. 1984; Shields et al. 1987). The reported functional outcomes of untreated isolated posterior cruciate ligament (PCL) tears are even better, with an 80%–86% rate of good to excellent results that usually include a full return to the preinjury level of sports participation (Cross and Powell 1984; Dandy and Pusey 1982; Degenhardt 1981; Longenecker and Hughston 1987; Parolie and Bergfeld 1986; Tietjens 1985).

The outcome is less favorable, however, when the cruciate ligament tear is combined with other ligamentous injuries (Barton and Torg 1985; Degenhardt 1981; Jackson et al. 1980). Also, eventual meniscal damage is thought to be an inevitable sequel to a conservatively treated cruciate ligament injury, especially a rupture of the ACL (Dejour et al. 1987; Dupont et al. 1986; Feagin and Curl 1976; Fetto and Marshall 1980; Kennedy et al. 1974; Mariani et al. 1983; Noyes et al. 1983; Satku et al. 1986). These knees are considered, in fact, to have a preosteoarthritic deformity (Hackenbroch and Wirth 1979).

Advocates of primary surgical stabilization consider the cruciate ligament-injured knee to be severely function-impaired. They also believe that surgical intervention is necessary to avoid the symptomatic instabilities that would otherwise ensue (Andersson et al. 1988; Barton et al. 1984; Cabaud et al. 1982; Cain and Schwab 1981; Clancy et al. 1983; Feagin and Curl 1976; Hughston and Degenhardt 1982; James et al. 1979; Jones 1963; Kannus and Järvinen 1987; Kannus 1988; Kennedy and Grainger 1967; Marshall et al. 1982; McMaster 1975; Noack and Schleicher 1983; Noack and Scharf 1987; Warren 1982). Several authors emphasize the need for autologous tendon augmentation of a repaired ACL midsubstance tear (Cabaud et al. 1980; Darby 1983; Ficat et al. 1975; James 1980; Paar 1985; Paulos et al. 1983; Tscherne et al. 1987). Augmentation makes the procedure technically more difficult and prolongs the operating time, but it provides significantly better functional stability (Wirth et al. 1984). An extraarticular lateral augmentation is usually added to protect the ACL repair (Ellison 1980; Ellison et al. 1976; Fox 1980; James 1980; Losee et al. 1978; Müller 1982; Opitz et al. 1985, etc.).

Nevertheless, even prospective randomized studies reach different conclusions in terms of the most appropriate therapy. In cases where cruciate ligament ruptures were managed by primary repair, the functional outcome was either found to be identical to that in nonoperatively treated knees (Murnaghan et al. 1988; Sandberg 1987) or superior to it (Andersson et al. 1988; Clancy et al. 1985; Odensten et al. 1985). The results of operative repairs of midsubstance tears of the PCL are rated as good in only about half of all cases (Bianchi 1983; Hughston and Degenhardt 1982; Loos et al. 1981; Strand et al. 1984).

Both the operative and nonoperative treatment of isolated cruciate ligament tears have advantages and disadvantages that can be summarized as follows: Nonoperative treatment avoids the immobilization insult to bone and soft tissues but inevitably leads to the stretching of secondary capsuloligamentous restraints and to degenerative articular changes. A prolonged muscle strengthening program is necessary to compensate for the ligamentous instability. Conversely, operative treatment is advantageous in that it preserves knee stability, but disadvantageous in that it requires prolonged rehabilitation of bone and soft tissues compromised by postoperative immobilization.

Indications for the Nonoperative Treatment of Cruciate Ligament Tears

Absolute Indications

1. Refusal of the patient to undergo surgery
2. Other life-threatening injuries
3. Contaminated or infected wounds about the knee
4. Lack of physician experience in the surgery of knee ligaments
5. Patient unwillingness or inability to cooperate with a postoperative rehabilitation program
6. Adequate muscular compensation of the instability

Relative Indications

1. Positive anterior drawer sign (Lachman test) with a weak pivot shift sign
2. Positive posterior drawer sign (knee flexed 90°) with no genu recurvatum and no varus/valgus instability in extension or 30° flexion
3. Patient over 40 years of age with no athletic ambitions
4. Cruciate ligament ruptures in children
5. Injury more than 14 days old

Concerning the relative indications for nonoperative care, we believe that a mild pivot shift in a knee with a ruptured ACL (Jakob and Stäubli 1987), especially when elicited under anesthesia, is a good prognostic sign in terms of muscular compensation and long-term knee function. With appropriate preoperative counseling, surgical intervention can be limited to the arthroscopic evaluation and excision of a meniscal tear, if present.

An isolated rupture of the PCL also can be managed conservatively in some cases, for the resulting instability is limited to the transverse plane and is not coupled with a rotational component. This type of instability can be well compensated by quadriceps tension.

These are particularly important considerations in patients over 40 years of age who have no athletic as-

pirations. Surgical intervention will generally be the preferred option in younger individuals.

Cruciate ligament ruptures are very rare in children. The open epiphyseal growth plates limit surgical options from a technical standpoint. Results of cruciate ligament repairs in children reported to date have been few and mostly poor, so an expectant approach is favored in the management of these cases (Blauth et al. 1988; Bradley et al. 1986; DeLee and Curns 1983; Matz and Jackson 1988). In children with combined injuries, however, operative treatment is still recommended (Kannus and Järvinen 1988).

Partial tears of the ACL are problematic and are increasingly identified by arthroscopy as a source of posttraumatic hemorrhage. The question of surgical repair, usually of the torn anteromedial bundle, has been settled by invasive arthroscopy.

Indications for the Operative Treatment of Cruciate Ligament Tears

1. Athletically active or performance-oriented patient under 40 years of age (high-demand knee)
2. Bilateral knee injuries
3. Complex capsuloligamentous injury
4. Displaced cruciate ligament avulsion fracture
5. Partial cruciate ligament tear
6. Deficient muscular compensation

As an intraarticular injury, the cruciate ligament avulsion fracture constitutes an absolute indication for surgery. All the other indications are relative, for even an active athlete can remain competitive with a knee brace; this has been demonstrated by alpine ski racers. Even a complete capsuloligamentous disruption in the knee can often heal to a remarkable level of stability with conservative therapy. Given the random nature of the outcome of conservative therapy, however, operative treatment is definitely preferred, especially in younger individuals. The same is true of capsuloligamentous injuries affecting both knees. In these cases it is important to restore ligamentous stability in at least one knee so that the patient can remain athletically active.

The possibility of performing an adequate reconstruction or repair of the cruciate ligament tear, perhaps with augmentation, is of course an essential factor in the decision to operate. If there is a coexisting, unstable, reparable meniscal tear (usually a peripheral longitudinal tear in the posterior horn), we feel that the cruciate ligament tear should be repaired concurrently. This is because we have seen the highest incidence of meniscal retearing or failure of meniscal healing in knees with persistent instability in the transverse plane (Wirth et al. 1988). Other authors express similar (Miller 1988) or opposing views (Sommerlath and Gillquist 1987).

If adequate muscular compensation for an initially nonoperatively treated cruciate ligament tear is not achieved within the first 6 months, the recommendation for secondary cruciate ligament reconstruction is justified.

Conclusions

There is diversity of opinion on the feasibility of conservative treatment or the necessity of operative treatment for cruciate ligament tears. The severity of the resulting instability, and especially the age and athletic ambitions of the patient, will generally dictate the individual therapeutic approach. It is our experience that nonoperative treatment with muscular training can achieve good intermediate-term results only in patients with a straight instability on the transverse plane, like that caused by an isolated tear of the anterior or posterior cruciate ligament. In the longer term, however, there will be a progressive deterioration of knee function due to meniscal damage and osteoarthritic changes; consequently a rationale exists for primary surgical treatment in athletically active patients under 40 years of age. With a multidirectional instability caused by a complex capsuloligamentous disruption, operative stabilization is needed if the patient intends to resume athletic activities.

References

Andersson S, Good L, Odensten M, Gillquist J (1988) Surgical or non-surgical treatment of acute rupture of the anterior cruciate ligament. A randomized study. Eska, Amsterdam

Arnold JA, Coker TP, Heaton LM, Park JP, Harris WD (1979) Natural history of anterior cruciate tears. Am J Sports Med 7: 305-313

Barton TM, Torg JS (1985) Natural history of the posterior cruciate ligament deficient knee. Am J Sports Med 13: 439

Barton TN, Torg JS, Das M (1984) Posterior cruciate insufficiency. A review of the literature. Sports Med 1: 419-430

Bianchi M (1983) Acute tears of the posterior cruciate ligament: Clinical study and results of operative treatment in 27 cases. Am J Sports Med 11: 308-314

Blauth M, Lobenhoffer P, Haas N (1988) Operative Behandlungsmöglichkeiten und -ergebnisse bei Kreuzbandverletzungen im Kindesalter. Hefte Unfallheilkd 200: 515-516

Bradley GA, Shives TC, Samuelson KM (1986) Ligament injuries in the knees of children. J Bone Joint Surg [Am] 61: 588-591

Cabaud HE, Feagin JA, Rodkey WG (1980) Acute anterior cruciate ligament injury and augmented repair. Am J Sports Med 8: 395-401

Cabaud HE, Feagin JA, Rodkey WG (1982) Acute anterior cruciate ligament injury and repair reinforced with a biodegradable intraarticular ligament. Am J Sports Med 10: 259-265

Cain TE, Schwab GH (1981) Performance of an athlete with straight posterior knee instability. Am J Sports Med 9: 203-208

Chick RR, Jackson DW (1978) Tears of the anterior cruciate ligament in young athletes. J Bone Joint Surg [Am] 60: 970-973

Clancy WG, Shelbourne DK, Zöllner GB, Keene JS, Reider B, Rosenberg TD (1983) Treatment of knee joint instability secondary to rupture of the posterior cruciate ligament. J Bone Joint Surg [Am] 65: 310-322

Clancy WG, Ray JM, Zoltan DJ (1985) Acute third degree anterior cruciate ligament injury: A prospective study of conservative nonoperative treatment and operative treatment with repair and patellar tendon augmentation. Am J Sports Med 13: 435-436

Cross MJ, Powell JF (1984) Long-term follow up of posterior cruciate ligament rupture: A study of 116 cases. Am J Sports Med 12: 292-297

Dandy DJ, Pusey RJ (1982) The long-term results of unrepaired tears of the posterior cruciate ligament. J Bone Joint Surg [Br] 64: 92-94

Darby TA (1983) The results of early and late management of anterior cruciate ligament tears. J Bone Joint Surg [Br] 65: 99

Degenhardt TC (1981) Chronic posterior cruciate ligament instability: Nonoperative management. Orthop Trans 5: 486-487

Dejour H, Walch G, Deschamps G, Chambat P (1987) Arthrosis of the knee in chronic anterior cruciate laxity. French J Orthop Surg 1: 85-97

DeLee JC, Curns R (1983) Anterior cruciate ligament injury insufficiency in children. Clin Orthop 172: 112-118

Dupont JY, Scellier C, Chaudières D (1986) The natural history of ACL ruptures. ESKA-Meeting, Basel

Ellison AE (1980) Pathogenesis and treatment of anterolateral rotatory instability. Clin Orthop 147: 51-54

Ellison AE, Wieneke K, Benton LJ, White ES (1976) Preliminary report: Results of extra-articular anterior cruciate replacement. J Bone Joint Surg [Am] 58: 736

Feagin JA, Curl WW (1976) Isolated tear of the anterior cruciate ligament. Five-year follow-up study. Am J Sports Med 4: 95-100

Fetto JF, Marshall JL (1980) The natural history and diagnosis of anterior cruciate ligament insufficiency. Clin Orthop 147: 29-38

Ficat P, Couzacq JP, Ricci A (1975) Chirurgie réparatrice des laxités chroniques des ligaments croisés du genou. Rev Chir Orthop 61: 89-100

Fowler PJ, Regan WD (1987) The patient with symptomatic chronic anterior cruciate ligament insufficiency. Results of minimal arthroscopic surgery and rehabilitation. Am J Sports Med 15: 321-325

Fox JM (1980) Extraarticular stabilization of the knee joint for anterior instability. Clin Orthop 147: 56-60

Gudde P, Wagenknecht R (1973) Untersuchungsergebnisse bei 50 Patienten 10-12 Jahre nach der Innenmeniskusoperation bei gleichzeitig vorliegender Ruptur des vorderen Kreuzbandes. Z Orthop 111: 369-372

Hackenbroch M, Wirth CJ (1979) Gonarthrose nach persistierender Kniegelenksinstabilität. Z Orthop 117: 753-761

Hughston JC, Degenhardt TC (1982) Reconstruction of the posterior cruciate ligament. Clin Orthop 164: 59-77

Jackson RW, Peters RJ, Marczyk RL (1980) Late results of untreated anterior cruciate ligament rupture. J Bone Joint Surg [Br] 62: 127

Jakob RP, Stäubli H-U (1987) Grading the pivot shift. J Bone Joint Surg [Br] 69: 294-299

James SL, Woods GW, Homsy CA (1979) Cruciate ligament stents in reconstruction of the instable knee. A preliminary report. Clin Orthop 143: 90-93

James SL (1980) Biomechanics of knee ligament reconstruction. Clin Orthop 146: 90-94

Jokl P, Kaplan N, Stovell P, Keggi K (1984) Non-operative treatment of severe injuries to the medial and anterior cruciate ligaments of the knee. J Bone Joint Surg [Am] 66: 741-744

Jones KG (1963) Reconstruction of the anterior cruciate ligament. A technique using the cental one-third of the patellar ligament. J Bone Joint Surg [Am] 45: 925-932

Kannus P (1988) Conservative treatment of acute knee distorsions - longterm results and their evaluation methods. Acta Univ Tamperensis 250: 1-71

Kannus P, Järvinen M (1987) Conservatively treated tears of the anterior cruciate ligament, long-term results. J Bone Joint Surg [Am] 69: 1007-1012

Kannus P, Järvinen M (1988) Knee ligament injuries in adolescents. J Bone Joint Surg [Br] 70: 772-776

Kennedy JC, Grainger RW (1967) The posterior cruciate ligament. Trauma 7: 367-377

Kennedy JC, Weinberg HW, Wilson AS (1974) The anatomy and function of the anterior cruciate ligament. As determined by clinical and morphological studies. J Bone Joint Surg [Am] 56: 223-235

Longenecker SL, Hughston JC (1987) Long-term followup of isolated posterior cruciate injuries. Am J Sports Med 15:628

Loos WC, Fox JM, Blazina ME, Del Pizzo W, Friedman MJ (1981) Acute posterior cruciate ligament injuries. Am J Sports Med 9: 86-92

Losee RE, Johnston TR, Southwick WD (1978) Anterior subluxation of the lateral tibial plateau. J Bone Joint Surg [Am] 60: 1015-1030

Mariani PP, Puddu G, Ferretti A (1982) Hemarthrosis treated by aspiration and casting. How to condemn the knee. Am J Sports Med 10: 343-345

Marshall JL, Warren RF, Wickiewicz TL (1982) Primary surgical treatment of anterior cruciate ligament lesions. Am J Sports Med 10: 103-107

Matz SO, Jackson DW (1988) Anterior cruciate ligament injury in children. Am J Knee Surg 1: 59-65

McDaniel WJ, Dameron TB (1980) Untreated ruptures of the anterior cruciate ligament. A follow-up study. J Bone Joint Surg [Am] 62: 696-705

McDaniel WJ, Dameron TB (1983) The untreated anterior cruciate ligament rupture. Clin Orthop 172: 158-163

McMaster WC, (1975) Isolated posterior cruciate ligament injury: Literature review - case reports. J Trauma 15: 1025-1029

Miller DB (1988) Arthroscopic meniscus repair. Am J Sports Med 16: 315-320

Müller We (1982) Das Knie. Form, Funktion und ligamentäre Wiederherstellungschirurgie. Springer, Berlin Heidelberg New York

Murnaghan JJ, Cameron JC, MacIntosh DL, Kellam JF (1988) Acute knee dislocations: 10-years-experience. ESKA, Amsterdam

Noack W, Scharf HP (1987) Aktueller Stand in der Therapie der vorderen Kreuzbandverletzungen. Sportverletzung Sportschäden 1: 13-18

Noack W, Schleicher (1983) Indikation zum vorderen Kreuzbandersatz - die Bedeutung für die Stabilität. In: Rahmanzadeh R, Faensen M (eds) Bandverletzungen am Schulter-, Knie- und Sprunggelenk. Schnetztor, Konstanz, S 151-153

Noyes FR, Mooar PA, Matthews DS, Butler DL (1983) The symptomatic anterior cruciate-deficient knee. Part I. The long-term functional disability in athletically active individuals. J Bone Joint Surg [Am] 65: 154-162

Odensten M, Hamberg P, Nordin M, Lysholm J, Gillquist J (1985) Surgical or conservative treatment of the acutely torn anterior cruciate ligament. A randomized study with short-term follow-up observations. Clin Orthop 198: 87-93

Opitz A, Schabus R, Wagner M (1984) Ersatzoperationen bei anterolateraler Knieinstabilität - Experimentelle und klinische Beobachtungen. Hefte Unfallheilkd 167: 279

Paar O (1985) Verstärkung der frisch geklebten oder genähten Ruptur des vorderen Kreuzbandes durch die Semitendinosussehne. Indikation und Frühergebnisse. Chirurg 56: 728-731

Parolie JM, Bergfeld JA (1986) Long-term results of nonoperative treatment of isolated posterior cruciate ligament injuries in the athlete. Am J Sports Med 14: 35-38

Paterson FW, Trickey EL (1983) Meniscectomy for tears of the meniscus combined with rupture of the anterior cruciate ligament. J Bone Joint Surg [Br] 65: 388-390

Paulos LE, Butler DL, Noyes FR, Grood ES (1983) Intra-articular reconstruction. Clin Orthop 172: 78-84

Puddu G, Ferretti A, Mariani P, La Spesa F (1984) Meniscal tears and associated anterior cruciate ligament tears in athletes: Course of treatment. Am J Sports Med 12: 196-198

Sandberg R, Balkfors B, Nilsson B, Westlin N (1987) Operative versus non-operative treatment of recent injuries to the ligaments of the knee. A prospective randomized study. J Bone Joint Surg [Am] 69: 1120-1126

Satku K, Kumar VP, Ngoi SS (1986) Anterior cruciate ligament injuries to counsel or to operate? J Bone Joint Surg [Br] 68: 458-461

Shields CL, Silva J, Yee L, Brewster C (1987) Evaluation of residual instability after arthroscopic meniscectomy in anterior cruciate deficient knees. Am J Sports Med 15: 129-131

Sommerlath K, Gillquist J (1987) Knee funktion after meniscus repair and total meniscectomy - A 7-year follow-up study. Arthroscopy 3: 166-169

Strand T, Molster AO, Engesalter LB, Raugstad TS, Alho A (1984) Primary repair in posterior cruciate ligament injuries. Acta Orthop Scand 55: 545-547

Tietjens BR (1985) Posterior cruciate ligament injuries. J Bone Joint Surg [Br] 67: 674

Tscherne H, Lobenhoffer P, Blauth M, Hoffmann R (1987) Primäre Rekonstruktion von Kapselbandverletzung des Kniegelenkes. Orthopade 16: 113-123

Warren LF (1982) Primary repair of the anterior cruciate ligament. Clin Orthop 172: 65-70

Wirth CJ, Jäger M, Kolb M (1984) Die komplexe vordere Knieinstabilität. Thieme, Stuttgart New York

Wirth CJ, Rodriguez M, Milachowski KA (1988) Meniskusnaht, Meniskusersatz. Thieme, Stuttgart New York

Indications for Cruciate Ligament Reconstruction: A Recapitulation

R. P. Jakob

In this chapter we shall again review the indications for the operative and conservative treatment of acute tears and chronic insufficiency of the anterior cruciate ligament (ACL) and posterior cruciate ligament (PCL). This review is based on the extensive literature of the past 10 years (see list of references in Wirth, p. 266 ff.). Besides being guided by technical arguments, the experienced knee surgeon will in time develop his own guidelines for patient selection that are unavailable to the less experienced operator. To facilitate patient selection, we have compiled some criteria that we consider to be important. Because these criteria carry different weight for the ACL and PCL, they need to be considered separately. The following specific questions are addressed:

- Should surgery be done?
- Who should have surgery?
- When should surgery be done?
- What should be operated on?
- How should the operation be done?

Anterior Cruciate Ligament

Should Surgery Be Done?

When we ask whether it is appropriate to operate on the ACL, we must pose two additional questions:

- How does the knee joint function shortly after rupture of the ACL?
- What are the long-term sequelae of an untreated rupture?

Both questions touch on the problems of the natural history of an untreated ACL rupture. To answer them, we must look at previously published data and reports that let us compare the results of nonoperative treatment (functional therapy or immobilization and splintage) or lack of treatment in undiagnosed cases with surgical intervention (though there may be substantial differences in terms of economic implications such as vocational and athletic disability and the costs of physical therapy and splints).

To answer the above questions, let us recall the typical course of an untreated ACL rupture:

Untreated instability of the ACL can cause a subjective feeling of instability that is manifested by episodes of giving way, i. e., a sudden buckling of the knee due to pathologic translation and a momentary loss of proprioceptive coordination at the joint. This causes very large peak loads and shear stresses to act upon the cartilage, menisci, and the peripheral capsule and ligaments. One result of this may be the "ACL syndrome" with cartilage erosion, meniscal lesions, and peripheral laxity. Late sequelae include postmeniscectomy and instability-related osteoarthritis.

It has also been observed that absence of the ACL is well tolerated by some patients, who can continue to perform their normal activities and even engage in sports without external support for 20–30 years. Other patients can remain asymptomatic by modifying their activities, such as changing to a less strenuous form of recreation. Finally there are patients who do very well with a knee brace and experience no instability problems. It remains unclear whether this asymptomatic or minimally symptomatic "conservative" group will remain free of long-term degenerative disease and retain full, permanent functional competence of the knee, or whether subthreshold, subclinical pathologic translations and rotations will lead to accelerated degenerative articular changes.

Classic studies, of which there are still far too few, provide some insight into this question (Dejour et al. 1987). The much-quoted study of McDaniel and Dameron (1983) describes virtually no impairment of knee function for the first 10 years despite a high incidence of meniscal and cartilage lesions, followed by a period of rapid deterioration with progressive functional disability. The development of osteoarthritis after meniscectomy also has been amply documented (Johnson et al. 1974).

Besides these valuable studies, we base our decision making on clinical impressions and, though tending to favor operative treatment, are continually amazed by patients whose do well for 30 years after an untreated ACL tear with a marked pivot shift sign and who develop no degenerative joint disease. Apparently there are still unexplained and little-understood factors that cause the ACL to assume a dominant stabilizing role in "ACL-dominant knees," while other joints do well without the ACL. The factors that account for this dominance include anthropometric variations such as the convexity of the lateral tibial plateau, the sagittal diameter of the lateral femoral condyle, the concavity of the medial plateau, the stiffness of the peripheral restraints, muscular guidance, etc.

Who Should Have Surgery?

In theory, our discussion on patient selection would be most meaningful if it were possible to select as surgical candidates the "at risk" group that will suffer objectively and subjectively from cruciate ligament insufficiency, and thus withhold surgery and its potential complications from individuals that will have normal knee function even without an ACL.

In this more philosophical than scientific debate (apparently there are no strictly scientific criteria to be applied), we must base our judgment on signs suggesting that one type of progression is more likely to occur than another in a given case.

Arguments that favor surgery are: youthful age of the patient, heavy manual labor or strenuous sports activity, high demands in terms of joint performance, inability or refusal to modify activities, preexisting meniscal and cartilage lesions, frequent instability with activities of normal living, recurrent swelling, feeling of instability 6 months after intensive rehabilitation, and a previous identical lesion in the opposite knee with the same outcome. We tend to favor conservative treatment in patients over 45 years of age and in less active patients with a sedentary job. If both patient and physician are reluctant to proceed with surgery, little will be lost by watching and waiting for 6–12 months, although one must be prepared for a possible intercurrent meniscal tear and the need for a meniscal repair and joint stabilization. In exceptional cases we have even operated on patients over 50 years of age. One such patient was a prolific deep-snow skier whose performance level and degree of incapacitation by his knee injury were more critical than in a 25-year-old nonathlete. Whether an extra-articular reconstruction alone would be satisfactory at this age must be decided on a case-by-case basis. The earlier question regarding possible subclinical insults in cases managed expectantly remains unanswered but is on par with that regarding complications after surgery that leaves potentially significant residual functional impairment. While every attending physician must ultimately make his own decision, we point out that we operate on approximately three-fourths of our patients with acute lesions. Despite isolated reports of acceptable results with a conservative approach, today the pendulum is definitely swinging to a preference for surgical treatment at centers all over the world.

When Should Surgery Be Done?

Until a few years ago, the standard treatment for a torn ACL in German-speaking countries was direct suture repair. It was felt that the best timing for the repair was during the "acute" phase within 10–14 days of the injury. Only about 40% of these operations yielded an objectively stable joint. Today it is generally agreed that this procedure is not worthwhile and that a primary repair requires autologous augmentation. The step from repair to augmentation, or the combination of both, extends our options somewhat in terms of timing the operation. The first 2 weeks postinjury are still preferred for utilization of the distal stump, both to preserve the blood supply and to maintain a degree of proprioception. But if an ideal placement requires resection of the cruciate stump, the timing of the surgery is no longer critical. The operation will be the same at 6 months or 1 year.

Timing is a more important concern for a meniscal repair, which we believe is more rewarding when done acutely than in the chronic stage. Thus, in cases where a nonoperative approach is agreed upon in the initial consultation, early arthroscopy should be performed to exclude a meniscal detachment. Positive cases are an indication for meniscal repair, which in turn would necessitate a cruciate ligament repair since residual instability would reduce the prospect for successful healing and salvage of the meniscus.

In the acute stage when the articular cartilage is still intact, the result of the ACL and meniscal repairs in terms of joint function and stability is better than in the chronic stage, although acute cases more often require manipulation under anesthesia and more arthroscopies to separate adhesions than chronic cases. In the U.S., this has fostered a trend to postpone surgery for an acute cruciate tear combined with a medial collateral ligament rupture by 4–6 weeks to give the patient a chance to recover articular motion. This is believed to lower the incidence of adhesions and reduce the need for manipulation.

The patient who still feels unstable after a conservative trial and is unhappy with restrictions on his athletic activities will generally request surgery. The instability is most likely to be manifested during sports activities that involve deceleration, acceleration, and cutting. The decision belongs to the patient, who, in the face of chronic symptoms, is asked to rate subjectively the quality of the nonsurgical result. He must decide for himself whether he can accept activity restrictions that avoid pivot-shift episodes or whether he would like to engage more actively in sports or the general activities of daily living. If the patient complains that his functional disability is interfering with his desired life style and he remains symptomatic after an individualized rehabilitation program, we recommend surgical treatment. It is our experience that an overly rigorous muscular strengthening program can create an unchecked, potentially harmful quadriceps muscle action that increases the risk of meniscal and cartilage damage. In this sense a rupture of the ACL is an indication for operative treatment in the short or long term. In the skeptical patient, it can be helpful to postpone surgery for 2–3 years until the patient himself becomes convinced of its eventual necessity.

What Should be Operated On?

In addressing this question, we must take into account all the structures that contribute to the essential stability of the joint: the ACL itself, the menisci, and the peripheral restraints.

There is no question about the need to preserve the meniscal tissue, which forms a stabilizing wedge interposed between the femoral condyle and tibial plateau. The preservation of this fibrous ring system also maintains a critical link with the peripheral restraints.

A concomitant rupture of the collateral ligament and capsule is less important in the acute stage if the ACL is stabilized to a degree that permits postoperative functional therapy of the joint. Several studies have proven the superiority of postoperative exercises over cast immobilization for tears of the medial collateral ligament (see chapter by Ballmer et al., p. 321 ff.). If there is a coexisting meniscal tear ("unhappy triad" pattern), we repair that tear but do not treat the torn collateral ligament. With a lateral-posterolateral lesion, we continue to advocate the meticulous repair of all structures.

In the advanced stage of chronic global anterior instability with pronounced anteromedial and anterolateral displacement of the tibial plateau, it must be asked whether surgery should be limited to the central pivot (i.e., the cruciate ligaments) or whether the periphery should also be repaired.

It is unlikely, of course, that reconstruction of the central pivot alone, an extra-articular repair, or their combination offers the most appropriate or technically optimum solution. Basic scientific principles and rational criteria still need to be worked out, and greater attention must be given to these aspects in future studies. For the present, however, we feel that an intraarticular reconstruction of the ACL with extra-articular augmentation is indicated when the following criteria are met:

- Chronic instability with a prior meniscectomy, often with multiple previous attempts at stabilization and a "salvage knee"
- A greater than 13 mm discrepancy in anterior translation
- 3 + pivot shift, pronounced in external rotation, often with a posterolateral component
- Morphotypic factors with constitutional ligamentous laxity and multiple positive tests: hyperextension of the knee, $> 25°$ hyperrotation of the knee, hypermobile patella, hyperextension of the 5th metacarpophalangeal joint $> 90°$, hyperextension of the thumb, pronounced valgus angulation and hyperextension at the elbow, positive shoulder sulcus sign (downward subluxation)
- High-demand knee in a youthful patient

How Should the Operation Be Done?

This last question focuses on the technique of intraarticular reconstruction that has given us the best results. Probably the key issue here is what provides for adequate stabilization in a structural sense following an ACL reconstruction: Is it the graft, is it the augmentation, or is it the overall mass of scar fibers that occupy the intercondylar notch? L. Johnson believes that it is the scar as a whole, and that the tension in its fibrous adhesions is the main force preventing excessive abnormal translation between the tibia and femur. Indeed, it is common during follow-up arthroscopy at about 1 year to find a scar that starts far anterosuperiorly, where the synovial plica normally attaches (not the expected gleaming cruciate ligament with its constituent bundles). At a deeper level the graft itself may indeed be attached at the anatomically correct "isometric" site corresponding to the surgeon's intention, but the functionally important scar fibers add new meaning to the traditional concept of isometry. Despite this sobering insight, it is reasonable to assume that a strong, accurately placed graft offers the best prospect for the development of a sound substitute ligament. Bathed by synovial fluid, the graft becomes revascularized at a variable rate. A graft attached by bone blocks inserted into osseous tunnels revascularizes in 6–10 months, which apparently is more rapid than the synovialization and revascularization of a graft that has been sutured directly to the bone (Arnoczky et al. 1982).

In animal experiments, the strength of the graft reaches approximately 80% that of the healthy ligament at 12 months (Clancy 1981). The results that we achieve today show that some 80% of our patients who come to operation for an intraarticular lesion of the ACL emerge with a stable, pivot-shift-free joint with less than a 3–4 mm Lachman-test discrepancy relative to the uninvolved side. We perform the reconstruction arthroscopically using a free patellar tendon graft attached by 2 bone blocks in bony tunnels, achieving an accuracy of femoral tunnel placement that we believe is superior to that of an open implantation. We manage even acute ruptures by primary reconstruction with a 10-mm-wide graft. A proximally avulsed cruciate ligament of good size can be engaged with sutures, pulled up and attached together with the graft. Using the same technique for acute and chronic situations simplifies the operation and enables the surgeon to gain experience more quickly. The graft, which is first attached to the femur and then brought out through the tibia, is measured throughout the range of joint motion to assess its isometry. We consider no more than 2–3 mm of anisometry to be an acceptable reconstruction.

During postoperative treatment, we take care to avoid unfavorable quadriceps contraction in the first 40° of flexion for the first 3 months and to train the patient quickly in co-contraction of the hamstrings. Crutches are generally discarded at 6 weeks. Full extension (0°) without hyperextension should be encouraged in "tight-jointed" individuals and discouraged in high-risk patients with extremely lax joints, thus supporting the concept of establishing an individualized treatment program. One should avoid the extremes of a gradual program with painful loss of motion and a stable joint versus a vigorous recovery of motion with a 30% incidence of a 1 + or 2 + pivot shift.

Posterior Cruciate Ligament

Should Surgery Be Done?

In dealing with tears of the PCL, we are faced with uncertainty regarding the natural history of the lesions and also with a technical inability to achieve a result even approaching that of ACL reconstructions. Besides patients who do well with nonoperative treatment, there are reports of a 50% incidence of medial osteoarthritic changes and meniscal tears (Clancy et al. 1983). The accompanying femoropatellar disorders are based on the mechanical overload of that joint resulting from the posteriorly subluxed position of the tibia. True instability symptoms with giving-way episodes are seen less frequently than with anterior instability and are usually based on a coexisting posterolateral component (reversed pivot shift).

It is difficult to account for the fact that the reattachment of a PCL avulsed from the tibia on a bone fragment yields almost perfect stability, whereas repair and augmentation of the ligament or its complete replacement by autologous tissue provides at best a 50% reduction of instability. This is all the more remarkable when we consider that a free ACL graft has a less favorable synovial fluid environment and should be more refractory to revascularization than a posterior cruciate graft, which is rapidly synovialized from the posterior capsule. These findings are probably attributable to the heavy load imposed upon the ligament by gravity. Should we take no action, then, when confronted by this lesion?

Who Should Have Surgery?

Let us first consider a straight posterior instability. We believe that surgery is indicated for an acute PCL tear sustained by a young athlete (up to 35 years of age) who exhibits more than 10 mm of posterior translation. We feel that this degree of displacement signifies peripheral involvement, which untreated would lead to a fairly rapidly progressive laxity with increased posterior translation. If the PCL tear coexists with a primary medial or lateral capsuloligamentous disruption, we recommend surgery even for patients over 35 years of age, for the associated injury implies a rapid worsening of the instability. We also favor operative treatment for combined lesions of the PCL and ACL. We sometimes see this combination as an isolated injury following a hyperextension trauma, a medial or lateral pentade, or a possibly unrecognized dislocation of the knee.

We would recommend surgical treatment for chronic instability in patients up to about 45 years of age who have complaints or a physically demanding life style in cases where signs of subjective instability are coupled with excessive loading of the medial compartment. If these signs are associated with evidence of medial osteoarthritis (i.e., medial joint-space narrowing), we do not hesitate to proceed with valgus osteotomy (frequently open-wedge), without addressing the ligament problem directly.

When Should Surgery Be Done?

The age of the patient has already been addressed. Would it be reasonable to recommend surgery in the acute stage or only after about a 6- to 12-month trial of conservative treatment?

The acute osseous avulsion of the tibial attachment of the PCL is perhaps the clearest indication for acute intervention. The decision depends on the time of the diagnosis, however. Because many PCL injuries are sustained in motor vehicle accidents where there are coexisting diaphyseal fractures of the lower extremity, first priority is given to managing these fractures. The ligament injury often remains undiagnosed for weeks, sometimes leading the patient and surgeon to conclude that the timimg for surgery is unfavorable. It is easy in such cases to adopt a wait-and-see approach, which makes sense from the standpoint of the overall problems that are involved.

If an isolated PCL tear is managed conservatively, treatment should include an intense rehabilitation program in which quadriceps-strengthening exercises are combined with quadriceps-stretching exercises to relieve pressure on the femoropatellar joint. So far we have had no success with external splintage or bracing, but we do encourage patients to lie in the prone position, at least at night, as this reverses the otherwise constant loading in posterior translation that is so disruptive to ligament healing. With chronic PCL insufficiency, the decision to operate is made secondarily when subjective instability problems develop or, rarely, when symptoms of a torn meniscus appear.

What Should Be Operated On?

In repairs and reconstructions of the PCL, the peripheral component is of disproportionately greater significance than with the ACL because of the constant gravity-induced tibial load. We believe that neglect of the peripheral component is one reason for the unfa-vorable results of PCL operations. With an acute PCL tear, then, repair of the central pivot should be combined with the restoration of torn peripheral structures, whether by suture repair or primary reconstruction of a torn popliteus tendon and arcuate ligament or a lateral collateral ligament. Having had unsatisfactory results in chronic instabilities treated by replacement of the PCL alone, we devote considerable time and effort to peripheral transfers, which are discussed in the chapter by Jakob and Warner, p. 463 ff. Once again, preservation of the menisci is an essential consideration.

How Should the Operation Be Done?

Disappointing results of repairs and reconstructions of the PCL can have several causes. Repair without augmentation is promising only if the PCL has been ruptured near its femoral attachment. The use of tenuous grafts that are not harvested on bone blocks is less favorable than a free patellar tendon graft at least 13 mm in width. Isometric placement is a critical concern that has been given too little attention. Our results have been significantly improved by the arthroscopic technique, which provides a clear view for drilling the tibial tunnel using an arthroscopic drill guide. Alternatively, an open operation allows for fairly reproducible positioning of the drill guide when performed by an experienced surgeon. A major error is placing the entrance of the tibial tunnel too high and placing the femoral tunnel too far anterior. We also advocate reinforcing the cruciate substitute with a thin synthetic ligament strip that will protect the ligament during the initial months of remodeling while eliminating the need for unphysiologic fixation methods such as olecranization. While the problems of "stress protection" by the augmenting strip are poorly understood, its use is an essential prerequisite for an acceptable outcome. It is uncertain whether a 50% reduction of posterior translation is a satisfactory result of a PCL reconstruction that justifies the cost of the surgery and rehabilitation. The patient will supply us with this answer 1–2 years after the operation, when he has fully returned to his occupational and recreational activities. The question of how the knee will function in 20 or 30 years, with or without operative treatment, cannot be answered by a single surgeon. The future will demonstrate the validity or invalidity of our decision-making criteria.

References

Arnoczky SP, Tarvon GB, Marshall JL (1982) Anterior crucia- te ligament replacement using patellar tendon: an evalua- tion of graft revascularization. J Bone Joint Surg [Am] 64: 217

Clancy WG Jr, Narenchiania RG, Rosenberg TD et al. (1981) Anterior and posterior cruciate ligament reconstruction in Rhesus monkeys: a histological microangiographic, and biomechanical analysis. J Bone Joint Surg [Am] 63: 1270-1284

Dejour H, Walch G, Deschamps G, Chambat P (1987) Ar- throse du genou sur laxité chronique antérieure. Rev Chir Orthop 73: 157-170

Clancy WG, Shelbourne DK, Zöllner GB, Keene JS, Reider B, Rosenberg TD (1983) Treatment of knee joint instability secondary to rupture of the posterior cruciate ligament. J Bone Joint Surg [Am] 64: 310-322

Johnson RJ, Kettlekamp DB, Clark W et al. (1974) Factors affecting late results after menisectomy. J Bone Joint Surg [Am] 56: 719-729

McDaniel WJ, Dameron TB (1983) The untreated anterior cruciate ligament rupture. Clin Orthop 172: 158-163

Acute Tears
of the Anterior Cruciate Ligament

Treatment of Acute Tears

We. Müller

Some authors still contend that a knee joint can function well without an anterior cruciate ligament (ACL), and some operators continue to excise a ruptured ACL without reconstruction.

While every experienced orthopedist has probably seen athletically sound knees without an ACL, he has had to counsel far more patients with ACL insufficiency who suffer from functional instability. There are also surgeons who, motived by negative experience, immediately replace the torn ACL after the initial injury. Even without treatment or after months of cast immobilization, a good result may have been achieved. Although earlier authors described good results with direct repairs of the ACL, from our current perspective it is difficult to see how their suture techniques could have yielded a positive result. Success in these cases may well have been due to extensive adhesions among the intraarticular folds, greatly reducing joint play and restraining anterior translation while still permitting recovery of knee motion in flexion-extension.

Experienced operators soon learned that surgical restoration of the ACL was a technically demanding task. Wittek (1929), for example, observed that the ruptured ACL, usually avulsed from the femur, was often slightly too short for direct reattachment. He solved this problem by suturing the sound remnant of the ACL far back on the posterior cruciate ligament (PCL) through a lateral approach. This gave a synovial attachment to the ACL that promoted rapid revascularization, permitting early functional loading and resulting in improved healing. We know from everyday experience, however, that a proximally avulsed ACL often gains such attachment spontaneously, without surgical intervention.

While this type of fixation cannot reestablish normal kinematic relationships, it can at least restore partial function to the torn ligament. Above all, it may arrest further deterioration of joint function due to progressive distention. Most patients can tolerate the relatively small residual knee instability by modifying their activities.

The demands of present-day life and the increasing incidence of cruciate ligament tears, most commonly sustained in sports-related injuries and motor vehicle accidents, are again causing this problem to become a focus of concern. Recreational and competitive sports play a major role in modern-day social life, and it is interesting to note that cruciate ligament injuries on the job still account for only a small percentage of all injuries.

Below are some basic theoretical considerations that are helpful in understanding the stability and disruption of knee ligaments:

No ligament in the knee is *exclusively* responsible for a certain stability or a specific direction of stabilization. Daniel (1987) drew the splendid analogy with a camping tent supported by 2 poles and multiple ropes stretched in all 4 directions. When the tent is properly erected, none of the ropes is stretched too tightly. A stormy wind will deform the tent, causing the ropes on the windward side to become very taut and the ropes on the lee side to become slack. If a rope breaks under the strain, the tent pole will lean further, the adjacent ropes will become even more taut, and the stability of the tent in a heavy wind will be seriously compromised, perhaps placing it in danger of collapse. As more ropes become torn, the residual stability becomes more precarious, the tent becomes more deformable, and there is a greater risk that additional ropes will break.

We reported previously on the synergism that exists among different ligamentous structures (We. Müller 1982) and on the various lines of resistance to deformation of the knee joint, e.g., in the anterior-posterior or varus-valgus direction. When primary bastions are breached, however, these lines of resistance become redirected.

In this situation the ligaments can no longer restrain the knee within the narrow confines of physiologic "joint play," and pathologic displacements can occur. The ligaments that are still functional now restrain joint motion within an expanded region. While normal joint play would correspond to a more constrained envelope or "inner shell" of stability, ligament deficiencies give rise to an expanded "outer shell" within which pathologic articular motion can occur.

Frank Noyes and his engineer Ed Grood contributed much to our understanding of this synergistic stabilizing action of the ligaments and the resultant freedom of motion of the joint members (Noyes et al. 1980). They coined the terms "primary restraints" and "secondary restraints" to denote the stabilizing functions of different knee ligaments according to the direction of the forces responsible for a momentary deformation.

Their conceptual model, which is based on a large volume of precise data, includes the concept of normal joint play allowed by intact ligaments. "Pathologic motion" refers to any motion beyond these limits resulting from the partial or complete disruption of one or more ligamentous restraints. The space within which the joint surfaces are free to move is called the "envelope of motion." The degree to which the envelope of pathologic motion exceeds the envelope of normal joint play enables us to predict how many ligaments are still functioning competently as passive restraints and how many are functioning incompetently or not at all.

The ACL as the Cardinal Restraint to Anterior Tibial Translation

We have said that the ACL is the essential primary restraint to anterior tibial translation in neutral rotation, especially in the near-extension position of the Lachman test. This is the best test for detecting a lesion of the ACL, because there are no other restraints that can effectively check anterior translation of the tibia (anterior drawer) in that position. This situation changes if the tibia is internally or externally rotated, as internal rotation places tension on the lateral femorotibial structures (anterolateral femorotibial ligament) and external rotation tenses the structures of the semimembranosus corner (Müller 1982).

The weaker these medial and lateral restraints are in stabilizing against anterior translation, the greater the likelihood of an "isolated" ACL lesion. The ACL is the dominant anterior stabilizer in this type of joint, and its disruption will have a particularly deleterious effect on joint function.

Experience with Repairs

Many years of experience have taught us that the greater the involvement of medial and lateral structures in acute injuries, the greater the need to diagnose and repair these lesions along with the torn ACL. With good repair of the peripheral restraints, most of these knees did well for years in a compensated state. An overt secondary anterior instability tended to develop late and rarely, if at all. By contrast, in putatively "simple" knee injuries with a torn ACL and little apparent peripheral disruption – a frequent arthroscopic diagnosis – significant secondary deterioration is more commonly seen in just 1–3 years. Its incidence is the highest among cases of secondary deterioration in our own series.

Thus, the more surgical attention is given to the peripheral restraints at the time of ACL repair, the more favorable the long-term result will be. Conversely, suture repair of the ACL *alone* is less effective in terms of long-term success.

In all the cruciate ligament injuries that we repair today, we make every effort to perform a concomitant repair or tightening of the medial and lateral supplementary restraints.

From studying our results now in progress, we are learning that it matters a great deal whether too much focus is placed on the "central pivot," or whether attention is given to peripheral auxiliary structures by repairing a detached meniscus and placing tension sutures in stretched peripheral ligaments (Biedert et al. 1988; chapter by Biedert et al., p. 401 ff.).

This study, whose results will be published elsewhere, also shows that, through experience and better duplication of anatomy, we have achieved superior results by augmenting our cruciate ligament reconstructions with the repair of injured peripheral restraints. The more cases we treat, the greater our tendency to manage unfavorable midsubstance tears by primary reconstruction with the patellar tendon, especially in cases of "isolated" rupture.

Based on our experience of recent years, there is no doubt that the better the central pivot has withstood the injury or the better it has been repaired, the better the peripheral structures can adapt and heal in the setting of a kinematically sound pattern of joint motion. Without a functionally competent and stable central pivot, this is not possible.

In all cases, however, there is a need to protect the repaired or reconstructed central pivot by a sound restoration of the primary restraints to valgus and varus deformation (medial collateral ligament; posterior oblique ligament; pes anserinus and medial collateral ligament; biceps, popliteus corner, and anterolateral femorotibial ligament). There is good reason to believe that this will significantly reduce stresses on the repaired, reconstructed, or synthetic ligament, protect it from premature failure due to fatigue and attrition, and significantly prolong its survival. The failure rate of synthetic cruciate ligaments due to premature rupture has been substantial.

Techniques of Repair and Reconstruction

Bony Avulsions

Proximal Bony Avulsion

To date we have seen only one case of a proximal bony avulsion of the ACL from its femoral attachment. The lesion was clearly visible on radiographs.

We repaired the avulsion with an over-the-top tension suture, which provided both reduction and fixation for bony union.

Distal Bony Avulsion

These cases are managed by transosseous suture repair (Fig. 1). For this we use a nonabsorbable no. 2 Novolene suture or occasionally braided steel wire if radiopacity is desired. This is useful for detecting rup-

ture of the wire due to unstable attachment of the fragment, which can cause adverse effects from the dissemination of small wire particles into the joint (Müller 1982).

Recently we have performed these repairs with polydioxanone suture material (PDS), which is absorbed at a slower rate than other synthetics. It has been reported elsewhere (Pfeiffer, personal communication) that osteolytic foci have occurred in bone fragments fixed with PDS in hand operations. Although we have not seen this problem in our patients, this possibility should be kept in mind.

In all bony avulsions, the substance of the ligament itself should be evaluated for possible stretching or interstitial tearing. Moreover, if the fragment is not ideally repositioned on the tibial plateau, the ligament will remain too lax, and there is a danger of subsequent partial ACL insufficiency.

If deficient ligament tension is noted despite an ideal reduction of the bone fragment, we recommend deepening the avulsion bed in the tibial plateau slightly before reattaching the fragment to restore correct tension to the ACL (see Fig. 1).

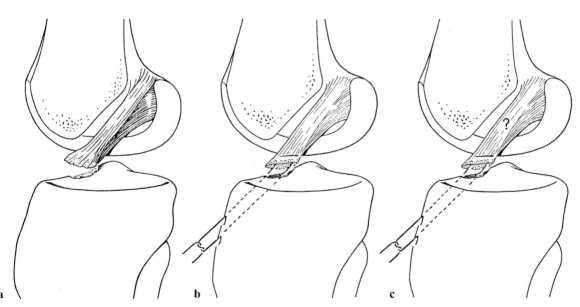

Fig. 1 a–c. Classic distal bony avulsion of the ACL. The fragment is small and displaced and must be stably reattached, e.g., with a transosseous suture. Attention should be given to possible internal tears within the ligament substance **(c)**

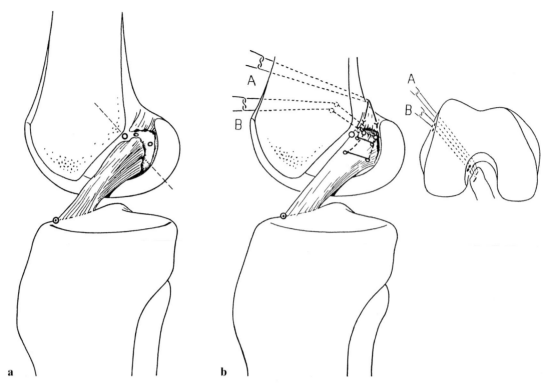

Fig. 2. a In a proximal ligament rupture, the bulk of the ligament has torn away intact, leaving a short remnant attached to the femur. **b** The ligament is sutured to the freshened avulsion bed. More than 2 pairs of sutures can be used. The final over-the-top suture imparts definitive tension to the repaired ligament. The holes for suture B at the avulsion site on the condyle must be placed behind the transition line (– – –) **(a)**

Ligamentous Tears

Proximal Detachment

Although a small remnant of the ligament is occasionally left on the femoral condyle, this injury should be treated separately from a true midsubstance tear. In adolescents, one will occasionally find that the ACL is still attached to the femur but is too far anterior because some collagen fibers at its lateral border are still adherent to the tense synovial covering of the condyle. The ligament is avulsed from behind forward, like wallpaper being torn from a wall; and like wallpaper, the ACL is partially stripped from the inner "wall" of the condyle while a portion still clings to the surface.

Similarly, these proximal ruptures may be connected by a synovial stalk to the midportion of the PCL. Thus, while the ACL is still present and functional to a degree, it is no longer attached to the femur, which bears no more than a remnant like that shown in Fig. 2.

These cases are a good indication for anatomic repair using 2 or 3 transcondylar sutures and a tension suture routed over or through the top. A better quality repair is obtained by first carefully freshening the attachment site on the femur. The placement of the transcondylar drill holes should be kept in mind while this step is planned and carried out. If the ligament is slightly elongated, tension can be improved by deepening the attachment site to create a slight bony recess into which the ligament is drawn.

Interstitial Stretching without a Grossly Visible Tear following an Acute Injury

Left alone, a traumatically stretched and elongated ACL will sag downward with healing, and there will be virtually no chance that it will become taut again as healing progresses. The force of gravity works against proximal tightening of the ligament, especially when motion-related stresses are also imposed.

For this reason we carefully weave an appropriate absorbable suture material (Dexon or PDS) into the cruciate ligament, without strangulating it, and gently pass the threads over the top (Fig. 3). The over-the-

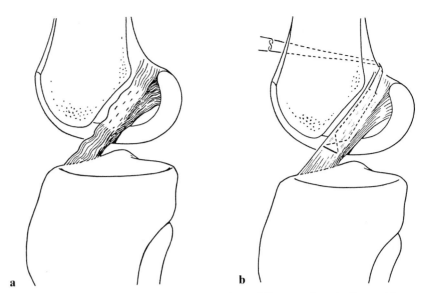

a   b

Fig. 3. a Grade I interstitial tear with preservation of continuity but marked laxness of the collagen fibers. **b** A nonstrangulating over-the-top suture is carefully woven into the ligament to restore its original length and tension

top route is preferred as long as there is no gross disruption at the actual femoral attachment of the ACL. This area should not be disturbed by transligamentous drill holes. But if these are necessary, it is least traumatizing to drill the holes with a smooth Kirschner wire; this prevents the winding of ligament fibers that might occur on a spiral drill bit.

If small sites are noted where fibers have been torn away from the femur, we feel that this transitional type of injury can be managed less traumatically with transosseous sutures. An appropriate drill sleeve should be used to provide soft tissue protection from the drill bit.

Midsubstance Tear

The more we see of these tears, the less we are inclined to regard them as pure burst ruptures through the middle of the ligament. Scrutiny with an experienced eye will very often reveal that some of the fiber bundles are ruptured distally while others match up with a short proximal stump.

In earlier years we repaired a number of these tears, again combined with a precise repair of the periphery, often by passing sutures in two different directions to reapproximate and restore tension to proximal and distal components of the tear. While many of these knees did well in subsequent years, some eventually developed insufficiency, causing us to adopt a skeptical attitude toward midsubstance injuries.

As early as 1974 we began managing certain of these "burst ruptures" by a primary over-the-top reconstruction with the patellar tendon and patellar galea aponeurotica. Even today there are a great many flawless long-term results of this older technique, even in competitive athletes.

Poor results, mostly in the hands of less experienced surgeons who watched us operate, kept us from popularizing this primary reconstruction technique. Since then, however, the technique of the ACL reconstruction has improved so greatly through many small steps that the advantages of primary replacement far outweigh the disadvantages in patients with difficult midsubstance tears.

For a time we augmented with a free 5-mm-wide strip of patellar tendon, but this technique proved too weak in some cases. This experience has led us to use our two-bundle reconstruction even for acute, unfavorable midsubstance tears of the ACL, employing a vascularized patellar tendon graft based on the fat pad prior to 1985, and using a free tendon graft thereafter (Drobny et al. 1986). Whenever possible we preserve the normal "foot" of the ACL on the tibia as well as synovial layers that can be attached to the graft from the proximal side. Distally based strands belonging to the original ACL are pulled proximally along with the through-the-top graft, using separate sutures. The results of this technique, even at 2–3 years, have been superior to those of suture repair alone. Long-term follow-up documentation is currently being compiled on these patients and has not yet been evaluated in detail.

Augmentation with Other Tissues

As long as the autologous or deep-frozen homologous augmentation tissue is sufficiently strong and is used in an anatomometrically correct fashion, there should be no biological or technical problems in the way of a successful augmentation. Until the results of large series can be analyzed, compared and published, it will be left to the individual surgeon to select the method with which he is most familiar based on his own experience, and which yields at least an 80% rate of good results. Any technique can only be as good as its application by the operator. Even a cylinder cast applied for a period of weeks postoperatively cannot help a poor augmentation, any more than it can remedy a deficient internal fixation, for example.

Anatomometric Two-Bundle Reconstruction

Drawing on the ideas of Clancy (1982), we have in the past 5 years developed our own anatomically oriented patellar tendon reconstruction of the ACL (Müller 1984). The patellar tendon consists anatomically of 2 different, completely separate fiber tracts (Drobny et al. 1986), one passing from the tibial tuberosity to the patellar apex and one ascending from the tibial tuberosity past the patella to blend with the quadriceps tendon (Figs. 4a, 5a). This arrangement is favorable for the construction of a two-bundle cruci-ate ligament substitute. The basic steps in the reconstruction are shown in Fig. 4.

This technique can employ either a vascularized graft based on the infrapatellar fat pad, which we used from 1981 to 1985, or a free graft, which has been standard since 1985.

The free graft is especially useful for an acute rupture in which significant, synovialized portions of the ACL still occupy the space between the condyles, leaving insufficient room for a fat-pad pedicle, which might cause a block to extension. Another major advantage of the free graft technique is that it permits an anatomic placement of the graft under ideal visual control. Both theory and practice teach us that this is better than using a transplant whose vascular pedicle results in graft malposition and unphysiologic tension.

During definitive attachment of the graft, care is taken that the patellar bone block, attached first, is inlaid absolutely flush with the femoral condyle. Both anchoring threads are tied securely to a mooring screw (Fig. 5) to prevent dislodgement of the block during subsequent manipulations. Next the graft is pulled into the upper tibia, its tension is adjusted, and the sutures in the tibial block are securely tied while care is taken that the femoral block stays in place. As the third step in the attachment procedure, the proximal end of the second bundle is routed "over the top" of the condyle and made tense. Inspection of the graft at this point will show distinct differences in the in-

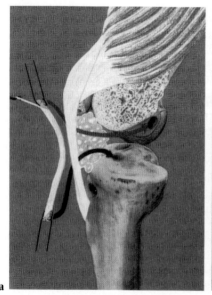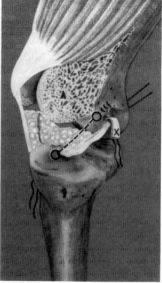

a   b

Fig. 4. a Two-bundle graft from the patellar tendon. The graft prior to transfer. **b** Pull-through of the graft bundles. The graft is free and no longer vascularized by the fat pad. The open circles and line indicate the most isometric course of the substitute

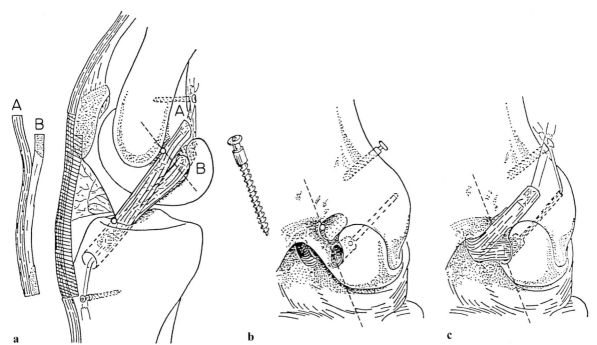

Fig. 5. a Removal of the free graft for the two-bundle technique. Note the isometric line between the *open circles* and the transition line – – – . **b** Location of the 4-mm trough through the femoral isometric point and the recess for the patellar bone block. None of the future ligament fibers should attach in front of the transition line. **c** Anatomometric placement of the graft, which is attached directly on and behind the transition line over an area of normal width. Two pairs of sutures are tied to each bone block for secure fixation (shown here with 1 pair of sutures for simplicity). Note the position of the transition line in all 3 views. (4.0 knee screw, Robert Mathys Co., 2544 Bettlach, Switzerland)

traarticular orientation and tension of the 2 bundles.

The portion of the graft that inserts far anteriorly on the tibia and passes through a 4.5-mm trough at the top of the femoral condyle is the most isometric bundle, and its sutures can be tied in any position of knee flexion. The part of the graft with the proximal bone block contains the fibers that are recruited as the knee approaches full extension (see chapter by Friederich and O'Brien, p. 78 ff.). Thus, if the femoral block is attached in flexion, its fibers will become tense prematurely and cause an extension deficit (this can be seen intraoperatively by an "indrawing" of the tibial end or tested with isometers).

We recommend leaving the free ends of the proximal anchoring sutures uncut so that they can be subsequently used for "rekaplanization," or refixation of the deep layer of the iliotibial tract to the femoral metaphysis to restore the primary restraints to varus deformation and anterolateral rotation.

Regarding the necessity of a notch plasty: With an acute rupture in a knee that shows no preexisting damage, it should not be necessary to debride normal tissue bordering the intercondylar space. This space needs to be large enough to accommodate a normal cruciate ligament substitute, but widening the notch would cause further intraarticular trauma leading to increased postoperative bleeding and adhesions while significantly reducing the femoral cartilage surface available for stress transfer to the tibial eminence.

This reasoning does not apply in previously injured joints in which secondary stenosing osteophytes already project into the intercondylar space from the femoral condyles, tibial eminence, and the upper end of Grant's notch. In these cases it is imperative to reestablish the original space that can accommodate the volume of a normal central pivot.

Alloplastic Reconstruction

Widespread optimism regarding the alloplastic augmentation or total alloplastic replacement of the acutely ruptured ACL has been cooled by the disappointing results obtained with available synthetic materials. There has been an unacceptably high failure rate due to premature rupture of the alloplastic implant within the first 2 years, despite hopes that the implant would provide a scaffold for endogenous scar tissue formation and the eventual development of a functionally sound secondary ligament. Given this fact, along with the substantial percentage of patients who develop a chronic irritative effusion and the fact that candidates for the procedure are in the third or fourth decades of life, we must still advise great caution in the use of synthetic implants. Fu et al. (1988) published an impressive report on pathologic changes in the synovial fluid incited by synthetic wear debris.

Despite evidence of improvements in implants and techniques, years of conscientious clinical research and testing are still needed before any general recommendations can be made.

Of course the results of autologous replacements and augmentations are not good in all cases; but with postoperative mobilization by the continuous passive motion principle (Salter 1989) and a nontraumatizing, anatomic operating technique, the secondary problems that develop in the knees of young patients are still far less threatening than the complications that can arise from a failed alloplastic implantation. The value of continuous passive motion in promoting healing of the ACL has also been confirmed experimentally in rabbits.

Homologous Reconstruction with Deep-Frozen Grafts

For the present these methods, too, are being practiced only in clinical research and testing centers. Their general use would be premature, although the concept of homologous reconstruction appears promising in terms of improving results. It is still too early to make a definitive assessment, however. In recent years the risks and problems of AIDS transmission have greatly curtailed developments in this area.

Review and Outlook

Inadequate and at times disappointing success rates, slow healing, and high rehabilitation costs are motivating a search for new options that can provide a rapid restoration of integral knee function with the ability to return to sports activity within a few weeks or months without exorbitant rehabilitation costs or general loss of strength. For the professional athlete, moreover, it is important to minimize absence from the team so that potentially vital career opportunities will not be missed.

Lateral Repair to Restore the First Line of Defense to Varus Deformation and Anterolateral Rotation

The hemorrhagic suffusions present in a fresh injury confirm the lesion that has occurred and suggest the type of repair that is required.

Figure 6 shows how unfavorable the lever arms of the central pivot are in terms of varus or valgus stabilization. If, as in Fig. 6a, the first line of defense to varus angulation is disrupted, the stresses on the ACL are immediately increased. The effects are particularly damaging to the freshly repaired or reconstructed cruciate ligament (Müller 1982).

This is why we always recommend performing the lateral/ anterolateral repair alluded to earlier. On incising the iliotibial tract system, the surgeon can distinguish at once between a superficial layer passing distally from the hip and a deeper femorotibial layer stretching mostly between the femoral metaphysis and the tubercle of Gerdy. An experienced surgeon, especially one familiar with regional anatomy from anatomic dissections, can readily see how the threads left projecting from the mooring screw can be used to reattach this deep, anti-varus lateral tension band to the femur (Müller 1982).

Nonoperative Treatment

Given the anatomy, kinematics, physiology, and problems of acute ACL disruptions, we see no real place for conservative treatment in restoring the joint to a high degree of function. Admittedly, we can by no means accomplish a 100% recovery in all operated cases using methods now available; we can achieve about a 80%–90% rate of good to excellent results, with success in younger patients approaching 90% owing to improved, anatomically refined techniques.

Nevertheless, we must not ignore everyday clinical experience. There have been a number of cases in which we withheld surgery from patients in the fourth or fifth decade of life with a known ACL rupture and managed the patients "only" by temporary fixation and muscular training. In some cases the results were unsatisfactory; the patients appeared resentful and complained that they could no longer go on weekend hikes through hilly and mountainous terrain as they once did, adding that they had particular trouble with downhill walking.

We know that when our otherwise proven surgical methods are applied in males and especially in females over 30 years of age, the course of rehabilitation tends to be more arduous and the outcome less

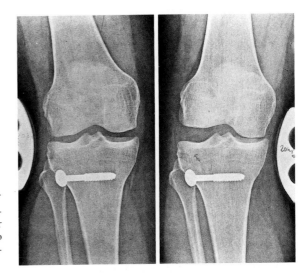

▷

Fig.6a. Varus instability following a lateral repair in an ACL-deficient knee. The varus angulation is so severe that it can tear or elongate the ACL. Without varus stabilization, there is no "first line of defense" for the ACL. The repaired or reconstructed ACL is equally unprotected against reinjury

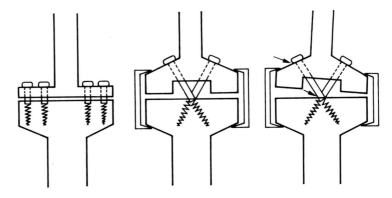

Fig.6b. Mechanical analogy with 4 screws

favorable. Some of these patients still underwent surgery at their own insistence. For these patients, systematic postoperative treatment starting immediately with continuous passive motion was critical to achieving a positive outcome.

Even so, it is difficult to give a definitive answer to the question of operative versus nonoperative treatment. We can say that with the arthroscopic diagnosis of an interstitially torn ligament (see Fig. 3a) or a distal bony avulsion, it is reasonable to treat conservatively by resting the limb and temporarily immobilizing it with a removable device. When a radiographically visible avulsion fragment is examined arthroscopically, there should be no gross cartilage fracture or at least no visible stepoff, and the avulsed fragment should be very wide before conservative treatment is considered. Even in these cases, however, the age and life style of the patient should be taken into account. In young, athletic patients who wish to return to strenuous activities, nearly all factors support the decision for surgical treatment, even

with an overstretched ligament or distal avulsion fracture.

Much will depend upon the abilities and personal experience of the attending physician.

At a center for the operative treatment of severe ligamentous injuries, it is certainly possible to extend the scope of indications for primary surgical intervention. However, the individual surgeon must carefully consider his selection criteria in the light of his own capabilities and weigh his decision carefully, especially since prospects are much improved today for a successful secondary reconstruction of the ACL.

References

Biedert R, Müller We, Hackenbruch W, Baumgartner R (1988) Comparative results of 163 anterior cruciate ligament injuries. In: Müller We, Hackenbruch W (eds) Surgery of the knee. Springer, Berlin Heidelberg New York Tokyo, pp 130–141

Clancy WG, Nelson DA, Reider B et al. (1982) Anterior cruciate ligament reconstruction using one-third of the patellar tendon. J Bone Joint Surg [Am] 64: 352–359

Daniel D (1987) The language of knee motion. In: Jackson DW, Drez D (eds) The anterior cruciate ligament deficient knee. Mosby, St. Louis Washington/DC Toronto

Drobny T, Müller We, Wentzensen A, Pevven SU (1986) Patellar tendon graft with a fat pad pedicle for anterior cruciate ligament reconstruction. In: Trickey EL, Hertel P (eds) Surgery and arthroscopy of the knee. Springer, Berlin Heidelberg New York Tokyo, pp 181–191

Fu F, Olson E, Kang J et al. (1988) The biochemical and histological effects of artificial ligament wear particles: In vitro and in vivo studies. Am J Sports Med 16/6: 558–570

Müller We (1982) Das Knie. Form, Funktion und ligamentäre Wiederherstellung. Springer, Berlin Heidelberg New York Tokyo

Müller We (1986) The technique of intraarticular cruciate reconstruction. In: Trickey EL, Hertel P (eds) Surgery and arthroscopy of the knee. Springer, Berlin Heidelberg New York Tokyo, pp 150–157

Noyes F, Grood E, Butler D, Paulos L (1980) Clinical biomechanics of the knee-ligament restraints and functional stability. AOSS-Symposium on the athet's knee, surgical repair and reconstruction. Mosby, St. Louis Toronto London

Salter R (1989) The biologic concept of continuous passive motion of synovial joints. Clin Orthop 242: 12–25

Wittek A (1927) Ueber Verletzungen der Kreuzbänder des Kniegelenkes. Dtsch Z Chir 200: 491–515

Primary Repair of Acute Ruptures

G. Blatter, F.B. Sprenger, and P. Burkart

Until a few years ago, primary suture repair of the torn anterior cruciate ligament (ACL) without augmentation was the accepted mode of treatment for an acute rupture. Poor long-term results, published increasingly in the 1970s, caused surgeons to abandon this technique. Recently, however, there have been several reports of arthroscopic repair or reattachment of the ACL without an augmentation procedure. Based on a follow-up study of 40 patients 10 years after ACL repair without augmentation, we shall demonstrate the inadequacy of this treatment and compare the results with those of 47 patients who underwent both repair and augmentation.

Materials and Methods

Of the patients who underwent surgery for a ruptured ACL at the Orthopedic Surgical Clinic of Kantonsspital St. Gallen between 1972 and 1985, 87 met the criteria for inclusion in our follow-up study:

- No previous injury or operation in the affected knee
- Acute rupture of the ACL
- Surgical treatment within 24 h
- Same operative technique and postoperative care
- No reconstruction until follow-up

Our first group comprised 40 patients who underwent repair of an acutely torn ACL without augmentation between 1972 and 1980. The average age of these patients at injury was 33 years (17–42 years). Follow-up examinations were performed in 1981 (average of 5 years after surgery) and in 1986 (average of 10 years after surgery).

A second group consisted of 47 patients whose ACL repair had been combined with semitendinosus tendon augmentation (1983 to 1986). They were examined in 1987, an average of 16 months after surgery (5–34 months). The average age at injury was 28 years (17–52 years).

All the patients were questioned and examined clinically, and radiographs were obtained in group 1. A questionnaire was used to assess instability or pain with activities of daily living and sports. The patients were also questioned about their occupational and athletic activities before and after the injury.

Two physicians performed the following tests separately in each patient:

- Lachman test in 20° of flexion
- Anterior drawer test in 80° of flexion
- Pivot shift test
- Varus-valgus stress test in 30° of flexion

Anterior drawer motion at 20° and 80° flexion and varus-valgus opening were compared with the healthy side, and the difference was recorded in mm. The pivot shift test was graded as negative, trace positive, or markedly positive. Both physicians compared their results and reexamined the patients together if a discrepancy was noted.

In all the patients from group 1 (repair without augmentation), AP and lateral radiographs were taken of both knees, and the healthy side was compared with the operated side for signs of osteoarthritis (joint-space narrowing, subchondral sclerosis, osteophytes, subchondral cysts).

Operative Technique and Postoperative Treatment in Group 1 (Repair without Augmentation)

At operation, absorbable and nonabsorbable sutures were woven into the longer portion of the ruptured ACL, passed through a 3.5-mm drill hole in the femoral condyle or proximal tibia (pull-through suture), and tied over a bone screw. Meticulous care was taken to obtain an anatomically correct placement of the drill hole.

The following associated injuries were noted at operation:

- Medial collateral ligament (21)
- Lateral collateral ligament (2)
- Medial meniscus (4)
- Lateral meniscus (1)
- Medial collateral ligament and medial meniscus (3)

- Medial collateral ligament and lateral meniscus (0)
- Medial and lateral collateral ligament (1)
- Medial and lateral meniscus (2)
- No associated lesions (7)

A torn or grossly stretched medial collateral ligament was repaired and reefed at operation. Meniscal tears were managed by partial meniscectomy.

Postoperatively the limb was placed in lateral and medial plaster splints with the knee flexed 30°. At 2 weeks this was converted to a cylinder cast for 5 weeks, again with the knee flexed 30°.

Operating Technique
and Postoperative Treatment in Group 2
(Repair with Semitendinosus Tendon
Augmentation)

As in group 1, sutures were woven through the longer stump of the ruptured cruciate ligament. The semitendinosus tendon was released proximally, pulled through 6-mm drill holes in the tibial plateau and femoral condyle, and attached proximally to a screw with nonabsorbable sutures. The sutures from the torn ACL were pulled through the same drill holes and also tied over a screw. Again, care was taken that the drill channels were anatomically positioned.

Associated injuries in this group were as follows:

- Medial collateral ligament (22)
- Lateral collateral ligament (3)
- Medial meniscus (2)
- Lateral meniscus (2)
- Medial collateral ligament and medial meniscus (4)
- Medial collateral ligament and lateral meniscus (2)
- Medial and lateral collateral ligament (1)
- Medial and lateral meniscus (1)
- No associated lesions (10)

These lesions were treated the same as in group 1. Postoperatively the limb was placed in plaster splints with the knee flexed 20°. At 4 days a removable splint was applied with the knee flexed 10°–20° and worn for 8–10 weeks. An intensive physical therapy program was maintained for 3 months.

Results

Group 1 (ACL Repair without Augmentation)

Questioning of the 40 patients yielded the following results at 5/10 years postoperatively:

	Preinjury level	Mildly impaired	Severely impaired
Job performance	21/16	10/12	9/12
Athletic performance	17/11	10/10	13/19
General performance	12/ 6	17/19	11/15
	None	Sporadic	Chronic
Pain or soreness	14/ 2	17/25	9/13
Swelling	18/20	9/11	13/ 9

Clinical examination yielded the following results at 5/10 years postoperatively:

	No difference between sides	5–10 mm	> 10 mm
Lachman test			40/40
Anterior drawer Neutral rotation	2/ 2	4/ 1	34/37
Joint-space opening			
Medial	12/11	15/14	13/15
Lateral	38/38	1/ 1	1/ 1
	Negative	Positive	
Pivot shift	16/10	24/30	

Radiographs showed early ostearthritic changes in 6 patients at 5 years postoperatively and in 12 patients at 10 years. The 2nd follow-up demonstrated severe osteoarthritis in 4 patients.

Group 2 (ACL Repair with Augmentation)

Questioning of the 47 patients yielded the following results an average of 16 months postoperatively:

	Preinjury level	Mildly impaired	Severely impaired
Job performance	46	1	0
Athletic performance	27	14	6
General performance	40	5	2
	None	Sporadic	Chronic
Pain or soreness	26	19	2
Swelling	43	2	2

Clinical examination indicated the following:

	No difference between sides	5–10 mm	> 10 mm
Lachman test	20	22	5
Anterior drawer	44	2	1
Internal rotation			
Neutral rotation	27	18	2
External rotation	33	13	1
Joint-space opening			
Medial	24	20	3
Lateral	45	2	
	Negative	Positive	
Pivot shift	46	1	

Radiographs were not obtained in this group due to the short length of follow-up.

Discussion

There is controversy as to whether an acute rupture of the ACL should be managed operatively or conservatively. In 1974 Kennedy et al. compared 19 patients whose ACL ruptures were operatively treated with 31 patients whose ruptures were untreated. The results at an average of 44 months were comparable: good or excellent in approximately 80% of cases. At 7 years postinjury, however (Kennedy 1981), degenerative arthritis of the knee was far more advanced in the untreated group. This led Kennedy to advocate surgical treatment for all acute ruptures. By contrast, McDaniel and Dameron (1980) and Balkfors (1982) reported that many patients could live a normal life without an ACL. Nevertheless, there is much recent evidence from long-term follow-ups and experimental animal studies to indicate that the knee instability caused by absence of the ACL predisposes to meniscal tears and osteoarthritis of the knee (Bergfeld et al. 1983; Clancy et al. 1982; Dettaven 1980; Eriksson 1976; Feagin and Curl 1976; Jacobsen 1977; McDevitt and Muir 1976; Marshall and Olsson 1971). Our results also confirm this. For example, 6 of the patients in group 1 (insufficiency) had to undergo meniscal surgery between the 1st and 2nd follow-ups (at 5 and 10 years postoperatively). Meniscal lesions developed exclusively in patients with a positive pivot shift. Additionally, we found osteoarthritis of the knee in 15% of the group 1 patients at 5 years and in 30% at 10 years. Seventy-five percent of these patients had previously undergone a partial meniscectomy, however. We found no apparent correlation between a positive pivot shift and the incidence of osteoarthritis.

The essential guide for deciding whether or not surgery is warranted for a torn ACL is the stability of the joint. The Lachman test is best for diagnosing a torn ligament (Torg et al. 1976), and the pivot shift test is best for detecting instability (Galway et al. 1972, 1980).

Our follow-ups confirm once more that patients with a positive Lachman test and absence of the ACL do not necessarily have a demonstrable pivot shift. Whereas the Lachman test was positive in all of our patients in group 1, a pivot shift was elicited in only 60%. Interestingly, only 80% of the patients with a positive pivot shift complained of instability problems. No patient with a positive Lachman test and negative pivot shift voiced such problems.

Based on our experience to date, we recommend the following protocol for patients with a suspected acute rupture:

– The injured knee should be carefully examined, if necessary under anesthesia. Arthroscopy is indicated for a clinically suspected rupture if there is also suspicion of an associated meniscal lesion (DeHaven 1980; Noyes et al. 1980).
– With a markedly *positive Lachman test* and a *positive pivot shift*, primary repair of the ACL is indicated.
– With a *positive Lachman test* and an unequivocally *negative pivot shift* (experienced examiner!), primary operative treatment is not indicated unless there is a coexisting, reparable meniscal tear. The ACL should be repaired at the time of the meniscal repair, even with a negative pivot shift. DeHaven showed in 1983 that a repaired meniscus retears in almost 30% of cases when the ACL is left deficient.
– With a *positive Lachman test* and a *trace pivot shift*, surgery should be recommended for all patients with an associated meniscal tear and all athletically active patients.

The question of whether a primary ACL repair should be performed with or without augmentation can be answered with confidence.

Feagin and Curl (1976) reported excellent results following primary ACL repairs without augmentation, but follow-up of these cases 5 years later showed evidence of functional instability in more than 90% of the patients. In 1979 Cabaud et al. showed experimentally in monkeys and dogs that a primarily sutured but unaugmented cruciate ligament had a low rupture strength and was readily torn. Further experiments (Cabaud et al. 1980) showed that augmentation of the repaired ligament with the patellar tendon substantially improved results.

In our series, all the patients in group 1 (primary repair without augmentation) developed instability. This demonstrates the importance of routinely augmenting every primary repair of the ACL. We have achieved excellent results by augmentation with the semitendinosus tendon. We do not believe it is critical whether the repair is augmented with the semitendinosus tendon or with a strip of patellar tendon, as Clancy recommended in 1985. Patellar tendon augmentations also have yielded good results at our center.

References

Balkfors B (1982) The course of knee ligament injuries. Acta Orthop Scand 53 [Suppl 198]: 7-99

Bergfeld JA, Fried JA, Werber GG (1983) Two to five year evaluation of anterior cruciate reconstruction using patellar tendon and Ellison iliotibial band transfer. AAOS Annual Meeting, Anaheim/CA

Cabaud HE, Rodkey WG, Feagin JA (1979) Experimental studies of acute anterior cruciate ligament injury and repair. Am J Sports Med 7: 18-22

Cabaud HE, Feagin JA, Rodkey WG (1980) Acute anterior cruciate ligament injury and augmented repair: Experimental studies. Am J Sports Med 8: 395-401

Clancy WG jr (1985) Intra-articular reconstruction of the anterior cruciate ligament. Orthop Clin North Am 16: 181-189

Clancy WG jr, Nelson DA, Reider B, Narechania R (1982) Anterior cruciate ligament reconstruction using one-third of the patellar ligament augmented by extra-articular tendon transfer. J Bone Joint Surg [Am] 64: 352-359

DeHaven KE (1980) Diagnosis of acute knee injuries with hemarthrosis. Am J Sports Med 8: 9-18

DeHaven KE (1983) Peripheral meniscus repair. Three to seven year results. Third Congress of the International Society of the Knee, Gleneagles, Scotland

Eriksson K (1976) Sports injuries of the knee ligaments: Their diagnosis, treatment, rehabilitation, and prevention. Med Sci Sports 8: 133-144

Feagin JA, Curl WW (1976) Isolated tears of the anterior cruciate ligament: 5 year follow-up study. Am J Sports Med 4: 95-99

Feagin JA, Abbott HG, Rokous JR (1972) The isolated tear of the anterior cruciate ligament. J Bone Joint Surg [Am] 54: 1340

Galway HR, MacIntosh DL (1980) The lateral pivot shift: a symptom and sign of anterior cruciate ligament insufficiency. Clin Orthop North Am 147: 45-50

Galway RD, Beaupre A, MacIntosh DL (1972) Pivot shift: a clinical sign of symptomatic anterior cruciate ligament insufficiency. J Bone Joint Surg [Br] 54: 763-764

Jacobsen K (1977) Osteoarthrosis following insufficiency of the cruciate ligaments in man. A clinical study. Acta Orthop Scand 48: 520-526

Kennedy JC (1981) Natural history, management of acute and chronic problems part V. Presented at AAOS Instructional Course. The Athletes Knee and Arthroscopy, Palm Beach, Florida

Kennedy JC, Weinbert HW, Wilson AS (1974) The anatomy and function of the anterior cruciate ligament as determined by clinical and morphological studies. J Bone Joint Surg [Am] 56: 223-235

Marshall JL, Olsson S-E (1971) Instability of the knee. A long-term experimental study in dogs. J Bone Joint Surg [Am] 53: 1561-1570

McDaniel WJ, Dameron TB jr (1980) Untreated ruptures of the anterior cruciate ligament. A follow-up study. J Bone Joint Surg [Am] 62: 696-705

McDevitt CA, Muir H (1976) Biochemical changes in the cartilage of the knee in experimental and natural osteoarthritis in the dog. J Bone Joint Surg [Br] 58: 94-101

Noyes FR, Basset RW, Grood ES, Butler DL (1980) Arthroscopy in acute traumatic hemarthrosis of the knee: incidence of anterior cruciate tears and other injuries. J Bone Joint Surg [Am] 62: 687-695

Torg JS, Conrad W, Kalen V (1976) Clinical diagnosis of anterior cruciate ligament instability in the athlete. Am J Sports Med 4: 84-93

Late Results after Primary Repair

P. M. Ballmer, W. C. Kipfer, B. Grünig, H.-U. Stäubli, R. Zehnder, and R. P. Jakob

The value of surgical repair of the acutely torn anterior cruciate ligament (ACL) remains controversial despite numerous studies (Feagin and Curl 1976; Feagin et al. 1972; Hughston and Barrett 1983; Järvinen and Kannus 1985; Liljedahl and Nordstrand 1969; Liljedahl et al. 1965; Lysholm et al. 1982; McDaniel and Dameron 1980; Marshall et al. 1979, 1982; O'Donoghue 1955; Palmer 1938; Solonen and Rokkanen 1967). Marshall et al. (1969, 1971) showed in their experimental studies that degenerative articular changes are a sequela of ACL insufficiency. Fetto and Marshall (1980) reported on clinical findings documenting the necessity of the ACL as a primary stabilizer of the knee joint and emphasized the importance of early, primary operative repair of ACL rupture. The progressive functional disability resulting from degenerative joint changes and secondary meniscal tears in the ACL-deficient symptomatic knee has been further documented by Noyes et al. (1983).

Aside from the basic question of whether acute ACL insufficiency warrants surgical intervention, there is diversity of opinion concerning the most appropriate operative technique. Liljedahl et al. (1965) reported good results following simple suture repair of the torn ACL. Marshall et al. (1982) also confirmed the value of primary ACL repairs in 61 patients evaluated an average of 29 months after surgery. The Lachman test was negative in 52% of the patients, and 48% had mild laxity but a firm anterior end point. This contrasts with the series of Lysholm et al. (1982) in which one-third of patients with repaired ACL ruptures either had to undergo reoperation for instability or showed ligamentous insufficiency at follow-up. Feagin and Curl (1976) reported instability rates as high as 94% following ligament repairs alone. These findings appear to contrast with the substantially better results noted when the repair was reinforced by primary augmentation (Cho 1975; Lipscomb et al. 1979; Puddu 1980; Zarins and Rowe 1986).

Because of the great diversity of ACL repair outcomes reported in the literature, we were interested in our own results. The present study is a retrospective analysis of acute ACL ruptures that were treated at the Orthopedic Clinic of Inselspital Bern by repair alone or by repair combined with an intra- or extraarticular augmentation procedure.

Clinical Material and Methods

A total of 241 acute, complete ruptures of the ACL were operatively treated from 1972 to 1982; 155 patients with a total of 160 ACL ruptures (= 100%) were available for follow-up after an average of 5 1/2 years (2–12 years). The remaining 81 cases were excluded from follow-up for various reasons: 4 patients had died, 63 could not be located or would not come for follow-up, and 14 (all with nonaugmented repairs) had undergone an ACL reconstruction since their initial surgery.

The following data were taken from the patients' case histories for our evaluation: cause and mechanism of the injury, pre- and intraoperative findings, type of surgery performed, complications, postoperative treatment, and clinical course. The patients consisted of 61% men and 39% women with an average age of 32 years (16–65 years) at the time of injury. The left knee was involved in 56%, the right knee in 39%, and both knees in 5%. Eighty-eight percent of the knee injuries came to operation within 1 week, and 12% between 1 and 5 weeks. The cause of the injury and the pattern of injury to the ACL and other ligaments are shown in Tables 1–3.

The technique of cruciate ligament repair varied considerably (Table 4). In 23% of cases (all operated after 1979) the repair was reinforced with an intra- and extraarticular strip of iliotibial tract using a modification of the through-the-top technique of MacIntosh and Darby (1976). Tears of the medial and/or lateral collateral ligament and of the posterior cruciate ligament were exposed and primarily repaired. Acute meniscal tears were present in a total of 35% of cases (21% medial, 11% lateral, 3% bilateral); 17% were repaired, 5% were managed by partial meniscectomy, and 13% by total meniscectomy.

Table 1. Causes of ligamentous injuries, by percent

Skiing	33
Soccer	20
Other sports	14
Vehicular accident	20
Accident on the job	6
Other activities	7

Table 2. Patterns of ligamentous injury, by percent

Isolated ACL	18
ACL + MCL	60
ACL + LCL	4
ACL + MCL + LCL	5
ACL + PCL + MCL	9
ACL + PCL + LCL	2 brace* 13
ACL + PCL + MCL + LCL	2

ACL = lesion of anterior cruciate ligament
PCL = lesion of posterior cruciate ligament
MCL = lesion of medial collateral ligament
LCL = lesion of lateral collateral ligament

Table 3. Types of ACL injury, by percent

Proximal third	71
Middle third	12
Distal third	4
Proximal and distal third	8
Distal bony avulsion	5

Table 4. Techniques of ACL repair, by percent

Femoral transosseous	57 (23 with augmentation)
Over the top	5
Femoral transosseous and over the top	21
Femoral and tibial transosseous	8
Intraligamentous repair	6
Tibial transosseous	3

Table 5. Subjective patient assessment, by percent

Excellent	18
Good	71
Fair	10
Poor	1

Table 6. Residual complaints, by percent

	None	Mild occasional	Severe, chronic
Pain	40	47	13
Swelling	76	24	–
Giving way	73	27	–

Table 7. Range of knee motion, by percent

Extension	Normal	58
	< 10° restriction	40
	> 10° restriction	2
Flexion	Normal	49
	< 20° restriction	48
	> 20° restriction	3

The average length of postoperative immobilization was 7 weeks, using a long leg cast in 86% and a cast brace in 14%. Regarding local complications, there was a 1% incidence of wound hematoma and a 1% incidence of deep infection *(Staphylococcus epidermidis)*. Three percent of the knees had to be manipulated under general anesthesia during rehabilitation to restore motion. A total of 7% of knees had undergone arthroscopy by the time of follow-up: 4% diagnostic and 3% for partial meniscectomy. Four percent of the knees were reoperated for femoropatellar problems.

Our follow-up encompassed subjective ratings and a clinical examination. Stability was tested by at least one of the authors and the project head, employing the usual grading system for frontal and sagittal stability (Hughston et al. 1976). The pivot shift and reversed pivot shift were graded as described by Jakob et al. (1987). Radiographs were obtained of both knees, the views consisting of an a.p. projection in the one-legged stance, a lateral projection, a tunnel view, and a patellar sunrise view in 45° of flexion. Four percent of the patients would not submit to radiography. The one-legged stance views were used to determine the femorotibial axis under weight bearing and evaluate for medial and/or lateral joint-space narrowing by the method of Hollingworth et al. (1982). Degenerative changes were evaluated according to the criteria of Ahlbäck (1968), Fairbank (1948), and Feagin et al. (1982). The method of Danielsson and Hernborg (1970) was used to determine the size of medial and lateral osteophytes.

Results

The subjective patient assessments, residual complaints, and range of motion on the operated side compared with the healthy side are summarized in Tables 5–7.

While 57% of the patients engaged in the same type of sport at the same level as before the injury, 27% experienced some impairment of their athletic performance, and 4% were no longer active in sports.

Table 8. Frontal stability, by percent

	Total population (n = 160)				Repair only (n = 123)				Repair with augmentation (n = 37)			
	0	1+	2+	3+	0	1+	2+	3+	0	1+	2+	3+
In extension:												
Medial	95	5	–	–	94	6	–	–	97	3	–	–
Lateral	97	3	–	–	98	2	–	–	95	5	–	–
In flexion:												
Medial	42	55	3	–	39	59	2	–	54	41	5	–
Lateral	78	19	3	–	79	20	1	–	78	16	6	–

Table 9. Sagittal stability, by percent

	Total population (n = 160)				Repair only (n = 123)				Repair with augmentation (n = 37)			
	0	1+	2+	3+	0	1+	2+	3+	0	1+	2+	3+
Lachman	20	71	9	–	21	67	12	–	19	81	–	–
Anterior drawer in NR	45	44	11	–	39	46	15		62	38	–	–
Posterior drawer in NR	85	14	1	–	84	15	1	–	92	8	–	–
Pivot shift	61	28	8	3	49	37	11	3	100	–	–	–
Reversed pivot shift Injured side	52	37	10	1	62	30	7	1	22	57	21	–
Healthy side	70	28	2	–	72	25	3	–	65	32	3	–

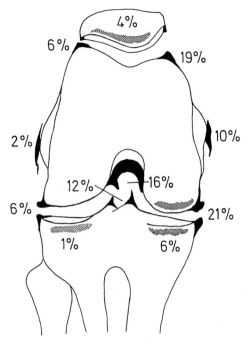

Fig. 1. Radiographic changes (1)

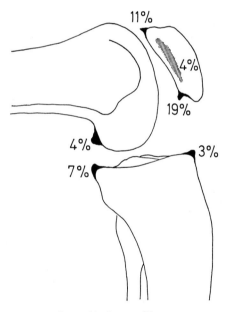

Fig. 2. Radiographic changes (2)

Twelve percent did not participate in sports before their injury. The results of frontal and sagittal stability testing are shown in Tables 8 and 9.

Radiographs in the one-legged stance showed a physiologic femorotibial axis (from −5° to −9°) in 22% of the operated knees and 19% of the opposite knees. The axis was between −1° and −4° in 44% of operated knees and 43% of opposite knees, and between 0° and +9° in 34% of operated knees and 38% of opposite knees. None of the patients showed obvious joint-space narrowing, but increased subchondral sclerosis of the patella was noted in 4%. Osteophytes were found on one or both patellar poles in 20%, and femoropatellar osteophytes were present in 22%. There was no instance of significant narrowing of the femorotibial joint space, i.e., narrowing of 50% or more relative to the opposite side. The medial subchondral bone was mildly sclerotic in 6%. There was minimal flattening of the femoral condyles in 6% (2% medial, 4% lateral), and slight depression of the tibial plateau was noted in 3% (2% medial, 1% lateral). Twenty-seven percent of joints showed osteophytes on the medial and/or lateral aspect of the tibia or femur (17% medial, 2% lateral, 4% medial and lateral), 11% posteriorly, and 3% anteriorly. Stenosis of the intercondylar notch was noted in 16% of cases, and peaking of the intercondylar eminence in 12%. Periarticular calcifications were observed in 12% of cases (10% medial, 2% lateral) (Figs. 1, 2).

Discussion

The 5-year study of Feagin et al. (1972), showing an instability rate of 94% and a 34% incidence of secondary meniscal tears following primary ACL repair, contrasts with the study of Marshall et al. (1982), who found no evidence of giving way symptoms or secondary meniscal tears at 2 1/2 years postoperatively. Despite the 93% rate of good to excellent subjective ratings by our patients after an average of 6 years, the objective test results of sagittal knee stability (79% positive Lachman test, 61% positive drawer in flexion, 48% positive pivot shift) after an unaugmented ACL repair must be judged unsatisfactory, especially when we consider that 35% of patients had an altered or absent anterior end point signifying functional incompetence of the ACL. The 21% negative Lachman tests versus the 52% rate found by Marshall et al. (1982) could, according to Odensten and Gillquist (1984), result from the anisometry of our cruciate ligament repairs. Most of the ACL tears were proximal, and many of them were probably reattached through femoral drill holes placed too far anterior; this would also account in part for the frequency of flexion deficits (51%).

We have achieved significantly better results by augmenting the ACL repair with an intra- and extraarticular transfer from the iliotibial tract. This procedure eliminates anterolateral rotatory instability (pivot shift), and maximum anterior drawer displacement in the Lachman and flexed-knee tests does not exceed 5 mm (1 +). The contribution of the extraarticular tenodesis effect to the anterior stability is difficult to assess, especially when we note the study of Zarins and Rowe (1986) in which two clinically stable joints were found to have lax intraarticular ligaments on arthroscopy. The authors attribute the good sagittal stability in those cases to the lateral extraarticular augmentation that imparted tension on the secondary restraints. The increased posterolateral instability in our augmented cases probably relates to the technique of MacIntosh and Darby (1976) and has not been mentioned in any study where the iliotibial tract was used for intra- and/or extraarticular transfers (Insall et al. 1981; Ireland and Trickey 1980; MacIntosh and Darby 1976; Nicholas and Minkoff 1978; Yost et al. 1981).

As other studies have demonstrated (Feagin and Curl 1976; Odensten et al. 1984), a sufficiently long follow-up period is needed in order to make favorable prognostic statements about joint stability following ACL repairs. While this requirement is satisfied by the 6 years' average follow-up (5–12 years) in patients who have undergone ACL repairs alone, only a relatively short follow-up of about 3 years (2–5 years) is currently available in patients with augmented repairs. Various studies point to the markedly increased rate of femorotibial osteoarthritis in the absence of the ACL (Fetto and Marshall 1980; Gudde and Wagenknecht 1973; Jacobsen 1977; Noyes et al. 1983). Our incidence of osteoarthritis (6% rate of increased femorotibial subchondral sclerosis) appears to be lower compared with untreated cruciate ligament tears, with Noyes et al. (1983) reporting a 21% incidence of significant degenerative changes at 9 years. Danielsson and Hernborg (1970) state that osteophytes alone are not a reliable predictor of future osteoarthritis.

Despite optimistic reports of full returns to athletic participation after untreated ruptures of the ACL (Giove et al. 1983; Jokl et al. 1984; McDaniel and Dameron 1980), the percentage of secondary meniscal lesions is relatively high. Clancy et al. (1982) found that 86% of patients undergoing ACL reconstruction had at least one torn meniscus, while 54% had significant degenerative articular changes. In our series, by contrast, we found only a 3% incidence of secondary meniscal lesions besides the 13% total meniscectomies that were performed for acute injury. We cannot conclusively evaluate the incidence of postmeniscectomy osteoarthritis, as this would require a follow-up period of more than 10 years (Appel 1970; Giove et al. 1983; Gudde and Wagenknecht 1973; Johnson et al. 1974).

Based on our results, we believe that an acute tear of the ACL should be surgically treated in physically active patients, especially if there are coexisting ligamentous lesions. This lowers the risk of functional disability, secondary meniscal tears, and osteoarthritic changes. Due to the frequency with which residual instability is noted after ligament repairs alone, we agree with Feagin (1979) and Feagin and Curl (1976) that primary repairs of the ACL should be reinforced by an appropriate augmentation. Because the varus morphotype predominates in our series compared with the normal population (Lerat 1977), we do not feel that the iliotibial tract transfer, with its lateral tension-band effect, is the optimum augmentation procedure. On the other hand, use of the semitendinosus tendon for ACL augmentation (Cho 1975; Lipscomp et al. 1979, 1981; Puddu 1980) may perhaps cause a significant relative weakening of the medial structures. Experience with secondary cruciate ligament reconstructions (Clancy et al. 1982) suggests that the patellar tendon may provide an ideal material for ACL augmentation and reconstruction, even in acute tears (Bilko et al. 1986; Montmollin and Le Coeur 1980).

References

Ahlbäck S (1968) Osteoarthrosis of the knee. A radiographic investigation. Acta Radiol [Suppl 277]

Appel H (1970) Late results after meniscectomy in the knee joint. Acta Orthop Scand [Suppl 133]

Bilko TE, Paulos LE, Feagin JA, Lambert KL, Cunningham HR (1986) Current trends in repair and rehabilitation of complete (acute) anterior cruciate ligament injuries. Am J Sports Med 14: 143–147

Cho KO (1975) Reconstruction of the anterior cruciate ligament by semitendinosus tenodesis. J Bone Joint Surg [Am] 57: 608–612

Clancy WG Jr, Nelson DA, Reider B, Narechania RG (1982) Anterior cruciate ligament reconstruction using one-third of the patellar ligament, augmented by extra-articular tendon transfers. J Bone Joint Surg [Am] 64: 352–359

Danielsson L, Hernborg J (1970) Clinical and roentgenologic study of knee joints with osteophytes. Clin Orthop 69: 302–312

Fairbank TJ (1948) Knee joint changes after meniscectomy. J Bone Joint Surg [Br] 30: 664–670

Feagin JA (1979) The syndrom of the torn anterior cruciate ligament. Orthop Clin North Am 10: 81–90

Feagin JA, Curl WW (1976) Isolated tear of the anterior cruciate ligament: 5-year follow-up study. Am J Sports Med 4: 95–100

Feagin JA, Abbot HG, Rokous JR (1972) The isolated tear of the anterior cruciate ligament. J Bone Joint Surg [Am] 54: 1340–1341

Feagin JA, Cabaud HE, Curl WW (1982) The anterior cruciate ligament: Radiographic and clinical signs of successful and unsuccessful repairs. Clin Orthop 164: 54–58

Fetto JF, Marshall JL (1980) The natural history and diagnosis of anterior cruciate ligament insufficiency. Clin Orthop 147: 29–38

Giove TP, Miller SJ, Kent BE, Sanford TL, Garrick JG (1983) Non-operative treatment of the torn anterior cruciate ligament. J Bone Joint Surg [Am] 65: 184–192

Gudde P, Wagenknecht R (1973) Untersuchungsergebnisse bei 50 Patienten 10–12 Jahre nach der Innenmeniskusoperation bei gleichzeitig vorliegender Ruptur des vorderen Kreuzbandes. Z Orthop 111: 369–372

Hollingworth P, Melsom RD, Scott JT (1982) Measurement of radiographic joint space in the rheumatoid knee: Correlation with obesity, disease duration, and other factors. Rheumatol Rehabil 21: 9–14

Hughston JC, Barrett GR (1983) Acute anteromedial rotatory instability. Long-term results of surgical repair. J Bone Joint Surg [Am] 65: 145–153

Hughston JC, Andrews JR, Cross MJ, Moschi A (1976) Classification of knee ligament instabilities. Part I: The medial compartment and cruciate ligaments. Part II: The lateral compartment. J Bone Joint Surg [Am] 58: 159–179

Insall J, Joseph DM, Aglietti P, Campbell RD (1981) Bone-block iliotibial band transfer for anterior cruciate insufficiency. J Bone Joint Surg [Am] 63: 560–569

Ireland J, Trickey EL (1980) McIntosh tenodesis for anterolateral instability of the knee. J Bone Joint Surg [Br] 62: 340–345

Jacobsen K (1977) Osteoarthrosis following insufficiency of the cruciate ligaments in man. A clinical study. Acta Orthop Scand 48: 520–526

Järvinen M, Kannus P (1985) Clinical and radiological long-term results after primary knee ligament surgery. Arch Orthop Trauma Surg 104: 1–6

Jakob RP, Stäubli H-U, Deland J (1987) Grading the pivot shift. J Bone Joint Surg [Br] 69: 294–299

Johnson RJ, Kettelkamp DB, Clark W, Leaverton P (1974) Factors affecting late results after meniscectomy. J Bone Joint Surg [Am] 56: 719–729

Jokl P, Kaplan N, Stoven P, Keggi K (1984) Non-operative treatment of severe injuries to the medial and anterior cruciate ligaments of the knee. J Bone Joint Surg [Am] 66: 741–744

Lerat JL (1977) Morphotypes des membres inférieurs. Chir Genou J Lyon 120–122

Liljedahl SO, Nordstrand A (1969) Injuries to the ligaments of the knee. Diagnosis and results of operation. Injury 1: 17–24

Liljedahl SO, Lindvall N, Wetterfors J (1965) Early diagnosis and treatment of acute rupture of the anterior cruciate ligament. A clinical and arthrographic study of forty-eight cases. J Bone Joint Surg [Am] 47: 1503–1513

Lipscomb AB, Johnston RK, Snyder RB, Brothers JC (1979) Secondary reconstruction of anterior cruciate ligament in athletes by using the semitendinosus tendon. Am J Sports Med 7: 81–84

Lipscomb AB, Johnston RK, Snyder RB (1981) The technique of cruciate ligament reconstruction. Am J Sports Med 9: 77–81

Lysholm J, Gillquist J, Liljedahl SO (1982) Long term results after early treatment of the knee injuries. Acta Orthop Scand 53: 109–118

Marshall JL (1969) Periarticular osteophytes. Initiation and formation of the knee of the dog. Clin Orthop 62: 37–47

Marshall JL, Olsson SE (1971) Instability of the knee. A long-term experimental study in dogs. J Bone Joint Surg [Am] 53: 1561–1570

Marshall JL, Warren RF, Wickiewicz TL, Reider B (1979) The anterior cruciate ligament: a technique of repair and reconstruction. Clin Orthop 143: 97–106

Marshall JL, Warren RF, Wickiewicz TL (1982) Primary surgical treatment of anterior cruciate ligament lesions. Am J Sports Med 10: 103–107

McDaniel WJ Jr, Dameron TB Jr (1980) Untreated ruptures of the anterior cruciate ligament. J Bone Joint Surg [Am] 62: 696–705

McIntosh DL, Darby TA (1976) Lateral substitution reconstruction. J Bone Joint Surg [Br] 58: 142

Montmollin B, Le Coeur P (1980) La rupture isolée fraîche du ligament croisé antérieur du genou. Rev Chir Orthop 66: 367–371

Nicholas JA, Minkoff J (1978) Iliotibial band transfer through the intercondylar notch for combined anterior instability (ITPT procedure). Am J Sports Med 6: 341–353

Noyes FR, Mooar PA, Matthews DS, Butler DL (1983) The

298   P.M. Ballmer et al.

symptomatic anterior cruciate-deficient knee. Part I: The long-term functional disability in athletically active individuals. J Bone Joint Surg [Am] 65: 154–162

Odensten M, Gillquist J (1984) Functional anatomy of the anterior cruciate ligament and a rationale for reconstruction. J Bone Joint Surg [Am] 67: 257–262

Odensten M, Lysholm J, Gillquist J (1984) Suture of fresh ruptures of the anterior cruciate ligament: a 5 year follow-up. Acta Orthop Scand 55: 270–272

O'Donoghue DM (1955) An analysis of end results of surgical treatment of major injuries to the ligaments of the knee. J Bone Joint Surg [Am] 37: 1–13

Palmer J (1938) On the injuries to the ligaments of the knee joint: a clinical study. Acta Chir Scand [Suppl 53]

Puddu G (1980) Method for reconstruction of the anterior cruciate ligament using the semitendinosus tendon. Am J Sports Med 8: 402–404

Ricklin P (1976) Spätergebnisse nach Meniscectomie. Hefte Unfallheilkd 128: 51–58

Solonen KA, Rokkanen P (1967) Operative treatment of torn ligaments in injuries of the knee joint. Acta Orthop Scand 38: 67–80

Tapper EM, Hoover NW (1969) Late results after meniscectomy. J Bone Joint Surg [Am] 51: 517–526

Yost JG, Chekofsky K, Schoscheim P, Nolan P, Slovin H, Scott WN (1981) Intraarticular iliotibial band reconstruction for anterior cruciate ligament insufficiency. Am J Sports Med 9: 220–224

Zarins B, Rowe CB (1986) Combined anterior cruciate-ligament reconstruction using semitendinosus tendon and iliotibial tract. J Bone Joint Surg [Am] 68: 160–177

Avulsion Fractures of the Intercondylar Eminence in Adolescents: Pathophysiology, Case Material, and Late Results

P. Bachelin

Ligamentous injuries in children are rare. A relatively common type is the avulsion fracture of the intercondylar eminence, whose causative mechanism is identical to that of cruciate ligament tears. It is the typical injury of the central pivot in the pediatric age group (Bachelin and Pirkls 1987; Baxter and Wiley 1988; Dejour 1982; Rigault et al. 1976; Seriat-Gautier 1983). The fracture is caused by the relatively high mechanical resistance of the cruciate ligaments compared with their bony sites of insertion. Nevertheless, isolated midsubstance ligament tears are occasionally encountered in adolescents whose growth plates have not yet closed (Bradley et al. 1979; Dejour 1982). Both types of injury – midsubstance tears and bony avulsions – are caused by similar mechanisms and present identical subjective symptoms and clinical signs on initial consultation. An early diagnosis is essential, therefore, especially since fractures of the intercondylar eminence are frequently overlooked or mistaken for a simple hemarthrosis (Rigault et al. 1976). The natural history of an untreated avulsion fracture of the intercondylar eminence is commonly marked by acute and chronic knee problems (recurrent episodes of instability, progressive distention of the capsule and ligaments). Most avulsion fractures of the intercondylar eminence are sustained in vehicular accidents, especially those involving bicycles and motorbikes (Meyers and McKeever 1970; Rigault et al. 1976). Recent developmental trends in sports are a social phenomenon that is bringing with it a growing number of tibial eminence avulsion fractures (Zifko and Gaudernak 1984).

The results in published series consistently indicate a very favorable prognosis for operatively or conservatively treated avulsion fractures. Nevertheless, it is difficult to single out a treatment method of choice because the comparative series are too small. The same is true of surgical procedures, which range from simple tunneling and snaring to rigid internal fixation with screws or Kirschner wires.

Pathophysiology

To aid in understanding the various types of fracture and their classification, we shall describe briefly the epiphyseal zone of the proximal tibia which bounds the articular surfaces of the tibial plateaus. The surface of each plateau is elevated centrally to form a tubercle, the lateral and medial tubercles together forming the intercondylar eminence. The cruciate ligaments generally do not insert on the tubercles themselves, but on the anterior and posterior intercondylar areas located in front of and behind the eminence. The anterior and posterior horns of the menisci also are attached in these areas. In an avulsion fracture of the intercondylar eminence, an osteochondral fragment breaks away from the site where the anterior cruciate ligament (ACL) inserts on the anterior intercondylar area. Generally this fragment is oval, in prolongation of the ACL fibers. The anterolateral margin of the fragment may extend beneath the anterior portion of the medial meniscus. The fragment, whose surface area is larger than the cross section of the ACL, represents a prolongation of the connective tissue fibers in the microtunnels, where the area of attachment is located (Seriat-Gautier et al. 1983). The bone fragments vary in size and extent. They are broad, smoothly contoured, and rarely involve just the articular surface. The size and displacement of the fragment in the lateral projection form the basis for radiographic classification of these fractures. The ACL is very rarely torn through its substance in this type of injury. The fracture most likely occurs at the end of the elastic phase of the strain curve of the ACL, i.e., at the critical point marking the onset of plastic deformation of the ligament.

The cause of the injury is always violent and complex (Baxter and Wiley 1988; Rigault et al. 1976; Seriat-Gautier et al. 1983). Reports from other authors and our own case material indicate that there are two principal causative mechanisms. The first is a posteroanterior force directed against the back of the lower leg with the knee flexed, driving both tibial plateaus forward. This may be caused by a fall from a

Table 1. Causes of avulsion fractures of the intercondylar eminence

	Meyers and McKeever (1959)	Rigault et al. (1976)	Zifko and Gaudernak (1984)	Our series Bachelin and Bugmann (1988)
Auto accidents	9	9	2	4
Bicycle accidents	24	10	6	6
Athletic injuries	6	2	13	16
Gymnastics			6	8
Skiing			7	8
Other causes	8	5	0	5
Total	47	26	21	31

bicycle or by certain athletic injuries sustained in soccer, football, or other contact sports. The direct blow generally produces an avulsion fracture in the anterior intercondylar area, since it causes the ACL to come under maximal tension with the knee flexed 90°. As the physical forces increase, the compliant phase is shortened due to elastic resistance, and the load increment becomes more rapid. The second causal mechanism is a rotational injury of the minimally flexed knee, like the "knee twist" injury in skiing. This causes the greatest damage to the posterolateral bundle of the ACL, which comes under maximum tension if the rotation is not checked. This mecha-

nism often produces a large avulsion fragment encompassing both the medial and lateral tubercles of the tibial eminence. The leading cause in the 1960s was bicycle injuries, followed closely by motor vehicle accidents. Comparing our series with those of other authors, we find that athletic injuries, especially those sustained in skiing and soccer, have become more prevalent over the years while vehicular injuries have shown a downward trend (Table 1).

Radiographic Assessment and Classification of Injuries

Two main classification systems have been utilized in the literature: that of Meyers and McKeever (1970), based on the degree of displacement of the bony avulsion fragment, and that of Rigault et al. (1976), which is geared toward pediatric knee pathology and is based on fragment displacement as well as the extent of involvement of the proximal tibial epiphysis. Three types of fracture are recognized in the Meyers-McKeever classification:

– Type 1: The avulsion fragment is minimally displaced, and there is slight elevation of its anterior margin.
– Type 2: The fragment is displaced for more than half its length ("beak-like" appearance on the lateral radiograph).
– Type 3: The fragment is completely separated from its bone bed. Its cartilaginous surface is markedly

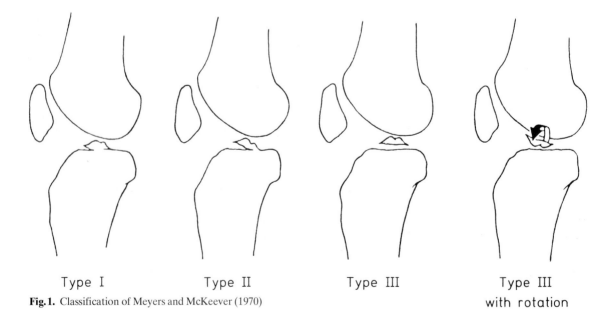

Fig. 1. Classification of Meyers and McKeever (1970)

Type I   Type II   Type III   Type III with rotation

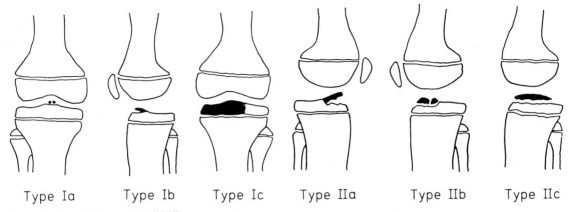

Type Ia   Type Ib   Type Ic   Type IIa   Type IIb   Type IIc

Fig. 2. Classification of Rigault et al. (1976)

displaced or may be rotated to face the eminence, resulting in a type 3b lesion.

Zaricny (1977) suggests adding a type 3c or type 4 lesion to allow for comminuted fractures, which may involve both the medial and lateral tibial plateaus.
In the classification of Rigault et al., two main groups of tibial eminence fracture are recognized (Fig. 2):

– Type 1a: Simple comminuted avulsion fracture with small osteochondral fragments, best appreciated on AP radiographs
– Type 1b: Minimally displaced fracture with anterior gaping at an angle not exceeding 10°
– Type 1c: Undisplaced epiphyseal fracture with involvement of the medial tibial plateau and intercondylar eminence, best appreciated on lateral radiographs

Type 1 fractures are characterized by an incomplete lesion with little or no osseous displacement.

– Type 2a: Avulsion of the intercondylar eminence with anterior gaping at an angle greater than 10°; the fragment retains intact posterior cartilaginous and fibrous attachments
– Type 2b: Large osteochondral fragments that are completely separated from the anterior epiphysis
– Type 3b: The anterior intercondylar area, tibial eminence, and posterior intercondylar area are avulsed and displaced.

The advantage of the first classification, based chiefly on fragment displacement, is its simplicity. It is the most widely used scheme in English-language publications. Occasionally it seems somewhat imprecise, especially in the assessment of type 2 and type 3 lesions.
The advantage of the Rigault classification is that it is precise and conforms to the radiographic appearance of the pediatric knee. The radiographic classification of these injuries is important, as it provides confirmation of the diagnosis, permits classification of the anatomic lesions, and establishes a more accurate basis for therapeutic decision making than that provided by clinical examination.

Case Material

From 1986 to 1988, 31 patients were treated at the Pediatric Surgical Clinic of the Kantonal Universitätsspital Genf for an avulsion fracture of the intercondylar eminence. Twenty patients were clinically examined between 6 months and 12 years after their injury (average 3 1/2 years) and followed radiographically. The radiographic follow-ups consisted of AP and lateral views in the one-legged stance, supplemented by active radiographic Lachman tests in both knees. Clinical follow-up evaluated knee stability, level of athletic participation, and subjective residual complaints.
The 20 patients were between 10 and 16 years of age (average 12 1/2 years) at the time of injury. Ten girls and 10 boys had sustained an avulsion fracture of the intercondylar eminence. When first examined, all the patients had a knee effusion which was pronounced in 12 cases and subtle in 6. A flexion deficit was noted in 8 cases. Examination was difficult in the remaining patients on account of pain. Twelve patients had a positive Lachman test, with pain preventing clinical examination in the rest. Positive dynamic subluxation tests could be elicited in only 3 patients initially.
An associated injury was found in 8 cases (5 involving the medial collateral ligament, 2 with a partial tear of the medial meniscus).

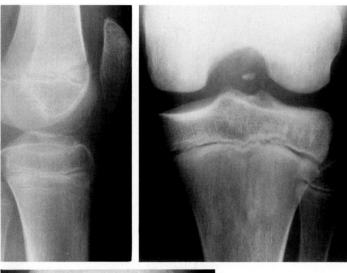
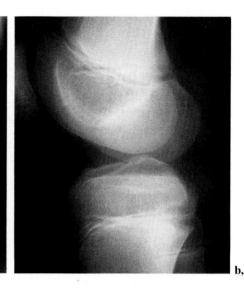

a

b, c

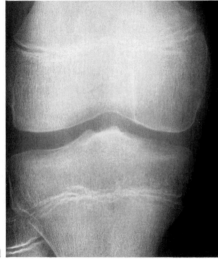

d

Fig. 3 a–d. Type R1 intercondylar eminence fracture, admission film **(a)** and films at 2nd, 3rd, and 4th follow-ups **(b–d)** over a 6-month course of conservative treatment

Radiographic evaluation using the classification of Rigault et al. (1976), which we chose for our series owing to its simplicity and precision, identified 8 injuries of the R1 type and 12 injuries of the R2 type (6 of which were type 2a, 4 type 2b, and 2 type 2c). The degree of anterior displacement or the prominence of the Lachman sign appeared to correlate with the fracture type: The 8 type R1 cases showed little or no anterior tibial displacement with respect to the femur, while the 12 R2 cases showed marked anterior displacement (Figs. 3, 4).

Treatment

In most published series, the radiographic classification of avulsion fractures of the intercondylar eminence serves as the main criterion for deciding between operative and nonoperative treatment.

Other authors (Rigault et al. 1976; Zifko and Gaudernak 1984) employ additional decision-making criteria. The clinical examination, supplemented by stability testing under anesthesia, permits a more accurate diagnosis of associated capsuloligamentous injuries. In general, however, the radiographic evaluation provides the basis for treatment.

Authors who use the classification of Meyers and McKeever (1970) favor conservative treatment for type 1 fractures, unless marked anteroposterior knee laxity is apparent clinically (Rigault et al. 1976; Seriat-Gautier et al. 1983). The treatment for type 2 lesions is surgical in most patients. Type 3 lesions are always managed surgically. Only Zifko and Gaudernak (1984) feel that conservative treatment is appropriate for type 2 and 3 lesions in which the osteochondral fragment encompasses the entire tibial eminence. They claim that this injury is amenable to closed reduction in hyperextension. If radiographs show inadequate reduction, the attempted closed reduction is followed by surgical intervention.

Authors who use the classification of Rigault et al. (1976) manage type R1 fractures conservatively except in cases where marked anterior tibial displacement is noted clinically. Type R2 fractures are generally treated operatively by open reduction of the osteochondral fragment. These criteria are not absolute, however; critical emphasis is placed on the clini-

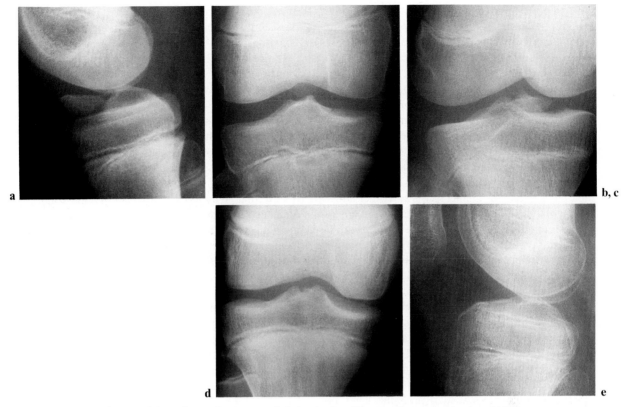

Fig. 4a–e. Type R2 intercondylar eminence fracture on admission **(a–c)** and 7 years after surgical treatment **(d–e)**

cal examination and especially on testing under anesthesia, the only truly relevant examination in terms of knee stability.

In our series 7 patients were treated conservatively by immobilizing the limb in a long cast for 6 weeks with the knee flexed approximately 0°–5°. The remaining 13 cases were managed by open reduction and stabilization. If the osteochondral fragment was larger than the insertion of the ACL, the fragment was snared with a U-shaped suture loop passed through 2.0-mm drill holes in the proximal tibia and secured on the anteromedial tibial metaphysis. For a smaller fragment, the transosseous suture was woven into the substance of the ACL (Fig. 5). Surgical treatment was always followed by cast immobilization and non-weight-bearing for 4–6 weeks.

Rehabilitation of the knee following cast removal presented no unusual problems after either operative or conservative therapy. Graduated weight bearing was commenced in the 6th postoperative week, and crutch weaning was accomplished within 1 week. For operatively treated patients, care was taken to avoid excessive stimulation of the quadriceps near extension during the rehabilitation period. An effort was made to achieve a range of 20°–90° knee flexion by

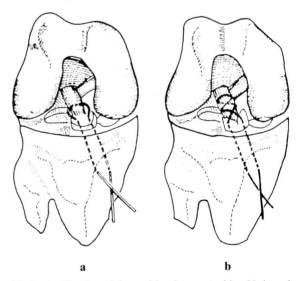

Fig. 5a, b. Fixation of the avulsion fragment with a U-shaped transosseous snare **(a)**, fixation with a suture woven into the ACL **(b)**

the 2nd postoperative month, and full extension was generally achieved at 3 months.

From 1980 to 1986, we conducted an initial clinical follow-up study of 13 patients according to strict criteria (Bachelin and Pirkla 1987). Since that time our population has increased by 10 patients, in whom we have applied a simple evaluation scheme. Eighteen patients had no subjective complaints of instability or unsteadiness and were fully satisfied with the condition of their knees. Two patients with an unsatisfactory result showed a positive Lachman sign and positive dynamic subluxation tests that prevented their participation in contact sports and other athletic endeavors. In patients who had other lesions coexisting with the avulsion fracture, there were 2 with detachment of the anterior horn of the medial meniscus and involvement of the medial collateral ligament, and 1 with a Salter type II proximal tibial epiphyseal fracture. In our series we found no correlation between results relating to mode of treatment or radiographic fracture type. In 15 cases the qualitative Lachman test showed a competent anterior restraint with a firm but delayed anterior end point. This clinically mild residual anterior laxity did not limit the sports activities of any of the patients, who continued to participate in sports at their preinjury level. Follow-up radiographs in the one-legged stance (frontal and sagittal planes) showed the following:

Bony consolidation was achieved in all cases. A slight elevation of the anterior margin of the anterior intercondylar area persisted in 6 cases, occasionally with small calcifications at the insertion of the ACL. Six patients showed subtle preosteoarthritic changes with flattening of the femoral condyles and slight narrowing of the medial joint space. Two patients who had lesions coexisting with the intercondylar eminence fracture showed mild degenerative articular changes on radiographs.

Objective Laxity Measurement (Active Lachman Test)

Radiographic Lachman tests were performed in 6 girls and 8 boys with an average age of 12.5 years. Eleven had been treated surgically and 3 conservatively by cast immobilization. The measurement of active anterior subluxation was based on a contour analysis of the knee joints in a lateral projection with perfect superposition of the posterior femoral condyles (Jacobsen 1981). In all cases we found a significant difference in anterior, active residual laxity between the injured and healthy sides. The difference averaged 3.34 mm in this small series (Figs. 6, 7). The persistent side-to-side difference in anterior residual laxity despite an anatomic reduction of the fracture (average of 2 1/2 years after surgery) has been previously noted by several authors (Bachelin and Bugmann 1988; Baxter and Wiley 1988; Zifko and Gaudernak 1984). This phenomenon can be explained by the strain behavior of the ACL up to the point at which the avulsion fracture occurs. Several authors have used the same experiment to demonstrate the phases of elastic and plastic deformation that precede definitive rupture of the ligament. We believe that an avulsion fracture of the intercondylar eminence in children and adolescents occurs at the moment when the strain curve makes the transition from elastic to plastic deformation; this occurs when the ACL has undergone an average elongation of 20%–25%. The consequent likelihood of permanent elongation of the ACL can account for the residual anterior laxity noted in the majority of our cases. Thus, in addition to reducing and stabilizing the osteochondral fragment, we now attempt to restore normal ligament tension by additional tightening of the fixation threads. This could also be accomplished by curetting the bone bed in the anterior intercondylar area and reattaching the fragment in a recessed position, but our results do not appear to justify this since the short-term effects of a moderately elongated ACL did not cause functional disability in our patients.

In agreement with the literature, the following points from our study may be emphasized:

Although the initial clinical examination varied from case to case according to the degree of pain, all patients were found to have hemarthrosis with functional incompetence of the knee joint. It is extremely important to inquire about the mechanism of the injury, as this provides a high index of suspicion for an avulsion fracture of the intercondylar eminence. This differential diagnosis should be considered in young patients who have been injured during sports, skiing, bike riding, etc. Early diagnosis is important, as neglected cases generally progress to a nonunion whose treatment carries a poor prognosis. It is also essential to verify the extent of associated lesions by a standard radiographic workup.

If the AP and lateral radiographs are inconclusive, a third view centered on the anterior intercondylar eminence should be obtained. This "intercondylar view" generally permits a diagnosis to be made. If there is still doubt as to the integrity of the central pivot, we feel that an examination under anesthesia is indicated. We believe that both classifications lead essentially to the same course of action in a given

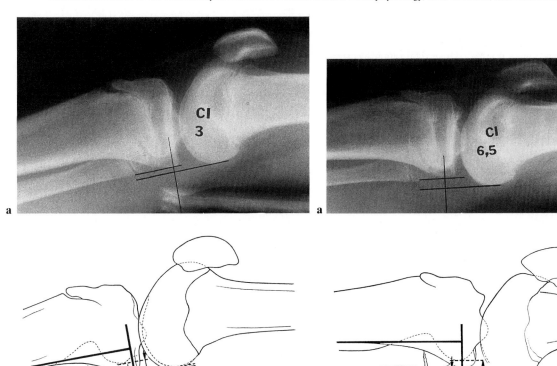

Fig. 6a, b. Normal knee joint of a 15-year-old girl, lateral projection in one-legged stance, showing 3-mm anterior subluxation of the medial compartment *(solid line)* and 8-mm anterior subluxation of the lateral compartment *(dashed line)*

Fig. 7a, b. Residual anterior laxity 18 months after surgical treatment of a Rigault type 2b avulsion fracture. Residual anterior subluxation is 6.5 mm in the medial compartment and 11 mm in the lateral compartment

case, and that examination under anesthesia can aid in deciding between operative or conservative treatment of a type R1 fracture or a type 1 or 2 fracture according to the Meyers-McKeever scheme. In the rare case of a type R2 fracture with a large osteochondral fragment, we recommend a conservative approach if the lateral radiograph in extension confirms perfect reduction of the fragment. At operation we enter the joint through a short medial arthrotomy and retract the infrapatellar fat pad laterally to obtain a clear view of the osteochondral fragment in the anterior intercondylar area. After probing the menisci with a hook to test their function, we anatomically reduce the avulsion fragment and secure it temporarily with a reduction clamp with the knee flexed 60°. After marking the proximal tibial and medial growth plate with a fine needle, we drill two parallel 2.0-mm holes from the proximal anteromedial tibial metaphysis toward the anterior intercondylar area. The osteochondral avulsion fragment is definitively stabilized with transosseous nonabsorbable 2/0 mersilene threads. We always check knee stability near extension and test ACL tension with a probing hook.

Postoperatively the limb is placed in a long cast for 4–6 weeks with the knee flexed 20°. After cast removal the knee is rehabilitated, taking care to avoid stresses on the ACL for the first 3 months after surgery.

The future probably belongs to arthroscopy, which can be used both to diagnose the avulsion fracture and to proceed immediately with surgical repair. For 1 year we have been treating avulsion fractures of the tibial eminence arthroscopically, using two threaded 2.0-mm Kirschner wires in a technique related to that recommended by McLennan (1982). It seems premature to report on the results of our arthroscopic repairs at the present time. Nevertheless, the fixation appears to be adequate, and there is less surgical morbidity than with a formal arthrotomy. The only disadvantage of this method is the necessity of a two-stage procedure for removal of the fixation material.

References

Bachelin P, Bugmann P (1988) Active subluxation in extension, radiographical, control in intercondylar eminence fractures in childhood. Z Kinderchir 43: 180–182

Bachelin P, Pirkla S (1987) Fractures des épines tibiales et rupture du ligament croisé antérieur chez l'enfant et l'adolescent. Med Hyg 45: 1656–1662

Baxter MP, Wiley JL (1988) Fractures of the tibial spine in children. J Bone Joint Surg [Br] 70: 228–230

Bradley GW, Shives TC, Samuelson KM (1979) Ligament injuries in the knees of children. J Bone Joint Surg [Am] 61: 558–591

Dejour H (1982) Le sport et les lésions du genou chez l'enfant. J Med Lyon 63: 103–109

Jacobsen K (1981) Gonylaxometry: stress radiographic measurement of passive laxity in the knee joint of normal subjects and patients with ligaments injuries. Acta Orthop Scand [Suppl 194]

McLennan JG (1982) The role of arthroscopic surgery in the treatment of fractures of the intercondylar eminence of the tibia. J Bone Joint Surg [Br] 64: 477–480

Meyers MH, McKeever F (1970) Fracture of the intercondylar eminence of the tibia. J Bone Joint Surg [Am] 52: 1677–1684

Rigault P, Moulies D, Padovani JP, Lesaux D (1976) Les fractures tibiales chez l'enfant. Ann Chir Inf 17: 137–250

Seriat-Gautier B, Frick M, Pieracci M (1983) Fractures des épines tibiales chez l'enfant. Rev Chir Orthop 69: 221–231

Zaricny B (1977) Avulsion fracture of the tibial eminence, treatment by open reduction and pinning. J Bone Joint Surg [Am] 59: 1111–1115

Zifko B, Gaudernak T (1984) Zur Problematik in der Therapie von „Eminentiaausrissen" bei Kindern und Jugendlichen. Unfallheilkunde 87: 267–272

Dislocation of the Knee

R. Johner, P. M. Ballmer, D. Rogge, H. B. Burch, R. P. Jakob, and H. Tscherne

Dislocation of the knee is the most severe form of ligamentous knee injury that involves rupture of the anterior cruciate ligament (ACL). The knee is said to be dislocated when the tibial and femoral articular surfaces have lost contact with each other or may have lost contact based on an existing instability. Knee dislocations are designated anterior or posterior according to the direction of tibial displacement with respect to the femur. Other forms such as medial, lateral, or rotary are far less common and are often combined with anterior or posterior dislocation. The massive displacement of the joint members during the dislocation causes extensive disruption of the joint capsule and ligaments. At least 3 of the 5 groups (central, medial, lateral, posterior, and anterior) of capsuloligamentous structures are damaged, sometimes 4, and occasionally all 5, rendering the joint totally unstable.

Knee dislocation is an ominous injury not just in terms of the extensive ligament damage. In 4 of 5 cases there are associated local and other injuries that worsen the prognosis. Approximately one-half of knee dislocations are open (Chapuis 1984; O'Donoghue 1960; Stäubli et al. 1983). Two-thirds of closed dislocations have concomitant severe local and distal injuries. Green and Allen (1977) found ischemia of the lower leg and foot in one-third of knee dislocations, and Jones et al. (1979) found peroneal nerve palsy in one-fourth.

Ligament Injuries

There is still uncertainty regarding the minimum amount of ligament disruption that must be present for a knee dislocation to occur. Rupture of the ACL is consistently reported in studies where knee dislocations were surgically explored. The posterior cruciate ligament (PCL), too, is generally described as torn. Meyers (1971) found that the ACL was invariably torn in 11 surgically treated dislocations, while the PCL was intact in 1 case; however, stability testing at follow-up suggested that the lesion had been missed initially. Honton et al. (1978) and Thomsen et al. (1984) found that both cruciate ligaments were ruptured in 12 explored joints. Reports vary concerning the damage to peripheral structures. The explored cases showed that the capsule and ligaments were torn on at least one side and frequently on both sides. Controversy on this point stems from the fact that the dislocated knee occasionally shows no medial-lateral instability in the postreduction state. This can be explained by noting that the collateral ligaments are sometimes "peeled" from the bone without true disruption. When the joint is reduced, the peeled structures reappose to their correct sites and appear intact on valgus-varus testing owing to their periosteal attachment (Kennedy 1963). Damage to the posterior capsule is also frequently reported, although we have not found a systematic study on this point. It is not uncommon for a posterior dislocation to involve the extensor apparatus, either in the form of a patellar fracture or damage to the patellar tendon (Kennedy 1963).

To our knowledge, the only experimental study on mechanisms of knee dislocation was performed by Kennedy (1963), who attempted to reproduce various types of dislocation in cadaver knees using a stress machine. Anterior dislocation was consistently produced in the specimens by hyperextension of the joint. The ligaments began to tear at approximately 30° of hyperextension. Generally the posterior capsule tore first, followed by rupture of the PCL and ACL. The collateral ligaments were generally torn on both sides, but occasionally just one ligament was torn, or the ligaments were peeled subperiosteally from the femur without rupture.

Kennedy was able to produce only 2 posterior dislocations, and only by greatly increasing the applied torque. In both cases there was an associated rupture of the patellar tendon. This led Kennedy to conclude that the extensor apparatus is a major tethering structure that restrains posterior displacement of the tibia.

Attempts to produce lateral dislocations caused fractures of the tibial plateau.

The experimental discoveries of Kennedy are consistent with clinical experience. Anterior dislocation is caused by hyperextension of the knee and is commonly seen in athletic injuries, crushing injuries (rock slides, cave-ins), or sudden hyperextension caused by stepping into a hole. Posterior dislocation is caused by an impact to the upper tibia in the flexed knee, typically sustained in an automobile or motorcycle accident.

Until the 1960s, ligamentous injuries in the dislocated knee were managed conservatively by months of immobilization in a plaster cast. The major problem was to prevent the unfavorable posterior tibial subluxation that is promoted by gravity and hamstring tension. Some tried to prevent this by casting the knee in full extension, a position that is unfavorable for neurovascular lesions. Others used Kirschner wires, Steinmann pins, and even medullary rods to immobilize the femur and tibia in the desired relation to each other. But these fixation methods did not gain wide acceptance because the implants were prone to bending, loosening, infection, or aggravating the joint injury. External skeletal fixation also was occasionally used (Honton et al. 1978; Jones et al. 1979).

When the operative treatment of ligamentous knee injuries became more popular in the early 1960s following the work of O'Donoghue (1960) and Kennedy (1963), the suture repair of ligaments became increasingly practiced in the management of knee dislocations. In 1971 Meyers and Harvey reported on 18 dislocations that they treated between 1965 and 1969. In 4 cases they repaired all the torn ligaments. Three of these cases had a good or excellent outcome. None of the 14 conservatively treated cases achieved a good result. In France, Geneste et al. (1972) and Honton et al. (1978) reported similar experience in 16 and 12 cases, respectively, where the repair of all disrupted ligaments yielded much better results than nonoperative treatment.

Vascular Injuries

The impairment of arterial blood flow is the most common and severe complication of knee dislocations. Even today, it jeopardizes the survival of the limb. In the 19th century, dislocation of the knee was considered life-threatening unless the leg was promptly amputated (Stäubli et al. 1983). But with increasing experience, shorter intervals from injury to treatment, and advances in vascular surgery, the incidence of amputation has steadily declined. By the 1960s the amputation rate had fallen to 20% (O'Donoghue 1960) and by the 1970s to 11% (Green and Allen 1977). In a review of 245 knee dislocations, Green and Allen (1977) found that amputation had been performed in 4 of 5 cases where the ischemic interval from injury to treatment was longer than 8 h. The vascular injury may range from decollement of the intima to a complete vascular rupture, depending on the degree of stretch injury to the vessel. Kennedy (1963) observed that the popliteal artery in cadaver knees ruptured at an average angle of 50° of hyperextension. Ischemia is immediate in the wake of a complete rupture, while partial lesions can produce a progressive ischemia that does not become evident for hours or days. Honton et al. (1978) described a cases in which ischemia was not manifested until 4 days after the injury.

Arterial damage is not always easy to diagnose clinically. Praefull (1975) reports that the pedal pulses are initially normal in 10% of knee dislocations with vascular injury. Green and Allen (1977) state emphatically that a warm leg with an intact microcirculation does not prove the absence of vascular damage in a dislocated knee. The crucial factor is not the microcirculation of the skin and subcutaneous tissue but the pedal pulses. If these pulses are absent or diminished, the physician should assume injury of the popliteal artery or its bifurcation and proceed with emergency exploration. If the vascular injury is not treated, most limbs will come to amputation, and the others will have incapacitating muscular fibrosis, contracture, and intermittent claudication. This finding is consistent with the experience of De Bakey and Simeone (1946) in World War II, who noted a 72% amputation rate following ligation of the popliteal artery. The use of angiography in dislocated knees is controversial. Honton et al. (1978) state that arteriography should be used sparingly, while Jones et al. (1979) support its liberal use. Green and Allen (1977) regard preoperative arteriography as a dangerous and needless waste of time because the damaged vessel is consistently located in the popliteal fossa. Chapuis (1984) shares this opinion and, like Jones et al. (1979), notes that the area that may contain a vascular injury can be completely explored through a medial incision, with no need for preoperative localization of the lesion. He agrees with Welling et al. (1981) that arteriography is unnecessary in clear cases, but recommends arteriography on the operating table in doubtful cases, noting that high-quality radiographs are obtained since timing of the study is not critical in the presence of a vascular obstruction.

Nerve Lesions

Injuries of the peroneal nerve are common. The tibial nerve is less frequently affected. The associated palsies are often definitive. Green and Allen (1977) observed 6 cases of peroneal nerve palsy in 18 knee dislocations, none of which had a return of function. In 4 explored cases there was 1 extensive stretch injury not accessible to resection and primary repair and 3 nerve ruptures with ragged ends. Meyers and Harvey (1971) reported on the unfavorable effect of casting in extension, which they consistently performed due to rupture of the PCL. The palsy persisted in the 6 cases immobilized in this way. In the series of Jones et al. (1979), 4 of the 5 patients with peroneal nerve palsy had a return of function.

Knee Dislocation and External Skeletal Fixation: An Analysis of 28 Cases

Honton et al. (1978) and Jones et al. (1979) mention the occasional use of external skeletal fixation in dislocated knees with severe soft-tissue disruption, without discussing the advantages and disadvantages of this method. In the 1970s we began using external skeletal fixation routinely for knee dislocations. The advantages are obvious. The reduction can be effected and securely maintained in any position desired. The full circumference of the extremity is accessible at all times, greatly facilitating the supervision of blood flow and the muscle compartments. The patient can stand, walk, and bear weight on the limb to the degree permitted by associated injuries. Our study was conducted to determine whether these advantages would outweigh the disadvantage of rigid fixation of the knee joint.

As of spring, 1984, external skeletal fixation was used in a total of 28 dislocated knees treated at the Trauma Clinic of Hannover Medical College, the Department of Orthopedic Surgery at the University of Bern, and the Department of Orthopedic Surgery of Kantonsspital Freiburg. Only patients who had a radiographically documented knee dislocation or a severe capsuloligamentous instability in the anterior, posterior, and medial or lateral direction (or both) consistent with a knee dislocation were enrolled in the study.

Fourteen of the 28 dislocations were sustained in vehicular accidents, 9 on the job, 4 during sports, and 1 due to a misstep on a flail joint. Five of the dislocations were anterior, 8 posterior, and the rest were unclear. Fifteen of the dislocations were closed,

13 were open. Using the grading system of Tscherne and Gotzen (1983), the soft-tissue damage in the closed injuries was rated as 0 in 4 cases, grade 1 in 2 cases (contusion), and grade 3 in 9 cases (extensive crushing of skin and muscle, Figs. 1, 2). Among the open dislocations, 1 patient had grade 1 soft-tissue damage (skin disruption without significant contusion), and the remaining 12 had grade 3 (extensive soft-tissue destruction, often with associated neurovascular injuries).

Five patients had no local associated injuries. Fifteen had ischemia distal to the knee (8 closed and 7 open dislocations). The ischemic period was 11 h in 1 patient, 8 h in 4, 6 h in 1, 5 h in 4, 2 and 3 h in 1 case each, and unknown in 1 case. Ten patients had peroneal nerve palsy, and 9 had 1–3 local associated fractures (Fig. 3). Sixteen patients had other coexisting injuries, and 9 had severe multiple injuries. The dislocated joint was surgically explored in 17 patients, and the detected ligament injuries are listed in Table 1. Both cruciate ligaments were injured in all patients, the medial ligaments in 13, the lateral structures in 12, the medial meniscus in 5, and the lateral meniscus in 3. Two patients sustained a complete avulsion of the extensor apparatus from the tibia, 1 with a closed dislocation had a partial avulsion, and 1 had a patellar fracture. In 9 cases damage to both cruciate ligaments was accompanied by involvement of both the medial and lateral capsuloligamentous structures. Three of these were closed dislocations. The 4 cases with extensor damage also fall within this group.

External skeletal fixation was applied in various forms. Initially a full frame was used, conforming to practices then current, and was sometimes combined with a half-frame device. Later an anterior or anterolateral half frame alone was used almost exclusively (see Figs. 1–3). A total of 3 full frames were used, 4 tent frames, and 20 half frames. The half frames were mounted anterolaterally in 2 cases, laterally in 1, and anteriorly in 17. In 12 cases a total of 4 Schanz screws were used, interconnected in 11 cases by 2 parallel rods and in 3 cases by 1 rod. The angle of knee flexion ranged from 15° to 70°, with an average of 36°. The varus-valgus position of the knee was correct in all 21 cases that could be evaluated. Reduction on the sagittal plane was evaluated by the criteria of Jacobson (1974, 1976). It was correct in 16 patients, and in 7 the error was less than 5 mm. In 2 patients the tibia was fixed with 11 and 18 mm of anterior drawer, and in 1 it was fixed with 9 mm of posterior drawer.

In 11 cases repairs were performed on all injured ligaments. In 2 cases only 1 of the cruciate ligaments was repaired, and in 2 cases only the collateral ligaments were repaired (Table 1).

The patients were mobilized as soon after surgery as possible. They were permitted to put the operated leg down and bear partial weight. The external fixation material was removed at 3–11 weeks (average 7 weeks). Follow-up examinations were conducted at 5–72 months (average 37 months). The patients were questioned, examined, and X-rayed. Their medical history, X-ray files, and operation reports were analyzed. The roentgen examination comprised a minimum of 8 films: both knees AP standing, lateral supine in 90° flexion, and anterior and posterior drawer lateral stress films near extension (Stäubli 1982). In some cases additional stress films were taken in 90° flexion and various rotational positions. The anterior and posterior drawers were measured and averaged using the anatomic reference points defined by Jacobsen (1974, 1976) for the medial and lateral compartments. The results were recorded on a 120-point questionnaire and evaluated on a personal computer.

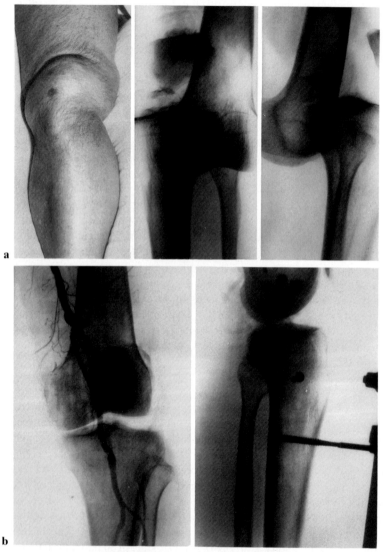

Fig. 1 a–c. Closed anterior dislocation of the knee in a 55-year-old man who collided with a ski-lift post at about 3:00 p.m. When admitted at 5:00 p.m., he had a cold leg with no pulses. The foot was paretic except along its lateral border (grade 3 soft-tissue injury). There were contusional marks over the patellar ligament (**a**). Hyperextension injury. The knee was re-duced 15 min after arrival in the emergency room. Since there were still no pedal pulses, the patient was taken to X-ray for arteriograms. Surgical treatment commenced at 10:00 p.m. The popliteal vessels were explored and a bypass performed using an interposed vein graft. Perfusion was reestablished at 11:15 p.m. (**b**). **c** see p. 311

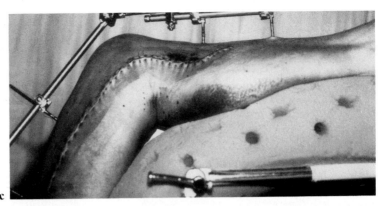

c

Fig. 1c. Next, for orthopedic treatment, an anteromedial arthrotomy was performed through the same incision plus a lateral skin incision. The torn posterior capsule was repaired at the level of the menisci. The posteromedial origin of the medial meniscus, avulsed on a bone fragment, was reattached; the torn lateral meniscus was resected; the PCL was reattached with transcondylar sutures; a midsubstance ACL tear was left alone; and bony avulsions of the medial and lateral capsule and ligaments were repaired using 2 screws and toothed washers per side. After the sutures for the posterior and central structures had been placed, the external fixation material was applied, and the joint was X-rayed and its position adjusted. Finally all sutures and screws were tightened. Surgery concluded at 3:15 a.m. **(c)** External skeletal fixation was maintained for 6 weeks, and the patient returned to work at 4 months. At 5 months the knee was painless and showed no signs of irritation. Thigh girth was reduced 3 cm and range of motion was 115–15–0, with good medial and posterior stability. There was moderate anterolateral instability. Overall the patient rated the knee at 50% of the uninjured knee. Arteriography in this case needlessly prolonged ischemia by 2 1/2 h to the critical 8h, leaving insufficient time to perform the complex ACL repair. Accordingly, the functional outcome was fair

▷

Fig. 2a–c. Eighteen-year-old foreign worker whose legs were pinned beneath 3 tons of spilled concrete mix at 9:00 a.m. Admitted at 10:30 a.m. with severe soft-tissue contusions on both legs, a grade 3 closed fracture of the right femur, and a grade 3 closed dislocation of the left knee with ischemia and peroneal nerve palsy. Arteriograms were taken of both legs in the X-ray unit. Surgery commenced at 1:00 p.m. in the prone position. Blood flow in the left leg was reestablished at 2:00 p.m. The posterior capsule, ruptured at the level of the joint line, was repaired along with both gastrocnemius heads. A below-knee posterior fasciotomy was done, and the patient was moved to the supine position. Fasciotomy of the peroneal compartment was done, and an external half frame was applied in 45° flexion. Angiography was repeated when left and right pulses did not return. Vascular exploration commenced at 7:00 p.m. on the left side and at 10:30 p.m. on the right, with subsequent compression plating through the same medial approach. Surgery concluded at 11:00 p.m. **a** Status after surgery and **b, c** 4 months later. Patient did not return to work and retired abroad, where 3 years later he was asymptomatic and needed no additional surgery. More than 2h were wasted by angiography, which dangerously prolonged the ischemic period

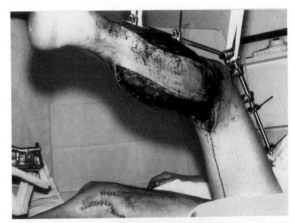

a

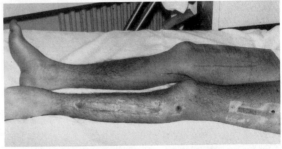

b

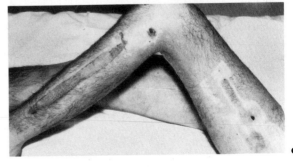

c

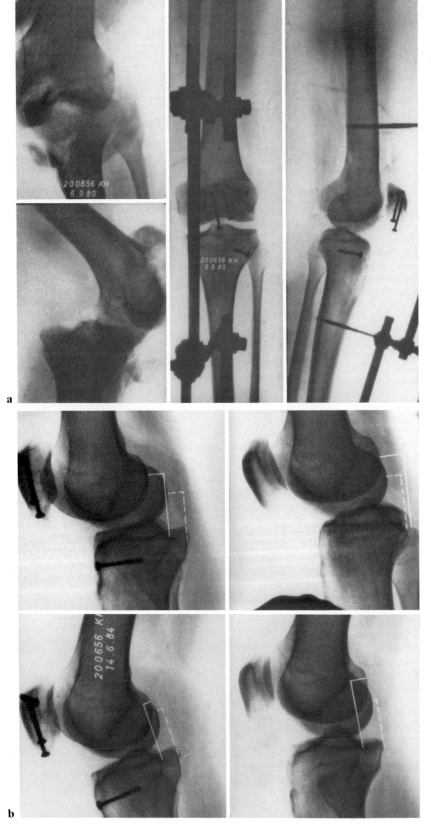

Fig. 3. Legend see p. 313

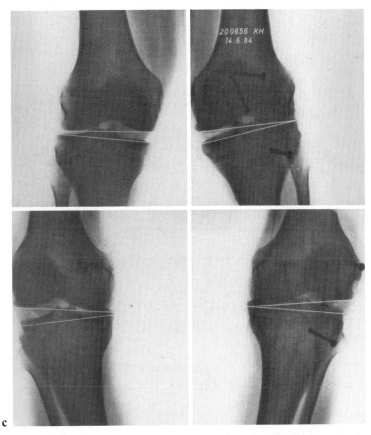

Fig. 3a–c. Motorcyclist 24 years of age with typical posterior, grade 3, widely open knee dislocation heavily contaminated with dirt. There is complete disruption of the central and peripheral ligaments and capsule, a fractured patella with severe patellar tendon damage, bony avulsion of the iliotibial tract, and abrasion of the lateral femoral condyle. Primary treatment consisted of debridement, internal screw fixation of the patella and Gerdy tubercle, and erection of an anterior half frame with good reduction of the slightly flexed knee since there was no posterior neurovascular damage **(a)**. The ligaments were not repaired. The postoperative course was uneventful. The half frame was removed at 6 weeks, followed by 2 weeks of passive mobilization on an electric splint, full weight bearing at 20 weeks, and full return to work as a bricklayer at 32 weeks. At 33 months the knee was painless and stable, and the patient could use it normally in work and recreation (squash). Overall patient rating was 90% of the preinjury value. Patient had no problem standing, walking, jogging, running straight ahead, zig-zag running, cutting, or stopping abruptly. He had slight difficulty with stair climbing and kneeling. The knee appeared free of irritation, had a + 2 cm circumference without effusion, a 2 cm thigh girth, and symmetrical drawer mobilities in the Lachman test **(b)**. Posterior drawer in flexion was 5 mm in NR and 10 mm in ER. Range of motion was 130–0–10°. This was by far the best result in patients who did not have ligament repairs

Results

Four of the 28 patients died, 1 from a pulmonary embolism, 1 from a severe head injury and burns, and 1 from septic pulmonary failure. One patient, who had sustained the knee dislocation in a suicide attempt, shot himself 5 months later (see Fig. 3). One patient was still in coma following a severe head injury. Two foreign workers had retired and left the country. Twenty patients were available for clinical and radiographic follow-up. Two were evaluated on the basis of a family physician's report and radiographs, and one was questioned by telephone. Thus, our follow-up covered all patients who were still alive. The average follow-up interval was 37 months after operation.

One patient had undergone amputation above the knee. The leg had been ischemic for 8 h prior to reconstruction. Two patients had postischemic and postcontusional damage, which in 1 case had been treated with an orthopedic device and in the second case led to early retirement. One patient had to have a below-knee amputation due to a concomitant burn with secondary infection of the ankle joint. In all cases the knee joint healed without infection. Six patients had pin tract infections, which in 2 cases were treated by

Table 1. Ligament injuries in 17 surgically treated knee dislocations. Following Tscherne, soft-tissue damage is graded *0–4* in closed dislocations and *4–6* in 1st- to 3rd-degree open dislocations. The *arrows* indicate the location of the ligament injury: → midsubstance tear; ↑ proximal, anterior, or peripheral injury; ↓ distal, posterior, or central tear; ! proximal, anterior tear; *F* fracture; + ligament injury not precisely defined. + in the "Repaired" column means that all the torn structures were repaired. (+) means that only some were repaired. * Preexisting damage, ? not described. An empty column means that the ligament was intact

Patient	Age	Dislocation		Central		Medial			Lateral					Meniscus		Extensor apparatus	Side	
		Type	Skin	ACL	PCL	MCL	MCap	PMC	LCL	Popl	Bcps	ITT	PLC	Med	Lat		Injured	Repaired
BM	21	a	0	←	←			←	↑	←	↑	↑	?	?	?		CML	+
GF	55	a	0	→	→		↑	↑	?	→	?	?	?	?	?		CML	+
EG	55	a	3	+	←	←	←		←	←	?	?	?	↑	←		CML	(+)
TH	72	a	3	*	↑	*	*	*						↑	←		CM	(+)
BP	28	a	6	↑	↑	↑	↑	↑	↑	↑			←				CML	+
WK	34	p	0	↑	←				↑	←				←			CL	+
SR	20	p	3	↑	↑		↑	←									CM	(+)
SE	22	p	3	→	←	↑		↑					↑				CL	+
WU	20	p	5	+	+	+	+	+	+	→		+	↑			→	CML	(+)
KH	24	p	6	+	+	+	+	+	+	←	?	→	+	?	?	F	CMLS	(+)
RH	54	?	1	←	←	→	←	↑	←	←		→	↑			(+)	CMLS	+
CP	18	?	3	+	+	↑	↑	↑	F	←	F			↑			CM	–
AI	18	?	6	↑	↑	→	→	↑		←		→					CML	+
GH	18	?	6	↑	←	→	←	↑	↑	↑		→	↑				CM	+
LB	20	?	6	↑	↑		↑	↑	F	?	F	→	↑	↑	?		CL	+
KC	24	?	6	↑	←	↑	→	↑	F	→			?	↑		?	CML	(+)
HL	32	?	6	→	→	→	→	→	→	↑			↑		↑	→	CML	+
Total				17	17	13	14	15	12	10	4	8	10	5	3	4		

ACL Anterior cruciate ligament
PCL Posterior cruciate ligament
MCL Medial collateral ligament
MCap Medial capsular ligament
PMC Posteromedial capsule

LCL Lateral collateral ligament
Popl Popliteus
Bcps Biceps
ITT Iliotibial tract
PLC Posterolateral capsule

C Central ligaments (ACL, PCL)
M Medial ligaments (MCL, MCap, PMC)
L Lateral ligaments and tendons (LCL, Popl, Bcps, ITT, PLC)
V Extensor apparatus

pin removal at 6 weeks. All the infections healed without sequelae.

The 4 peroneal nerve ruptures were all treated secondarily by sural nerve grafting, which in all cases was unsuccessful. Of the 6 patients with peroneal axonotmesis, 2 recovered completely and 1 had partial recovery at 13 months; in 2 cases paresis persisted, and in 2 the result was unknown.

Full weight bearing was regained at 4 months on average, with a range from 6 weeks to 6 months. Patients returned to work after an average of 25 weeks, disregarding the cases with severe associated injuries.

The average range of knee motion was 112° (70°–130°). Extension was no problem. Only 4 patients had an extension deficit, which was less than 10° in all cases. Six patients had less than 100° of flexion, and 5 of these had sustained severe local soft-tissue injuries. The achieved range of motion bore no relation to the flexion angle during external skeletal fixation, or the duration of external skeletal fixation, or whether or not the ligaments had been repaired.

On the other hand, the treatment of the ligament injuries and especially of the cruciate ligaments had a significant impact on the functional result. The ligaments had been surgically repaired in 12 patients, 7 with a closed and 5 with an open dislocation. Nine of the patients showed little or no residual instability, 1 had moderate instability, and 2 had marked instability. The radiographic measurements showed 5 mm of anterior drawer and 4 mm of posterior drawer. Ten patients were fully able to return to work, with 2 requiring some retraining. One patient was 25% disabled for work, and 1 was still unable to return to work; there were no premature retirements. One patient rated overall function compared with the uninjured knee at 100%, 3 at 90%, 2 at 75%, and 6 at 50%.

The ligament ruptures had been treated conservatively in 11 patients, 7 with a closed and 4 with an open dislocation. Four patients had little or no residual instability, and 3 had significant instability. Two patients were treated with a brace, and 2 others were reoperated for instability, 1 after a recurrence of the dislocation. Anterior drawer in the non-reoperated patients averaged 5 mm, as in the operated group, but the posterior drawer was significantly greater, averaging 9 mm. The average total drawer was 13 mm as opposed to 9 mm in the repaired group. Four patients were fully able to return to work, 2 after retraining; 3 were unable to return to work or retired, and 1 was already retired at the time of injury. One patient rated overall function at 90%, 2 at 75%, 1 at 50%, and 2 at 25%.

Radiographs showed osteoarthritic changes in patients who had sustained their dislocations a long time before. These changes were most common about the patella. On the whole the changes were not very pronounced, and they were less conspicuous in patients with a stable knee than in patients with a lax joint.

Discussion

Today there is no longer any doubt that dislocation of the knee is associated with complete insufficiency of both cruciate ligaments and the capsuloligamentous structures on at least the medial or lateral side. The pathology may involve midsubstance ruptures, detachments, subperiosteal separations, equivalent fractures, or preexisting laxities. Our surgically explored cases indicate involvement of both the medial and lateral sides in more than half of the cases, resulting in a massive, global instability. In 30% of these cases there is an associated injury of the extensor apparatus. Unfortunately, injury to the posterior capsule is not systematically documented in our study or in the literature. Based on stability descriptions and radiographic findings, however, we must assume that the posterior capsule was torn at least on one side and probably on both sides in the majority of cases.

Our study is consistent with other publications in demonstrating the superiority of the primary repair of torn ligaments over treatment without ligament repair. Indeed, suture repair is almost essential to achieve a good functional outcome. The case shown in Fig. 1 is an exception that leaves room for hope in cases where primary ligament repair is considered too risky. We see several potential reasons for withholding primary ligament repair:

- A widely open dislocation that is heavily contaminated
- Severe soft-tissue contusions or burns
- Long ischemic interval of more than 4–6 h
- Large skin defects that require grafting for coverage
- Poor general condition of the patient
- Lack of a competent surgeon

It must be realized that the decision for ligament repair implies a significant prolongation of operating time. It is our experience that 2–4 h are required for reduction, skin preparation, draping, vascular repair, debridement, fasciotomy, external skeletal fixation, internal fixation of accompanying fractures, and intraoperative radiographs. The repair of all ligaments takes another 2–4 h, resulting in a total operating time of 6 h or more.

We did not find that the longer operating time increased the risk of infection, nor has this been reported in the literature. On the contrary, it is remarkable that no instance of joint infection occurred despite the high percentage of open grade 3 dislocations, half of which were treated by ligament repair, and the large number of young surgeons. The infection rate of 8% cited by Shields et al. (1969) is also low. Nevertheless, in patients with risk factors the surgeon should carefully consider how much he should repair and how well. Often, with systematic planning, some ligament injuries can be satisfactorily repaired in a short time with a few coapting sutures. Whenever possible, however, an attempt should be made to repair as many injured structures as possible during the first operation. As in other areas of reconstructive and trauma surgery, it has been found that the meticulous repair of all injuries in the dislocated knee affords the best result in the shortest amount of time. Secondary operations on the ligaments are frequently compromised by contaminated pin sites and other local or general complications. In several of our patients we planned secondary procedures for subsequent weeks during the primary operation but did not follow through. In 2 cases a ligament reconstruction was performed 2 months later due to incapacitating instability.

The amputation rate of 4% in our series is considerably lower than in other studies. We believe that this can be credited to the use of external skeletal fixation, which provides excellent access for monitoring circulatory and muscle-compartment status. External skeletal fixation offers a decisive advantage in this regard over cast immobilization.

Peroneal nerve palsy is a complication that shows a decidedly poor regenerative tendency in our patients and in the literature. Even sural nerve grafting appears unable to help the situation.

When we began using external skeletal fixation in the treatment of knee dislocations, we feared cartilage damage of the kind described by Salter of Toronto, Canada, in the immobilized limbs of animal models. Initially we maintained the fixation for only a few weeks but later increased this to 6–7 weeks. In the subsequent rehabilitation period, we frequently observed patellar chondropathy in a setting similar to that seen in patients with cruciate ligament repairs who had an equally long immobilization in a long cylinder cast. We do not know whether the osteoarthritic changes noted years later are attributable to the external skeletal fixation or more to the residual instability. It would be useful to have an external fixation device with an articulated connection that would permit progressive flexion-extension of the knee. Combined with partial weight bearing, such a device could eliminate the major disadvantage of excessively rigid fixation.

Amputation, with an incidence of 4%, has become a rare complication in our practice. Besides shorter intervals from injury to treatment, we attribute this largely to improvements in vascular surgical techniques. It has been shown that the damaged vascular segment must be excluded by resection or bypass, since intimal damage in the stretched portion of the vessel can predispose to recurrent thrombosis. We would add that besides the 1 patient in our series who required amputation, there were 2 other patients who were unable to work or had to retire because of postischemic changes. All 3 patients had ischemic periods of 5 h or longer. Thus, it cannot be overemphasized that every effort must be made to reestablish perfusion as expeditiously as possible. Especially in closed dislocations, the urgency of the situation is easily underestimated by those involved. Emergency admission and evaluation are not conducted with the necessary haste. Like Green and Allen (1977), we feel it is a serious mistake to move the patient to X-ray for arteriograms when there is suspicion of circulatory impairment or incipient compartment syndrome. This often delays surgery by 1–2 h. Another 1–2 h pass in the operating room until perfusion is reestablished in the limb. Adding to this the transport time from the accident scene, the critical 6-h limit is rapidly approached. This limit may be even lower in patients with soft-tissue injuries, depending on the degree of compromise of the periarticular collateral circulation. Vascular surgeons, moreover, tend to underestimate the urgency of the situation because they mostly see older vascular patients who have developed a competent collateral circulation prior to the acute obstruction and thus can better tolerate occlusion of the major vessel. It is understandable that they would wish to document the lesion and believe there is time to move the patient to X-ray for arteriograms. Thus, it may be incumbent on the orthopedist to stress the urgency and see to it that, after immediate life-saving measures have been instituted, blood drawn, and standard radiographs obtained, the patient is taken at once to the operating suite and the knee reduced under anesthesia. If normal pedal pulses do not return after this maneuver and there is doubt as to the underlying lesion, transfemoral arteriography can always be performed on the operating table. In the absence of pedal pulses, however, we agree with Green and Allen (1977), Jones et al. (1979), and Chapuis (1984) that preoperative arteriograms should be omitted altogether so that no time is lost. In any case the popliteal artery must be inspected as far as the bifurcation and excluded from the circulation in accordance with gross findings.

Recommendations for Operative Treatment

The first step in the anesthetized patient is to reduce the dislocated knee and then carefully test its stability on all planes. Because the structures are damaged on at least 3 sides, including the posterior capsule, the surgeon must approach the joint from 3 sides and wait for the proper moment to apply and adjust the external skeletal fixation material. All this must be taken into account during the tactical planning stage. It is important to appreciate the existing pattern of injury and repair all injuries in the shortest possible time with minimum repositioning, which may cause breach of asepsis. We have had the best results with the following procedure:

Starting with the patient in the supine position, a small area is prepared and sterilely draped for the insertion of 2 short Schanz screws each into the tibia and femur. The patient is then moved to the lateral position, the entire leg and hip are prepped and sterilely draped, and the popliteal artery is explored. As soon as blood flow has been reestablished, sutures are placed for repair of the posterior capsule and PCL. Then the patient is returned to the supine position, and the remaining ligament sutures are placed. At this point the rods are mounted on the Schanz screws, the knee is reduced with the aid of an image intensifier, and the rods are interconnected. The knee is fixed at the flexion angle that is most appropriate for the soft-tissue lesions, preferably at about 20° to permit weight-bearing ambulation. Two AP and lateral radiographs are taken, some while contrast medium is injected into the artery. If the reduction is not acceptable, it is corrected at this time, and more X-rays are taken. Finally, all the preplaced sutures are tightened and tied, a meticulous hemostasis is effected, and the soft tissues are closed. The leg can now be suspended by the external fixation material and supported on a splint so that the soft-tissue status, blood flow, and sensation can be continuously monitored all around the limb. Blood flow should be checked hourly for the first few days, regardless of whether or not vascular surgery has been performed.

Dislocation is the most severe soft-tissue injury of the knee joint and always carries the implicit threat of above-knee amputation. But with a highly organized, competent operating team that can be swiftly mobilized, today amputation can be avoided and a satisfactory functional result achieved in the majority of traumatically dislocated knees.

References

Chapuis G (1984) Les lésion vasculaires associées au traumatisme du genou. Helv Chir Acta 51: 575–580

De Bakey ME, Simeone FA (1946) Battle injuries of the arteries in World War II. Ann Surg 123: 534–579

Geneste R, Senegas J, Gautier D, Liorzou G (1972) Les luxations traumatiques du genou. Bordeaux Med 16: 2051–2058

Green NE, Allen BL (1977) Vascular injuries associatet with dislocation of the knee. J Bone Joint Surg [Am] 59 236–239

Honton JL, Le-Rebeller A et al. (1978) Luxation traumatiques du genou. Traitement précoce. À propos de 12 cas. Rev Chir Orthop 64: 213–219

Jacobson K (1974) Area intercondylaris tibiae: Osseous surface structure and its relation to soft tissue structures and applications to radiography. J Anat 117/3: 605–618

Jacobson K (1976) Stress radiographical measurement of the anteroposterior, medial and lateral stability of the knee joint. Acta Orthop Scand 47: 335–344

Jones RE, Smith EC, Bone GE (1979) Vascular and orthopedic complications of knee dislocation. Surg Gynecol Obstet 149: 554–558

Kennedy JC (1963) Complete dislocation of the knee joint. J Bone Joint Surg [Am] 45: 889–904

Meyers MH, Harvey JP (1971) Traumatic dislocation of the knee joint. J Bone and Joint Surg [Am] 53: 16–29

Myles JW (1967) Seven cases of traumatic dislocation of the knee. Proc R Soc Med 60/1: 279–281

O'Donoghue DH (1960) Surgical treatment of injuries to the knee. Clin Orthop 18: 11–36

Prafull V et al. (1975) Civilian arterial injuries. New York Medical college

Salter R. Field P (1960) The effect of continuous compression on living articular cartilage. Bone Joint Surg [Am] 42: 31–49

Shields L, Mohinder M, Cave EF (1969) Complete dislocation of the knee. Experience at the Massachusetts General Hospital. J Trauma 9/3: 192–215

Stäubli H-U, Noesberger B, Jakob RP (1983) The drawer sign of the knee in extension. A prospective study. Orthop Trans 7/3: 585

Taylor AR, Arden GP, Rainey HA (1972) Traumatic dislocation of the knee. J Bone Joint Surg [Br] 54: 96–102

Thomsen PB, Rud Bjarne, Jensen UH (1984) Stability and motion after traumatic dislocation of the knee. Acta Orthop Scand 55: 276–283

Tscherne H, Gotzen L (1983) Fraktur und Weichteilschaden. Hefte Unfallheilkd 162

Welling RE, Kakkasseril J, Cranley JJ (1981) Complete dislocation of the knee with popliteal vascular injury. J Trauma 21/6: 450–453

Injuries of the Collateral Ligaments and Menisci

Instability of the Medial Collateral Ligament: Operative or Nonoperative Treatment?

P. M. Ballmer and R. P. Jakob

Introduction

Based on favorable long-term results, O'Donoghue (1950, 1955) and later Hughston and Eilers (1973) advocated the operative treatment of injuries of the medial collateral ligament (MCL) of the knee. But the 98% success rate reported by Ellsasser et al. in 1974 following the conservative treatment of isolated medial collateral ligament tears led to renewed interest in the nonoperative management of this common ligamentous injury, which became the subject of further investigations (Bergfeld 1979; Derscheid and Garick 1981; Fetto and Marshall 1978; Hastings 1980; Indelicato 1983; Jones et al. 1986; O'Connor 1979). Although the outcomes in these studies are quite convincing, there are significant discrepancies in terms of diagnosis (especially the grading of injuries by severity), treatment methods, and follow-up criteria.

The purpose of this prospective study was to compare the results of two different methods of nonoperative treatment in precisely defined and documented complete MCL injuries.

Patients and Methods

Our study included all isolated lesions of the MCL that showed grade III instability and 2 + medial opening by the classification of Hughston et al. (1976). Grade I in this classification is a mild sprain (slight tenderness over the ligament attachment, no instability), grade II is a moderately severe sprain (marked collateral ligament tenderness, no instability), and grade III is a complete ligament tear resulting in 1 + to 3 + instability (where 1 + denotes up to 5 mm of medial opening, 2 + 6–10 mm, and 3 + more than 10 mm).

The clinical and radiologic assessments included stability testing of both knees under spinal anesthesia and an arthroscopic evaluation. The radiographic study (valgus stress film in 20°–30° flexion) provided objective documentation of the severity of the injury, while arthroscopy served to exclude intraarticular injuries (cruciate ligaments, menisci, cartilage). Treatment alternated between the use of an elastic wrap (latex-coated cotton bandage) for 8 weeks (group A) or immobilization in a plaster cast for 4 weeks followed by an elastic wrap for another 4 weeks (group B). In both groups only 10–15 kg of partial weight bearing was permitted on the injured limb for the first 4 weeks. The patients in group A were placed as soon as possible on a knee rehabilitation program consisting of muscle strengthening and range-of-motion exercises. The same rehabilitation program was started in the group B patients after the cast was removed.

Of the 23 patients (8 women, 15 men) who were seen from March, 1985, to December, 1986, with an isolated grade III tear of the MCL (2 + opening), 20 patients were followed for an average of 1 1/2 years (8–30 months). Their average age was 29.5 (16–51) years. In all patients the injury represented an initial, acute insult with a normal opposite knee. The injury was sports-related in 16 cases, and 4 injuries were sustained in other types of activity. In 19 cases arthroscopy of the knee was performed after an average of 7 (0–14) days, and in 1 case the workup was limited to examination under anesthesia and radiographic documentation.

During clinical examination under anesthesia, medial opening in extension was negative in 13 cases and positive (1 +) in 7. At 30° of flexion, there was 2 + medial opening in 20 cases. All the patients retained sagittal knee stability with a firm end point in flexion and near extension. The valgus stress radiographs showed an average increase of 7 mm of medial opening (minimum 6, maximum 10 mm) compared with the opposite side. In 9 cases arthroscopy disclosed a tear in the meniscotibial ligament complex measuring up to 20 mm, and in 5 cases it confirmed a tear in the meniscofemoral ligament measuring up to 10 mm. No additional intraarticular injuries (cruciate ligaments, menisci, cartilage) were present. Ten knees each were treated according to the group A and group B protocols. There were no significant differences between the two groups in initial clinical

Table 1. Subjective assessment

Excellent:	No pain No swelling No giving way Full return to preinjury activities
Good:	Nonrestricting pain with strenuous activity No swelling No giving way Full return to preinjury activities
Fair:	Pain at rest after strenuous activity Moderate swelling after strenuous activity Occasional giving way Return to preinjury activities, but at lower performance level
Poor:	Pain at rest unrelated to activity Severe swelling Giving way Return to different/less strenuous activities

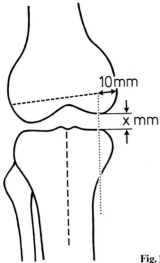

Fig. 1. Method of measurement

findings (including valgus stress radiographs) or arthroscopic findings.

All follow-up examinations were conducted by the authors themselves. Follow-up consisted of a subjective assessment (Table 1), a clinical examination including stability testing, and AP radiographs of both knees in 20° and 30° flexion during application of a 20-kp valgus stress. The amount of valgus opening was measured as the distance between the femoral condyle and the anterior border of the tibial plateau on the medial side. The measurement was performed 1 cm lateral to the medial border of the medial femoral condyle, on a line parallel to the long axis of the tibia (Fig. 1).

Results

Of the total of 20 patients, 8 in group A and 7 in group B had an excellent subjective result. The remaining 5 patients rated the result as good, i.e., they experienced nonrestricting pain during strenuous activity. Valgus testing in extension showed no abnormal medial opening in any patients of either group. In 30° flexion the clinical stability was identical to the opposite side in 3 patients of group A and 2 patients of group B, and 1 + medial opening was found in 7 patients of group A and 8 patients of group B. The valgus stress radiographs showed no right-left differences in 6 group A patients and 2 group B patients. A maximum of 3-mm medial opening was noted in 4 group A patients and 7 group B patients (in 1 patient radiographs were contraindicated due to pregnancy) (Table 2). Sagittal stability in flexion and near extension was normal in all cases, and equal ranges of motion were measured on both sides. There was no evidence of meniscal damage except in 1 patient demonstrating tenderness over the lateral meniscus. All patients who had participated in sports before the injury could return to full participation with no decline in performance and no external bracing or taping. No subsequent injuries have occurred. The average disability time was 6 1/2 weeks for group A and 9 1/2 weeks for group B.

Table 2. Medial instability (in 30° flexion) at the time of final follow-up

Group	Clinical		Radiographic	
	A	B	A	B[a]
0 (0–2 mm)	3	2	6	2
1 + (3–5 mm)	7	8	4	7
2 + (6–10 mm)	–	–	–	–
3 + (>10 mm)	–	–	–	–

[a] One patient did not undergo radiographic examination due to pregnancy.

Discussion

The anatomy of the MCL and its function are well documented in various studies (Hughston and Eilers 1973; Warren and Marshall 1979). Whereas nonoperative treatment is generally advocated for mild sprains of the MCL (grades I and II of Hughston et al. 1976), opinions differ as to the ideal treatment for a grade III injury. The difficulty of comparing published materials is compounded by differences in nomenclature and grading methods. There is no question that good long-term results are achieved by surgical repair (Hughston and Eilers 1973; O'Donoghue 1950, 1955). On the other hand, there are reports describing nonoperative approaches in the treatment of this lesion. An important factor in this regard is the division of cases into 1 + to 3 + to express the degree of instability. Fetto and Marshall (1978) show in their study that complete anatomic and functional ligament insufficiency (3 +) is combined in 78% of cases with concomitant internal derangement that require an operation. Thus, grade III lesions that are associated with no more than 10 mm of medial opening (1 + and 2 +) justify discussion with regard to the best mode of treatment. Besides the study of Ellsasser et al. (1974), the prospective study of Indelicato (1983) offers an important comparison of operative and nonoperative treatment results. Since nonoperative treatment is found to give equally good results with a significantly shorter rehabilitation period, a preference is stated for managing these injuries without surgery. Our late results support this position, although many patients have a minimal residual instability.

Due to the great variation in conservative treatment methods described in previous studies, and because none of the studies compare different treatments for lesions of identical grades (Derscheid and Garrick 1981; Ellsasser et al. 1974; Hastings 1980; Indelicato 1983; Jones et al. 1986), we selected 2 different treatment modalities. Our late follow-ups show no significant difference in subjective or objective results in patients mobilized early (group A) and patients immobilized in plaster for 4 weeks (group B). On the other hand, the earlier rehabilitation is reflected indirectly in the length of disability time, which is an average of 3 weeks shorter in group A. Besides the known advantages of early functional therapy in injuries of the locomotor system, the use of a supportive bandage saves time and money and is comfortable for the patient.

The arthroscopically confirmed tear of the deep layer of the MCL in our patients corresponds to the capsular defect described by Fritschy (1984). We can also confirm the good healing potential of this peripheral meniscal lesion, even with early mobilization. Moreover, grade III lesions that permit up to 10 mm of valgus opening probably do not cause significant damage to the posterior oblique ligament leading to anteromedial rotatory instability and pathology of the posterior horn of the medial meniscus (Biedert 1986).

In summary, we believe that early functional therapy is appropriate not just for an isolated grade I or grade II injury of the MCL but also for complete grade III lesions that permit up to 10 mm medial opening. While a mild degree of instability (1 +) in 30° flexion does not warrant further investigation, we believe that examination under anesthesia and diagnostic arthroscopy are indicated when the instability is 2 + (6–10 mm) or greater. Owing to the high diagnostic precision of arthroscopy in the acutely injured knee, associated lesions (cruciate ligaments, menisci, cartilage) that critically affect therapeutic decision making can be confidently excluded (Haftgoli-Bakhtiari 1981; Noyes et al. 1980). In no case did we find secondary sagittal instability, although Jones et al. (1986), in a prospective study of MCL ruptures not evaluated by arthroscopy, reported one case in which a tear of the ACL had been missed. Fetto and Marshall (1978) found that the very rare isolated grade III MCL injury with 3 + medial opening did equally well with nonoperative and operative treatment. This further underscores the value of nonoperative therapy for the complete lesion of the MCL.

References

Bergfeld J (1979) First-, second-, and third-degree sprains. Am J Sports Med 7: 207–209

Biedert R (1986) Spezielle Verletzungen des Semimembranosusecks. Schweiz Z Sportmed 34: 87–91

Derscheid GL, Garrick JG (1981) Medial collateral ligament injuries in football: Nonoperative management of grade I and grade II sprains. Am J Sports Med 9: 365–368

Ellsasser JC, Reynolds FC, Omohundro JR (1974) The nonoperative treatment of collateral ligament injuries of the knee in professional football players: An analysis of seventy-four injuries treated non-operatively and twenty-four injuries treated surgically. J Bone Joint Surg [Am] 56: 1185–1190

Fetto JF, Marshall JL (1978) Medial collateral ligament injuries of the knee: A rationale for treatment. Clin Orthop 132: 206–218

Fritschy D (1984) L'entorse méniscale moyenne. Schweiz Z Sportmed 32: 108–110

Haftgoli-Bakhtiari J (1981) Déchirure isolée du ligament croisé antérieur et arthroscopie. Med Hyg 39: 1621–1622

Hastings DE (1980) The non-operative management of collateral ligament injuries of the knee joint. Clin Orthop 147: 22–28

Hughston JC, Eilers AF (1973) The role of the posterior oblique ligament in repairs of acute medial (collateral) ligament tears of the knee. J Bone Joint Surg [Am] 55: 923–940

Hughston JC, Andrews JR, Cross MJ, Moschi A (1976) Classification of knee ligament instabilities, Part I: The medial compartment and cruciate ligaments. J Bone Joint Surg [Am] 58: 159–172

Indelicato PA (1983) Non-operative treatment of complete tears of the medial collateral ligament of the knee. J Bone Joint Surg [Am] 65: 323–329

Jones RE, Henley MB, Francis P (1986) Nonoperative management of isolated grad III collateral ligament inju-

324   P. M. Ballmer and R. P. Jakob

ry in high school football players. Clin Orthop 213: 137–140

Noyes FR, Bassett RW, Grood ES, Butler DL (1980) Arthroscopy in acute traumatic hemarthrosis of the knee: Incidence of anterior cruciate tears and other injuries. J Bone Joint Surg [Am] 62: 687–695

O'Connor GA (1979) Collateral ligament injuries of the joint. Am J Sports Med 7: 209–210

O'Donoghue DH (1950) Surgical treatment of fresh injuries to the major ligaments of the knee. J Bone Joint Surg [Am] 32: 721–737

O'Donoghue DH (1955) An analysis of end results of surgical treatment of major injuries to the ligaments of the knee. J Bone Joint Surg [Am] 37: 1–124

Warren LF, Marshall JL (1979) The supporting structures and layers on the medial side of the knee: An anatomical analysis. J Bone Joint Surg [Am] 61: 56–62

Treatment of Combined Injuries of the Anterior Cruciate Ligament and Medial Collateral Ligament Complex

P.M. Ballmer, F.T. Ballmer, and R.P. Jakob

Methods for the treatment of acute injuries of the anterior cruciate ligament (ACL) and medial collateral ligament (MCL) range from purely conservative management to repair of the MCL complex alone or the concomitant repair of both ligaments (Fetto and Marshall 1978; Hughston and Barrett 1985; Jokl et al. 1984; Warren and Marshall 1978b). Fetto and Marshall (1978) state that the good late results following the nonoperative or operative treatment of isolated MCL lesions depend mainly on the integrity of the ACL, so they emphasize the importance of repairing the ACL in addition to the MCL for combined injuries of both structures. Warran and Marshall (1978a, b) also place restoration of the cruciate ligament above the repair of the extraarticular restraints.

Thus, in the relatively frequent cases where injury of the MCL complex is associated with a tear of the ACL, the question arises whether reconstruction of the ACL alone would be sufficient to achieve stable healing of the MCL injury.

The goal of our prospective study was to analyze the results of ACL reconstruction alone in patients with complete ruptures of the ACL and MCL.

Materials and Methods

From January to April, 1988, 14 patients (5 women and 9 men) presented at the Department of Orthopedic Surgery of the University of Bern with a complete rupture of the ACL combined with a grade III lesion of the MCL. Ten of the patients had sports-related injuries, 4 were injured on the job. The average age of the patients was 30 (19–56) years. Clinical stability testing with comparison of both sides was supplemented by instrumented stressradiography under epidural anesthesia using a machine-applied stress of 20 kp (anterior and posterior drawer displacement and varus-valgus opening in 20°–30° flexion) (Figs. 1, 2). In all cases the injury was a first-time occurrence, and the opposite knee was uninjured except in 1 case where there was a contralateral lesion of the MCL.

The preoperative clinical and radiographic stability findings were graded using the standard classification system (Hughston et al. 1976; Jakob et al. 1987) and are summarized in Tables 1 and 2.

Preoperatively 13 patients had a midsubstance rupture of the ACL, which in 13 cases was repaired by arthroscopically assisted intraarticular ACL using the central one-third of the patellar tendon (see chapter by Ballmer and Jakob, p.437ff.; Clancy et al. 1982). One bony tibial ACL avulsion was reattached and augmented with the semitendinosus tendon. In 8 cases a deep tractopexy was added for lateral reinforcement. Of 4 patients with meniscal lesions, 2 underwent partial medial meniscectomy, 1 partial lateral meniscectomy, and 1 medial tear was sutured. All knees were mobilized early with unlimited flexion and an extension deficit of 5°–10° for the first 6–8 weeks. Eight patients wore an elastic wrap for 7–8 weeks of partial weight-bearing ambulation, and 6 wore a posterior plastic splint. Except for 1 below-

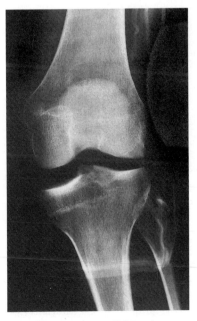

Fig. 1. Preoperative medial opening

326   P.M. Ballmer, F.T. Ballmer, and R.P. Jakob

Table 1. Preoperative clinical stability (n = 14)

		Frontal plane in 30° flexion		Sagittal plane in 30°, 70° flexion		Dynamic	
		Medial	Lateral	Anterior	Posterior	Pivot shift	Reversed pivot shift
0	(0–2 mm)	–	12	–	14	–	13
+	(3–5 mm)	–	2	–	–	4	1
+ +	(6–10 mm)	10	–	4	–	5	–
+ + +	(>10 mm)	4	–	10	–	5	–

Table 2. Preoperative radiographic stability (n = 14) (stress radiographs at 20 kp)

		Frontal plane in 20°–30° flexion		Sagittal plane in 20°–30° flexion	
		Medial	Lateral	Anterior	Posterior
0	(0–2 mm)	–	12	–	13
+	(3–5 mm)	–	2	–	1
+ +	(6–10 mm)	11	–	1	–
+ + +	(>10 mm)	3	–	13	–

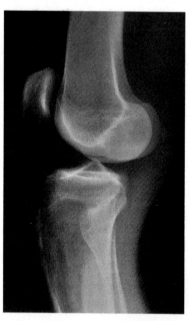

Fig. 2. Preoperative anterior drawer

knee thrombosis, there were no postoperative complications. The average hospital stay was 8 days. Follow-up included a subjective assessment in addition to a clinical examination of the knee joint, giving particular attention to stability. We also obtained instrumented stress radiographs at 20 kp (anterior drawer displacement and valgus opening in 20°–30°

flexion). The overall result was rated according to the scheme of Warren and Marshall (1978b).

Results

All the patients were followed for an average of 14 months (12–19 months). Twelve patients had no subjective complaints, while 2 reported minimal pain after strenuous physical activity. None of the patients complained of giving-way episodes or recurrent swelling. All athletically active patients returned to their preinjury level of participation.

Objectively, all the knees were free of effusion. Twelve patients had equal range of knee motion on both sides. One showed an extension deficit of 8° and another had 5° extension and flexion deficits relative to the opposite side. No patients exhibited meniscal symptoms. The clinical and radiographic stability data (Figs. 3, 4) for the ACL and MCL are summarized in Tables 3 and 4. Lateral opening, posterior drawer displacement, and reversed pivot shift corresponded to preoperative findings. The overall result was rated excellent in 11 cases, good in 2 cases, and fair in 1 case.

Discussion

Whereas grade III isolated tears of the MCL are now generally managed by nonoperative treatment (Ballmer and Jakob 1988; Ellsasser et al. 1974; Fetto and Marshall 1978; Indelicato 1983), there is diversity of opinion regarding the management of combined injuries affecting both the ACL and the MCL complex (Fetto and Marshall 1978; Hughston and Barrett 1983; Jokl et al. 1984; Shelbourne and Baele 1988; Warren and Marshall 1978b). Although the present study is preliminary in nature due to the small case numbers and relatively short follow-up, the results

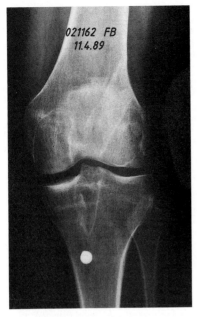

Fig.3. Medial opening 14 months postoperatively

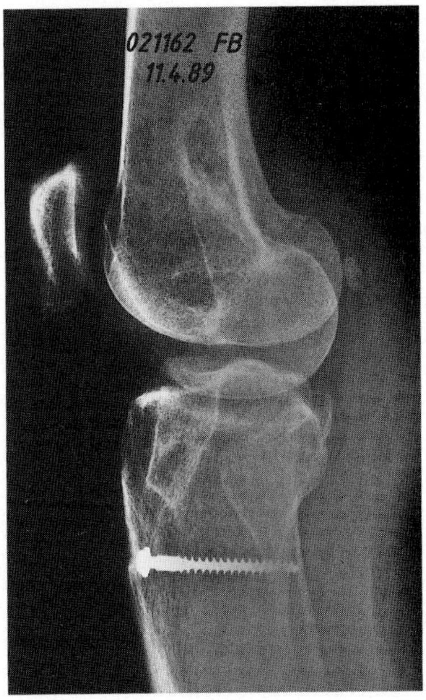

Fig.4. Anterior drawer 14 months postoperatively

Table 3. Preoperative clinical stability (n = 14)

		Medial opening in		Anterior tibial translation in mm		Pivot shift
		Extension	30° Flexion	30° Flexion	70° Flexion	
0	(0–2 mm)	14	12	9	13	13
+	(3–5 mm)	–	2	4	1	1
+ +	(6–10 mm)	–	–	1	–	–
+ + +	(>10 mm)	–	–	–	–	–

Table 4. Postoperative radiographic stability (n = 13)[a]

		Medial opening in 20°–30° flexion	Anterior tibial translation in 20°–30° flexion
0	(0–2 mm)	10	8
+	(3–5 mm)	3	4
+ +	(6–10 mm)	–	–
+ + +	(>10 mm)	–	–

[a] One patient did not undergo radiographic examination due to pregnancy.

support certain trends in the treatment of ligamentous knee injuries.

All the patients in our series were virtually asymptomatic at follow-up with no significant functional disability, reflecting good knee function with adequate ligament stability, a largely normal range of knee motion, and good muscular rehabilitation. In cases where combined ACL and MCL ruptures were managed nonoperatively, Jokl et al. (1984) observed functional problems in 30% of patients within only 6 months after the injury.

The medial opening measured in our series corresponds to the collateral ligament stability achieved under nonoperative treatment with an undamaged ACL and after surgical treatment with reconstruction of the ACL. This underscores the excellent healing potential of the torn MCL in the presence of a competent ACL (Ballmer and Jakob 1988; chapter by Ballmer et al., p.321ff.; Ellsasser et al. 1974; Fetto and Marshall 1978). With an isometric placement of the ACL substitute, postoperative functional therapy leads to no significant losses of sagittal stability; this is especially noteworthy when one considers the additional stress imposed on the graft in our series by initial absence of restraint by the MCL. The anterior tibial translation in flexion and near extension measured in our patients is very close to that measured after similar cruciate ligament reconstruction procedures (Clancy et al. 1982; Jakob et al. 1988). An important advantage of immediate knee rehabilitation is seen in the excellent range of knee motion, which can remain limited for years in knees that have been immobilized in a plaster cast or initially restricted in their motion (chapter by Ballmer et al., p. 293 ff.; Jakob et al. 1988).

The retrospective study of Shelbourne and Baele (1988) confirms our experience. The authors compared 13 reconstructions of the ACL and concomitant MCL repairs with 14 ACL reconstructions in which the torn MCL was treated nonoperatively. While stabilities were the same in both groups, they found a markedly more rapid rehabilitation with better knee function in the patients who underwent ACL reconstruction alone. The 3-year length of follow-up in their series suggests that our results will not change significantly with further passage of time.

In summary, we feel that reconstruction of the ACL alone in patients with combined injuries is sufficient to ensure stable healing of the untreated MCL lesion. Knee rehabilitation is accomplished through an early exercise program without significant loss of stability. Limiting factors in our present study are the relatively short follow-up period and the small patient population.

References

Ballmer PM, Jakob RP (1988) The non operative treatment of isolated complete tears of the medial collateral ligament of the knee. A prospective study. Arch Orthop Trauma Surg 107: 273–276

Clancy WG, Nelson DA, Reider B, Narechania RG (1982) Anterior cruciate ligament reconstruction using one-third of the patellar ligament augmented by exta-articular tendon transfer. J Bone Joint Surg [Am] 64: 352–359

Elsasser JC, Reynolds FC, Omohundro JR (1974) The nonoperative treatment of collateral ligament injuries of the knee in professional football players: an analysis of seventy-four injuries treated non-operatively and twenty-four injuries treated surgically. J Bone Joint Surg [Am] 56: 1185–1190

Fetto JF, Marshall JL (1978) Medial collateral ligament injuries of the knee: a rationale for treatment. Chir Orthop 132: 206–218

Hughston JC, Barrett GR (1983) Acute anteromedial rotatory instability. Long-term results of surgical repair. J Bone Joint Surg [Am] 65: 145–153

Hughston JC, Andrews JR, Cross MJ, Moschi A (1976) Classification of knee ligament instabilities I. The medial compartment and cruciate ligaments. J Bone Joint Surg [Am] 58: 159–172

Indelicato PA (1983) Non-operative treatment of complete tears of the medial collateral ligament of the knee. J Bone Joint Surg [Am] 65: 323–329

Jakob RP, Stäubli H-U, Deland J (1987) Grading the pivot shift. Objective tests with implications for treatment. J Bone Joint Surg [Br] 69: 294–299

Jakob RP, Kipfer W, Klaue K, Stäubli H-U, Gerber C (1988) Étude critique de la reconstruction du ligament croisé antérieur du genou par la plastie pédiculée sur le Hoffa à partir du tiers médian du tendon rotulien. Rev Chir Orthop 74: 44–51

Jokl P, Kaplan N, Stovell P, Keggi K (1984) Non-operative treatment of severe injuries to the medial and anterior cruciate ligaments of the knee. J Bone Joint Surg [Am] 66: 741–744

Shelbourne KD, Baele JR (1988) Treatment of combined anterior cruciate ligament and medial collateral ligament injuries. Am J Knee Surg 1: 56–58

Warren RF, Marshall JL (1978a) Injuries of the anterior cruciate and medial collateral ligaments of the knee: A retrospective analysis of clinical records. Part I. Clin Orthop 136: 191–197

Warren RF, Marshall JL (1978b) Injuries of the anterior cruciate and medial collateral ligaments of the knee. A long-term follow-up of 86 cases. Part II. Clin Orthop 136: 198–211

Meniscus Repairs

B. Moyen, J. L. Lerat, and H. Muller

The importance of the menisci and especially of the medial meniscus has been amply documented. The concept of meniscus repair has gained an established place as an alternative to meniscectomy.

The menisci transmit about half of the contact force in the medial compartment and even more in the lateral compartment (Walker and Erkman 1975). Seedhom and Hargreaves (1979 a,b) showed that the removal of 16%–34% of the meniscal tissue increases the contact forces between the articular surfaces by approximately 350%.

A number of studies (Gudde and Wagenknecht 1973; Johnson et al. 1974; Lynch et al. 1983; Lipscomb and Anderson 1986; Neyret et al. 1987) have shown that the incidence of degenerative changes is high (68%–88%) following meniscectomy in knees with a deficient anterior cruciate ligament (ACL).

The concept of meniscal repair dates back to 1863 (see Annandale 1985). King in 1936 demonstrated the importance of vascularity in the healing of meniscal tears. Recently Arnoczky and Warren (1982) showed that the peripheral 1/4 to 1/3 of the meniscus in adults is vascular and that 10%–20% of the periphery can undergo cicatricial healing. Clark and Ogden (1983) showed that the vascularized portion of the meniscus is relatively large until 14 years of age. Henning et al. (1987) estimate that approximately 20% of meniscal lesions occur within an area of potential scar formation; DeHaven (1985) estimates 15%–20%.

Measures That Promote Healing

Four primary approaches have been taken:

- Resection of the meniscal rim to a bleeding capsular bed (Cassidy and Shaffer 1981; DeHaven 1983). Henning et al. (1987) found that patients who had this procedure developed degenerative changes at a more rapid rate than patients with partial meniscectomy. Apparently this is because the meniscus is recessed away from contact with the load-bearing portion of the femoral condyle.

- Vascular access channels. This principle was originally developed by Scott et al. (1986), who showed that making perforations in the meniscus with a biopsy needle produced a slight but insignificant improvement of healing. This idea was adopted and experimentally confirmed by Zhongnan et al. (1986), who showed that radially placed vascular access channels 1.5 mm in diameter extending from the periphery of the meniscus to the longitudinal tear led to healing within 8 weeks in non-immobilized dogs.

- Use of a parameniscal synovial flap. Henning et al. (1986) use an arthroscopic rasp for parameniscal synovium abrasion. The arthroscope is passed through the intercondylar notch between the medial femoral condyle and posterior cruciate ligament to visualize the posterior horn of the medial meniscus. The rasp is introduced through a posteromedial arthrotomy. The inferior parameniscal synovium is broadly abraded under arthroscopic control. The middle third of the medial meniscus is approached through an anteromedial portal, and the lateral meniscus through a posterolateral arthrotomy. Henning et al. noted a 9% incidence of retearing at 6- to 13-month follow-up. This series can be compared to the peripheral rim resection technique, where the author found a 22% incidence of failures in 240 cases.

- Use of a fibrin clot. In 1988 Arnoczky et al. found in experimental dogs that a 2-mm defect in the avascular portion of the meniscus can consolidate when filled with a fibrin clot. The clot appears to function as a scaffolding for fibrous connective tissue proliferation. The reparative tissue differs from normal meniscal tissue but is morphologically identical to the scar tissue that forms in the vascular portion of the meniscus. This technique can easily be combined with others.

Arthroscopic Techniques

In most techniques the meniscus is repaired from "inside-to-outside" using a system of curved needles. Henning et al. (1986) use a needle with a slightly curved tip. They perform the repair with sutures introduced from the undersurface of the meniscus. Clancy and Graf (1983) use a flat double-lumen cannula interconnected by a channel so that 2 needles, linked by a single suture, can be passed simultaneously through the meniscus. Blackwood (personal communication) uses 2 curved needles that are introduced through a double cannula. The instrument is operated with 1 hand. Jakob et al. (1988) use a single needle that is passed through cannulas of varying curvature. The same needle is used to pass the suture a second time through the meniscal rim over a freely selected bridge of intact menuscus. Defrere and Franckart (1988) use Teflon-coated double cannulas whose ends are curved to match the selected approach to the torn meniscus. Rosenberg et al. (1986) use curved needles introduced through curved, malleable cannulas that can be adapted to different anatomic conditions. Morgan and Casscells (1986) prefer an outside-to-inside technique that avoids the risk of neurovascular damage during suturing of the posterior horn.

Open Techniques

DeHaven (1985) advocates careful preparation of the peripheral meniscal rim in the vascular zone. He repairs the meniscus with absorbable sutures placed at 3- to 4-mm intervals. The repair may be intra- or extracapsular, though DeHaven prefers the intracapsular technique. Gillquist and Oretorp (1982), Cassidy and Shaffer (1981), and Dolan (1983) prefer to tie the sutures outside the capsule. Bousquet et al. (1985) repair the meniscus with horizontal extracapsular sutures.

Healing Rates

A survey of recent publications shows that several factors appear to affect the healing rate of meniscal repairs. Healing proceeds at a markedly slower rate in an unstable knee (DeHaven 1985; Hamberg et al. 1983). Stone (1979) believes that the length of the meniscal tear has an unfavorable effect, although Rosenberg et al. (1986) question this. Stone (1979) insists on the importance of an anatomic coaptation of the sutured meniscus, stating that tears over 10 mm long should be repaired with sutures passed from the superior and inferior surfaces. The presence of multiple longitudinal tears is an unfavorable factor in terms of meniscal healing (Henning et al. 1986; Stone 1986).

Stone (1979) considers it advantageous to use nonabsorbable suture material, as this secures effective coaptation for a longer time. The sutures are placed at about 5-mm intervals. Jakob et al. (1988) use absorbable sutures in the central areas of the meniscus and nonabsorbable sutures in the periphery. These authors state that repair is probably not justified in patients over 35–40 years of age or in competitive athletes, who have a 12%–22% risk of retearing. Pouget (1988), Defrere and Franckart (1988), and Henning (1986) believe that the results are more favorable for the lateral meniscus, although their series are small.

Arthroscopy or Arthrotomy?

Two aspects must be considered in addressing this question: safety and efficacy.

DeHaven (1985) states that the time required for maturation of collagen healing is the same whether the repair is open or arthroscopic. On the other hand, the recommended postoperative immobilization tends to offset the theoretical advantage of arthroscopy over arthrotomy, especially since the use of a posterior counterincision is strongly recommended for safety in arthroscopic repairs.

Hazards of the Arthroscopic Technique

The following serious complications have been observed:

– Damage to the popliteal artery
– Peroneal and saphenous nerve palsy
– Deep venous thrombosis in the leg
– Infection, even in the hands of experienced arthroscopists

It is strongly recommended that a posterolateral or posteromedial counterincision be used so that the sutures can be tied directly over the capsule and not over the skin.

Efficacy of the Arthroscopic Technique

The results are variable: clinical, arthroscopic, arthrographic, and follow-up at 3–39 months. A series of 11 recent publications (1986–1988) report the occurrence of 48 reruptures in 294 cases (10.5%) over an average period of 22.5 months. The reported incidence of technical problems is 7.7%. The most common are saphenous nerve lesions and loss of joint motion, necessitating manipulation under anesthesia.

Favorable factors noted by several authors are:

– Repair of the lateral meniscus
– Repair in young patients
– Repair in a stable knee joint (with an intact or reconstructed ACL)

Most authors agree on the need for a posterior counterincision, which brings the procedure closer to an open repair. Jakob et al. (1988) note that a long tear with a relatively wide peripheral rim can be difficult to repair in an open operation.

On the medial side, transillumination is helpful for identifying the saphenous nerve. Jakob et al. (1988) suggest using a femoral distractor to expand the joint compartment and facilitate placement of the repair sutures.

The outside-in arthroscopic technique, though technically demanding (Morgan and Casscells 1986), can be useful for suturing the posterior horns due to the neurovascular risk and also for repairing the anterior horns due to the special technical difficulties encountered in that area.

Efficacy of Open Repair

This technique is the oldest (DeHaven 1981). The initial series from 1981 reports on 55 cases with 2 ruptures over a follow-up period of 12–48 months. In 1985 DeHaven published 155 cases managed by open repair and claimed that only 15%–20% of meniscal tears are suturable. He found no neurovascular complications. DeHaven recommends the use of vertical intracapsular sutures of absorbable material (4/0) placed at 3- to 4-mm intervals with a small, well curved needle. The limb is cast in 45° flexion for 2 weeks, then knee motion is limited to 30°–65° for another 2 weeks. Crutch ambulation with non-weight-bearing is continued for 7–8 weeks. DeHaven notes that the failure rate is 38% in cases where the ACL is absent and 5% in knees with a reconstructed ACL; 4% of repairs do not heal in cruciate ligament-stable joints.

Bousquet et al. (1985) report an 80% success rate in a series of meniscal repairs (starting in 1976). These authors immobilize the limb in plaster but allow full weight bearing, followed by rapid restoration of motion from 0 to 160° flexion.

Hamberg et al. (1983) report that 84% of 50 patients had clinically apparent healing of the sutured meniscal tear after a mean follow-up of 18 months. The operated limbs were cast in 30° flexion for 5 weeks with no weight bearing. At repeat arthroscopy, done in 67% of cases, all tears were found to be healed. In 35 repaired old tears, there was an 11% incidence of rerupture at the initial suture site and a 9% incidence of new tearing in an unsutured area.

Sommerlath (1988) showed that a repaired meniscus has the same prognosis as an intact meniscus in an unstable knee following cruciate ligament repair. Eighty-seven percent of the menisci were still intact after 7 years. Half of the tears were successfully repaired. This study in knees with residual laxity seems to imply that stabilization is not absolutely necessary to get a good prognosis for the repaired meniscus.

Activity reduction, good muscle function, and avoiding undue stress on the knee are equally important factors in ensuring a good outcome of open meniscal repairs.

Bornert and Pasquier (1987) found a 90% clinical success rate in 44 patients followed for 26 months.

Conclusions

Meniscus repair is a logical solution that can be performed by open or arthroscopic technique. Arthroscopic repairs are usually performed from the inside out. The failure rate at 2 years averages 10% or more.

This type of repair involves neurovascular risks, which are avoidable by employing appropriate techniques and aids. Another potential complication is the danger of postoperative joint stiffness.

Cicatricial healing is facilitated by a peripheral location of the meniscal tear.

The repair must effect a good coaptation of the torn edges. This is simple with a short meniscal tear. Tears longer than 1 cm require the use of nonabsorbable sutures passed from the superior and inferior surfaces. Various techniques such as radial perforations, parameniscal synovial flaps, and the use of a fibrin clot are currently being developed to improve the healing rate of meniscal repairs and extend the indication to the avascular portion of the meniscus. Repair is contraindicated in patients over 35 years of age and in patients engaging in vigorous competitive sports.

Most authors feel that there is a greater prospect of success when the repair is performed in a cruciate ligament-stable joint.

References

Annandale T (1985) An operation for displaced semi-lunar cartilage. Br Med J 1: 799

Arnoczky SP, Warren RF (1982) Microvasculature of the human meniscus. Am J Sports Med 10: 90-95

Arnoczky S, Warren RF, Spivak JM (1988) Meniscal repair using an exogenous fibrin clot. J Bone Joint Surg [Am] 70: 1209-1217

Bornert D, Pasquier G (1988) Réinsertion méniscale par arthrotomie. Journées Arthroscopiques d'ESNEUX, avril 1988

Bousquet G, Passot JP, Girardin P, Relave M, Gazielly D, Charmion L (1985) La réinsertion ou suture méniscale. 100 cas avec un recul de 12 ans. Rev Chir Orthop 71 [Suppl 2]: 119-120

Cassidy RE, Shaffer AJ (1981) Repairs of peripheral meniscal tears. Am J Sports Med 9: 209-214

Clancy N, Graf B (1983) Arthroscopic meniscal repair. Orthop Surg 6: 1125-1129

Clark CR, Ogden JA (1983) Development of the menisci of the human knee joint: morphological changes and their potential role on childhood meniscal injury. J Bone Joint Surg [Am] 65: 538-547

Defrère J, Franckart A (1988) Résultats des sutures méniscales par arthroscopie. Journées Arthroscopiques d'ESNEUX, avril 1988

DeHaven KE (1981) Peripheral meniscal repair: an alternative to meniscectomy. J Bone Joint Surg [Br] 63:463

DeHaven KE (1985) Meniscus repair open versus arthroscopic. Arthroscopy 1/3: 173-174

Dolan W (1983) Peripheral meniscus repair. A clinical and histopathologic study. Presented at AAOS annual meeting, Anaheim/CA

Gillquist J, Oretorp N (1982) Arthroscopic partial meniscectomy. Technique and long term results. Clin Orthop 167: 29-33

Gudde P, Wagenknecht R (1973) Untersuchungsergebnisse bei 50 Patienten 10-12 Jahre nach der Innenmeniskusoperation bei gleichzeitig vorliegender Ruptur des vorderen Kreuzbandes. Z Orthop 3: 369-372

Hamberg P, Gillquist J, Lysholm J (1983) Suture of new and old peripheral meniscus tears. J Bone Joint Surg [Am] 65: 193-197

Henning C, Clark J, Lynch M (1986) Closed meniscal repair with posterior incision. Read at AAOS New Orleans

Henning C, Lynch M, Clark R (1987) Vascularity for healing of meniscus repairs. Arthroscopy 3/1: 13-18

Jakob RP, Stäubli HU, Zuber K, Esser M (1988) The arthroscopic meniscal repair. Techniques and clinical experience. Am J Sports Med 16: 137-142

Johnson RS, Kettelkamp D, Clarke N, Leaverton P (1974) Factors affecting late results after meniscectomy. J Bone Joint Surg [Am] 56: 719-729

King D (1936) The function of the semi-lunar cartilages. J Bone Joint Surg [Am] 18: 1069-1076

Lipscomb AB, Anderson AF (1986) Tears of the anterior cruciate ligament in adolescents. J Bone Joint Surg [Am] 68: 19-28

Lynch M, Henning C, Glick K (1983) Knee joint surface changes long term follow up meniscus tear treatment in stable anterior cruciate ligament reconstructions. Clin Orthop 172: 148-152

Morgan C, Casscells W (1986) Arthroscopic meniscus repair: a safe approach to the posterior horns. Arthroscopy 2/1: 3-12

Neyret P, Dejour H, Walsh G, Trillat A (1987) La méniscectomie intra-murale d'Albert Trillat. Résultats fonctionnels et radiologiques à plus de 20 ans. SOFCOT, Paris

Pouget G (1988) 4 ans ½ de réinsertion méniscale sous arthroscopie. Journées Arthroscopiques d'ESNEUX, avril 1988

Rosenberg T, Scott S, Coward D, Dunbar W, Ewing J, Johnsons L, Paulos L (1986) Arthroscopic meniscal repair evaluation with repeat arthroscopy. Arthroscopy 2/1: 14

Ryu R, Dunbar W (1988) Arthroscopic meniscal repair with two years follow up. Arthroscopy 4/3: 168-173

Scott GA, Jolly BL, Henning CE (1986) Combined posterior incision and arthroscopic intra-articulair repair of the meniscus. J Bone Joint Surg [Am] 68: 847-861

Seedhom BB, Hargreaves DJ (1979a) Transmission on the load in the knee with special reference to the role of the menisci. Part I: Anatomy, analysis and apparatus. Eng Med 8: 207-219

Seedhom BB, Hargreaves DJ (1979b) Transmission on the load in the knee with special reference to the role of the menisci. Part II: Experimental results discussion and conclusions. Eng Med 8: 220-228

Seedhom BB, Donson D, Wright V (1974) Functions of the menisci. A preliminary study. J Bone Joint Surg [Br] 56: 381-382

Sommerlath K (1988) The prognosis of repaired and intact menisci in instable knees. A comparative study. Arthroscopy 4: 93-95

Stone RG (1979) Peripheral detachment of the menisci of the knee: a preliminary report. Orthop Clin North Am 10: 643-657

Walker PS, Erkman MJ (1975) The role of the menisci in force transmission across the knee. Clin Orthop 109: 184-190

Warren R (1985) Arthroscopic meniscus repair. Arthroscopy 1/3: 170-172

Zhonghan Z, Yinkan X, Wenming Z, Zhibua Z, Shihuan O (1986) Suture and immobilization of acute peripheral injuries of the meniscus in rabbits. Arthroscopy 2/4: 227-233

Meniscus Repair with Special Reference to Arthroscopic Technique

R. P. Jakob, P. M. Ballmer, K. Zuber, and H.-U. Stäubli

One of the most important challenges to reconstructive knee surgery is the preservation of a maximum amount of healthy meniscal tissue. The degenerative changes in the knee joint that follow total meniscectomy were vividly described by Fairbank in 1948, and "Fairbank's changes" were subsequently confirmed by other authors (Fairbank 1948; Jackson 1968; Krause et al. 1976; Tapper and Hoover 1969). Fairbank was the first to question the appropriateness of total meniscectomy. One of the most impressive studies to date is that of Johnson et al. (1974). In their study of patients 17 years after meniscectomy, 40% showed marked signs of osteoarthritis while only 6% showed similar changes in the opposite, nonoperated knee.

Ideally, conservative meniscus surgery should limit the resection to the damaged portion of the meniscus. Cox and Cordell (1977) showed in experimental animals that degenerative changes after partial meniscectomy are directly proportional to the extent of the meniscal resection, implying that partial meniscectomy has less serious consequences than complete meniscectomy. This observation has since been confirmed in studies of partial arthroscopic meniscectomies in humans (Jackson and Dandy 1976; Dandy 1978; Northmore-Ball and Dandy 1982; Tapper and Hoover 1969; Wirth 1981).

Attempts to preserve meniscal tissue have a long history. The first account of meniscal reattachment was published by Annandale in 1889 (quoted by Heatley 1980). King, in 1936, succeeded in reattaching a meniscus in a canine knee. This led him to conclude that a peripheral meniscal tear extending to the synovial boundary would heal well, whereas a central tear extending to the free border of the meniscus would not heal. This conjecture has since been confirmed to some degree. Cabaud et al. (1981), who sutured radial meniscal cuts in Rhesus monkeys, observed complete healing in 38% of the animals and partial healing in 56%.

The peripheral portion of the meniscus is well vascularized, so longitudinal tears through this area heal well. This good healing potential is confirmed by our experience with open meniscal surgery, which we use routinely for meniscal tears associated with peripheral capsuloligamentous injuries. Vertical repair sutures lead to stable healing in the majority of cases. Other authors confirm these good long-term results, provided there is no coexisting deficiency of the central pivot, i.e., of the cruciate ligaments (Cassidy and Schaffer 1981; DeHaven 1981, 1983, 1985a,b, 1988; Hamberg et al. 1983). If the repaired meniscus is exposed to the effects of recurrent subluxation episodes associated with a deficient anterior cruciate ligament (ACL), the prognosis is guarded, especially for lesions of the posterior horn, where stresses are particularly high.

A fresh meniscal tear is more amenable to repair than an older tear, although, with preliminary debridement, lesions several weeks or months old can be successfully repaired (Hamberg et al. 1983). With advances in arthroscopic meniscal surgery, efforts have been made in recent years to repair isolated meniscal tears from inside the joint. Several authors have recommended techniques that involve the use of specially designed instruments (Barber and Stone 1985; Clancy and Graf 1983; Henning 1983; Hendler 1984; Morgan and Casscells 1986; Rosenberg et al. 1985; Tiling and Röddecker 1986). We have done considerable work on the technical and practical problems of meniscus repair and since 1982 have sought to develop a simplified arthroscopic technique. In the present article we shall review current techniques, present our own technique, and review our clinical experience over the past 6 years. The technique of open repair is discussed in the chapter by Rodriguez (p. 343 ff.).

Current Techniques of Arthroscopic Meniscus Repair

Henning has the greatest experience with the arthroscopic repair technique. He uses a slightly curved Keith needle passed with a needle holder specially modified for arthroscopic use (Henning 1983; Scott

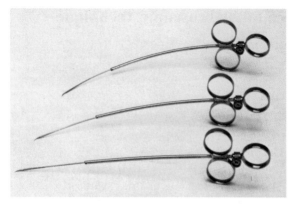

Fig. 1. Our arthroscopic meniscus repair system consists of 3 cannulas of varying curvature with needles 1.2 mm in diameter whose distal end fastens to a metal thumb ring. (From Jakob et al. 1988)

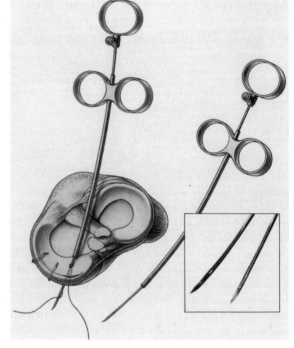

▷

Fig. 2. Technique of meniscus repair using the principle of the sewing-machine needle

et al. 1986). He emphasizes the importance of passing the sutures through the superior and inferior surfaces of the meniscus and recommends bringing the sutures out through a posteromedial and posterolateral incision in the skin and subcutaneous tissue and tying them over the intact capsule. A special spoonlike retractor is inserted behind the capsule to protect neurovascular structures. In our view, techniques that do not employ a posterior skin incision are obsolete and apt to cause serious complications. Henning also places much importance on preparation of the tear site by extensive debridement and synovial abrasion at the upper and lower surfaces to evoke a pannus-like synovial response.

Clancy and Graf (1983) use a double-lumen cannula through which 2 fine suture-armed needles are passed posteriorly through the meniscus. One problem with this apparently simple technique is that the meniscal posterior horn is difficult to reach in a small knee, due in part to the fixed channel that interconnects the 2 lumens of the instrument.

Rosenberg et al. (1985) have developed a special instrument set whose main feature is a doubly bent cannula that slips over the intercondylar eminence when inserted from the opposite side. The cannula is designed to facilitate the repair of posterior horn tears.

All these techniques, in which the needle pierces the meniscus from inside the joint and is retrieved on the outside ("inside-out"), offer the advantage of good visibility and simple manipulation of the pierced meniscus. We have developed a new instrument set to supplement these techniques (Jakob et al. 1988). Our objective was to find an instrument that can be operated with one hand, permits the use of thin cannulas of varying curvature for access to the posterior horn, and has a sharp tip that can accommodate different types of suture material. Our system consists of 3 cannulas of varying curvature with needles 1.2 mm in diameter that can be locked in a distal thumb ring (Fig. 1). The needle is perforated 15 mm from the tip to accept the suture material. The threaded needle pierces the meniscus and capsule from the inside, and the end of the suture is grasped in the posterior incision and held with a clamp. The needle is then retracted and readvanced through the meniscus and capsule over an intact meniscal bridge of 6–8 mm, producing a stitch similar to that of a sewing-machine needle. The second suture end is unthreaded from the needle and tied to the first end over the intact capsule (Fig. 2).

We shall illustrate this technique for the repair of a bucket-handle tear of the medial meniscus:

1. A lateral arthroscopic portal is established next to the patellar tendon, and a second portal is placed just medial to the tendon. A probe is inserted through this portal, and the meniscus is reduced; the blunt obturator may be used to assist this maneuver. The width of the peripheral meniscal

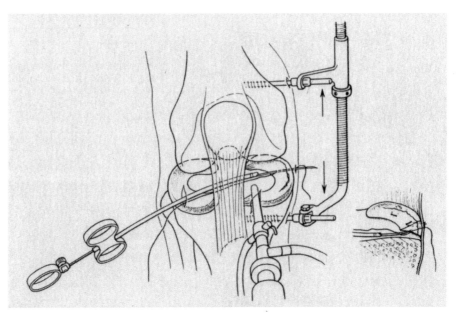

Fig. 3. Use of the ASIF distractor. (From Jakob et al. 1988)

rim is determined, and residual meniscal stability is assessed. The tear is classified as to type, giving attention to a possible 2nd bucket-handle tear or an unstable meniscal rim. The meniscus is debrided with a shaver passed through the anteromedial portal or a separate posteromedial portal until both margins of the tear are smooth. The synovium is freshened and abraded above and below the meniscus with the shaver or the special meniscal rasp developed by Henning.

2. The posteromedial or posterolateral approach is prepared. The saphenous nerve is identified on the medial side, and the peroneal nerve may be identified laterally, as the dissection is carried to the capsular surface. A retractor is inserted posteriorly to protect the neurovascular structures.

3. If necessary, the ASIF distractor or an external fixation device is applied across the joint (Fig. 3). This is done by inserting two Schanz screws, one proximally into the adductor tubercle of the femur and one 3 cm distal to the joint line. The device is mounted on the screws, and the proper amount of distraction is carefully applied. If the screws are inserted no deeper than 30 mm, there is no danger of laceration of the medial collateral ligament. We have observed in cadaver tests that the proximal Schanz screw loosens when excessive, forcible distraction is applied. The distraction improves visualization of the meniscal posterior horn, permitting a more accurate suturing technique and avoiding cartilage scoring from instrument man-

ipulations. Use of the distractor, considered by some to complicate the procedure unnecessarily, may be superfluous for experienced operators and in lax knee joints. It should be noted, however, that use of the distractor spares the assistant from having to hold the compartment open during the procedure.

4. Posterior horn sutures are placed using the most curved needle and cannula, which are passed through the ipsilateral portal. Sutures can be placed up to about 15 mm from the attachment of the posterior horn through this approach. The middle third of the medial meniscus is sutured with a less curved needle (Nos. 1, 2) introduced from the lateral portal. Four or 5 sutures are passed from the top surface of the meniscus and 3 or 4 sutures from the undersurface. The scope is used to confirm an anatomic repair (Figs. 4, 5).

5. The distractor is released, and the efficacy of the repair is checked by pulling on the sutures, which then are definitively tied over the capsule with moderate tension. The subcutaneous tissue and skin are closed.

We prefer to use nonabsorbable size 0 monofilament suture material (Dermalon) for the peripheral part of the meniscus, and absorbable material for more centrally placed sutures.

Postoperatively, we follow Henning's recommendations and immobilize the knee for 6 weeks in slight flexion with 20 kg of weight-bearing to exert a pe-

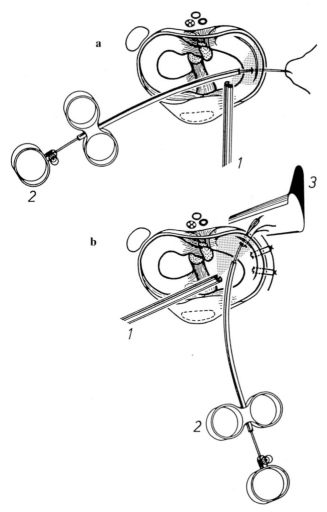

Table 1. Clinical material

Type of tear	Cases
Length 1–3 cm, meniscus displaceable anteriorly	41
Length 1–3 cm, meniscus not displaceable	12
Bucket-handle tear not involving the anterior horn	34
Bucket-handle tear involving the anterior horn	6
Total	93

Table 2. Suture materials used for the repairs

Suture material	Cases
Absorbable	35
Nonabsorbable	37
Combined	14
Unknown	7
Total	93

Table 3. Subjective results (n = 67)

	0	(+)	1+	2+
No complaints	48	–	–	–
Sensitivity to weather changes	–	3	7	–
Difficulty climbing stairs	–	2	2	–
Pain	–	7	1	1
Swelling	–	7	1	–
Locking	–	1	1	–

Fig. 4. Introduction of the needle through a contralateral (**a**) and ipsilateral (**b**) portal. (From Jakob et al. 1988)

ripherally directed force on the repaired meniscus. Lately we have changed to a 20°–80° limited motion regime. Sports participation is prohibited for 4 months.

Clinical Material (Table 1)

We repaired 93 menisci from 1982 to 1987. The average patient age was 28 1/2 years (13–60 years). Seventy-one tears involved the medial meniscus, 22 the lateral meniscus; 87 lesions were in the posterior horn or middle third, and only 6 involved the anterior horn. All lesions were longitudinal tears involving the peripheral 5 mm of the meniscus. We did not repair horizontal or transverse tears. The types of suture material used are listed in Table 2.

Sixty-seven patients had an isolated meniscal tear. Eighteen patients had an acute or chronic lesion of the anterior cruciate ligament that was repaired by open or arthroscopic surgery at the time of the meniscus repair or several weeks later. Eight patients were found to have a partial tear of the anterior or posterior cruciate ligament, which was not repaired.

Results

Sixty-seven patients (without reoperation) with a minimum postoperative course of 6 months were available for follow-up after an average of 20 months (6–51 months). Forty-eight of the patients (72%) were completely asymptomatic; the symptoms in the remaining 19 patients are listed in Table 3.

Follow-up arthrography performed in 29 patients 4 months after the repair disclosed 7 cases of incomplete healing. Only 4 of these patients had occasional complaints.

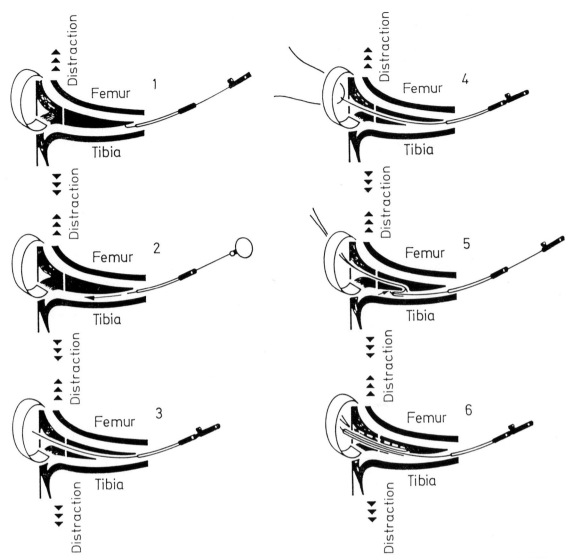

Fig. 5. Technique of arthroscopic repair in which the needle pierces the undersurface of the meniscus. (From Jakob et al. 1988)

Retearing occurred in 15 cases (18%). Nine were caused by mild trauma sustained 2 1/2–24 months postoperatively, and 6 by a significant injury occurring after the repair. Eleven of the 15 tears involved the medial meniscus, 4 the lateral meniscus.

Thirteen of the 15 reruptures were treated by partial meniscectomy, and 2 by a second repair; both were successful.

With regard to the functional status of the operated knees, we found that 28 patients could participate freely in sports, while 24 could participate at a reduced level. Fifteen patients did not engage in sports activities.

Discussion

Our results over an average 20-month follow-up indicate an overall healing rate of 82% with a rerupture rate of 18%. These results are comparable to those of Henning (1983). It should be noted, however, that Henning routinely performed follow-up arthrography 2–4 months postoperatively and found clinical and arthrographic healing in 59% of cases, no healing in 23%, and partial healing in 18% although the latter menisci were clinically stable and indolent. It may be assumed that our series also includes several clinically stable cases that would show incomplete healing by arthrography and thus would be subject to an in-

Table 4. Factors that affect healing

Age of patient	
Type of meniscal tear:	Longitudinal, transverse, horizontal, medial, lateral
Suture preparation and technique:	Debridement, synovialization, fibrin clot, distraction, vascular access channels
Suture material:	Absorbable, permanent
Associated lesions:	Anterior and posterior cruciate ligament, collateral ligament
Postoperative care:	Immobilization vs. mobilization
Activities:	Occupational and recreational

creased risk of retearing. Our age distribution matches that of Henning's population, with a peak between 15 and 30 years.

With regard to healing rate, Henning (1983; Scott et al. 1986) states that the lateral meniscus, though affected less frequently, shows a somewhat better healing potential.

Factors affecting the course and rate of meniscal healing are listed in Table 4.

Patient Age

Scapinelli (1968) and Arnoczky and Warren (1982) have shown that 10%–25% of the peripheral portion of the meniscus has a blood supply. Clark and Ogden (1983) found a gradual age-dependent decrease in meniscal blood flow. Whereas the fetal meniscus has a rich vascularity that extends into the central third, by 11 years of age few remaining blood vessels can be found in the central areas. Thus, one would likely find a better blood supply in the menisci of 20- to 30-year-old patients than in the 50-year-old or older cadaveric menisci examined by Arnoczky and Warren. This assumption is also supported by the observations of Stone (1979), who found a blood supply up to 6 mm from the periphery in his patients, who averaged 28 years of age.

Although the incidence of reruptures is no higher in our older patients, we would repair only very peripheral meniscal detachments in patients over 40 years of age, first because the vascularity is reduced after age 40 and second because postmeniscectomy degenerative changes develop over a period of 15–20 years.

Type of Meniscal Tear

Longitudinal and radial tears have been repaired in experimental animals. Henning (1983) recognizes a very broad scope of indications, repairing longitudinal tears with a peripheral white rim up to 5 mm. He sutures radial tears provided there is an intact outer bridge of 3 mm, and lateral meniscal tears if resection would sacrifice more than 1/4 of the whole meniscus. We take a more cautious approach, limiting repairs to longitudinal tears that are at least 15 mm long and have no more than a 3- to 4-mm white rim.

Suture Preparation and Technique

One mechanism of meniscal healing is based on intramural scar formation induced by the meniscal vascular network and thus is restricted to the peripheral 25% of the meniscal cross section that is vascularized (Arnoczky 1984; Arnoczky and Warren 1982). Although there is evidence in animal models that the placement of vascular access channels can stimulate the vascularization of more central areas, the healing produced by this mechanism is probably less stable. Additionally, it has been observed that a more mechanically effective reparative process proceeds from the upper and lower surfaces through the formation of a stabilizing synovial pannus on the sutured meniscus (Fabbriciani 1986). Attention should be given to both healing processes during preparation of the repair site. Intramural healing is possible only if the meniscus is adequately debrided and cleared of loose debris. The goal is to create fresh bleeding surfaces, which is especially important in lesions several weeks old. A fine basket forceps or small shaver head can be passed through an anterior or posterior portal to the rupture site. Generally this is easier once the bucket-handle tear has been reduced. Second or third tears should be sparingly resected.

Synovialization, as recommended by Henning, is induced by roughening the synovium at the meniscal border with a special arthroscopic rasp or with a small basket forceps and shaver until bleeding surfaces are obtained.

Henning (1983) and Arnoczky (1984) advocate the insertion of a fibrin clot into the repair site to stimulate and support a reparative response. The clot is prepared by precipitating clot material in a flask, rinsing and blotting the clot on sterile compresses, and injecting it into the tear with a special syringe before the sutures are tightened. In Europe, this complicated process can be replaced by the use of fibrin adhesive (Milachowsky et al. 1985). Jonson (1985) prefers to open the tourniquet and cause blood to flow through the tear by holding the suction tip at that site to promote the formation of a fibrin clot.

It is of critical importance to obtain an anatomic repair; this is essential if the meniscus is to perform its complex functions. When the first 2 sutures are placed, care is taken that the meniscal rim is accurately apposed to the periphery. This is accomplished by passing sutures from the superior and inferior surfaces of the meniscus and testing their action by carefully applying tension to the threads before they are tied. The difficulty of this maneuver, especially for the less experienced surgeon, makes use of the distractor worthwhile. Although arthroscopists are hesitant to use this device, we emphasize the value of this technique, also recommended by Henning, during instruction. There are 2 reasons why we take this position: First, the repair is technically easier owing to the enhanced exposure of the posterior horn. The upper and lower meniscal surfaces can be visualized during placement of the sutures, which can be spaced more closely at intervals of about 8–10 mm. The distractor also reduces instrumental scoring of the cartilage, which can cause permanent damage to the lamina splendens.

Suture Material

Initially we used absorbable suture material exclusively, but increasingly we have come to favor permanent material for peripheral lesions. A review of our patients showed a significantly greater incidence of retearing when absorbable material had been used. Of our 15 reruptures, 10 had been sutured with absorbable material, 1 with nonabsorbable material, and 2 with a combination of both; in 2 cases the suture material had not been specified. Today we tend to use nonabsorbable size 0 suture material for the periphery of the meniscus and absorbable material for the center. It is conceivable that nonabsorbable material on the meniscal surface might damage the articular cartilage, but we find no evidence for this in the literature. Barber and Stone (1985) contend that permanent suture material is not harmful.

Associated Lesions

Compared with the literature, we have by far the largest series of isolated meniscal tears. Henning (1983) reports on 37 isolated meniscal lesions and 140 coexisting with ACL insufficiency. This discrepancy results from the fact that, until mid-1987, we per-

formed cruciate ligament repairs and reconstructions by open arthrotomy and also performed meniscus repairs by an open or arthroscopy-like technique using the arthroscopic suture set. This eliminates many "combined" meniscal tears.

The intact ACL "guards" the posterior horns of the menisci. Conversely, the chronically deficient ACL subjects the intact posterior horn to excessive stresses, frequently resulting in tears of that segment. A well-known phenomenon in this setting is Finochietto's sign, caused by entrapment of the posterior horn of the meniscus during the anterior drawer test. Theoretically, then, the arthroscopic or open meniscus repair becomes a high-risk procedure when the ACL is deficient. Indeed, a significantly higher rerupture rate is seen after posterior meniscal repairs, as DeHaven (1985a, b, 1988) in particular has emphasized.

We would go so far as to state that a detached meniscus should be considered repairable only if the patient is ready to accept reconstruction of the ACL. Otherwise the cost/benefit ratio of 6 weeks' immobilization and 4 months' activity restriction is unacceptable due to the risk of retearing. Technically, 2 options are available in these cases. First, the meniscus can be arthroscopically repaired and the ACL reconstruction performed 2 weeks later. Today we do both procedures simultaneously using arthroscopic technique. In exceptional cases it may be decided to combine meniscal repair with an extraarticular ACL reconstruction in the patient with a complete peripheral meniscal detachment and an acutely torn ACL. These therapeutic eventualities should be discussed with the patient in advance whenever possible. Epidural anesthesia is advantageous in this regard, as it enables the surgeon to discuss intraoperatively the procedure that is best for the patient.

In acute "unhappy triad" injuries with complete rupture of the medial collateral ligament, detachment of the medial meniscus, and rupture of the ACL, we have introduced a further simplification by reattaching the meniscus and reconstructing the ACL (patellar tendon transfer) arthroscopically while leaving the medial collateral ligament alone. The limb is carefully mobilized during the first 6 weeks. Results to date with this method are encouraging.

Immobilization

Postoperatively we have always favored immobilizing the limb in a posterior splint for 5–6 weeks. We believe that continued motion of the knee, even over a limited range of 20°–60° as practiced by some authors, cannot serve to promote healing. Recent studies by Arnoczky (1984) show that during the healing process, a thin layer of fibrin is laid down within the rupture site and becomes organized and stabilized into a fibrinous callus. Arnoczky contends that absolute immobility is more conducive to undisturbed healing and strengthening of this callus than mobilization. The limb should be immobilized in a slightly flexed position, as this provides sufficiently close contact between the femoral condyles and tibial plateau to press the meniscus toward the periphery.

Activity

We have our patients refrain from sports activities for 4 months after surgery. This appears to be adequate for the slow progression of stable collagen healing.

Complications

The American literature initially contained reports of neurovascular damage caused by perforation of the needle into the popliteal fossa. Later this complication became far less common owing to the use of a posterior counterincision, protection of the posterior structures with a finger or special retractor, the use of curved needles, and warnings issued at arthroscopic conferences and courses. No instances of this problem have been reported in the past 2 years. Nevertheless, great care should still be taken to avoid complications. The saphenous nerve and vein must be protected on the medial side, and the popliteal vessels and nerves are vulnerable during the placement of posterior horn sutures. On the lateral side, sutures placed posterior to the fibular head pose a risk of peroneal nerve injury. Once again, the distrac-

tor can reduce the risk of lesions by permitting better visualization of endangered structures.

Aware of the hazards of inside-out repair techniques, Warren (quoted by Morgan and Cascells 1986) introduced an outside-in technique that has become increasingly accepted and utilized in recent years. The technique is as follows (Fig. 6): The meniscus is punctured with 2 spinal needles inserted through a posteromedial or posterolateral incision that exposes the capsule; the needles, spaced about 6 mm apart, should pierce the central portion of the torn meniscus. Sutures are passed through the needles so that a suture end emerges from one needle and a loop of suture through the other. A grasping tool is then passed into the joint through an anterior portal, and the suture end is pulled through the loop under arthroscopic vision. Finally the loop is withdrawn, bringing the suture end outside the capsule, where it is tied (Fig. 6). A somewhat more convenient technique, which requires the use of absorbable material but is attractive for its simplicity (we use it mainly on the anterior horn), is the button suture technique described by Tiling and Röddecker (1986) (Fig. 7). Again, a spinal needle is used to pass a suture through the torn meniscus from outside to inside. The suture end is retrieved inside the joint with a grasping forceps and brought out through a second portal. There, several small buttons are threaded over the suture to form a cone-shaped disk, which is pulled back into the joint against the meniscus to hold the stitch in place. The suture is tied to a second, adjacent suture placed 1 cm away.

Anyone who performs these two techniques, especially the first one, will quickly realize that they are more technically difficult than they appear. Problems arise during the correct placement of the needle (which can easily score the articular cartilage surfaces), during anatomic reduction of the tear due to

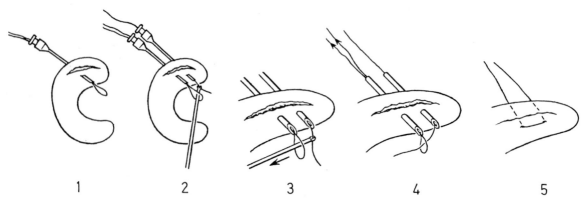

1   2   3   4   5

Fig. 6. The outside-in technique of Warren (quoted in Morgan and Casscells 1986)

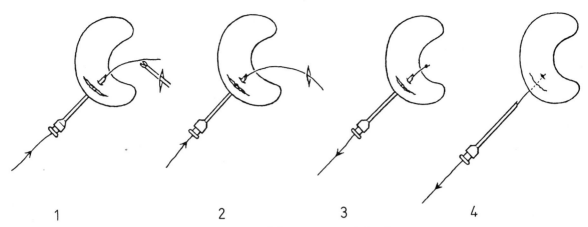

Fig. 7. Outside-in technique of Tiling and Röddecker (1986) (button suture technique)

the tendency of the needle to push the meniscus into the joint, and during the difficult intraarticular thread manipulations. Anyone who masters both the inside-out and the outside-in techniques will soon realize that repairs can be effected more quickly in most situations by the one-handed inside-to-outside technique. Individual experience with both techniques should be taken into consideration, however. We recommend using a combination of both techniques; the outside-in technique is excellent for the extreme posterior horn and the anterior horn.

Future studies are needed to compare arthroscopic and open techniques for the repair of isolated meniscal tears. Basically, it probably does not matter whether the meniscus is repaired from the outside or inside, as long as the surgeon can anatomically reduce and secure the meniscus with an equal number of stitches without sacrifice of meniscal tissue. We believe that arthroscopic repair is most advantageous for a longitudinal tear located 3–4 mm from the peripheral rim. Open repair is difficult in these cases, because the 3- to 4-mm white rim hampers exposure and impedes access to the central portion of the torn meniscus. It would be wrong to improve exposure by resecting the white rim and pulling the thin central portion of the meniscus outward, as this would significantly alter meniscofemoral congruity and thus defeat the purpose of the repair. Arthroscopic meniscus repair, moreover, is a logical next step for the surgeon who has mastered arthroscopic resection techniques. Since the arthroscope and instrument portal are already in place, following the arthroscopic diagnosis of a repairable meniscus tear, it is a simple matter technically to extend the procedure to a meniscus repair. For a peripheral meniscal tear, open repair is less demanding in terms of instrumentation and operator skill, and the repair can be accomplished more quickly in some circumstances. We doubt that the broad capsular incision necessitated by open repair is a disadvantage. Analogous to the perimeniscal synovial abrasion that is so important in arthroscopic repairs, the arthrotomy can be viewed as advantageous in that it creates a more favorable healing environment. We believe that both techniques should be applied with appropriate care, and we caution the arthroscopic surgeon against "making do" with 1–3 repair sutures, a temptation for the novice due to the technical difficulty of the procedure. An inadequate suture line is the pivotal factor behind the trend toward somewhat less favorable results of arthroscopic repairs. We again emphasize the value of the femoral distractor in this technically challenging situation.

Advocates of arthrotomy contend that the posterior open approach to the meniscus is simpler than the arthroscopic approach. Having practiced both techniques in the past, we believe that every surgeon should select the technique that appears to be the simplest yet still produces gratifying results.

The results of open and arthroscopic repairs are comparable, each showing a rerupture rate of 15%–20%. Several studies cite somewhat better statistics for open repairs. This may stem from the fact that the arthroscopist is more apt to repair a "borderline case," such as a tear with a 4- to 5-mm peripheral white rim, which would be sacrificed in an open operation.

It remains to be determined whether the benefits of meniscus repair, whether open or arthroscopic, justify its substantial cost. We still know little about the quality of the repaired meniscus. Can it adequately perform its intended functions of shock absorption, lubrication, congruity enhancement, and stabilization, or will the meniscus-stabilizing synovial pannus, which can significantly alter the surface of the meniscus, incite the development of degenerative joint changes like those following partial or complete meniscectomy? Follow-ups of 10–20 years will be needed, along with additional basic research, before this question can be answered.

The authors thank Mr. C. Langenegger (Figs. 4, 5), Department of Instructional Media, University of Bern and Inselspital Bern, and Mr. K. Oberli, Bern, for providing the illustrations.

References

Arnoczky SP (1984) Meniscal healing, regeneration, and repair. Adv Orthop Surg 7: 244–252

Arnoczky SP, Warren RF (1982) Microvasculature of the human meniscus. Am J Sports Med 10: 90–95

Barber FA, Stone RG (1985) Meniscal repair, an arthroscopic technique. J Bone Joint Surg [Br] 67: 39–41

Cabaud HE, Rodkey WG, Fitzwater JE (1981) Medial meniscus repair, an experimental and morphologic study. Am J Sports Med 9: 129–134

Cassidy RE, Shaffer AJ (1981) Repair of peripheral meniscus tears, a preliminary report. Am J Sports Med 9: 209–214

Clancy WG, Graf BK (1983) Arthroscopic meniscal repair. Orthopedics 6/9: 1125–1129

Clark CR, Ogden JA (1983) Development of the menisci of the human knee joint: morphological changes and their potential role in childhood meniscal injury. J Bone Joint Surg [Am] 65: 538–547

Cox JS, Cordell LD (1977) The degenerative effects of medial meniscus tears in dogs' knees. Clin Orthop 125: 236–242

Dandy DJ (1978) Early results of closed partial meniscectomy. Br Med J I: 1099

DeHaven KE (1981) Commentary. Repair of peripheral meniscus tears, a preliminary report. Am J Sports Med 9: 213–214

DeHaven KE (1983) Peripheral meniscus repair — 3–7 year results. Orthop Trans 7/3: 576

DeHaven KE (1985a) Meniscus repair — open versus arthroscopic. Arthroscopy 1: 173–174

DeHaven KE (1985b) Meniscus repair in the athlete. Clin Orthop 198: 31–35

DeHaven KE (1988) Meniscal repair, introductory lecture. Third Congress of the European Society of Knee Surgery and Arthroscopy, May 16–20, 1988, Amsterdam

Fabbriciani C (1986) Experimental meniscal repair lecture. 2nd Congress of the European Society of Knee Surgery and Arthroscopy, May 1986, Basel

Fairbank TJ (1948) Knee joint changes after meniscectomy. J Bone Joint Surg [Br] 30: 664–670

Hamberg P, Gillquist J, Lysholm J (1983) Suture of new and old peripheral meniscus tears. J Bone Joint Surg [Am] 65: 193–197

Heatley FW (1980) The meniscus — can it be repaired? An experimental investigation in rabbits. J Bone Joint Surg [Br] 62: 397–402

Hendler RC (1984) Arthroscopic meniscal repair, surgical technique. Clin Orthop 190: 163–169

Henning CE (1985) Arthroscopic repair of meniscus tears. Orthopedics 6/9: 1130–1132

Jackson JP (1968) Degenerative changes in the knee after meniscectomy. Br Med J 2: 525–527

Jackson RW, Dandy DJ (1976) Partial meniscectomy. J Bone Joint Surg [Br] 58: 142

Jakob RP, Stäubli H-U, Zuber K, Esser M (1988) The arthroscopic meniscal repair, techniques and clinical experience. Am J Sports Med 16/2: 137–142

Johnson L (1985) Diagnostic and surgical arthroscopy, 3rd edn. Mosby, St. Louis

Johnson RJ, Kettlekamp DB, Clark W et al. (1974) Factors affecting late results after meniscectomy. J Bone Joint Surg [Am] 56: 719–729

King D (1936) The healing of the similunar cartilages. J Bone Joint Surg 18: 333–342

Krause WR, Pope MH, Johnson RJ et al. (1976) Mechanical changes in the knee after meniscectomy. J Bone Joint Surg [Am] 58: 599–604

McGinty JB, Geuss LF, Marvin RA (1977) Partial or total meniscectomy. A comparative analysis. J Bone Joint Surg [Am] 59: 763–766

Milachowsky KA, Wiesmeier K, Wirth CJ et al. (1985) Die Meniskopexie — tierexperimentelle Untersuchungen zur Naht und Fibrinklebung der frischen und veralteten Meniscusläsion. Hefte Unfallheilkd 174: 94–96

Morgan CD, Casscells SW (1986) Arthroscopic meniscus repair: a safe approach to the posterior hours. Arthroscopy 2/1: 3–12

Northmore-Ball MD, Dandy DJ (1982) Long-term results of arthroscopic partial meniscectomy. Clin Orthop 167: 34–42

Northmore-Ball MD, Dandy DJ, Jackson RW (1983) Arthroscopic, open partial and total meniscectomy. A comparative study. J Bone Joint Surg [Br] 65: 400–404

Rosenberg T, Scott S, Paulos L (1985) Arthroscopic surgery: repair of peripheral detachment of the meniscus. Contemp Orthop 10/3: 43–50

Scapinelli R (1968) Studies on the vasculature of the human knee joint. Acta Anat 70: 305–331

Scott GA, Jolly BL, Henning CE (1986) Combined posterior incision and arthroscopic intra-articular repair of the meniscus. An examination of factors affecting healing. J Bone Joint Surg [Am] 68: 847–861

Stone RG (1979) Peripheral detachment of the menisci of the knee: A preliminary report. Orthop Clin North Am 10: 643–657

Tapper EM, Hoover NW (1969) Late results after meniscectomy. J Bone Joint Surg [Am] 51: 517–526

Tiling T, Röddecker K (1986) Knieinstabilität und Meniskusschaden, Bd II. Enke, Stuttgart

Wirth CR (1981) Meniscus repair. Clin Orthop 157: 153–160

Open Meniscus Repair:
Technique, Postoperative Treatment, and Results

M. Rodriguez

In recent years there has been a growing appreciation of the menisci as an important component of the healthy knee joint. Whereas for decades meniscectomy was deemed the treatment of choice for all meniscal lesions, today there is a trend toward reconstructive knee surgery that seeks to preserve a maximum amount of meniscal tissue, despite initial skepticism regarding meniscus repair. The major impetus for meniscus salvage has been proof that the subtotal or total removal of a meniscus leads to the long-term sequelae of *osteoarthritis* and *instability*.

Numerous long-term follow-ups after meniscectomy in diverse populations using various criteria have shown that meniscectomy is almost invariably followed by a unilateral and asymmetrical compartmental osteoarthritis (85% according to Tapper and Hoover 1969; 82% according to Schreiber and Dexel 1979; 70% according to Ricklin et al. 1980; 97% according to Puhl et al. 1981; 18.3% according to Allen et al. 1984). This is due to the fact that meniscectomy alters the pattern of stress transfer within the joint (Fairbank 1948; Böhler 1955; Jackson 1968; Kettelkamp and Jacobs 1972; Cotta and Puhl 1976) and leads to a reduced contact area with increased loading of the tibial plateau. These effects are directly proportional to the extent of the meniscal resection (Kettelkamp and Jacobs 1972; Hehne et al. 1981; Maquet 1984; Bourne et al. 1984; Barat et al. 1986).

Knee instability also has been demonstrated clinically and experimentally as a sequel to meniscectomy (e.g., Johnson et al. 1974; Hughston 1975; Oretorp et al. 1978; Müller 1982), appearing not just as an increase of rotation in the affected compartment but also as an increase of varus-valgus laxity (Wang and Walker 1974; Bracker et al. 1982).

The rationale for total meniscectomy was based on the belief that the residual rim would form a nidus for subsequent formation of a regenerative meniscus (Möller 1920; Mandl 1929; Smillie 1944; Courvoisier 1959; Elmer et al. 1977; Arnoczky et al. 1985). The best that could be hoped for, however, was the formation of a thin "pseudoregenerate" composed of non-cartilaginous connective tissue, as Dietrick (1931), King (1936), and Will-Hofmann (1985) demon-strated. The functional incompetence of this tissue is manifested by the subsequent development of meniscoprival degeneration and instability.

The reparative salvage of a torn meniscus can be accomplished by open arthrotomy or a closed arthroscopic technique. It is generally agreed that the lesion most amenable to repair is a peripheral longitudinal tear in the vascularized outer third of the meniscus (King 1936; Stone 1979; Heatley 1980; Cabaud et al. 1981; Arnoczky et al. 1980; Krackow and Vetter 1980; Veth et al. 1983b). Contrary to the findings of King (1936), it was shown by Veth et al. (1983a), Ghadially et al. (1986), Fabricciani et al. (1986), and Scheuer et al. (1986) that tears in the central "degenerative zone" of the meniscus could be repaired by bridging the tear site with vascularized synovial flaps; Melanotte and Baldovin (1986) reported on initial clinical results using this technique. Arnoczky et al. (1986) achieved good experimental results with these lesions by transfixing the torn surfaces with fibrin pins.

In recent years, initial results in large clinical series have furnished definitive proof of the value of meniscus repair as an alternative to conventional meniscectomy (C. R. Wirth 1981; Cassidy and Shaffer 1981; Marshall 1982; Hamberg et al. 1983; Rodriguez 1983, 1985, 1986; C.J. Wirth et al. 1984; Lemaire 1984; Schreiber and Rodriguez 1984, 1986; DeHaven 1985, etc.).

Diagnosis

We agree with Rüttimann and Kieser (1974), Jäger and Wirth (1979), Langlotz and Dexel (1980), Levinsohn and Baker (1980), Insall (1984), Lemaire et al. (1984) and others that arthrography is still the most accurate noninvasive diagnostic technique for evaluating the meniscus, especially the peripheral posterior horn region where reparable tears are most commonly encountered. We use arthrography routinely, despite the widely held but incorrect belief – fostered by modern imaging procedures and especially the rise of arthroscopy – that it is outmoded and un-

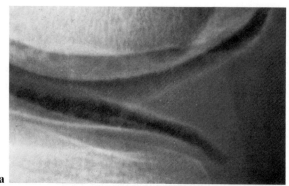

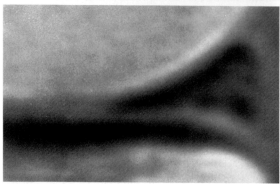

Fig. 1a, b. The meniscus appears arthrographically normal at the level of the posterior oblique ligament, with no evidence of traumatic or degenerative change **(a)**. The MR image (magnified) of the same meniscus shows marked structural degeneration **(b)**

reliable. The truth is that, in experienced hands, arthrography is a fast, minimally invasive, uncomplicated, and diagnostically precise method whose capabilities go well beyond the comprehensive depiction of meniscal pathology.

It may be added that in 93.2% of our meniscus repair cases, arthrography has yielded an astonishing 97.7% rate of true-positive diagnoses, with only 3 false-positive cases (1.6%). As in any diagnostic procedure, the critical factors that determine accuracy are a high-quality apparatus, an experienced examiner, and the meticulous interpretation of findings.

Arthroscopy is superior for evaluating a detached meniscal fragment and especially the character of its surfaces. Arthrography is useful to a degree for structural characterization, although this can be done more precisely by MRI, which more clearly depicts sites of meniscal degeneration (Fig. 1) and is more useful for assessing the prospects of a successful repair (Jung et al. 1988).

Open Meniscus Repair

Preoperative Measures

As in practically all knee operations, we begin by fitting a long posterior plaster splint to the leg with the knee flexed 30°. The splint is immediately oven-dried and padded. This avoids the troublesome problems that can result from applying the splint in the immediate postoperative period, i.e., wetness, breakage, nonuniform flexion angles, and especially abrupt knee movements. The knee is gently shaved and the whole leg wrapped overnight in an antiseptic dressing (Braunoderm, Betadine, etc.).

The operation is performed under general or spinal anesthesia, using a pneumatic tourniquet to obtain a bloodless field.

Operating Technique

General

When the meniscal tear coexists with a ligamentous injury, the meniscus is concurrently repaired through a large arthrotomy. With an isolated meniscal tear, a classic anteromedial or anterolateral arthrotomy can give exposure of all meniscal segments. Practically the entire joint can be inspected through the anterior arthrotomy, and tears in the anterior horn or middle third of the meniscus are easily repaired through this approach. For the frequent posterior horn tear, it is necessary to open the corresponding posteromedial or posterolateral compartment.

The *posteromedial* dissection is performed with the knee maximally flexed and the affected leg crossed over the opposite limb. Sparing the infrapatellar saphenous nerve branch and saphenous vein, the joint capsule is exposed subcutaneously and the second incision made immediately behind the posterior oblique ligament, parallel to the tibial axis (Fig. 2).

On the *lateral* side it is sufficient to flex the knee 90° over the edge of the table, and the arthrotomy is made parallel and posterior to the lateral collateral ligament and anterior to the arcuate ligament while sparing the popliteus tendon. No special measures are taken to protect the peroneal nerve or biceps tendon, because these structures are lax and are located well back of the area of dissection.

We used to repair posterior horn tears through direct arthrotomies, sometimes using 2 separate approaches. We finally abandoned this practice due to limitations of exposure and frequent local healing problems, and today we use only the classic anteromedial or anterolateral arthrotomy.

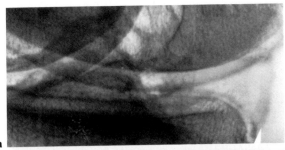

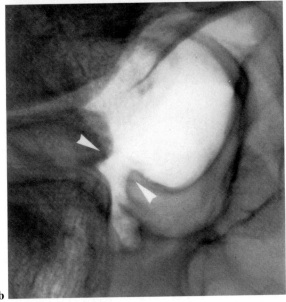

Fig.2a, b. The vertical posterior horn tear in the medial meniscus **(a)** gapes widely with increasing knee flexion **(b)**. The same phenomenon is seen with a posteromedial arthrotomy

Tears of the medial meniscus located at the level of the collateral ligament also can present a problem. The technique for demonstrating these tears is described below. Often it will be necessary to excise nearby hypertrophic, yellowish, scarred synovium to obtain a clear view.

The next step is debridement of the tear to create a "fresh" injury. Besides excision of synovium as described, we use a curette to debride both surfaces of the tear until the meniscus "sings." The tear is repaired with absorbable suture material (2/0 Dexon S, 65 cm, on a TT-20 needle).

The sutures are placed perpendicular to the tear line at intervals of 5 mm. It is imperative that the sutures fully encompass both portions of the meniscus from the superior to the inferior surface to ensure that all portions of the tear are securely approximated.

The sutures are passed inside-to-outside for posterior horn repairs, backward-to-forward for other segments, and tied so that the knots are proximal to and outside the tear. If there is a concomitant ligament repair, the meniscus sutures are tied just before definitive tensioning and fixation of the repaired or reconstructed ligament. Tangential sutures that are oblique or parallel to the torn surface are very difficult to place and cannot ensure a precise, stable coaptation (Fig.3).

Following copious joint irrigation and the insertion of an intraarticular suction drain, the posterior arthrotomy is closed with plication of the capsule, or the anterior arthrotomy is closed in layers, and the leg is immobilized on the plaster splint constructed earlier.

Suture Technique

Following established general surgical principles, the procedure involves the simple suture repair of an inherently simple lesion whose major difficulty is one of access and visualization. Accordingly, different meniscal segments call for different suture techniques, as will be explained later in detail.

The principle of the repair is to *visualize* the lesion, *debride* it, and *repair* it with sutures that *encompass* the tear.

Visualization of the posterior horn through the relatively small capsulotomy can be very frustrating for the inexperienced operator. Indeed, a tear located more than 4 mm from the periphery can be clearly visualized only by adjusting the rotational position and flexion angle of the lower leg. Exposure of the tear is greatly aided by the use of a probe or "nerve" hook. With very few exceptions, and invariably with peripheral tears, we have been able to visualize the lesion without difficulty.

Repairs of the Medial Meniscus (Fig.4a)

Anterior horn. Anterior horn tears are very uncommon (3.5% in our series); most are true avulsions that are not difficult to visualize or repair.

Middle third. Tears at the level of the collateral ligament are occasionally somewhat difficult to repair from an anterior or posteromedial arthrotomy. Curettage is performed from the anterior side. Accurate visualization and repair generally requires 2 longitudinal incisions of the collateral ligament at the level of the meniscal rim. The meniscus is then repaired with vertically placed sutures. When the sutures are tied, care is taken not to entrap the collateral ligament as this would hamper its gliding. We have had poor results with horizontal sutures passed through the collateral ligament and tied outside the ligament; they cannot ensure stable fixation of the tear, and their restraint of free ligament gliding hinders postoperative mobilization of the knee.

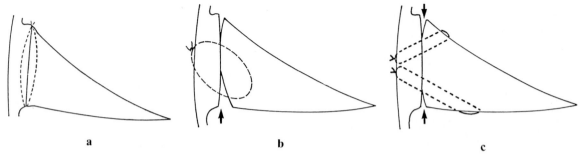

Fig. 3a–c. Only vertically placed sutures can effect a complete, stable coaptation of the torn surfaces **(a)**. The edges gape when the tear is repaired openly with horizontal sutures **(b)** or arthroscopically with oblique sutures **(c)**

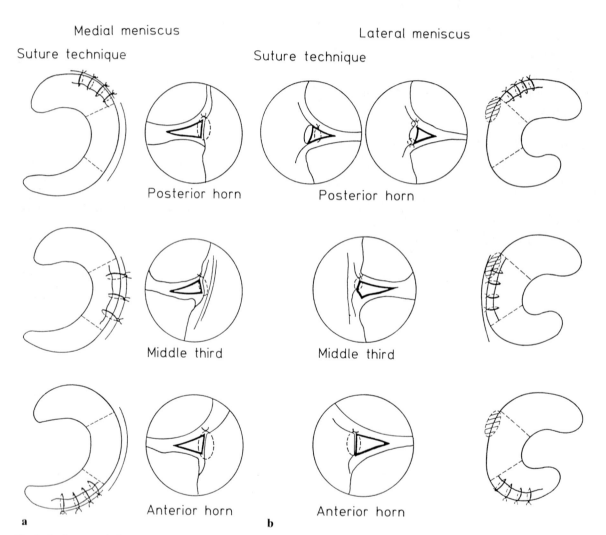

Medial meniscus

Lateral meniscus

Suture technique

Suture technique

Posterior horn

Posterior horn

Middle third

Middle third

Anterior horn

Anterior horn

a

b

Fig. 4a, b. Suture techniques. (From Wirth et al. 1988)

Fig. 5. Typical incomplete posterior horn tear of the medial meniscus. The tear, which may be degenerative, is favorably situated for suture repair ▷

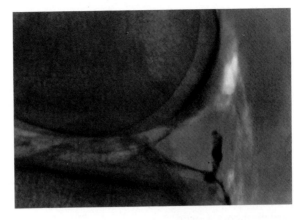

Fig. 6 a, b. Tear of the lateral meniscus extending along the course of, and central to, the popliteal hiatus **(a)**. Follow-up arthrogram **(b)** demonstrates complete healing with an anatomically repaired hiatus and no tendon constriction ▽

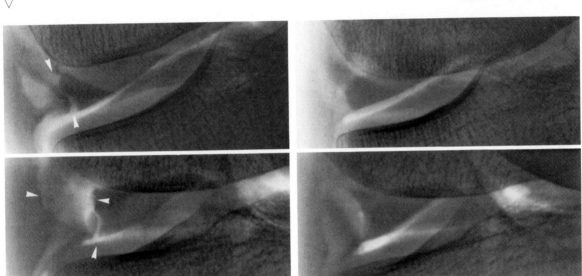

a

b

Posterior horn. Longitudinal tears at the junction of the peripheral and middle thirds of the body of the meniscus can prove problematic. Some cases may require oblique suturing or, as in the arthroscopic technique, passing the needle through the front of the posterior horn and retrieving it in the posterior compartment. A special case is the incomplete peripheral tear, which usually runs obliquely upward and outward from the inferior meniscal surface, leaving the upper surface intact (Fig. 5). Tears of this kind are plainly demonstrated by arthrography but can be difficult to detect arthroscopically, even by an experienced examiner. The debridement of this lesion includes completing the tear by sharp division of the meniscal surface.

Repairs of the Lateral Meniscus (Fig. 4 b)

Anterior horn. The suture technique is analogous to that for the medial meniscus.

Middle third. Middle-third tears require attention to the special anatomy of the meniscus, especially the loose capsular attachment of the meniscus and the peculiar anatomy of the popliteal hiatus and tendon. The suture is all-layer anterior to the tendon, but at the hiatus level it incorporates only the upper surface of the meniscus.

Posterior horn. As in the central portion, accurate repair of the popliteal hiatus is required without constricting the tendon or catching it with the suture. Very centralized tears are repaired with all-layer sutures like those used for the medial meniscus. Longitudinal tears of the lateral meniscus often do not run in continuity with the hiatus but immediately within and along it. They are repaired in standard fashion with all-layer sutures (Fig. 6).

Special Types of Tear

In cases where, say, peripheral tears are combined with flap tears, radial tears, or fish-mouth lesions that are largely degenerative in nature, the necessary partial resection is carried out before the periphery is repaired.

In isolated cases with full-thickness horizontal tears through the inferior meniscal surface, we have obtained the best results by dividing the meniscus back into the posterior horn at the periphery, suturing its undersurface through a posteromedial arthrotomy, reducing the meniscus, and then carrying out a standard peripheral repair.

Postoperative Treatment

As Table 1 indicates, our postoperative regimen emphasizes early functional therapy in which the knee is immobilized for just 1 week postoperatively on the plaster splint. During this time the patient performs isometric muscle exercises while local and systemic anti-inflammatory agents are given. During week 2 the knee is alternately mobilized on a motion splint and by active assisted exercises, increasing to a maximum range of $90°-15°-0°$; the plaster splint is worn only at night to avoid undesired full extension or abrupt rotation. Meanwhile the patient ambulates on crutches and is discharged once the desired degree of wound healing has been achieved; weight bearing at this time is restricted to approximately 20 kg. During the next 4 weeks the knee is progressively mobilized to $110°-0°-0°$, weight bearing is increased, and muscle strengthening exercises are performed. By initial follow-up at 6 weeks postoperatively, the patient generally has regained full knee extension and full weight bearing. At that time the patient may discard his crutches and continue his rehabilitation at home. Return to work will of course depend on the demands placed on the knee joint in the work setting.

In theory, limited sedentary work can be resumed immediately after discharge, while higher-demand professions should not be resumed until the 6th–8th postoperative week. The patient is instructed to avoid squatting and other extreme positions of knee flexion for at least 3 months. Athletic participation is proscribed, although we do allow moderate swimming and bicycling starting in the 2nd postoperative month. Competitive athletics, skiing, and other sports that are very stressful to the knee are permitted after 2 months in patients with good musculature and an asymptomatic knee joint.

Arthrographic follow-ups of meniscal healing were initially performed in almost all patients after 2 months. This was done not only to document and confirm the result of the surgery but also to guide the decision whether to permit resumption of normal activities (Fig. 7). Based on the excellent results of our first 100 cases, today we obtain follow-up arthrograms only in patients who are still doing poorly months after the operation. Clinical follow-ups are routinely scheduled for the 3rd, 6th, and 12th postoperative months.

Case Material

From 1979 to February of 1988, 200 meniscus repairs were performed in a total of 191 patients, predominantly males (68.5%), at the Balgrist University Orthopedic Clinic. The youngest patient was 14 at the time of operation, the oldest 62 (average 28.2 years).

Table 1. Postoperative treatment regimen (in weeks)

Hospitalization	2
Posterior plaster splint	1
Motorized splint	1
Outpatient physiotherapy	4
Crutch ambulation	4–6
Time away from work	4–8
Sports abstinence	12
First follow-up at	4
Final follow-up at	12
Follow-up arthrograms if progress is poor	

Table 2. Clinical material (August 1978–February 1988)

Patients	191
Men	131
Women	60
Age at operation 14–62 years (average 28.2 years)	

Meniscus repairs (200 total)	
Fresh	46
Old	154
Isolated	128
Associated lesions	72
Right	113
Left	87
Medial	159
Lateral	41 (11 bilateral)

Associated ligament injuries	
Anterior cruciate ligament	37
Posterior cruciate ligament	3
Medial collateral ligament, semimembranosus corner	19
Lateral collateral ligament	1

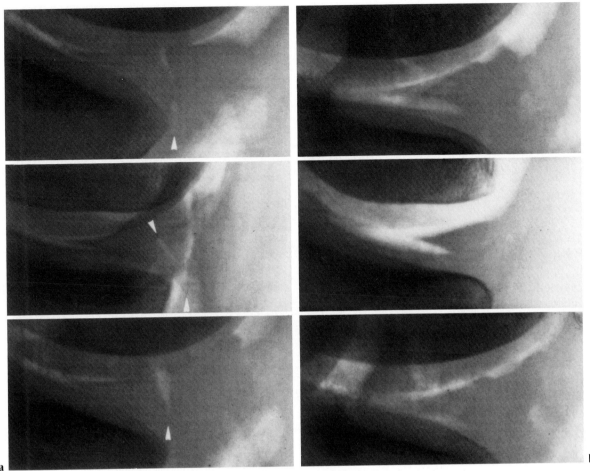

Fig. 7 a, b. Tear involving the entire outer third of a medial meniscus. The rim is partially detached, and the main portion of the tear extends partly into the degenerative zone (a). Follow-up arthrogram confirms complete reattachment (b)

Most of the lesions were old (77%) and isolated (64%) tears of the right (56.5%) medial meniscus (79.5%) involving the posterior horn. Fresh or old tears of the anterior cruciate ligament were concomitantly repaired in 37 cases, of the posterior cruciate ligament in 3, and of the medial collateral ligament including the semimembranosus corner in another 19. The 1 lateral collateral ligament tear was part of an extremely complex injury involving practically all knee structures including both menisci (Table 2).

The fresh lesions had been sustained an average of 6.6 days before treatment. Old injuries sustained (or first noticed) 4–24 months previously constituted the main group, accounting for 65.5% of cases. Eleven patients had repairs of both menisci.

Complications

The only complications involved 1 knee that had to be mobilized under general anesthesia and arthroscopic guidance 8 weeks after repair of the medial meniscus and intraarticular reconstruction of the anterior cruciate ligament, and a second knee requiring evacuation of a posteromedial subcutaneous hematoma due to anticoagulant hemorrhage. Two additional knees required needle aspiration of an irritative effusion. In contrast to conventional partial or total meniscectomy (even by arthroscopic technique), it is noteworthy that irritative effusion was extremely rare in the postoperative period following meniscal repairs.

The most plausible explanation for this, we believe, is the atraumatic operating technique, the careful closure of the synovium, and especially the complete immobilization of the joint for the first postoperative week. Certainly another factor is the precise coapta-

Table 3. Results

Subjective		187	
Excellent	73		86.7%
Good	89		
Fair	13		6.95%
Poor	12		6.41%
Objective		184	
Good	164		89.1%
Fair	11		5.9%
Poor	9		4.8%
Follow-up arthrography		110 of 200 repairs (55%)	
Healing			
Complete	96		87.2%
Partial	7		6.3%
Absent	7		6.3%
Reruptures	6		(3%)
Reoperations	15		(7.5%)

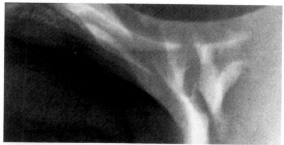
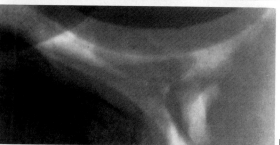
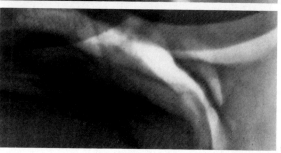

Fig. 8 a–c. Unsuccessful repair of an old crush injury of a lateral meniscus posterior horn. Analysis of the lesion shows that the main damage involves the middle third of the body of the meniscus (**a**). Arthrographic follow-ups confirm healing of the peripheral tear with anatomic repair of the popliteal hiatus (**c**) but persistence of the lesion in the central degenerative zone (**b**). In retrospect, resection of the central lesion should have preceded repair of the peripheral tear

tion of the peripheral vascularized portion of the meniscus, which is not left within the joint as an open wound.

Results (Table 3)

Some 187 (97.9%) patients were examined clinically during the 3rd postoperative month as part of the first routine follow-up. Of these, 86.7% rated the outcome as good to excellent; 12 patients (6.4%) were dissatisfied with the result.

In all, 110 meniscus repairs (55%) were evaluated by follow-up arthrography, which showed absence of healing in 7 (6.3%) of the reexamined cases (Fig. 8). In the final series of 100 repairs, only 12 follow-up arthrograms were required for persistent problems months after surgery; these showed absence of meniscal healing in only 1 case. In 3 cases the subjective complaints were consistent with meniscal degeneration, although this could not be confirmed arthrographically.

Based on a very strict, objective evaluation of the clinical and radiographic findings (especially arthrography), we rated the final result as poor in 9 of the cases (4.8%).

Analysis of the cases given a poor subjective rating shows that the patient dissatisfaction usually related to pain associated with a preexisting degenerative arthritis or chondropathic complaints, even though arthrographic follow-up confirmed healing of the repair site. Residual instabilities in joints with healed menisci were another source of patient dissatisfaction. Four cases with unhealed repair sites were given a poor objective rating even though the patients were subjectively pleased. This implies that the reason for

dissatisfaction in some cases is based less on the meniscus than on an uncorrected instability or preexisting degenerative disease. Proper counseling is invaluable in selected patients with an apparently good clinical and arthrographic outcome.

We reoperated 4 confirmed new ruptures of the repair site and partially resected another meniscus due to degeneration. Two other arthrographically confirmed ruptures have remained asymptomatic. Seven of our meniscus repairs were completely or partially removed elsewhere; it is unclear whether these represented true recurrences of the tear. Assuming that this is the case with the most rigorous critera applied, this would signify a total recurrence rate of 6.5%. Reruptures were confirmed and arthrographically documented in only 6 cases (3%), however.

Fifteen of the menisci required reintervention

(7.5%), one-third due to ligament injuries caused by new trauma. In 2 cases we were able to resuture the meniscus, but the other cases required a partial to subtotal resection. It is noteworthy that 5 of the repaired menisci either remained intact during repeat trauma causing anterior cruciate ligament disruption, or else sustained a tear central to the repair site. This is consistent with the reports of Hamberg et al. (1983), DeHaven (1985), and Schmid et al. (1988), who found that approximately half of new ruptures occurred outside the area of the repair.

Discussion

Indication

It is our experience that meniscal repairs have a reasonable prospect of success only when performed in the vascularized outer third of the meniscus (Fig. 9). Farther centrally, within the "degenerative zone,"

there is a poorer chance of vascular invasion, as King (1930) first demonstrated. One advantage of arthroscopic fixation may be that tears located centrally in the meniscal substance can be repaired better than by arthrotomy, or may be reparable only by the arthroscopic technique. These more centrally located tears, however, are prone to recurrence (Table 4). DeHaven (1985) believes that penetration of the avascular portion of the meniscus with the repair sutures creates sites of predilection for tearing in subsequent stress situations. Indeed, our own experience has shown us that tears located in the middle third of the body of the meniscus do not heal; at the same time, most of the lesions are not true longitudinal tears but incomplete arcuate or flap tears ("longuette posterieure" of Trillat 1962) that will eventually propagate to the free border of the meniscus. In cases of this kind we perform a minimal arthroscopic meniscal resection rather than deal with the risks of a probable rerupture.

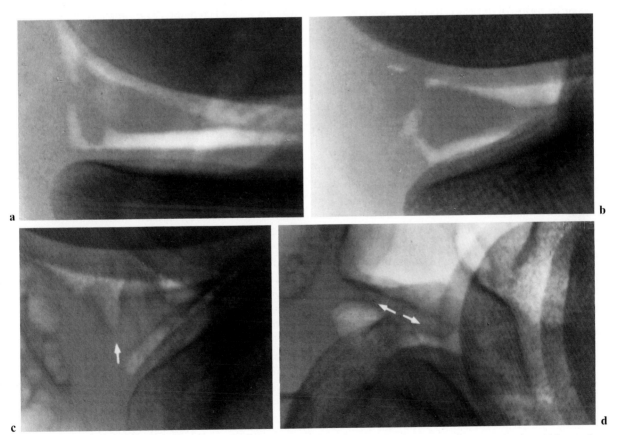

Fig. 9 a–d. Noncomplex peripheral tears in a structurally undamaged meniscus **(a, b)** are ideal for a successful repair. The incomplete tear presenting arthrographically as a "deep upper ridge" **(c, d)** usually appears with increasing knee flexion as an elongation of the meniscal-capsular attachment and is associated clinically with a Finochietto-like instability. It is repaired by synovial excision and meniscocapsular sutures

Table 4. Reruptures after meniscal repairs (follow-ups of more than 50 cases)

	Number of cases	Rerup-tures	Percent-age
Open technique			
Hughston (1975)	68	0	0
Hamberg et al. (1983)	50	8	8
Lemaire et al. (1984)	78	23	30
Rodriguez (1985)	60	3	5
DeHaven (1985)	55	3	6
Wirth et al. (1988)	459	32	6.9
Arthroscopic technique			
Stone and Miller (1985)	52	3	6
Scott et al. (1986)	178	38	21
Morgan and Casscells (1986)	70	1	1.5
Jakob et al. (1988)	54	12	22

Operating Technique and Suture Material

The view expressed by some authors that meniscus repair is a technically difficult operation is misleading. In an open repair, the only critical factor is adequate exposure of the lesion through a posterior arthrotomy; the rest falls within the scope of routine general surgery.

The surgeon must free the lesion of all scar tissue so that the debrided surfaces of the tear can acquire a new vascular supply. As Fig. 3 demonstrates, the sutures must incorporate the complete height of the meniscal rim to effect accurate coaptation of the torn surfaces. As in the surgical treatment of many other structures, the knots are left inside the joint. We agree with DeHaven (1985), who employs the same method, that other more complex techniques and extraarticular knots are needlessly complicated and offer no advantages.

We have had good results with 2/0 Dexon S suture material on a TT-20 needle. Equally good is Vicryl with a UR-6 size needle. We use absorbable material exclusively based on our excellent results in initial follow-ups. We have had no negative experiences in those cases, or in our clinical population as a whole, that would motivate a change to different materials. Moreover, the use of nonabsorbable sutures has been associated with a small but definite incidence of granulomas and foreign body reactions.

Postoperative Treatment

In the belief that a meniscus repair was like the repair of a capsuloligamentous injury, we initially followed an aftercare regimen like that for a ligament repair or reconstruction, i.e., 6 weeks' immobilization in a cylinder cast. However, initial follow-ups showed us that even repairs which, for whatever reason, had received little or no immobilization healed just as well as repairs that had been immobilized in plaster for several weeks. At the same time, the muscular atrophy that invariably accompanies prolonged casting significantly delayed postoperative rehabilitation and the resumption of normal activities. For these reasons we gradually reduced the period of cast immobilization for isolated meniscus repairs and since 1983 have limited it to a single week. When the meniscus has been repaired concomitantly with other injuries, we of course tailor the aftercare regimen to those injuries, although we still try to institute functional rehabilitation at the earliest possible time.

A review of the literature quickly reveals that, while there is general agreement as to the type and duration of immobilization needed after ligament operations, there is no such consensus regarding meniscus repairs. Recommendations range from 4 weeks' immobilization (Henning 1983; DeHaven 1985; Karpf 1986; Melanotte 1986) to 5 weeks (Hamberg 1983) to up to 6 weeks (Hendler 1984; Barber 1985; Morgan 1986; Marshall 1988) or a compromise solution (4–6: Defrere 1988; Schmid 1988; 5–6: Jakob 1988), depending on whether the meniscal tear is isolated or coexists with other injuries. The knee flexion angle during immobilization is another point of dispute, with some advocating full extension (Morgan 1986), 15° flexion (Karpf 1986), 30° flexion (Hamberg 1983; Melanotte 1986; Jakob 1988), or 45° flexion (Hendler 1984; DeHaven 1985; Barber 1985; Marshall 1988). Others immobilize the joint in 45° flexion for 3 weeks and then permit limited motion for another 3 weeks (30°–60°: Barber 1985; 30°–90° Marshall 1988). Lemaire (1984) tests the stability of the repair and apparently does not immobilize the joint.

One senses that some authors make their decision largely on empirical grounds. We, too, originally advocated prolonged immobilization in the belief that, as with other knee structures, ample time must be allowed for healing of the poorly vascularized and relatively mobile meniscus. But the results of stringent follow-ups have made us realize that this is not the case, and we have concluded that early functional aftercare, like that currently employed in ligament operations, is most appropriate.

Summary

In collaboration with the Munich University Orthopedic Clinic, we analyzed our meniscus repairs up to 1986, evaluated them using a complex scoring system that places special emphasis on possible causes of recurrence, and published our findings in a monograph (Wirth et al. 1988).

Our analysis showed that old meniscus injuries can heal with about the same frequency as fresh tears. There is some propensity for recurrence in patients with a concomitant capsuloligamentous reconstruction, but this is also seen with isolated tears. Meniscal healing is not significantly affected by the age, gender, and physical constitution of the patient or by the age, length, or location of the tear. On the other hand, preexisting degenerative joint changes and persistent instabilities are significant deleterious factors, at least with regard to the subjective treatment outcome.

On the whole, it can be said that a traumatic or degenerative meniscal tear located in the peripheral third of the meniscus is an indication for suture repair. It does not matter whether the open or closed technique is used; each has its advantages and disadvantages, but each is equivalent to the other in experienced hands.

References

Allen PR, Denham RA, Swan AV (1984) Late degenerative changes after meniscectomy. Factors affecting the knee after operation. J Bone Jt Surg [Br] 66: 666–671

Arnoczky SP, Marshall JL, Joseph A, Jahne C, Yoshioka M (1980) Meniscal nutrition – An experimental study in the dog. Trans Orthop Res Soc 26: 127

Arnoczky SP, Mc Devitt CA, Warren RF, Spivak J, Allen A (1986) Meniscal repair using an exogenous fibrin clot. An experimental study in the dog. Referat, 32nd Annual Trans Orthop Res Soc, New Orleans/LA

Arnoczky SP, Warren RF, Kaplan N (1985) Meniscal remodeling following partial meniscectomy. An experimental study in the dog. Arthroscopy 1: 247–252

Baratz ME, Fu FH, Mengats R (1986) Meniscal tears: The effect of meniscectomy and of repair on intraarticular contact areas and stress in the human knee. Am J Sports Med 14: 270–275

Barber AF, Stone RG (1985) Meniscal repair, an arthroscopic technique. J Bone Jt Surg [Br] 67: 39–41

Böhler L (1955) Behandlung, Nachbehandlung und Begutachtung von Knieverletzungen. Erfahrungen an 1000 operierten Fällen. Langenbecks Arch Klin Chir 282: 264–276

Bourne RG, Finlay B, Papadopoulos P, Andrea P (1984) The effect at the medial meniscectomy on strain distribution in the proximal part of the tibia. J Bone Jt Surg [Am] 66: 1431–1437

Bracker W, Götte S, Wirth CJ (1982) Zur Frage der Kniebandinstabilität nach Meniskektomie. Z Orthop 120: 501

Cabaud HE, Rodkey WG, Fitzwater JE (1981) Medial meniscus repair: An experimental and morphological study. J Sports Med 9: 129–134

Cassidy E, Shaffer AJ (1981) Repair of peripheral meniscus tears. Sports Med 4: 209–214

Cotta H, Puhl W (1976) Pathophysiologie des Knorpelschadens. Hefte Unfallheilkd 127: 1–22

Courvoisier E (1959) Sur la régénération des ménisques du genou après méniscectomie. Helv Chir Acta 26: 358–374

Defrère J, Franckart A, Bassleer R (1988) Meniscus repair by arthroscopy. In: Müller We, Hackenbruch W, (eds) Surgery and arthroscopy of the knee. Springer, Berlin Heidelberg New York Tokyo, pp 306–316

DeHaven KE (1981) Peripheral meniscus repair: An alternative to meniscectomy. J Bone Jt Surg [Br] 63: 463

DeHaven KE (1985) Meniscus repair in the athlete. Clin Orthop 198: 31–35

Dietrich H (1931) Die Regeneration des Meniskus. Chirurg 230: 251–260

Elmer RM, Mastowitz RW, Franckel VH (1977) Meniscal regeneration and post-meniscectomy degenerative joint disease. Clin Orthop 124: 304–310

Fabbricciani A, Schiavonne-Panni A, Oransky M (1986) The repair of meniscus lesions by synovial flaps: An experimental study. In: Trickey EL, Hertel P (eds) Surgery and arthroscopy of the knee. Springer, Berlin Heidelberg New York Tokyo, pp 96–100

Fairbank TJ (1948) Knee joint changes after meniscectomy. J Bone Jt Surg [Br] 30: 664–670

Ghadially FN, Wedge JH, Lalonde JM (1986) Experimental methods of repairing injured menisci. J Bone Jt Surg [Br] 68: 106–110

Hamberg P, Gillquist J, Lysholm J (1983) Suture of new and old peripheral meniscus tears. J Bone Jt Surg [Am] 65: 193–197

Heatley FW (1980) The meniscus – can it be repaired? J Bone Jt Surg [Br] 62: 397–402

Hehne HJ, Riede UN, Hausschild G, Schlageter M (1981) Tibiofemorale Kontaktflächenmessungen nach experimentellen partiellen und subtotalen Meniskektomien. Z Orthop 119: 54–59

Hendler RC (1984) Arthroscopic meniscal repair. Clin Orthop 190: 163–169

Henning CE (1983) Arthroscopic repair of meniscus tears. Orthopedics 69: 1130–1132

Hughston JC (1975) A simple meniscectomy. J Sports Med 3: 179–187

Insall JN (1984) Surgery of the knee. Churchill-Livingstone, New York

Jackson JP (1968) Degenerative changes in the knee after meniscectomy. Br Med J 2: 525–527

Jäger M, Wirth CJ (1978) Kapselbandläsionen. Thieme, Stuttgart

Jakob RP, Stäubli H-U, Zuber K, Esser M (1988) The arthroscopic meniscal repair. Techniques and clinical experience. J Sports Med 16: 137–142

Johnson RJ, Kettelkamp DB, Clark W, Leaverton P (1974) Factors affecting late results after meniscectomy. J Bone Jt Surg [Am] 56: 719–729

Jung T, Rodriguez M, Augustiny N, Friedrich N, Schulthess O von (1988) 1,5-T-MRI, Arthrographie und Arthroskopie in der Evaluation von Knieläsionen. Fortschr Röntgenstr 148: 390–393

Karpf PM, Aigner R, Gradinger R (1986) Meniskusverletzungen. In: Lange M, Hipp OE (Hrsg) Hrsg Lehrbuch der

Orthopädie und Traumatologie, Bd 3. Enke, Stuttgart, S 446–452

Kettelkamp DG, Jacobs AW (1972) Tibiofemoral contact area-determination and implications. J Bone Jt Surg [Am] 54: 349–356

King D (1936) The healing of semilunar cartilages. J Bone Jt Surg 18: 333–342

Krackow KA, Vetter WL (1980) Surgical reimplantation of the medial meniscus and repair of meniscal lacerations: An experimental study in dogs. Trans Orthop Res Soc 5: 128

Langlotz M, Dexel M (1980) Wie zuverlässig ist die intraoperative Untersuchung des medialen Meniskushinterhornes? Diskrepanz zwischen Arthrographie und Arthrotomie. Z Orthop 118: 868–873

Lemaire M, Combelles F, Miremad C, Van Vooren P (1984) Les désinsertions ménisco-capsulaires postéro-internes associées aux instabilités chroniques du genou par rupture du ligament croisé antérieur. Rev Chir Orthop 70: 613–622

Levinsohn EM, Baker BE (1980) Prearthrotomy diagnostic evaluation of the knee: Review of 100 cases diagnosed by arthrography and arthroscopy. AJR 134: 107–111

Mandl F (1929) Regeneration des menschlichen Kniegelenkzwischenknorpels. Zentralbl Chir 56: 3265–3268

Maquet PGJ (1984) Biomechanics of the knee. Springer, Berlin Heidelberg New York

Marshall DJ (1982) Meniscopexie: The reattachment of peripherally detached menisci. J Bone Jt Surg [Br] 64: 119–120

Marshall SC (1988) Combined arthroscopic - open repair of meniscal injuries. In: Müller We, Hackenbruch W (eds) Surgery and arthroscopy of the knee. Springer, Berlin Heidelberg New York Tokyo, pp 317–327

Melanotte PL, Baldovin M (1986) Surgical repair of chronic meniscal injury: Plastic meniscus surgery. In: Trickey EL, Hertel P (eds) Surgery and arthroscopy of the knee. Springer, Berlin Heidelberg New York Tokyo, pp 336–340

Möller W (1930) Luxation eines nach Exstirpation nachgebildeten Kniegelenksmeniskus. Zentralbl Chir 57: 2790–2792

Morgan CD, Casscells SW (1986) Arthroscopic meniskus repair: a safe approach to the posterior hours. Arthroscopy 2/1: 3–12

Müller We (1982) Das Knie. Springer, Berlin Heidelberg New York

Oretorp N, Alm A, Exström H, Gillquist J (1978) Immediate effects of meniscectomy on the knee joint. The effects of tensile load on knee joint ligaments in dogs. Acta Orthop Scand 49: 407–414

Puhl W, Niethard F, Braun M, Hubert W (1981) Das meniskektomierte Kniegelenk. In: Hohmann D, Rausch E (Hrsg) Das Knie. Stork, Bruchsal, S 451–458

Ricklin P, Rüttimann A, Del Buono MS (1980) Die Meniscusläsion. Thieme, Stuttgart

Rodriguez M (1985) Möglichkeiten und Grenzen der Meniscopexie bei veralteten Meniscusrissen. In: Jäger M (Hrsg) Weichteilschäden und Weichteilverletzungen. Praktische Orthopädie, Bd 15. Stork, Bruchsal, S 231–240

Rodriguez M, Schreiber A (1986) Meniscus sutures for old tears - Report on over 100 cases. In: Trickey EL, Hertel P

(eds) Surgery and arthroscopy of the knee. Springer, Berlin Heidelberg New York Tokyo, pp 102–108

Rodriguez M, Zollinger H (1983) Die Naht basisnaher Meniskusrisse. In: Chapchal G (Hrsg) Sportverletzungen und Sportschäden. Thieme, Stuttgart, 161–164

Rüttimann A, Kieser C (1974) Die Bedeutung der Arthrographie nach Traumen des Kniegelenkes. Orthopade 3: 166–177

Scheuer J, Lies A, Müller KM (1986) Die Meniskusnaht — eine tierexperimentale Studie. Hefte Unfallheilkd 181: 251–256

Schmid A, Schmid F, Tiling T (1988) Electron microscopical observations on sutured meniscus tears. In: Müller We, Hackenbruch W (eds) Surgery and arthroscopy of the knee. Springer, Berlin Heidelberg New York Tokyo, pp 328–334

Schreiber A, Dexel M (1979) Gonarthrose nach Meniskektomie und Meniskektomie bei Gonarthrose. Chirurg 50: 618–625

Schreiber A, Rodriguez M (1984) Traitement conservateur des lésions méniscales. Rev Chir Orthop 70: 119–120

Schreiber A, Rodriguez M (1986) Chirurgie conservative des lésions du ménisque. Chirurgie 112: 155–162

Scott GA, Jolly BL, Henning CE (1986) Combined posterior incision and arthroscopic intra-articular repair of the meniscus. J Bone Jt Surg [Am] 68: 847–861

Smillie JS (1944) Observations on the regeneration of the semilunar cartilages in man. Br J Surg 31: 398–401

Stone RG (1979) Peripheral detachment of the menisci of the knee: A preliminary report. Orthop Clin North Am 10: 643–657

Stone RG, Miller GA (1985) A technique of arthroscopic suture of torn menisci. Arthroscopy 1: 226–232

Tapper EM, Hoover NM (1969) Late results after meniscectomy. J Bone Jt Surg [Am] 51: 517–526

Trillat A (1962) Lésions traumatiques du ménisque interne du genou. Classement anatomique et diagnostic clinique. Rev Chir Orthop 48: 551–560

Veth RPH, Den Heeten GJ, Jansen HWB, Nielsen HKL (1983a) Repair of the meniscus. An experimental investigation in rabbits. Clin Orthop 175: 258–262

Veth RPH, Den Heeten GJ, Jansen HWB, Nieslen HKL (1983b) An experimental study of reconstructive procedures in lesions of the meniscus: use of synovial flaps and carbon fiber implants for artificially made lesions in the meniscus of the rabbit. Clin Orthop 181: 250–254

Wang CJ, Walker PS (1974) Rotatory laxity of the human knee joint. J Bone Jt Surg [Am] 56: 161–170

Will-Hofmann H (1985) Reparationsvorgänge der Binnenstrukturen des Kniegelenks nach Meniscektomie. Experimentelle Studie am Kniegelenk des Kaninchens. Z Orthop 123: 957–961

Wirth CJ, Jäger M, Kolb M (1984) Die komplexe vordere Knie-Instabilität. Thieme, Stuttgart

Wirth CJ, Rodriguez M, Milachowsky KA (1988) Meniskusnaht - Meniskusersatz. Thieme, Stuttgart

Wirth CR (1981) Meniscal repair. Clin Orthop 157: 153–160

Chronic Insufficiency
of the Anterior Cruciate Ligament

Autologous or Allogeneic Reconstruction?

A. Gächter

The surgical treatment of tears of the anterior cruciate ligament (ACL) dates from the year 1895, when Mayo Robson performed the first documented cruciate ligament repair. The first reconstructions of the ACL were described by Hey Groves in 1917 and by Alwyn Smith in 1918. Both replaced the ligament with a strip of fascia lata. Also at this time, initial attempts were made to develop a synthetic substitute. Corner tried strands of wire, while Alwyn Smith used multiple silk threads (Burnett and Fowler 1985). Neither method proved successful. The first extra-articular "repairs" were performed during the 1920s using free strips of fascia lata (Cotton, Morrison, Bosworth). In 1936 Campbell described the intraarticular use of patellar tendon grafts. As early as 1938, Ivar Palmer confirmed that cruciate ligament reconstructions were difficult, time-consuming, and risky and usually did not bring about a full recovery. At that time Palmer developed a drill guide for the more accurate placement of the graft. The importance of the ACL for knee stability was emphasized in 1950 by O'Donoghue and later by Jones, Slocum and Larson, and Nicholas. As early as 1918, Alwyn Smith recommended electrostimulation to avoid postoperative quadriceps atrophy, while Mauck recommended a long leg cast hinged at the knee for postoperative treatment (quoted in Burnett and Fowler 1985).

Thus, many discoveries in the area of cruciate ligament reconstruction are not as new or significant as a survey of the recent literature would suggest. One might expect that the problems involved in the treatment of a recent or old rupture of the ACL would have been solved in the interim, yet we all know that this is not the case. There is not even a consensus with regard to graft selection, let alone operating technique or postoperative care. In the present article we shall review briefly the ACL substitutes that have been recommended in the literature, confining our attention to the use of autologous, allogeneic, or xenogeneic materials (see chapter by Munzinger, p. 518 ff., for a discussion of prosthetic ligaments).

The selection of a suitable graft depends to a large extent on the operating technique. As a rule, different demands are placed on extraarticular cruciate substitutes than on intraarticular reconstructions. Noyes (Noyes et al. 1984) conducted biomechanical tests comparing different connective-tissue structures about the knee that might serve as ACL substitutes with the properties of a normal ACL from young and older adults. Prepatellar retinacular tissue and thin fascia lata strips were found to be too weak. The semitendinosus and gracilis tendons displayed somewhat better properties, but the strongest substitute by far was the central or medial one-third of the patellar tendon. On the negative side, patellar tendon was approximately 3–4 times stiffer than the normal ACL; the pes anserinus tendons most closely approximated normal ACL stiffness. The data published by Noyes et al. (1984) are not undisputed, however.

Below I shall discuss the tissues most commonly used for replacement of the ACL.

Meniscus

Following cruciate ligament tears, it is not uncommon to find an incarcerated bucket-handle fragment of the medial or lateral meniscus within the joint. Early on, this inspired attempts to utilize the "superfluous" meniscal tissue as a cruciate ligament substitute. However, these menisci are already subject to degenerative processes, and the tissue is bradytrophic. Seiler et al. (1985) examined 20 patients in whom meniscal tissue had been used as an autograft. The results at 2 years were poorer than with a conventional repair or extraarticular reconstruction. Even so, the authors recommend that this method be kept in mind as a possible "mini-reconstruction" technique for the ACL in selected cases. More recent trends favor preserving the menisci at their anatomically correct sites whenever possible rather than using them to construct a ligament substitute of inferior quality.

Pes Anserinus Tendons

Particularly since the work of Lindemann, the gracilis and semitendinosus tendons have consistently been recommended as an ideal substitute. These tendons may be used intraarticularly, singly, doubly, "dynamically," or even extraarticularly. Another technique is to combine pes anserinus tendons with strips of the iliotibial tract. In this method the semitendinosus tendon is detached proximally, routed over the top of the lateral femoral condyle with the distally based strip of iliotibial tract, and both grafts are passed down through an osseous tunnel and sutured together (Zarins and Roew 1986). This technique is claimed to have restored functional stability in 90% of the operated patients.

Best known is the technique of Lindemann, in which 1 or 2 of the pes anserinus tendons are used "dynamically," i.e., some of the pes muscular contraction force is used to stabilize the tibia against anteroposterior displacement. Villiger (1984) states that the results of 1- to 8-year follow-ups of 250 dynamic reconstructions were good or excellent in 89% of cases. Comparable results are reported with the modified technique of Lindemann-Bousquet (Pasquali-Lasagni 1981). Ellera-Gomes and Marczyk (1984) obtained approximately 85% good results using a looped semitendinosus tendon graft. Pes anserinus tendon release is a technically simple procedure, usually requiring a tendon stripper or a relatively long incision. Despite the proximity of the saphenous nerve and vein, the pes anserinus cruciate reconstruction holds much promise for the future, especially in arthroscopic procedures. The highly elastic tendon tissue can be augmented if desired by the additional use of synthetic material (e.g., LAD). Perhaps a more familiar procedure is the extraarticular pes anserinus transfer originated by Slocum and Larson (1968). As the pes anserinus is released distally and transposed proximally, it loses mechanical efficiency as a flexor but gains efficiency as an internal rotator. At least in theory, the effect can be likened to the wearing of a Lenox-Hill brace: By checking external rotation of the tibia, the transfer reduces the degree of anterior drawer. This effect is at best highly questionable, however. It is likely that the broad detachment of the pes anserinus impairs its proprioceptive capabilities. Easy to harvest, the pes anserinus is suitable for arthroscopic ACL reconstructions.

Fascia Lata

Following the initial use of fascia lata strips for extraarticular repairs (McIntosh), various modifications and combined techniques were developed in which fascial strips were usually routed "over the top" of the condyle, through the intercondylar notch, and through the tibial plateau. Today the ACL is seldom reconstructed using an extraarticular procedure alone. The advantages of technical simplicity and swift rehabilitation are offset by the poor long-term efficacy of the repair (Hefti et al. 1982). The extraarticular procedures are, however, used as adjuncts to reinforce and augment an intraarticular reconstruction (Simonet and Sim 1984). Another approach is to use synthetic materials such as plastics or carbon fibers and interpose them with fascia lata to construct a cruciate ligament substitute. This composite has 2 functions: First, it helps eliminate contact between the synthetic material and moving joint parts, which could generate potentially harmful wear debris. Second, the interposed connective tissue could assume the biologic function of a cruciate ligament substitute following "breakdown" of the synthetic with passage of time. Another method, published by Lenox Hill Hospital (Scott and Schlosheim 1983), involves the intraarticular transfer of the iliotibial muscle-tendon unit. This dynamic stabilization apparently yields very high success rates but robs the knee of an essential stabilizer. The removal of broad tendon strips has its own pathology, which includes muscle herniation and unsightly scars.

Cutaneous and Periosteal Flaps

Dissected and undissected skin flaps have found use as ligament substitutes for decades. Enneker (1985) stresses the technical simplicity of these operations. Kuner (1978) showed in reoperations (removal of internal fixation material, etc.) that vascularized flaps of periosteal tissue could remodel into ligament-like structures in various joints such as the ankle and acromioclavicular joint. Willenegger (Müller et al. 1975) advocated the use of free autologous grafts in the management of the unstable knee. The main purported advantage of these methods is that they do not sacrifice important tissue structures about the knee. On the other hand, it may be more difficult to achieve adequate, nontraumatizing fixation of the graft. Finally it should be added that reconstructive materials that have proven effective outside the joint are not necessarily suitable for intraarticular use.

Biceps Tendon

Decades ago the very powerful biceps tendon was recommended for use in transfer operations (Trillat). Even recent publications have recommended detaching the tendon from the fibular head on a bone fragment, passing it beneath the lateral collateral ligament, and reinserting it anteriorly on the tibia. Less traumatizing procedures detach only part of the biceps tendon, free or on a pedicle, for use in lateral repairs. The very thickness of the biceps tendon should tell us that this is a powerful and important muscle that cannot be arbitrarily transposed without negative consequences.

Quadriceps Tendon

Quadriceps tendon strips with or without a patellar bone block are sometimes used as an intraarticular substitute. This may take the form of a full-thickness or partial-thickness transfer. When the patellar tendon is used, the graft can be extended up into the quadriceps tendon. This makes it possible to route even relatively short patellar tendon strips "over the top" and even augment the reconstruction with a lateral stabilizing procedure.

Patellar Tendon

Patellar tendon grafts have been used as cruciate ligament substitutes for many years (Campbell, quoted in Burnett and Fowler 1985). Perhaps the best known technique is that of Jones (1980) in which the patellar tendon is left attached distally and is brought up to the femur through a tibial tunnel. Although this provides an elegant solution to the problem of graft attachment, it does not permit an isometric placement of the substitute. Also, the sharp angle between the graft and its bony attachment can predispose to retearing. The studies of Noyes et al. (1984) have shown that a strip of patellar tendon removed on proximal and distal bone blocks provides the strongest cruciate ligament substitute. A major advantage of this method is that it permits solid, bone-to-bone healing of the graft (Eriksson 1986; Friedman et al. 1985; Johnson et al. 1984). The procedure does not significantly weaken the residual patellar tendon, which in fact can regenerate in 4–6 months to the point where another graft can be harvested at the same site (personal observation).

The original Jones method has been substantially modified. A major discussion point in recent years has been whether a vascularized patellar tendon graft might be the optimum solution. The concept of this technique, advanced most strongly by Clancy (1985), is to maintain a blood supply to the graft by preserving the vascular pedicle connecting the patellar tendon with the infrapatellar fat pad. This greatly complicates the operating technique, and to our knowledge it has not yet been proven that the pedicle can ensure a permanent blood supply in humans. It is generally acknowledged that a graft must go through the stages of remodeling, restructuring, and revascularization. Noyes et al. report that 8 months after ACL reconstruction with a patellar tendon graft, the substitute exhibits about 80% of the mechanical properties of a healthy ligament in human patients. Today the rationale for a vascularized replacement has shifted more toward the concept that improved vascularization (which is still questionable in humans due to the technical difficulties of the operation) may be useful in shortening the phase of softening and edema. The remodeling phase, when the graft is susceptible to secondary elongation, is repeatedly cited as a cause of poor outcomes. Other opinions favor tacking fat pad tissue to an otherwise free graft as a relatively simple means of providing a vascular supply. The experimental studies of Drobny (see chapter by Drobny et al., p. 370 ff.) in sheep indicate that the fat pad pedicle provides only a minimal head start in graft vascularization. The technical effort of preserving a vascular pedicle would be justified only if the rupture strength of the substitute were markedly greater than that of a free graft. Basing the graft at its site of origin on the tibia over the bone block does not in itself provide a blood supply. Revascularization of the graft usually proceeds in a proximal to distal direction (Arnoczky et al. 1986). Ginsburg et al. (1980) showed in experimental animals that the diffusion of nutrients from the synovial fluid is more important for graft nutrition than a direct blood supply.

It remains to be proven whether the vascularization of a graft is the most important factor in long-term stability. Isometric graft placement appears to be at least of equal importance. The disadvantage of the patellar tendon graft is that, unlike the pes anserinus tendons, it can become frayed even during the operation. Aberrant graft fibers can become interposed between articular surfaces, causing a mechanical irritation that leads to hypertrophy of intraarticular structures, which in turn can cause locking and extension deficits. In one of our own series, we found that patellar tendon grafts with a fat pad pedicle offered no advantages and in fact were disadvantageous. In particular, the incidence of graft hypertrophy was markedly higher than when free grafts had been used. The patellar tendon has advantages (availability, strength, bone blocks at both ends, approach) but also potential disadvantages (stiffness, hypertrophy, patella infera).

Miscellaneous Tendon Grafts

Plantaris tendons and pedal extensor tendons have been used for cruciate ligament reconstruction (Zaricznyj 1983), but these grafts offer no advantages either on the donor side or in terms of subsequent rupture strength.

Deep-Frozen Allografts

Deep-frozen allogeneic tendons and ligaments (possibly with bone plugs attached) would seem to offer an ideal solution to the problem of weakening knee structures by autograft removal. Concern about the AIDS problem has eroded the popularity of these grafts, however, and animal studies have shown that their rupture strength at 6–10 months is well below the normal range for the ACL. In experiments on dogs, Curtis et al. (1985) performed histological and mechanical follow-up tests of freeze-dried allografts implanted up to 24 weeks earlier to function as a stent for fibrous tissue ingrowth. They found that the rupture strength of the grafts was approximately two-thirds that of a normal ACL. Shino et al. (1984) compared autologous patellar tendon grafts with deep-frozen allografts in dogs. Microangiographic studies showed that the allografts began to revascularize in the 6th week and later developed a vascularity conforming to the vascular pattern of normal cruciate ligaments. Histologic examination showed the development of a fibrous mesh scaffolding in the allografts similar to that in a normal ligament. Mechanical testing showed no significant differences between the deep-frozen allografts and the directly transplanted autografts (see also Webster and Werner 1983).

Xenografts

Specially prepared kangaroo tendons have been utilized for decades, and calf tendons were introduced several years ago amid great enthusiasm. Zich-ner (1985), while removing internal fixation material from human patients, obtained histologic specimens of previously implanted calf tendons. He found that joint stability was satisfactory after an average of 26 months' implantation. Histologic examination showed no evidence of remodeling or collagenation. It must be assumed that xenografts, like synthetics, are subject to eventual fatigue and rupture with passage of time. These assumptions are supported by the practical studies of Teitge (personal communication). Other difficulties are a relatively high incidence of infection, graft fixation problems, and the relative thickness of the implant.

Lyophilized Dura

Lyophilized dura has been used with varying degrees of success in various modes of application. A major use of this material is for repairing dural defects following neurosurgical operations. In assessing its value for cruciate reconstructions, a distinction must be drawn between extra- and intraarticular use. The studies of Wirth and Jäger (1980) indicate that lyophilized dura used extraarticularly in experimental animals undergoes the highest rate of incorporation and remodeling, which are complete by only 12 weeks postimplantation. When the material is used as an intraarticular cruciate substitute, this process takes roughly twice as long, and dura inside an osseous tunnel do not show completion of remodeling even after 40 weeks.

Comparisons

There have been few studies to date comparing the results of different materials as cruciate ligament substitutes. Ascherl et al. (1985) published comparative results in experimental animals. Friedmann et al. (1985) confirm that cruciate reconstructions with the patellar tendon, semitendinosus tendon, gracilis tendon, iliotibial tract, and meniscus have a success rate of 75%–85% during the first 3 years.

Before such comparisons can be made, however, we feel that a precise and comparable evaluation system must be devised. This is probably one of the main reasons why it has not yet been possible to define an objectively "best" solution for cruciate ligament replacement. It is extremely difficult to conduct a prospective study based on comparable instabilities, ages, and degrees of joint stress. Hefti et al. (1982)

conducted a retrospective comparative study evaluating different methods of cruciate ligament reconstruction. The results, compared according to subjective and objective criteria, were carefully analyzed. The authors found that the "lateral repair" alone led to the shortest rehabilitation time but was associated with markedly higher grades of instability than intraarticular procedures. Carbon fiber implants yielded unsatisfactory results due to the high incidence of retearing and because the hoped-for ingrowth of mechanically sound connective tissue failed to occur. Clancy (1985), comparing 200 free patellar tendon grafts with 300 vascularized patellar tendon grafts in human patients, found that functional stability in the pivot shift test was essentially the same in both groups. However, a definite improvement in the Lachman test was noted in the group with a vascularized patellar tendon graft. It is possible, of course, that the favorable Lachman results were due merely to the greater bulk of the vascularized graft (as, for example, with the relatively thick Gore-Tex ligament and calf tendons).

Summary

It will probably be several years before we can answer the question of whether synthetic, autologous, or other biological grafts are best for ACL reconstruction. Synthetic materials have the known advantages of simpler operating technique, less surgical trauma, and faster rehabilitation. Implants that succumb to fatigue failure can generally be replaced. Autologous replacements usually involve additional traumatization caused by harvesting the graft, and the operative technique is more demanding, but graft fixation usually presents fewer difficulties, as illustrated by patellar tendon grafts with a bone block at each end. Reportedly, the main disadvantage of autologous replacements is that their initially good stability decreases within a few months due to graft remodeling. Usually this phenomenon is transient. But excessive loading of the graft during this period can lead to elongation or even failure. A major concern, then, is to bridge this period of restructuring, either by applying external measures such as splintage or by the use of temporary synthetics. Care should be taken that these materials do not create a "stress shielding" effect that renders the autograft superfluous, leading to its resorption. Finally, it should be emphasized that success depends not just on graft selection but also on a meticulous operating technique and proper patient selection. The donor site might also have its own pathology, such as patellar infera after removal of parts of the patellar tendon. Arthroscopic techniques in particular would benefit from prefabricated grafts. Another essential factor, which will become increasingly important in the future due in part to financial concerns, is an optimum postoperative treatment program, which should be as brief as possible and involve a minimum period of immobilization.

References

Arnoczky SP, Warren RF, Ashlock MA (1986) Replacement of the anterior cruciate ligament using a patellar tendon allograft. An experimental study. J Bone Joint Surg [Am] 68/3: 376-85

Ascherl R, Siebels W, Kobor B et al. (1985) Comparative experimental studies with biologic materials for replacement of the anterior cruciate ligament. Unfallchirurgie 11/6: 278-88

Burnett QM, Fowler PJ (1985) Reconstruction of the anterior cruciate ligament: historical overview. Orthop Clin North Am 16/1: 143-57

Clancy WG jr (1985) Intra-articular reconstruction of the anterior cruciate ligament. Orthop Clin North Am 16/2: 181-189

Curtis RJ, DeLee JC, Drez DJ jr (1985) Reconstruction of the anterior cruciate ligament with freeze dried fascia lata allografts in dogs. A preliminary report. Am J Sports Med 13/6: 408-14

Ellera-Gomes JL, Marczyk LRS (1984) Anterior cruciate ligament reconstruction with a loop or double thickness of semitendinosus tendon. Am J Sports Med 12/3: 199-203

Enneker C (1985) Kombinierte Plastik des vorderen Kreuzbandes mit gestieltem Periostlappen und Kutisstreifen. Unfallchirurgie 2/5: 235-237

Eriksson E (1986) Stalked patellar tendon graft in reconstruction of the anterior cruciate ligament. Orthopedics 9/2: 205-211

Friedmann MJ, Shermann OH, Fox JM (1985) Autogenic anterior cruciate ligament (ACL) anterior reconstruction of the knee: A review. Clin Orthop 196: 9-1

Ginsburg JH, Whiteside LA, Piper TL (1980) Nutrient pathways in transferred patellar tendon used for anterior cruciate ligament reconstruction. Am J Sports Med 8/1: 15-18

Hefti F, Gächter A, Jenny H, Morscher E (1982) Replacement of the anterior cruciate ligament. A comparative study of four different methods of reconstruction. Arch Orthop Trauma Surg 100: 83-94

Johnson RJ, Eriksson E, Haggmark T, Pope MH (1984) Five- to ten-year follow-up evaluation after reconstruction of the anterior cruciate ligament. Clin Orthop 183: 122-140

Jones KG (1980) Results of use of the central one-third of the patellar ligament to compensate for anterior cruciate ligament deficiency. Clin Orthop 147: 39-44

Kuner EH (1978) Der gestielte Periostzügel als Möglichkeit des Außenbandersatzes am oberen Sprunggelenk. Hefte Unfallheilkd 133: 191-195

Lambert KL (1983) Vascularized patellar tendon graft with rigid internal fixation for anterior cruciate ligament insufficiency. Clin Orthop 172: 85-89

Müller J, Willenegger H, Terbrüggen D (1975) Freie autologe

Transplantate in der Behandlung des instabilen Knies. Hefte Unfallheilkd 125: 109-116

Noyes FR, Butler DL, Grood ES, Zernicke RF, Hefzy MS (1984) Biomechanical analysis of human ligament grafts used in knee-ligament repairs ad reconstructions. J Bone Joint Surg [Am] 66/3: 344-52

Pasquali-Lasagni M (1981) Reconstruction of the anterior cruciate ligament according to Lindemann-Bousquet in chronic anterior slackness of the knee. Minerva Orthop 32/12: 943-948

Scott WN, Schlosheim PM (1983) Intra-articular transfer of the iliotibial muscle-tendon unit. Clin Orthop 172: 97-101

Seiler H, Hager D, Kayser M, Flory PJ (1985) Ist der Meniscusersatz am vorderen Kreuzband tatsächlich eine historische Methode? Unfallchirurgie 88/7: 315-321

Shino K, Kawasaki T, Hirose H et al. (1984) Replacement of the anterior cruciate ligament by an allogeneic tendon graft. An experimental study in the dog. J Bone Joint Surg [Br] 66/5: 672-681

Simonet WT, Sim FH (1984) Repair and reconstruction of rotatory instability of the knee. Am J Sports Med 12/2: 89-97

Slocum DB, Larson RL (1968) Pes anserinus transplantation. A surgical procedure for control of rotatory instability of the knee. J Bone Joint Surg [Am] 50: 226-242

Trillat A, Dejour H, Bousquet G (1969) Laxité ancienne isolée du ligament croisé antérieur. Etudes des resultats de différentes methodes reconstructives ou palliatives. Rev Chir Orthop 55: 163

Villiger KJ (1984) Erfahrungen bei 250 dynamischen, proximal muskulär gestielten, vorderen Kreuzbandplastiken (Lindemann). Chirurg 55/11: 710-716

Webster DA, Werner FW (1983) Freeze-dried flexor tendons in anterior cruciate ligament reconstruction. Clin Orthop 181: 238-43

Wirth CJ, Jäger M (1980) Tierexperimentelle Untersuchungen zum Ein- und Umbau lyophilisierter Bindegewebe in Abhängigkeit vom Transplantatlager. In: Jäger M, Hackenbrock MH, Refior HJ (Hrsg) Osteosynthese, Endoprothetik und Biomechanik der Gelenke. Thieme, Stuttgart New York

Zariczynyj B (1983) Reconstruction of the anterior cruciate ligament using free tendon graft. Am J Sports Med 11/3: 164-176

Zarins B, Rowe CR (1986) Combined anterior cruciate-ligament reconstruction using semitendinosus tendon and iliotibial tract. J Bone Joint Surg [Am] 68/2: 160-77

Zichner L (1985) Kreuzbandersatz mit heterologen Bindegewebsstrukturen. Unfallchirurgie 11/5: 238-241

Arthroscopically Assisted Reconstruction of the Anterior Cruciate Ligament. Preoperative Planning: Two-Tunnel Technique

H.-U. Stäubli and S. Spörri

The precise placement of the tibial and femoral osseous tunnels for an anterior cruciate ligament (ACL) reconstruction requires a knowledge of the three-dimensional anatomy of the ACL. The reconstruction must replicate the geometry of the normal ACL attachment sites on the tibia and femur in order to achieve reproducible results.

We base our preoperative planning on anatomic studies by other authors supplemented by our own analysis of the geometry of the cruciate ligament attachments. In their investigation of the geometry of the ACL insertions on the femur and tibia, Girgis et al. (1975) described the femoral area of attachment as a semicircular segment at the medial border of the lateral femoral condyle located high up in the intercondylar notch. The tibial area of attachment of the ACL was located in the anterior intercondylar area, and its extent was defined.

Odensten and Gillquist (1985) described an oval-shaped femoral attachment site and defined the tibial attachment in relation to the anterior tibial border and the medial and lateral intercondylar tubercles.

Good et al. (1987) recommended using a drill guide with a single-tunnel technique for open reconstruction of the ACL. Use of the drill guide led to better reproducibility of the femoral attachment than when the insertion sites were selected by hand.

Sidles et al. (1988) drew attention to the broad-based natural areas of ACL insertion, which allow for discretion in varying the placement of the attachment sites. Using the MAS technique, they found differences in ligament length and tension relationships from the center to the periphery of the anatomic insertion sites. Hefzy et al. (1989) identified the "most isometric" areas of femoral attachment.

Purpose of Study

The present study is concerned with the preoperative planning of an arthroscopically assisted reconstruction of the ACL. The goal of preoperative planning is to achieve a reconstruction that closely replicates the normal anatomy of the ACL at operation.

Planning of the 2-tunnel technique is based on the analysis of standard X-ray films. The individualized planning allows for a morphologically precise reconstruction of the ACL in 3 planes (Stäubli 1988) that takes into account the functionally "most isometric" zones of ligament attachment.

Three-Dimensional Geometry of the ACL Attachment Sites: Experimental Findings

We performed experiments to investigate the three-dimensional arrangement of the ACL attachments and the anatomic course of the ligament.

The anatomic attachment sites were marked in cadaveric knee joints using lead wires and small lead plates and then analyzed radiographically in relation

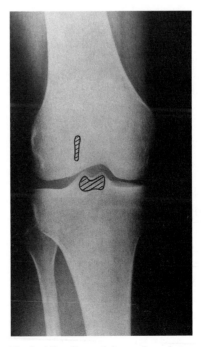

Fig. 1. AP radiograph in one-legged stance, showing the areas of ACL attachment on the frontal plane

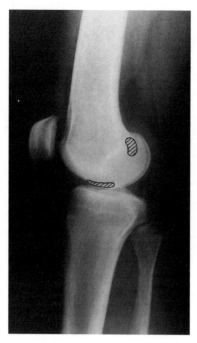

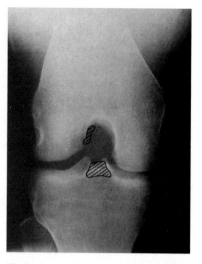

Fig. 3. Areas of ACL attachment as projected on the intercondylar "tunnel" view with the knee flexed 45°

Fig. 2. Lateral radiograph in one-legged stance, showing the areas of ACL attachment on the sagittal plane

to designated landmarks and standard reference lines. The areas of attachment were analyzed using standard radiographic projections (AP, lateral, tunnel views). The relationship of the marked attachment sites to known reference lines served as the basis for anatomic planning of the reconstruction. These findings were transferred to macerated bone models and analyzed micrometrically with respect to standard contours and reference lines.

The femoral and tibial attachment sites of the ACL are shown schematically on the frontal plane in Fig. 1 and on the sagittal plane in Fig. 2. Figure 3 shows the areas projected on the tunnel view in 45° flexion, and Fig. 4 shows the sites on the sagittal plane in 90° flexion.

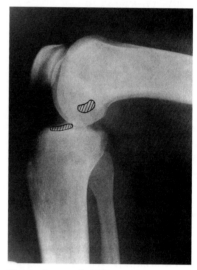

Fig. 4. Areas of ACL attachment as projected on a lateral radiograph with the knee flexed 90°

Preoperative Planning of the Arthroscopically Controlled Reconstruction

Preoperative planning of the arthroscopially assisted reconstruction is based on an analysis of the following standard X-ray films, which are obtained in both knees.

Standard Radiographic Series

The standard series consists of an AP view of the knee in the one-legged stance (20 × 40-cm cassette, see Fig. 1), a lateral view of the knee in the one-legged stance (20 × 40-cm cassette, see Fig. 2), a lateral view of the knee in 90° flexion (see Fig. 4), an intercondylar tunnel view in 45° flexion (see Fig. 3), and a patellar sunrise view in 30° flexion.

Stressradiographs Under Anesthesia

Stressradiographs are taken to document the antero-posterior limits of motion, which define the degree of femorotibial subluxation. The direction, limits, and type of displacement are important criteria in selecting candidates for reconstruction.

Definition of the Anatomic Tibial and Femoral Areas of Attachment

We based our planning on anatomic studies by Girgis et al. (1975), Van Dijk et al. (1979), Arnoczky (1983), Arnoczky and Warren (1988), Odensten and Gillquist (1985), Good et al. (1987), Hefzy et al. (1989), and Sidles et al. (1988). We also referred to functional anatomic studies by Kennedy et al. (1974), Norwood and Cross (1979), Ellison and Berg (1985), and technical planning guidelines for arthroscopic surgery published by Purnell et al. (1988) and Rosenberg et al. (1988).

Normal Anterior Cruciate Ligament

On the frontal plane the ACL ascends from the anterior intercondylar area toward the lateral half of the intercondylar notch. The femoral insertion site is located in the posterosuperior portion of the intercondylar aspect of the lateral femoral condyle. For functional definition of the areas of attachment, contour maps were plotted and transferred to the macerated bone. Known radiographic landmarks and reference lines were marked with lead wires and small lead plates to aid in understanding the anatomic definition of the attachment sites. Analysis of the knee contours, knowledge of the location of the projected attachment sites, and the location of anatomic landmarks and reference lines formed the basis for individualized planning of the reconstruction.

Tibial Area of Attachment

The tibial area of attachment (TAA) of the ACL is determined on the preoperative radiographs as follows. The anteroposterior knee film in the one-legged stance or the tunnel view is used to define the center of the TAA on the *frontal plane*. This point is located in the anterior intercondylar area, anterior to the intercondylar eminence and posterior to the transverse knee ligament between the central borders of the medial and lateral tibial plateaus, which are bounded by the tubercles of the intercondylar eminence. The course of the ACL is directed anteromedially to posterolaterally (see Figs. 1, 3). On the *sagittal plane*, the TAA is projected as a line 10–12 mm long immediately in front of the intercondylar eminence. In the extended knee, the ACL runs along the posterior border of the intercondylar roof (see Figs. 2, 4).

Femoral Area of Attachment

The femoral area of attachment (FAA) and its center are located in the posterosuperior portion of the intercondylar surface of the lateral femoral condyle. As the degrees of freedom of knee flexion increase, the area of the "most isometric" femoral attachment becomes smaller (Hefzy et al. 1988). Because a knee flexion angle of 135° or more is desired after surgery, the central isometric attachment site is reduced to a very narrow, bandlike area whose longitudinal axis forms an angle of 37.6° +/− 5.4° with the slope of the intercondylar roof in 90° flexion under an anterior stress of 100 N (Hefzy et al. 1989).

Accordingly, the anterior border of the femoral osseous tunnel must be placed so that the central portion of the graft coincides with this bandlike region where there is less than 2 mm change in tibiofemoral distance from extension to 120° flexion (the "2-mm region").

Three-Dimensional Orientation of the Graft

Frontal Plane

The graft passes through the center of the TAA and the lateral half of the intercondylar notch to its attachment site on the femur (Fig. 5).

Sagittal Plane

The graft passes through the geometric center of the TAA and along the inferior edge of the intercondylar roof toward the attachment site of the anteromedial bundle on the intercondylar aspect of the lateral femoral condyle (see Fig. 6).

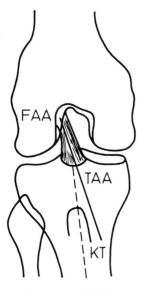

Fig. 5. The transtibial Kirschner guidewire *(KT)* is inserted at a 15° anteromedial angle toward the geometric center of the tibial area of attachment *(TAA)* and toward the center of the femoral area of attachment *(FAA)*, corresponding to the normal course of the ACL

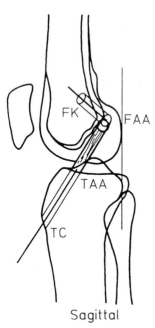

Sagittal

Fig. 6. The tibial Kirschner wire at the center of the tibial tunnel *(TK)* is directed toward the center of the tibial area of attachment *(TAA)* and along the lower edge of the intercondylar roof. The femoral Kirschner wire at the center of the femoral tunnel *(FK)* points to the center of the femoral area of attachment *(FAA)*

Transverse Plane

On the transverse plane the ACL takes an anteromedial-to-posterolateral course with respect to the intercondylar notch.

Orientation of the Tibial Kirschner Guidewire

Frontal Plane

On the frontal plane the Kirschner guidewire approaches the center of the TAA at a 15° angle from the anteromedial side. It points to the center of the lateral half of the intercondylar notch and toward the attachment of the anteromedial bundle on the lateral femoral condyle (see Fig. 5).

Sagittal Plane

The Kirschner guidewire passes through the geometric center of the TAA 3–5 mm caudal to the superior border of the intercondylar roof (Blumensaat's line) toward the center of the FAA (region of the anteromedial bundle) (see Fig. 6).

Transverse Plane

Viewed on the transverse plane, the tibial Kirschner guidewire enters the joint at a 15° angle from the medial tibial condyle. It is directed through the lateral half of the intercondylar notch toward the center of the anteromedial bundle at the femoral attachment site (Fig. 7).

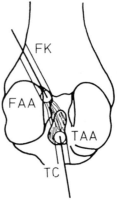

Horizontal

Fig. 7. A view on the transverse plane shows the tibial tunnel *(TK)* directed toward the center of the TAA and the femoral tunnel *(FK)* directed toward the FAA

Orientation of the Femoral Kirschner Guidewire

Frontal Plane

On the frontal plane the transfemoral Kirschner wire for a 2-tunnel reconstruction by the "inside-out" technique passes through the anteromedial portal above the transverse knee ligament through the lateral half of the intercondylar notch toward the attachment of the anteromedial bundle of the ACL (Fig. 8).

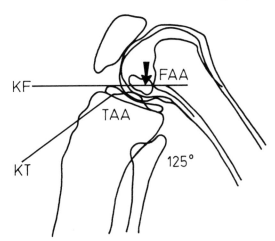

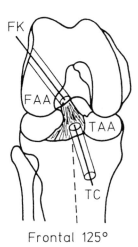

Fig. 8. The osseous tunnels are directed toward the tibial and femoral areas of attachment (*TAA, FAA*)

Sagittal Plane

For the inside-out technique, the transfemoral Kirschner guidewire is inserted directly above the superior margin of the transverse knee ligament or medial meniscus anterior horn with the knee flexed 125°. At this flexion angle the wire runs in a slightly ascending, posterolateral direction toward the center of the proposed femoral attachment site. It must pass through the condyle, which is not possible if the knee is flexed only 90°–100°. The center of the femoral attachment site of the anteromedial bundle is located 4–5 mm anterior and 4–5 mm caudal to the point of intersection of the intercondylar roof tangent and distal femoral metaphyseal line. The most isometric femoral attachment is located in the band-shaped, flexion-dependent "2-mm region" of length change as described by Hefzy et al. (1989). This attachment site coincides with the functionally most-isometric areas of attachment described earlier in this book by Friederich and O'Brien (p. 78 ff.). The exit point of

Fig. 9. The transtibial Kirschner wire (*KT*) is directed toward the center of the TAA, and the femoral Kirschner wire (*KF*) (for the inside-out technique) is inserted above the anterior horn of the medial meniscus toward the attachment of the anteromedial bundle in the FAA (knee must be flexed 125°). *Arrow:* point of entry into the bone

the transfemoral tunnel is cranial to the lateral intermuscular septum on the sagittal plane (Fig. 9).

Transverse Plane

On the transverse plane the transfemoral Kirschner wire ascends at a 35° angle from the anteromedial side, medial to the border of the patellar ligament, directed toward the lateral half of the intercondylar notch. Passing along the central aspect of the synovial sheath of the posterior cruciate ligament (PCL) toward the intercondylar border of the femoral attachment high up on the lateral femoral condyle, the wire penetrates the condyle and emerges on the femoral metaphysis, showing little tunnel divergence with respect to the transtibial Kirschner wire (Fig. 10).

Arthroscopic and Radiographic Position Check and Orientation of the Kirschner Guidewires

Emergence of the tibial Kirschner wire at the center of the tibial attachment site is easily accomplished from the anterolateral portal under arthroscopic guidance using a 30° scope. To avoid later impingement of the graft against the intercondylar roof in full knee extension, the position of the tibial guidewire is checked arthroscopically in the extended knee with correct femorotibial alignment. If the Kirschner wire is too far anterior, it will impinge on the inferior bor-

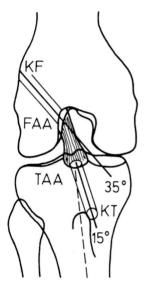

Fig. 10. For the 2-tunnel inside-out technique, the transfemoral Kirschner wire *(KF)* is oriented at a 35° angle from antero-medial to superolateral on the frontal plane. *KT*, Tibial Kirschner guidewire; *KF*, femoral Kirschner guidewire; *TAA*, tibial area of attachment; *FAA*, femoral area of attachment

der of the anterior intercondylar roof. A special aiming device and parallel drill guide can be used to achieve a posterior offset of the central transtibial Kirschner wire to avoid anterior impingement in extension, medial impingement against the PCL, and lateral impingement against the intercondylar aspect of the lateral condyle.

The position of the femoral Kirschner guidewire is difficult to assess in 125° flexion with the arthroscope in the anterolateral portal. A more accurate method is to check the position of the tip of the Kirschner wire on the sagittal plane using an image intensifier in the transverse projection. This can avoid placement of the guidewire too far anterior or posterior, which would result in primary anisometry of the ligament substitute. Use of the image intensifier guarantees reproducible attachment sites owing to the controlled placement of the Kirschner guidewires.

Tibial Tunnel Size and Orientation

The size of the graft is determined in advance in accordance with the arthroscopically confirmed position of the tibial Kirschner wire, intercondylar notch clearance, patient morphology (size, weight), demand level, and constitutional ligamentous laxity. We generally employ a graft 8–12 mm wide and 6–8 mm thick with a distal trapezoidal bone block in the region of the patellar base when we use the quadriceps

tendon for autologous replacement. For a graft 8 mm wide, we drill the tunnel with an 8-mm cannulated reamer. For a moderately thick graft we use a 10-mm reamer, and for grafts of greater diameter we enlarge the tibial attachment site with a curette.

Femoral Tunnel Size and Orientation

The diameter of the femoral tunnel is determined by the configuration of the proximal end of the quadriceps tendon graft. Generally we drill an 8-mm femoral tunnel in small individuals and a 10-mm tunnel in patients of normal or large stature.

When the ACL is replaced by the central one-third of the patellar tendon with bone blocks from the tibial tuberosity and patellar apex, the eccentric insertion of the graft on the bone block can be oriented so as to produce a posterior or anterior orientation of the graft within the femoral tunnel; this provides a means of adjusting isometry secondarily after the tunnels have been drilled.

Discussion

The three-dimensional planning and intraoperative position check of the Kirschner guidewires that define the centers of the tibial and femoral tunnels and their exit sites in the knee joint are important. The goal of planning is to achieve an anatomic reconstruction of the ACL that reproduces the natural states of tension within the ligament. Engebretsen et al. (1988) have shown that as the normal knee is extended from 45° flexion, the tension of the ACL gradually increases beyond 20° of flexion. An isometric progression of ACL tension like that described by Odensten and Gillquist (1985) does not seem physiologic and does not correspond to the normal states of tension in the ligament. For this reason we consider it important to achieve graft isometry between 130° and 20° of knee flexion. In the range from 15° flexion to full extension, the ligament is physiologically anisotonic, i.e., the state of ACL tension increases as the knee extends.

According to Hunter et al., this calls for a superoposterolateral placement of the femoral attachment combined with a geometrically centered tibial attachment (Engebretsen 1988). The goal of the reconstruction is an anatomic replication of the ACL, which requires an almost isometric (constant-length) and isotonic (constant-tension) graft state from 120° to about 20° of flexion. From 15° to 0° flexion, ligament tension should be slightly anisometric as well as anisotonic, increasing as the joint nears full extension. This is accomplished by *placing the tibial attachment in the anteromedial portion of the anatomic insertion site in the anterior intercondylar area* while *placing the femoral attachment at the insertion site of the anteromedial bundle* on the femur. The exact placement of the graft depends on the nature and thickness of the selected replacement material. Graft selection and the individual morphology of the joint call for an individualized anatomic planning of the reconstruction. Accurate, reproducible placement of the tibial and femoral attachments are guaranteed by preoperative planning, arthroscopy, and intraoperative image intensification control. Graft tension should be adjusted so that, as the knee approaches full extension (in the neutral position), the ligament becomes increasingly tense with an associated physiologic recruitment of a maximum number of graft elements.

The increase of ligament tension near extension can be checked arthroscopically by visual inspection and with a probing hook in various joint positions during definitive fixation of the graft.

References

Arnoczky SP (1983) Anatomy of the anterior cruciate ligament. Clin Orthop 172: 19–25

Arnoczky SP, Warren RF (1988) Anatomy of the cruciate ligaments. In: Feagin JA (ed) The crucial ligaments. Churchill Livingstone, New York Edingburgh London Melbourne, pp 179–195

Van Dijk R, Huiskes R, Selvik G (1979) Technical note: Roentgenstereophotogrammetric methods for the evaluation of the three dimensional kinematic behaviour and cruciate ligament length patterns of the human knee joint. J Biomech 12: 727–731

Ellison AE, Berg EE (1985) Embryology, anatomy and function of the anterior cruciate ligament. Orthop Clin North Am 16: 3–14

Engebretsen L, Lew WD, Lexis JL, Hunter RE (1988) Knee joint motion and ligament force before and after augmented primary repair of acute anterior cruciate ligament rupture. Acta Orthop Scand

Girgis FG, Marshall JL, Al Monajem ARS (1975) The cruciate ligaments of the knee joint: Anatomical, functional and experimental analysis. Clin Orthop 106: 216–231

Good L, Odensten M, Gillquist J (1987) Precision in reconstruction of the anterior cruciate ligament. Acta Orthop Scand 58: 658–661

Graf B (1987) Isometric placement of substitutes for the anterior cruciate ligament. In: Jackson DW, Drez D (eds) The anterior cruciate deficient knee. Mosby, St. Louis Washington/DC Toronto, pp 102–113

Hefzy MS, Grood ES, Noyes FR (1988) Factors affecting the region of most isometric femoral attachments Part II: The anterior cruciate ligament. Am J Sports Med 17: 208–216

Hunter RE, Lewis JL, Lw WD, Kowalzy KC, Settle W (1988) Biomechanics of ACL reconstructions: The effect of initial graft length. 14th Annual Meeting of the American Orthopedic and Sports Medicine Society (abstract)

Kennedy JC, Weinberg HW, Wilson AS (1974) The anatomy and function of the anterior cruciate ligament as determined by clinical and morphological studies. J Bone Joint Surgery [Am] 56: 223–235

Norwood LA, Cross MJ (1979) Anterior cruciate ligament: Functional anatomy of its bundles in rotatory instabilities. Am J Sports Med 7/1: 23–26

Odensten M, Gillquist J (1985) Functional anatomy of the anterior cruciate ligament and a rationale for reconstruction. J Bone Joint Surg [Am] 67: 257–262

Penner DA, Daniel DM, Wood P, Mishra D (1988) An in vitro study of anterior cruciate ligament graft placement and isometry. Am J Sports Med 16/3: 238–243

Purnell ML, Odén RR, Berkeley ME (1988) Arthroscopic anterior cruciate ligament reconstruction. A. I. Guide surgical technique. Johnson & Johnson, Aspea/CO

Rosenberg TD, Paulos LE, Abbott PJ (1988) Arthroscopic cruciate repair and reconstruction: An overview and descriptions of technique In: Feagin JA (ed) The crucial ligaments. Churchill Livingstone, New York Edingburgh London Melbourne, pp 409–423

Sidles JA, Larsen RV, Garbini JL, Matsen FA (1988) Ligament length relationships in the moving knee. University of Washington

Stäubli H-U (1988) Preoperative Planning to determine anatomic attachment areas in anterior cruciate ligament reconstruction. ACL study group conference, Snowmass, Aspen/CO, March 19–26th, pp 37–38

Reconstruction of the ACL with a Patellar Tendon Graft Based on the Infrapatellar Fat Pad: An Experimental Study in Animals

T. Drobny, We. Müller, U. Munzinger, and S. M. Perren

The experimental groundwork for the present study was laid during the 1980s, when it was already generally known that the McIntosh type of extraarticular cruciate ligament repair was of only short-term benefit, and that reconstruction of the anterior cruciate ligament (ACL) had to involve restoration of the central pivot. The Jones technique using a distally based strip of patellar tendon (Jones 1963) and the free patellar tendon graft (Brückner 1972) were the procedures that we used most frequently. Now as before, there is no question that the patellar tendon is the material best suited for ACL replacement owing to its histomorphologic and biomechanical properties (Noyes and Butler 1984). The groups of Clancy (Clancy 1983) and Noyes (Paulos et al. 1983) have advocated a technique of maintaining vascularity to the patellar tendon graft by carefully preserving its attachment with the infrapatellar fat pad as a "vascular pedicle." Following suitable dissection and mobilization, the vascularized patellar tendon graft can be transposed into the joint to function as an ACL substitute. The rationale for using a pedicled graft was to overcome the known disadvantages of a free graft and promote faster and more reliable graft healing. The increased technical difficulty of the operation seemed a reasonable price to pay. This attitude was reinforced when our initial experiments with disulphine blue vital staining in sheep confirmed vascularization of the patellar tendon graft through the fat pad pedicle (Fig. 1). The fact that the metabolic turnover in bradytrophic tissue is relatively low suggested that even partial retention of the microcirculation in the pedicle graft could contribute significantly to its survival as a cruciate substitute. To test this assumption, we conducted a long-term study in the knee joints of sheep, comparing the healing of free and pedicled grafts during the first postoperative year by means of microangiography and tensile testing.[1]

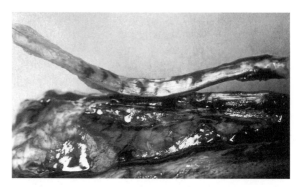

Fig. 1. Patellar tendon in the sheep knee joint, mobilized as a graft with a fat pad pedicle, 5 min after injection of disulphine blue into the femoral artery. Because the fat pad pedicle is the only tissue attaching the graft to the endogenous circulation, the blue staining of the graft confirms perfusion via the fat pad

Method

We divided 18 female Swiss mountain sheep into 2 groups of 9 animals each. Under general anesthesia and aseptic conditions, the ACL of the right knee joint was excised by open arthrotomy and immediately replaced with a graft from the central one-third of the patellar tendon. A free graft was used in one group, and in the other the graft was left attached to a fat pad pedicle. The operating technique is largely identical to that in the human knee. Postoperatively the knees were immobilized with a laterally applied AO/ASIF external fixation device in 90° flexion, which is the neutral position in sheep. The external skeletal fixation was removed 3 weeks postoperatively, and the animals were permitted to move about freely. During the immobilization period, the animals were kept in a standing position by a trapeze-like sling apparatus suspended from the ceiling of their stall. This ensured that the aftercare regimen was identical for all animals.

Seven sheep from each group were selected for microangiographic study. The first animal was killed immediately after surgery to assess the initial situation, and the others were sacrificed at 2, 4, 6, 8, 26,

---

[1] The experimental work was performed at the Swiss Research Institute for Experimental Surgery in Davos under the direction of S. M. Perren.

and 52 weeks postoperatively. In this way we were able to trace systematically the revascularization processes occurring in both groups during the first postoperative year.

The animals were killed using a standardized technique. Under intubation anesthesia, the femoral artery was exposed in the inguinal region, and 500 ml of 30% barium sulfate, filtered to a 1-μm particle size, was infused into the artery through a cannula. A special pump system maintained a constant infusion pressure of 140 mm Hg, corresponding to the systolic

blood pressure in sheep. The animals were fully heparinized (500 U/kg b.w.) before the infusion was started. Death was induced by the barium infusion itself or by an overdose of pentobarbital. After completion of the barium infusion, the knee segment was amputated in toto and deep frozen at -20° C. Two days later the central pivot was excised from the deep-frozen specimen with a band saw. The block, measuring approximately $2 \times 5 \times 10$ cm, was fixed in 4% formalin and decalcified in 6% formic acid. Finally the decalcified specimens were embedded in

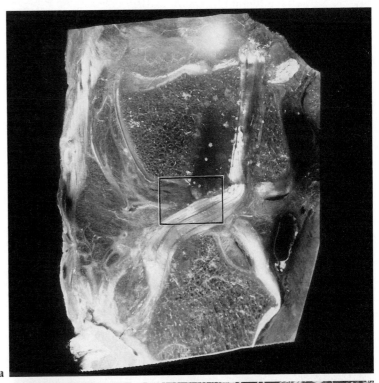

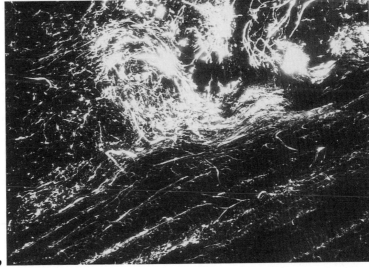

Fig. 2 a,b. Free patellar tendon graft 2 weeks postoperatively. **a** Longitudinal section through the knee joint on the sagittal plane clearly demonstrates the structure and course of the graft, the position of the fat pad, the distal femur, and the proximal tibia. **b** Microangiogram of the *boxed area* in **a** shows abundant longitudinally oriented capillaries within the graft. Some of the vessels appear to originate from the fat pad, which is directly in front of the graft

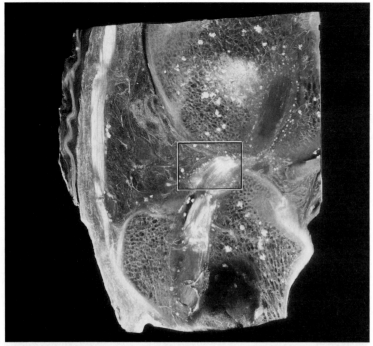

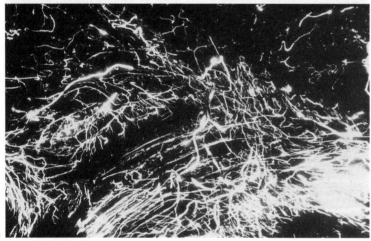

Fig.3a,b. Patellar tendon graft based on the fat pad 2 weeks postoperatively, plain section (**a**) and microangiogram (**b**, *boxed area* in **a**). The anatomic orientation is the same as in Fig.2. The vascularity of the graft is clearly visible

methylmethacrylate and cut into 1-mm-thick sagittal sections with a tissue slicer. Microangiograms were obtained in the sections by the use of high-resolution glass plates.

Two sheep from each group were selected for tensile testing of the graft at 1 year after ACL replacement. Immediately after the animals were killed, the knee joints were dissected free, and the gross appearance of the graft was documented photographically. After removal of all surrounding soft tissues, the femur-graft-tibia specimens were clamped in an Instron-like tensile testing machine, and the biomechanical properties of the specimens (stiffness, yield point, rupture point) were tested using a strain rate of 2 cm/min.

Results

Microangiography in Group A (Free Graft)

Not surprisingly, the free patellar tendon graft appeared as an avascular tissue band on the immediate postoperative microangiogram.

In the animal killed at 2 weeks, the microangiogram already showed extensive revascularization of the graft (Fig.2). Additional angiograms taken during the course of the first postoperative year showed the similar appearance of a well-vascularized graft, although we had the impression that the density of the capillary network decreased somewhat over time.

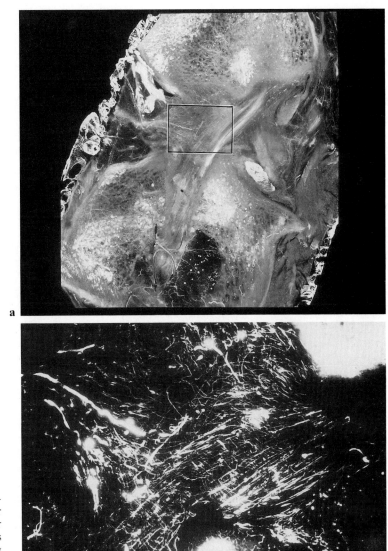

Fig. 4a,b. Plain section (**a**) and microangiogram (**b**, *boxed area* in **a**) of a patellar tendon graft based on the fat pad, 1 year postoperatively. The angiogram shows good perfusion of the graft with capillary attachments between the fat pad and graft

Microangiography in Group C (Graft with Fat Pad Pedicle)

Despite the standardized technique of the barium sulfate infusion, a technical error was committed in the first sheep of this group resulting in underfilling of the vascular network throughout the specimen. Hence the specimen could not be used to assess perfusion of the pedicled graft in the immediate postoperative period.

Because the next specimen at 2 weeks showed marked vascularity of the graft, similar to that in the other group (Fig. 3), we felt that a meaningful assessment could be made without having to repeat the immediate postoperative study.

The additional microangiograms in the pedicle group showed the same pattern of an abundant capillary supply in the graft with attachments between the fat pad and graft at the capillary level (Fig. 4).

Tensile Tests

The results of tensile tests on the free and pedicled grafts 1 year postoperatively are shown graphically in Figs. 5 and 6. The shaded areas mark the region that tends to contain the rupture curve of a normal ACL in the sheep. Because a strip of patellar tendon behaves much the same as the ACL in tensile tests, it is desirable to achieve values that are within the shaded range.

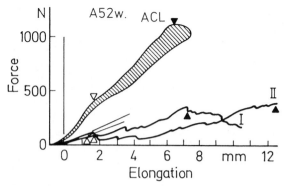

Fig. 5. The *open triangles* mark the yield points, beyond which the collagen undergoes irreversible strain. The *filled triangles* mark the points of complete rupture. Curves I and II clearly show that the stiffness and maximum load of the free grafts at 1 year postoperatively are well below the desired range *(shaded area)*

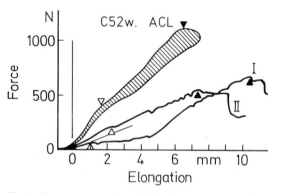

Fig. 6. Rupture curves (I and II) of the grafts with a fat pad pedicle at 1 year postoperatively (see also Fig. 5 and text)

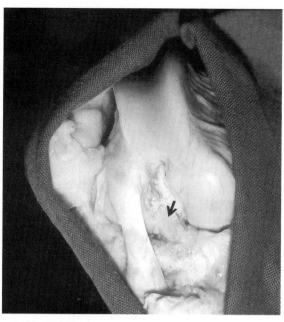

Fig. 7. The surgically exposed free graft appears as a strong, functionally sound neoligament 1 year postoperatively. Tensile testing of the graft leaves much to be desired, however (see also Fig. 5, curve II)

Discussion and Clinical Relevance

The results of the microangiograms and tensile tests in this study show no significant differences between the free and pedicled patellar tendon grafts. Both grafts had a blood supply by 2 weeks after surgery, indicating that graft revascularization occurred during the first 2 weeks regardless of whether a free or pedicled graft was used. Even beyond the first postoperative year, there was no difference in further revascularization and healing of the grafts in the sheep. Since the case numbers in this study are small, we advise caution in interpreting the results. Especially in the rupture tests, one might gain the impression that the pedicled grafts achieved somewhat better values than the free grafts, though probably not by a significant factor. One should also be cautious about applying the results to humans. The fat pad in the ovine knee is much larger than in the human knee and completely covers a free graft following joint closure. Thus, even if the graft is not left attached to the fat pad, the anatomic apposition of the fat pad to the graft tends to facilitate its revascularization. The situation may be quite different in humans.

The "blood supply" of the pedicled graft, as demonstrated by vital staining in Fig. 1, cannot be interpreted as a true circulation with arterial inflow and venous drainage, but only as a kind of graft perfusion at the capillary level – probably in a very reduced form.

The gross appearance of the grafts at 1 year is good, as we can see by the example of a free graft in Fig. 7. The discrepancy between the favorable appearance of the healed graft at 1 year and its biomechanical properties (see Fig. 5, curve II) leads us to conclude that the outward appearance of a cruciate ligament graft, as seen during arthroscopy, for example, is a poor indicator of its mechanical quality. Nevertheless, such a graft can still be functionally sound and even stress-competent to a degree, despite its inferior mechanical quality, as a result of static compensation by the synergists and dynamic compensation by the musculature.

We know that the initial biomechanical quality of both the free and pedicled grafts is not yet restored at 1 year postoperatively despite the potentially good appearance of the substitute ligament. We do not know, however, whether the mechanical quality of the grafts improves during subsequent years, remains the same as in the "snapshot" at 1 year, or deteriorates over time. Further long-term studies are needed to resolve this issue.

The operating technique for mobilizing a patellar tendon graft based on the infrapatellar fat pad is more demanding than that for a free graft. This extra effort is justified only if the results of the pedicled reconstruction are decidedly superior to those of the free graft. A retrospective comparison of patients at the Wilhelm Schulthess Hospital in Zurich who underwent ACL reconstructions with a free or pedicled patellar tendon graft has clearly shown that, as in our animal study, both techniques lead to essentially identical results. The long-term results do not confirm that the extra effort of the "vascularized" reconstruction is definitely worthwhile, but neither do they indicate a negative effect (Drobny et al. 1987).

On the other hand, there have been reports of negative effects associated with the pedicled technique, such as the potential for graft hypertrophy leading to an extension deficit caused by graft impingement in the notch of Grant (Gächter 1988). We have not encountered this problem in our own follow-ups.

Conclusion

The disadvantages of autologous ACL reconstruction with a free patellar tendon graft are the rather exacting surgical technique, the uncertainty of graft healing and thus of the long-term outcome, pro-longed rehabilitation, and prolonged occupational disability.

Animal experiments and clinical observations indicate that basing the patellar tendon graft on the infrapatellar fat pad eliminates none of these disadvantages. It compounds the technical complexity of the procedure and requires a higher degree of surgical skill than the free graft technique.

We conclude that the free patellar tendon graft, owing to its relative technical simplicity, which ultimately benefits precision, should be acknowledged as the procedure of choice. When atraumatic operating technique is used, when isometric principles are known and obeyed, and when the graft is provided with synovial coverage, the free patellar tendon graft should provide satisfactory and reproducible results in reconstructions of the ACL.

References

Brückner H, Brückner H (1972) Bandplastiken im Kniebereich nach dem Baukastenprinzip. Zentralbl Chir 97: 65–77

Clancy WG (1983) Anterior cruciate ligament functional instability. A static intra-articular and dynamic extra-articular procedure. Clin Orthop 172: 102–106

Drobny TK, Munzinger UK, Müller We (1987) Does the vascularised patellar tendon graft really produce better results? Semin Orthop 2/1: 35–43

Jones GK (1963) Reconstruction of the anterior cruciate ligament. A technique using the central one third of the patellar tendon. J Bone Joint Surg [Am] 925–932

Noyes FR, Butler DJ (1984) Biomechanical analysis of human ligament grafts used in knee-ligament repairs and reconstruction. J Bone Joint Surg [Am] 66: 344–352

Paulos LE, Butler DJ, Noyes FR, Grood ES (1983) Intra-articular cruciate reconstruction. II Replacement with vascularised patellar tendon. Clin Orthop 172: 78–84

Use of the Semitendinosus Tendon for Anterior Cruciate Ligament Reconstruction

J.-L. Meystre

Although the patellar tendon provides a graft material whose value is widely acknowledged, the following arguments can be advanced for use of the semitendinosus tendon:

– Operative removal of the semitendinosus tendon has fewer deleterious effects.
– The thin, regular cross section of the graft allows for simple arthroscopic placement. A notch plasty is usually not required.
– The thin cross section facilitates graft nutrition by the diffusion of synovial fluid, reducing the risk of necrosis until the graft is revascularized.
– Clinical and laboratory tests have shown that the semitendinosus graft is at least equivalent to the patellar tendon graft in its biomechanical properties.

Biological and Mechanical Properties of Autografts

We shall begin by comparing the properties of the semitendinosus tendon and the central one-third of the patellar tendon.

Biological Properties

Clinical and experimental studies demonstrate good survival of the grafts within the joint (Arnoczky et al. 1982; Chiroff 1975; Clancy et al. 1981; Drobny et al. 1984; Johnson 1986), although we do not yet have precise data on adaptation, possible metaplasia, or long-term mechanical properties.

Nutrition of the collagenous tissue relies mainly on the diffusion of nutrients from the synovial fluid (Peacock 1959; Potenza 1964) and also on circulatory pathways. Vascularization begins directly adjacent to the tunnel openings and through the newly formed synovial envelope (Arnoczky et al. 1982; Clancy et al. 1981; Drobny et al. 1984).

Pedicled and nonpedicled grafts do not differ significantly in their viability and revascularization. A free graft is easier to use, the absence of a pedicle facilitating placement. Both types of graft attach to the bone in approximately 6 weeks (Arnoczky et al. 1982; Clancy et al. 1981; Forward and Cowan 1963; Johnson 1986; Luhiston and Walmsley 1960).

In both cases the strength of the bony attachment increases fairly rapidly until about the 3rd postoperative month. There is then a transient decline, probably due to a progression of revascularization that later leads to metaplasia.

The strength of the graft declines greatly in the initial postoperative months and then increases again (Clancy et al. 1981; Drobny et al. 1984; Roth and Kennedy 1980). At its low point, the strength of the semitendinosus tendon graft is only 15% the strength of the normal ACL (Roth and Kennedy 1980), and that of the patellar tendon graft is 26% (Clancy et al. 1981).

If the semitendinosus tendon is looped to double its effective thickness, it approximates the value for the patellar tendon graft (30% vs. 26%).

Mechanical Properties

The mechanical properties of various human graft tissues were investigated in detail by Noyes et al. (1984). Here we shall cite comparative values for the following structures: the anterior cruciate ligament (ACL), the central one-third of the patellar tendon with bony attachments, and the semitendinosus tendon.

We are specifically interested in the values of cross-sectional area, rupture strength (maximum load), elasticity, and energy to failure; these are stated as a percentage of the values for the ACL.

The *cross-sectional area* measures 114% for the patellar tendon and 32% for the semitendinosus tendon relative to the ACL.

Various studies have shown that the core of the patellar tendon graft is prone to necrosis. Because graft nutrition depends on diffusion, the conditions should be more favorable in the thinner semitendinosus tendon (Johnson 1986; Potenza 1964). Also, the small cross-sectional area of this tendon eliminates or reduces the need for a notch plasty during placement of the graft.

The *rupture strength* values relative to the ACL are as follows: patellar tendon 168%, semitendinosus tendon 70%, and looped semitendinosus tendon 140%.

The strain (elasticity) of the semitendinosus tendon varies greatly depending on whether it is measured locally between 2 points in the tendon or between the tissue ends.

The strains measured in the patellar tendon and ACL are more similar because the functional length is defined by the bony ends.

Thus, the high elasticity of the semitendinosus tendon determined by grip-to-grip measurements is based on the greater length of the tendon and the occurrence of slippage within the grips. Therefore we shall consider the local strain values measured between points within the tendon.

The elasticity of the grafts measures 27% for the patellar tendon, 55% for the semitendinosus tendon, and approximately 27% for the looped semitendinosus tendon relative to the ACL over the linear range.

The *energy to failure* is 100% for the patellar tendon, 78% for the semitendinosus tendon, and 156% for the looped semitendinosus tendon.

In summary, the mechanical test values indicate superiority of the looped semitendinosus tendon over the patellar tendon.

Anatomy of the Semitendinosus Tendon
(Fig. 1)

The overall length of the tendinous portion of the semitendinosus, measured in 120 grafts, is 25–31 cm. The proximal part of the tendon is broad, flat, and shows a uniform thickness when the muscular portion is removed. It is followed by a more or less cylindrical, regular tendon segment 4–5 mm in diameter, completely ensheathed by peritendineum. This segment is 13–16 cm long and branches at its distal end, sending a larger expansion to the aponeurosis of the

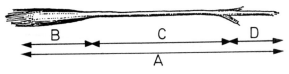

Fig. 1. Anatomy of the semitendinosus tendon. *A* = Overall length, *B* = proximal part, *C* = middle part, *D* = distal part

medial gastrocnemius muscle and a tapering tendon of insertion to the pes anserinus.

These anatomic properties allow for simple removal of the tendon through a small incision centered on the distal insertion of the pes anserinus.

The semitendinosus tendon is detached as far distally as possible and freed by scissor dissection to a point above its branches. The rest of the tendon is harvested as far as the muscular portion using a tendon stripper.

Functional Consequences of Graft Removal

The quadriceps is the extensor muscle of the knee, also controlling knee abduction and adduction. Removing one-third of the quadriceps tendon with its bony attachments and proprioceptors, and the associated scarring of the patellar tendon and infrapatellar fat pad, produces long-term anatomic and functional changes about the knee that cannot be overlooked – especially since the majority of patients with a chronically unstable knee have preexisting pathology of the extensor apparatus, including patellar chondromalacia, at the time of operation.

Although the removal of a tendon with a stripper leads to minimal problems of scarring, the complete removal of a pes anserinus muscle tendon still has consequences (Bousquet 1979; Lipscomb and Anderson 1986; Mott 1983).

The semitendinosus, which functions simultaneously as a flexor and internal rotator, also controls abduction of the knee. Its contribution to flexion is slight, accounting for less than 10% of the total force of all the flexors. Its function, then, is easily compensated by hypertrophy of the remaining flexors.

As an internal rotator, the semitendinosus muscle generates little force up to 40° of flexion, but thereafter its force progressively increases along with the semimembranosus, sartorius, gracilis, and popliteus. Because the total muscle mass is less than that of the flexors, removal of the semitendinosus has a greater impact. The semitendinosus muscle is responsible for 20% of the total force of internal rotation.

Except for the popliteus, the same muscles are used in the control of abduction. They are aided in this by the quadriceps, which acts strongly through the capsule fibers that pass directly from the vastus medialis to the medial tibial plateau.

Investigations have shown that use of the semitendinosus tendon does not significantly decrease the strength of knee flexion or internal rotation as measured by the Cybex dynamometer after full rehabilitation. This reduction is markedly less than that of the quadriceps, which was not damaged by the operation (Lipscomb and Anderson 1986). This finding is probably explained by scarring of the muscle body on the aponeuroses and tendons of the adjacent agonists or simply by the hypertrophy of these muscles.

In summary, we favor the semitendinosus tendon as an ACL substitute owing to its good biologic and mechanical properties. The anatomic form of the graft allows for simple implantation under arthroscopic control, and we have found that the graft can be taken with minimal trauma. It is likely, moreover, that the peritendineum promotes synovialization of the graft.

Surgical Technique

Because the intraarticular graft undergoes a significant, sustained strength loss postoperatively, we protect it by adding an extraarticular anterolateral stabilizing procedure of the type described by Lemaire.
The operation begins through a medial longitudinal incision. In our first patients this incision gave sufficient access for harvesting the graft, performing a medial arthrotomy, clearing the intercondylar space, and drilling 2 tibial tunnels.
Today the arthrotomy has been replaced by arthroscopy, so the medial incision is used only for removing the graft and drilling the tibial tunnels under arthroscopic guidance. The incision is centered on the pes anserinus and is 5–6 cm long. A second lateral incision is made over the proximal part of the lateral femoral condyle. This incision, approximately 7 cm long, gives access for detaching a fascia lata strip, drilling the transcondylar osseous tunnel, and introducing the intraarticular and extraarticular grafts.
The operation proceeds as follows: The sartorius tendon is exposed through the medial incision, and the interval between the gracilis and semitendinosus is identified by palpation. At this level the sartorius tendon is incised at the proximal border of the semitendinosus tendon in line with its fibers. In this way the distal part of the graft is dissected free. The expansions to the gracilis and to the gastrocnemius are cut. Then the tendon is freed as far as its muscular portion with a stripper and removed.
The proximal end is cleaned of all muscle fibers, and nonabsorbable suture material is woven through both ends over a length of 5–6 cm. Then either a medial arthrotomy is performed, or the arthroscope is inserted. The intercondylar space is cleared of osteophytes and any scar tissue that is present. A pair of

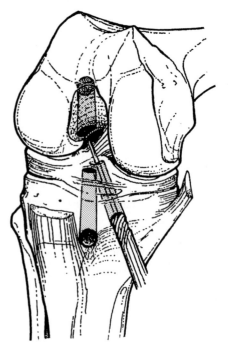

Fig. 2. Drilling the osseous tunnel

2 mm Kirschner wires are inserted through the tibia. These wires enter the tibia proximal to the pes anserinus at points spaced 2 cm apart. The tips of the wires converge within the joint in the posterior portion of the normal distal insertion site of the ACL.
When these wires have been accurately positioned, they are overdrilled with a 6-mm cannulated reamer to produce the 2 tibial tunnels (Fig. 2).
Moving to the lateral incision, the surgeon mobilizes a strip of iliotibial tract for the extraarticular transfer. He then exposes the condyle posterior and proximal to the insertion of the lateral collateral ligament. At that site a wire is inserted to a point fairly high in the intercondylar notch, in the proximal part of the normal femoral insertion site of the ACL. This wire is overdrilled with the 6-mm reamer to create the femoral tunnel. A suture is passed through the transcondylar tunnel, grasped inside the joint with an arthroscopic forceps, and pulled out through the anterior tibial tunnel. Each end of the suture is secured with a clamp wedged against the bone at the tunnel openings. At this time the knee is moved through flexion and extension to check the isometry of the selected placement.
A small curette is used to make necessary adjustments in the position of the transcondylar tunnel, which in any case must be widened before the double graft is introduced.
A thread or metal loop is placed at the proximal end

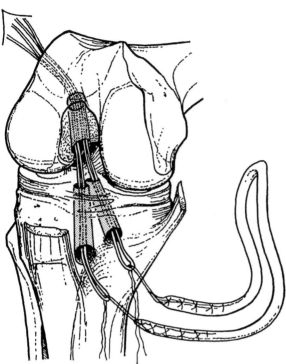

Fig. 3. Insertion of the graft

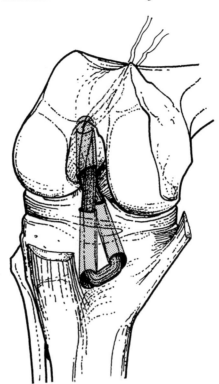

Fig. 4. Definitive graft position

of the suture and pulled through the transcondylar and first transtibial tunnel. Then a second loop is pulled through the condylar and second tibial tunnel (Fig. 3). The sutures previously woven into the tendon ends are passed through the protruding loops and are drawn through the tunnels to form a U-shaped graft (Fig. 4).

In all cases operated to date, the excess graft length emerging from the femoral tunnel was 3–5 cm. Thus, the weakest parts of the graft – the suture-woven ends – are inside the transcondylar tunnel, while the strongest, cylindrical portion is inside the joint cavity and at the tibial insertion. The graft is made slightly tense and fixed with either a metal clip (after Richards) or a screw with a polyethylene washer. The ends are sutured to the border of the iliotibial tract (Fig. 5). The extraarticular transfer is performed in the same sitting, and finally the tract is carefully closed by repairing the Kaplan fibers.

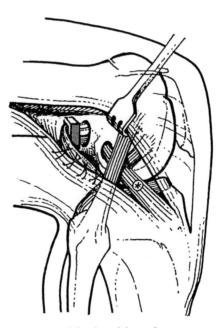

Fig. 5. Lateral fixation of the graft

Postoperative Rehabilitation

The knee is protected for 5 weeks by a removable splint in approximately 15° of flexion. Rehabilitation begins after removal of the drains, i.e., on the 2nd postoperative day. The program includes careful active mobilization with support, starting at 10°–40° and increasing by about 25° every 2 weeks until a range of 0°–150° is reached by the end of 12 weeks.

Isometric and electrogymnastic exercises are performed with the goal of neutralizing the anterior drawer component produced by isolated quadriceps contraction near extension. Intensive flexor exercises are initiated at an early stage. The quadriceps works against a resistance at the proximal tibia or together with the flexors. The knee must bear no weight during the first 7 weeks, and weight-bearing is gradually resumed thereafter.

Proprioceptive training is progressively introduced after 10 weeks, first in a sitting posture, then in bipedal stance, and finally in monopedal stance. Cycling is allowed after 10 weeks, and swimming after 12 weeks. Sprinting and nonstrenuous athletic activities may be gradually resumed after 6 months. Strenuous sports are proscribed before 12 months.

Clinical Population and Method

All patients operated during the period from December, 1984, to December, 1987, were available for follow-up 3–6 years postoperatively. They consisted of 28 males and 28 females ranging from 17 to 51 years of age.

Preoperative knee instability in all the patients was severe enough that they were unable to participate in sports. In 23 cases the knee was also unstable during walking. Laxity according to the Lysholm scale (Lysholm and Gillquist 1982) was 2 + to 4 + in the Lachman test, 2 + to 4 + for pivot shift, and 1 + to 4 + for anterior drawer in 90° flexion.

Six patients showed evidence of osteoarthritis, 2 requiring a corrective osteotomy that was done at the time of the ligament reconstruction.

Many of the patients had already had previous operations:

- Medial meniscectomy in 17
- Medial and lateral meniscectomy in 2
- Ligament repair in 9
- Ligament reconstruction involving the ACL in 10

Results

Postoperative follow-ups were conducted monthly during the first 6 months, then at 9, 12, 18, and 24 months, and finally once a year.

The *protocol* for the follow-up examination covered the following points:

- *Subjective assessment* (pain, swelling, functional deficits, stability, overall performance)
- *Trophic status* (effusion, inflammatory signs, muscle atrophy, degenerative changes including crepitus, clicks, and radiographic signs of osteoarthritis)
- *Instability*. This was assessed relative to the healthy knee according to the Lysholm score (where + / − indicates 2–3 mm of motion).

The following parameters were assessed: lateral laxity (varus, valgus), Lachman sign, pivot shift, reversed pivot shift, drawer in 90° flexion, passive external rotation in 90° flexion.

Here we shall consider only the results that relate to the technique described, i.e., laxity and overall result. The latter was frequently marred by degenerative changes such as chondromalacia, osteoarthritis, or other lesions unrelated to the operation.

The result is rated *excellent* if the knee is completely asymptomatic with a stability equal to or greater than that of the normal contralateral knee. The result is rated *good* in asymptomatic knees that show trace pathologic signs or laxity (+ / −) on examination. A *fair* result denotes a knee that becomes symptomatic during strenuous or prolonged exertion outside the scope of normal daily activities, with no subjective instability. These knees show mild pathologic signs or instability (1 +) on examination. The result is rated *unsatisfactory* in knees that are moderately symptomatic during the activities of daily living, cannot tolerate strenuous activity, are sometimes unstable, and display clinical signs or moderate laxity (1 + to 2 +). There is no "poor" outcome, i.e., a knee showing frequent instability or unable to function during daily activities.

Table 1 summarizes the results in patients whose reconstructions were performed by arthrotomy. They were evaluated 49–72 months after the operation. Table 2 shows the results in arthroscopically operated patients evaluated 37–63 months after surgery. The cases are arranged chronologically in each table.

Table 1. Patients operated by arthrotomy, 39–62 months after surgery

Case	Crepitus	Osteo-arthritis	Stiffness	Lachman test	Pivot shift or reversed pivot shift	Drawer 90°	Other laxities	Laxity result	Overall result
1	–	–	–	–	– / –	–	–	Excellent	Excellent
2	–	–	–	–	– / –	–	–	Excellent	Excellent
3	+	+	–	+	– / +	–	Postero-lateral	Fair	Unsatisfactory
4	±	–	–	–	– / –	±	–	Good	Good
5	±	–	–	–	– / –	±	–	Good	Good
6	+	–	–	–	– / +	±	Valgus	Fair	Fair
7	+	–	5° Extension deficit	–	– / –	±	–		Fair
8	–	–	–	–	– / –	–	–	Excellent	Excellent
9	–	–	10° Flexion deficit	–	– / –	–	–	Excellent	Good
10	±	–	–	+	– / –	±	–	Fair	Fair
11	+	–	–	±	– / –	±	–	Good	Fair
12	+	–	5° Flexion deficit	–	– / –	–	–	Excellent	Good
13	–	–	–	–	– / –	–	–	Excellent	Excellent
14	+	+	15° Flexion deficit	+	– / +	+	Postero-lateral	Unsatisfactory	Unsatisfactory
15	–	–	–	+	– / –	±	–	Fair	Fair
16	+	–	–	–	– / +	–	Varus	Good	Fair
17	±	–	–	–	– / –	–	–	Excellent	Excellent
18	±	–	–	–	– / –	–	–	Excellent	Excellent
19	±	±	5° Flexion deficit	–	– / –	±	Valgus	Good	Fair
20	+	–	–	–	– / –	–	–	Excellent	Good
21	+	±	–	–	– / –	–	–	Excellent	Good
22	+	–	–	+	– / ±	±	–	Fair	Fair
23	+	–	–	–	– / –	–	–	Excellent	Good
24	–	–	–	±	– / –	±	Valgus	Good	Good
25	+	–	–	+	– / +	+	–	Fair	Unsatisfactory
26	+	–	–	±	– / –	–	–	Good	Fair

Arthroscopic Follow-ups

Nineteen knees were examined arthroscopically (Fig. 6 a,b). Two of the knees had unsatisfactory stability; 2 were fair, 8 good, and 7 excellent.

In 15 cases the substitute ligament had healed well and had good synovial coverage. Thickness and tension were normal.

In 3 cases arthroscopy revealed a mass of amorphous scar tissue that had no tension but was attached at both insertion sites. One other case showed similar findings but had no significant femoral attachment. The results in these 4 cases were fair in 3 (perhaps owing to the extraarticular procedure) and unsatisfactory in 1.

Histologic Findings

In 10 patients, biopsies were taken from the midportion of the graft under local anesthesia using thin arthroscopic forceps 4–58 months postoperatively. The stability of these 10 cases was good. Nine biopsies showed normal ligamentous tissue with moderate hypercellularity, decreasing over time, below a thin synovial membrane. Some thin vessels were seen in 2 cases, but most biopsies were avascular. Only one biopsy showed a small area of subnecrotic hyaline tissue. These findings confirm that vascularity is not necessary to the viability of the graft. The tendinous tissue already shows hypercellularity and signs of metaplasia at 4 months, without any vascular development and without necrosis.

Table 2. Patients operated arthroscopically, 27–53 months after surgery

Case	Crepitus	Osteo-arthritis	Stiffness	Lachman test	Pivot shift or reversed pivot shift	Drawer 90°	Other laxities	Laxity result	Overall result
27	±	–	–	–	–/–	±	–	Good	Good
28	±	–	–	+	–/+	±	Valgus	Fair	Fair
29	±	–	–	+	–/+	+	–	Fair	Fair
30	±	–	–	–	–/–	–	–	Excellent	Good
31	–	–	–	–	–/–	–	–	Excellent	Excellent
32	±	–	–	–	–/–	–	–	Excellent	Excellent
33	+	–	–	+	±/–	±	Varus	Fair	Fair
34	+	±	10° Flexion deficit	–	–/–	±	–	Good	Unsatisfactory
35	+	–	10° Flexion deficit	–	–/–	–	–	Good	Fair
36	±	–	–	–	–/–	–	Postero-lateral	Good	Good
37	–	–	–	–	–/–	–	–	Excellent	Excellent
38	–	–	–	–	–/–	–	–	Excellent	Excellent
39	–	–	–	±	–	–	Good	Good	
40	±	–	–	–	–/–	±	–	Good	Good
41	–	–	–	–	–/–	–	–	Excellent	Excellent
42	–	–	–	–	–/–	–	–	Excellent	Excellent
43	±	–	–	–	–/–	–	–	Excellent	Good
44	–	–	–	–	–/–	–	–	Excellent	Excellent
45	–	–	–	±	–/–	–	–	Good	Good
46	–	–	–	±	–/–	–	–	Good	Good
47	–	–	–	±	–/–	–	Valgus	Good	Good
48	±	–	–	–	–/–	–	–	Excellent	Good
49	–	–	–	–	–/–	–	–	Excellent	Excellent
50	–	–	5° Flexion deficit	±	–/–	–	–	Good	Good
51	±	–	–	–	–/–	–	–	Excellent	Good
52	±	–	–	+	–/+	+	–	Fair	Fair
53	+	±	–	–	±/+	±	Varus	Fair	Unsatisfactory
54	–	–	–	–	–/–	–	–	Excellent	Excellent
55	±	–	–	±	–/–	–	–	Good	Good
56	–	–	–	±	–/–	–	–	Good	Good

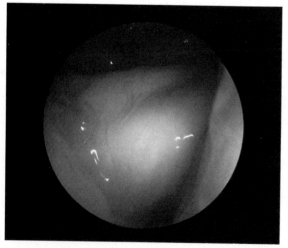

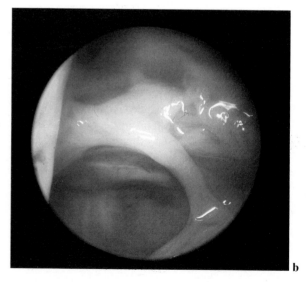

Fig. 6. a Arthroscopic view of a 4-month-old graft. **b** Arthroscopic view of a 24-month-old graft

Discussion

Two cases (3 and 14) from Group 1 were set aside for critical consideration and comparison. Both showed an old instability causing osteoarthritis that should be treated by osteotomy.

Table 3 shows a summary of the results after exclusion of these 2 cases.

The results of both methods are approximately the same in terms of joint laxity. However, the overall results in the patients operated by arthrotomy are significantly poorer as a result of trophic and functional disturbances caused by the surgical procedure.

The postoperative course was less eventful in Group 2: pain, inflammatory processes, effusions, and rehabilitation problems were greatly reduced, which is significant in terms of graft healing and the reduction of inflammatory elements in the synovial fluid.

A detailed analysis of the unsatisfactory results shows that preoperative problems (severe or complex instability, degenerative changes) or technical deficiencies play a greater role than the quality of the graft or the operative method.

Looking at the results listed chronologically in Tables 1 and 2, we observe no tendency for joint stability to decrease with passage of time.

In summary, we may say that the semitendinosus tendon can be removed as graft material without causing significant scarring or functional deficits. This tendon provides a biologically and mechanically sound graft for intraarticular reconstruction of the ACL. The surgical procedure, which can be performed under arthroscopic control, is relatively painless and is associated with minimal functional and trophic sequelae.

Table 3. Percentage distribution of results by groups

	Laxity result		Overall result	
	Group 1	Group 2	Group 1	Group 2
Excellent and good	79%	83%	58%	77%
Fair	21%	17%	38%	16%
Unsatisfactory	–	–	4%	7%

References

Arnoczky SP, Tarvin GB, Marshall JL (1982) Anterior cruciate ligament replacement using patella tendon. J Bone Joint Surg [Am] 64: 217

Bousquet G (1979) Chirurgia del ginocchio. Verduci, Rom, p 191

Chiroff RT (1975) Experimental replacement of the anterior cruciate ligament. J Bone Joint Surg [Am] 57: 1124

Cho KO (1975) Reconstruction of the anterior cruciate ligament by semitendinosus tenodesis. J Bone Joint Surg [Am] 57: 608

Clancy WC, Narechania RG, Rosenberg TD, Gmeiner J-G, Wisnefske DD, Lange TA (1981) Anterior and posterior cruciate ligament reconstruction in Rhesus monkeys. J Bone Joint Surg [Am] 63: 1270

Drobny TK, Wentzensen A, Müller We, Perren SM (1984) Anterior cruciate ligament replacement using patellar tendongraft–Experimental study on the knee of the sheep. First European Congress of ESKA, 1984

Ellison AE, Wieneke K, Benton JL, White ES (1976) Preliminary report: Results of extraarticular anterior cruciate replacement. J Bone Joint Surg [Am] 58: 736

Forward AD, Cowan RJ (1963) Tendon suture to bone. J Bone Joint Surg [Am] 45: 807

Johnson LL (1986) Arthroscopic surgery, principles and practice. Mosby, St. Louis

Laboureau JP, Testelin GM (1983) La plastie d'emblée dans les lésions fraîches du ligament croisé antérieur. Rev Chir Orthop 26: 263

Laboureau JP, Testelin GM, Benoist JP, Guth A (1981) Une plastie personnelle intraarticulaire du ligament croisé antéro-externe utilisant semi-tendineux et droit interne. Exposé à la SOFCOT, Paris

Lemaire M (1983) Résultat de la plastie extraarticulaire palliative de la rupture du ligament croisé antérieur. Rev Chir Orthop 69: 278

Lipscomb AB, Anderson AF (1986) Tears of the anterior cruciate ligament in adolescents. J Bone Joint Surg [Am] 68: 19

Luhiston TB, Walmsley R (1960) Some observations on the reaction of bone and tendon after tunneling of bone and insertion of tendon. J Bone Joint Surg [Br] 42: 377

Lysholm J, Gillquist J (1982) Evaluation of the ligament surgery results with special emphasis on use of scoring scale. Am J Sports Med 10: 150

Manske PR (1978) Nutrient pathways of flexor tendons within the flexon sheath. 33e Annual Meeting of the American Society for Surgery of the Hand, 1978

Mott HW (1983) Semitendinosus anatomic reconstruction for cruciate ligament insufficency. Clin Orthop 172: 90

Noyes FR, Butler DL, Grood ES, Zernicke RF, Hefzy MS (1984) Biomechanical analysis of human ligament grafts used in knee-ligament repairs and reconstructions. J Bone Joint Surg [Am] 66: 344

Peacock EE (1959) A study of the circulation in normal tendons and healing grafts. Ann Surg 149: 415

Potenza AD (1964) The healing of autogenous tendon grafts within the flexor digital sheath in dogs. J Bone Joint Surg [Am] 46: 1462

Roth J-H, Kennedy JC (1980) Intraarticular reconstruction of the anterior cruciate ligament in rabbits. Orthop Transact 4: 399

Whiston TB, Walmsley R (1960) Some observations on the reaction of bone and tendon after tunneling of bone and insertion of tendon. J Bone Joint Surg [Br] 42: 377

Anterior Cruciate Reconstruction Through a Transligamentous Approach

A. Gächter

Introduction

Research involving the anterior cruciate ligament (ACL) began with Palmer (1938), but many years passed before his discoveries regarding the importance of the central pivot and its associated structures were practically applied. The results of an ACL reconstruction technique first described by Jones (1970) were not ideal, although use of the patellar tendon to replace the ACL appeared logical and technically feasible. For a time there were arguments raised in favor of extraarticular reconstruction alone (technical simplicity, relatively short rehabilitation). Now, however, the trend is toward surgical procedures on the central pivot (Hefti et al. 1982). It makes sense to repair "in situ" a lesion that causes such a profound biomechanial imbalance. External reconstructions such as the biceps tendon transfer, lateral repair, and pes anserinus transfer are drastic procedures that can "decenter" the knee with the passage of time. The displacement of the center of rotation of the knee predisposes to cartilage damage from peak loads, distention of the capsule and ligaments, and meniscal pathology.

There are several criteria that a central (intraarticular) reconstruction of the ACL must satisfy:

- It should provide anatomic guidance of the articular surfaces while respecting the principle of isometry. This means that the substitute should maintain an approximately uniform tension in all degrees of flexion.
- It should be possible to attach the graft securely and initiate weight bearing as soon as possible.
- The operative technique should not be difficult and should be reproducible.
- The length of rehabilitation should be as short as possible (cost factor).

Success in meeting these requirements depends largely on appropriate graft selection and the use of a minimally invasive operating technique. In recent years a variety of techniques have been devised in an effort to meet these requirements:

- Cruciate ligament reconstruction with arthroscopic guidance (use of pes anserinus and/or synthetic ligaments)
- Use of synthetic ligaments or the synthetic augmentation of an autologous graft ("ligament augmentation device" of Kennedy 1983)
- ACL reconstruction with a strip of patellar tendon

At the present time, there seems to be no compelling rationale for arthroscopic reconstructions. While arthroscopy is very good for monitoring the attachment of the graft to the femur, conventional open surgery is still needed to harvest the graft. Only pes anserinus tendons can be harvested through a relatively small incision using a tendon stripper. The relatively thin prosthetic ligaments can be implanted arthroscopically, but their longevity within the joint is questionable.

We have attempted to combine the advantages of arthroscopic guidance with a minimally invasive open procedure. The basis of this reconstruction technique is a preliminary arthroscopic examination to evaluate any associated intraarticular pathology. Meniscal lesions and cartilage damage can be treated at this time using standard arthroscopic techniques. The subsequent open operation through a transligamentous route, while providing only limited exposure of the knee joint, gives an optimum view of the intercondylar notch region.

Technique

Following preliminary arthroscopy, the leg is positioned on a rest with the knee flexed approximately 70°. It is important to apply the tourniquet while the knee is flexed, for otherwise the quadriceps may be injured during subsequent isometric testing. We have used a parasagittal approach routinely since 1976. Care is taken that the incision runs lateral to the tibial tuberosity. The patellar tendon is exposed together with the patella and tibial tuberosity, and the central one-third of the patellar tendon is excised leaving a patellar and tibial bone block attached at its proximal and distal ends (Fig. 1). The bone blocks are not completely excised at this time, so the graft remains temporarily in situ. In patients with poor connective-tissue quality, lax ligaments, and in patients over 40, reinforcement of the patellar tendon strip may be advised. This can be done with the "ligament augmentation device" (LAD) of Kennedy (Fig. 2), a propylene band 6–8 cm long with heat-sealed ends that is inserted into the tendon strip prior to graft mobilization. The periosteal layer is undermined from the tibial end of the graft, and a soft-tissue sleeve is developed with a slender knife blade or chisel as far as the anterior patellar surface. This is relatively easy to do, as the fibers are not cut but merely pushed aside by blunt dissection. The LAD is pulled through the sleeve from the distal end with a suture, pulled taut, and 2 nonabsorbable sutures are passed through the

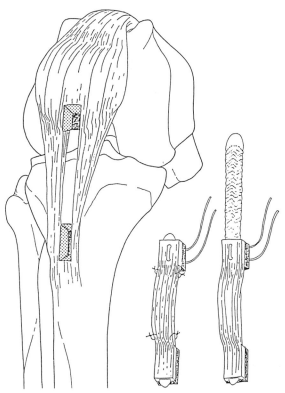

▷

Fig. 1. Removal of the central one-third of the patellar tendon with a bone block at each end. The infrapatellar fat pad is detached from the tibial plateau and retracted upward (transligamentous approach). The free graft is shown at right, reinforced with a standard-length Kennedy LAD and with a long LAD for over-the-top use (drawing by F. Freuler, Basel)

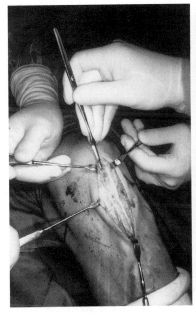
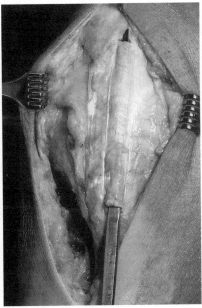
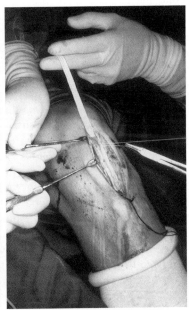

a   b   c

Fig. 2a–c. Before the graft has been mobilized, it can be reinforced if necessary (e. g., connective-tissue weakness) with a ligament augmentation device (LAD). **a** A slender blade inserted from the proximal or distal side dissects a subperiosteal sleeve through the graft, which is still partially attached at its bony ends. **b** Completed dissection of the subperiosteal sleeve. **c** The LAD, with its rounded and heat-sealed ends, is drawn into the pocket with a suture until it is completely ensheathed within the graft. The LAD is also secured to the graft with proximal and distal sutures ("hot dog" technique)

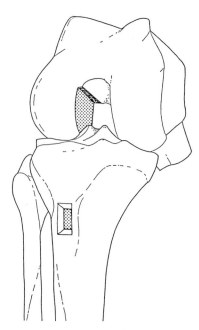

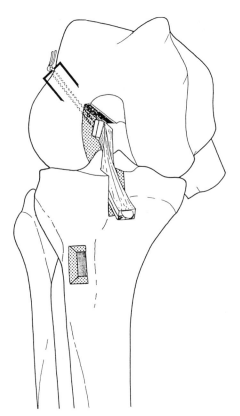

Fig. 3. With the knee flexed 90° (on the thigh rest), the intercondylar notch is widened by gouging material from the medial surface of the lateral femoral condyle. The extent of the notch plasty should match the width of the proximal bone plug (drawing by F. Freuler, Basel)

Fig. 4. First the proximal end of the graft is attached to the femur with through-the-top sutures. This can be done with non-absorbable threads or with steel wire if radiopacity is desired. The sutures can be anchored by tying them over titanium staples. The distal end of the graft is fitted into a prepared bone trough that runs below the intermeniscal ligament and is outside the weight-bearing zone. After graft isometry has been tested, the previously removed bone wedge can be placed back into the trough and stapled in place. This establishes direct contact between the graft and surrounding bone (drawing by F. Freuler, Basel)

proximal and distal patellar tendon as well as the bone blocks. The small proximal and distal bone blocks are now completely detached with a chisel, and the free graft, armed with the invisible LAD, is prepared for implantation. The patellar bone plug, which generally has a good cancellous bone layer, is slightly rounded at its proximal end, and 2 holes are drilled through it that converge toward the cancellous bone in V-shaped fashion. One thread of absorbable and one of nonabsorbable suture material (No. 2) are looped through the holes, taking care that the sutures encompass both the cancellous bone and the LAD. With the knee flexed 70°–90°, the infrapatellar fat pad is now sectioned vertically. At this point Langenbeck retractors at the wound margins should give excellent exposure of the intercondylar region. Clumped remnants of the old ACL are removed, and a notch plasty is performed. Only enough bone is removed to permit attachment of the proximal cancellous bone block without impingement (Fig. 3). A drill guide (e. g., the ASIF/AO drill guide) is now used to drill a 3.2-mm hole from the lateral surface of the lateral femoral condyle to the original attachment site of the ACL. A loop of suture is pulled through the drill hole for subsequent positioning of the proximal graft end. From the medial side, just adjacent to the patellar tendon insertion on the tibial tuberosity,

a 4.5-mm hole is drilled as far as the posterior border of the tibial attachment of the ACL, and a 0.5 Simal chisel is driven into the hole. Initially the chisel is left in place, then the entire wedge, including its superior and anterior tibial surfaces, is levered out in one piece (Fig. 4), sparing the anterior horn attachment of the medial meniscus. The bone trough thus created is outside the weight-bearing area of the joint, so it should cause no problems in this regard. Now the graft is pulled up into the joint, and the proximal plug is tentatively fixed by traction on the through-the-top sutures. An additional over-the-top suture may enhance the fixation. The distal plug is pulled down through the tibial bone trough until the graft is taut, and an impactor is used to seat the block as deeply as possible and avoid excessive anterior protrusion (Fig. 5). The joint is now moved through flexion-ex-

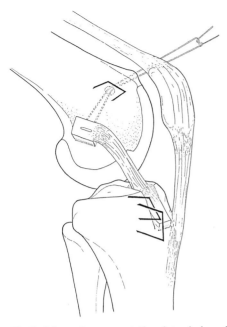

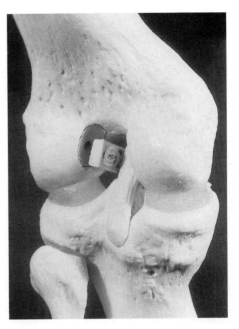

Fig. 5. Schematic representation, lateral view, showing details of the proximal "through-the-top" fixation. The cancellous portion of the bone plug seats directly against the freshened cancellous bone of the original cruciate ligament attachment site. The graft is twisted 90° about its longitudinal axis because the cancellous side of the distal plug faces posteriorly. This torsion is desired, as it simulates the normal helicoid course of the ACL (drawing by F. Freuler, Basel)

Fig. 6. Posterior view. The proximal bone plug is positioned over the notch plasty, prior to its through-the-top fixation to the femoral condyle. The bone plug must not be too large, or it might interfere with the posterior cruciate ligament

tension to test the isometry of the graft. Particular care is taken that the graft does not impinge on the condylar roof in extension. If isometry is unsatisfactory, it is adjusted by repositioning the proximal drill hole. When good isometric function is achieved, the proximal sutures are tied over a titanium staple driven into the lateral surface of the femoral condyle (Fig. 6). The distal end of the graft also is secured in its groove using titanium staples or screws over washers. Any cruciate ligament remnants are combed into the groove to round its edges. The bone wedge previously removed from the tibia is trimmed to a smaller size and "stacked" over the distal graft end. Leftover cancellous bone is packed into the donor sites in the patella and tibia. The patellar tendon defect is closed with absorbable sutures, and the tibial incision is closed. Power insertion of the titanium staples with a Shapiro stapler is advantageous as it is well tolerated and provides secure fixation (Fig. 7).

Postoperative Treatment

Postoperatively the knee is placed on a prefabricated splint. After swelling has subsided, a removable plastic splint is worn that immobilizes the knee in 5°–10° flexion. The patient can now perform full weight-bearing ambulation with or without crutches. No limits are placed on flexion during physical therapy (according to pain tolerance). Only assisted motion is permitted during the first 6 weeks. We do not use dynamic splints due to the risk of anterior tibial subluxation in extension. At 6 weeks a tunnel-view radiograph is taken to evaluate healing. Generally this film will show good bony consolidation of the femoral end of the graft. Anti-inflammatory agents are administered routinely for several days after surgery. Anticoagulant medication is started on the 2nd postoperative day and continued for 6 weeks.

Discussion

To date we have employed a similar procedure in more than 800 patients, using a modification of the technique described by Eriksson (1976). The proximal bone plug of the patellar tendon graft was fixed

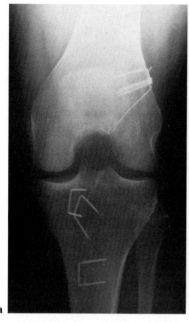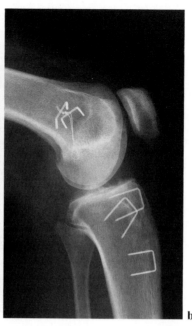

a   b

Fig. 7 a, b. Radiographs taken 6 weeks after graft implantation and postoperative functional therapy. The tunnel view demonstrates correct placement and healing of the proximal plug. The wire suture serves both as a marker and as attachment for the proximal graft end. The lateral view shows the through-the-top fixation at the correct site on the femur

with 2 transcondylar sutures or with braided wire for radiopacity. So far we have either left the graft attached distally to the tuberosity, transplanted it as a free graft, or perserved a vascular pedicle. Comparative results covering a period of several years were previously published (Hefti et al. 1982). We have found no advantages to using a graft with a fat pad pedicle (and the same transligamentous approach) and in fact have noted a significant incidence of pain in the fat pad area on full extension. There also seems to be a higher incidence of graft hypertrophy (Gächter and Kohler 1988). The transligamentous approach has proven effective in shortening rehabilitation time. Because the surgery inflicts minimum neurovascular trauma, there should also be less compromise of proprioceptive function. We have seen no problems relating to detachment and retraction of the fat pad; in particular, there have been no instances of patellar dystrophy (see Alm and Strömberg 1974).

References

Alm A, Strömberg B (1974) Vascular anatomy of the patellar and cruciate ligaments. Acta Chir Scand [Suppl] 445: 25–35

Arnoczky SP, Travin GB, Marshall JL (1982) Anterior cruciate ligament replacement using patellar tendon. An evaluation of graft revascularization. J Bone Joint Surg [Am] 64: 217

Bair GR (1980) Effects of early mobilization vs. casting on A.C.L. reconstruction. Proc Orthop Res Soc, Atlanta, Georgia, p 108

Clancy WG, Rosenberg T, Gmeiner J, Narchania RG, Wisnesfke D (1979) Anterior cruciate ligament reconstruction in primates and man: A biomechanical and microangiographic evaluation of patellar tendon substitution. Ist Congress of the International Society of the Knee, Lyon (Communication)

Clancy WG, Nelson DA, Reider B, Narechania RG (1982) Anterior cruciate ligament reconstruction using one-third of the patellar ligament, augmented by extra-articular tendon transfers. J Bone Joint Surg [Am] 64: 352

Eriksson E (1976) Reconstruction of the anterior cruciate ligament. Orthop Clin North 7: 167–179

Gächter A, Kohler O (1988) Transplantathypertrophie nach vorderer Kreuzbandplastik. In: Beck E (Hrsg) Fortschritte in der Arthroskopie, Bd 4. Enke, Stuttgart

Hefti F, Gächter A, Jenny H, Morscher E (1982) Replacement of the anterior cruciate ligament. A comparative study of four different methods of reconstruction. Arch Orthop Traumatol Surg 100: 93–94

Jones KG (1970) Reconstruction of the anterior cruciate ligament using the central one-third of the patellar ligament. J Bone Joint Surg [Am] 52: 1302–1308

Kennedy JC (1983) The use of a ligament augmentation device (L.A.D.) in the anterior cruciate deficient knee. Presented at the American Academy of Orthopaedic Surgeons, Anaheim

Palmer I (1938) On the injuries to the ligaments of the knee joint. A clinical study. Acta Chir Scand [Suppl 53] 81: 237

Palmer J (1957) Injuries to the crucial ligaments of the knee joint as a surgical problem. Wiederherstellungschirurgie und Traumatologie (Basel). Reconstr Surg Traumatol 4: 181–196

Modification of the Clancy Patellar Tendon Reconstruction of the ACL: Analysis of Three-Year Results

W. C. Kipfer, P. M. Ballmer, H.-U. Stäubli, B. Grünig, R. Zehnder, and R. P. Jakob

Introduction

Intraarticular replacement of the anterior cruciate ligament (ACL) with a strip of patellar tendon has, since Brückner (1966) and Jones (1963, 1970), become an established technique. First recommended by Palmer in 1938, the histomorphologic and biomechanical principles of the method have since been advanced and refined by numerous clinical and experimental studies (Alm and Strömberg 1974; Arniczky et al. 1982; Butler et a. 1979; Clancy et al. 1981; Drobny et al. 1984; Jakob 1985; Kieffer et al. 1984; Noyes et al. 1984; Odensten and Gillquist 1985; Paulos et al. 1983; Scapinelli 1968; Shino et al. 1984). Based on the observations of Scapinelli (1968) on the blood supply in the human knee joint, Alm and Strömberg (1974), Arnoczky (1983), Arnoczky et al. (1982), Clancy (1983), Clancy et al. (1981), and Drobny et al. (1984) investigated the revascularization of the patellar tendon graft in both vascularized and free transfers. A significant contribution was made by Butler et al. (1979), who showed that the patellar tendon is the mechanically strongest of the biologic tissues available for ACL substitution. Its value is enhanced by the fact that removing a strip from the central one-third of the patellar tendon does not significantly affect knee stability.

On the basis of these experimental studies, Clancy (1983) advocated a technique for preserving the microcirculation from the infrapatellar fat pad. He reasoned that preserving a vascular pedicle between the fat pad and graft would accelerate graft revascularization during the remodeling period.

Between 1981 and 1985, a slightly modified form of the Clancy technique was applied at the Orthopedic Surgery Clinic of the University of Bern. The modification involves a different technique for dissecting the vascular pedicle to the infrapatellar fat pad. By developing the vascular pedicle through the window formed in the patellar tendon, it is possible to preserve both the medial and lateral branches of the inferior genicular artery.

The goals of our retrospective study were as follows:

– To report our experience with this technique
– To offer a critical analysis of the 3-year results in the first 50 cases with regard to stability, motion, and tolerance of functional loading

Materials and Methods

From January of 1981 to January of 1984, 56 patients with symptomatic chronic anterior knee instability underwent ACL reconstruction using our modification of the Clancy technique (Clancy 1982, 1983). Fifty of these patients were followed during 1984/85. Six patients were lost to follow-up (4 could not be located and 2 refused to present). On average, the patients were evaluated 33 months after the operation with a range from 23 to 48 months.

Clinical Material

The demographic group most heavily represented in our clinical population was young males (Table 1).

On average the ACL was replaced 26 months after the initial trauma. All patients had sustained their injury more than 5 weeks preoperatively, and in 2 cases the interval from injury to operation was more than 10 years. All patients but 6 sustained their injury during sports activities (Table 2), with contact sports (ball games) predominating. Only 2 patients were injured while working.

The exact mechanism of the injury could not be ascertained in 22 patients, but all cases involved a dy-

Table 1. Clinical population: general data (n = 50)

Sex:	Female:male	8:42	
Age (years):	Operation	15–48	(n = 27)
	Follow-up	18–51	(n = 30)
Affected side:	Right: left	29:21	

Table 2. Causes of injury

Soccer	20	
Skiing	10	
Other ball games	9	Sports = 44
Tennis, gymnastics	3	
Other types of sport	2	
Motor vehicle	4	
Work	2	

Table 3. Mechanisms of injury

Valgus, flexion, external rotation	20
Varus, flexion, internal rotation	5
Hyperextension	2
Deceleration	1
Uncertain	22

Table 4. Stability I (n = 50)

/ Not documented	
0 = 0–3 mm	2 + = 5–10 mm
1 + = 3–5 mm	3 + = >10 mm

Drawer displacement

		Preoperative	Postoperative
Near extension (Lachman test)			
	/	1	–
	0	–	18
	1 +	4	30
	2 +	34	2
	3 +	11	–
Near flexion (70°–90°)			
Neutral	/	2	–
rotation	0	–	27
	1 +	7	22
	2 +	35	1
	3 +	6	–
External	/	2	–
rotation	0	–	12
	1 +	5	32
	2 +	27	6
	3 +	16	–
Internal	/	3	–
rotation	0	9	43
	1 +	33	7
	2 +	5	–

Table 5. Stability II (n = 50)

Pivot shift test	Preoperative	Postoperative
/	4	–
0	–	45
1 +	5	5
2 +	31	–
3 +	10	–

Table 6. Intraoperative findings (n = 50)

Anterior cruciate ligament absent or deficient		50
Posterior cruciate ligament intact		38
	unknown	12
Meniscal damage	Isolated medial	22
	Isolated lateral	10 } 41
	Medial and lateral	9
Cartilage damage	Patella	27
	Femoral condyle medial	17
	lateral	2
	Tibial plateau	5

namic force acting on a statically loaded or uncontrolled limb. Twenty-five patients described a valgus-varus stress occurring in various positions of flexion and rotation (Table 3).

Twenty-five of the 50 knees had had previous surgery, some on multiple occasions. Twelve patients had previous capsuloligamentous surgery, including 4 primary repairs of the ACL and 3 secondary reconstructions. There were 18 previous meniscectomies, 2 of which were bilateral.

All patients complained of debilitating pain on exertion, especially stair climbing and walking uphill. Thirty-one described frequent episodes of giving way or a feeling of instability during normal daily activities and sports.

Examination of 90% of the cases under anesthesia showed increased anterior subluxation near extension in 49 patients (positive Lachman test; Rosenberg and Rasmussen 1984; Torg et al. 1976). In 1 case this finding was not documented; comparison with stress radiographs was not routine at that time. In 48 patients, increased anterior displacement was detected in flexion as well (Table 4). Forty-six knees had a positive pivot shift test (Galway and McIntosh 1980) (Table 5), and in 4 patients this test was not documented.

Intraoperative findings. In all patients the ACL was absent or represented by a functionally deficient band of scar tissue, which was resected. Forty-one patients had meniscal pathology involving previously untreated lesions or the sequelae of meniscectomy. In 22 cases only the medial meniscus was affected, and in 10 cases only the lateral meniscus. Cartilage changes were found mainly on the medial femoral condyle and the undersurface of the patella (Table 6).

Surgical Technique

All 50 knees were operated on by the same surgeon or under his supervision (R. P. J.). All ACL reconstructions employed a vascularized strip from the central one-third of the ipsilateral patellar tendon.

The anesthetized patient was positioned supine, the leg supported on an adjustable lateral rest with the knee flexed 30°–40°. A pneumatic thigh tourniquet was inflated to 320–400 mm Hg.

The joint is entered through an anterolateral skin incision and anteromedial arthrotomy. This gives access for an adjunctive extraarticular procedure in the posterolateral quadrant. Access to the posteromedial quadrant may require making an additional posteromedial incision.

After the joint has been entered, the intraarticular structures are carefully and atraumatically explored with a probe, giving particular attention to the cruciate ligaments, menisci, and cartilage surfaces. Relavant findings are documented, especially if they might interfere with the postoperative course and rehabilitation.

First, meniscal lesions are repaired or resected, giving preference to suture repair whenever possible. The sutures for the meniscal repair are preplaced, and they are tied after the ACL reconstruction has been completed.

Preparation of the bone tunnels for attachment of the graft, and especially of the entry sites in the lateral femoral condyle and tibial plateau, is the most important phase of the operation. These sites define the anatomic reference points for an isometric ligament reconstruction (Jakob 1985; Odensten and Gillquist 1985). Their location affects the biomechanics of the joint and ultimately determines the outcome of the operation.

The tibial insertion of the graft is defined by the ACL remnant that is still present. If there is no remnant, a Kirschner wire positioned against the intercondylar notch and perpendicular to the femoral axis on the tibial plateau with the knee flexed 90° will point to the center of the attachment site (Fig. 1).

Once the site has been established, a threaded 2.5 mm Kirschner guidewire is driven into the upper tibia along the ligament axis so that its point emerges at the center of the ACL insertion in front of the intercondylar eminence. The definitive tunnel is made by overdrilling the Kirschner wire with cannulated reamers of 8 and 10 mm diameter (Fig. 2).

Before the femoral tunnel is drilled, the width and arch of the intercondylar notch are checked, and any obstructing osteophytes are removed. A minimum notch width of approximaly 20 mm is desired (Odensten and Gillquist 1985).

To view the posterior aspect of the intercondylar notch and femoral attachment, the knee is flexed 110°

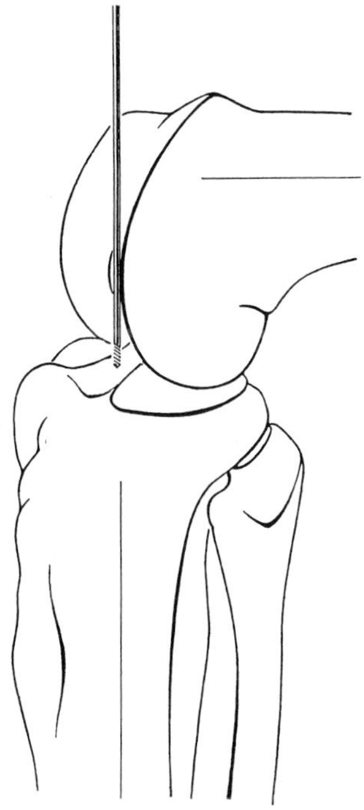

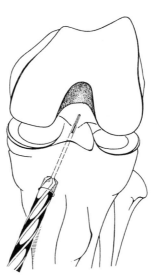

Fig. 1. Determination of the distal insertion site of the ACL in 90° flexion. The Kirschner wire is tangential to the intercondylar notch and perpendicular to the tibial plateau (from Jakob et al. 1988)

Fig. 2. Drilling the tibial tunnel: The direction of the tunnel is defined beforehand with a threaded Kirschner wire (2.5 mm) (from Jakob et al. 1988)

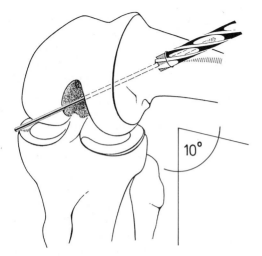

Fig. 3. Drilling the femoral tunnel: A threaded Kirschner wire is drilled from the inside out and overdrilled outside-in with an 8- to 10-mm cannulated reamer from a posterolateral entry site (from Jakob et al. 1988)

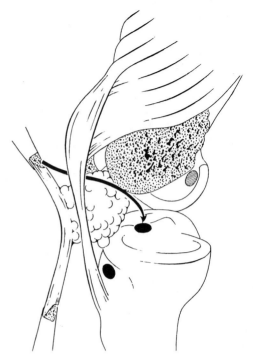

Fig. 4. Mobilized patellar tendon graft with a fat pad vascular pedicle. The patellar portion is within the tibial tunnel (from Jakob et al. 1988)

with the hip externally rotated. The center of the tunnel is located 2–3 mm anterior and inferior to the posterior border of the lateral femoral condyle. Again, the tunnel axis is marked with a threaded Kirschner wire driven out through the condyle from inside the intercondylar notch. The guidewire is overdrilled in the opposite direction (from the outside in) to avoid iatrogenic damage to the cartilage of the medial condyle and meniscus. Before the tunnel is drilled, the vastus lateralis is mobilized and the posterolateral aspect of the lateral femoral condyle is exposed. The exit hole of the tunnel is level with the distally tapering lateral lip of the linea aspera (Fig. 3).

After the edges of the intraarticular entrance holes have been smoothed and rounded, a trial prosthetic ligament is passed through the tunnels to test isometry, and necessary corrections are made. The scarred remnants of the original ACL are resected, unless they contribute to the revascularization of the graft.

After this preparatory phase is completed, the central 8–10 mm of the patellar tendon is removed along with a corticocancellous bone block from the diatal patella and the proximal tibia, each measuring 20–25 mm in length. Before the bone blocks are detached, 3 holes are made through each block with a 2.0-mm drill bit; these holes are for the nonabsorbable sutures (Ethibond 3) used to anchor the graft to the distal femur and proximal tibia. The bone blocks are then trimmed and the diameters of the plugs checked with a calibration sleeve of 8–10 mm inside diameter.

The tibial end of the graft is mobilized first. Then the fat pad is detached from the distal patella. While the medial and lateral branches of the inferior genicular artery are protected, the vascular pedicle is carefully dissected from the fat pad to the posterior surface of the graft. The whole graft is then inverted 180°, turning the patellar end distally and the tibial end proximally. The distal bone plug is pulled into the tibial tunnel until it is completely inside it, with no part projecting into the joint. The plug should not be placed too far distally, however, as this might tear the vascular pedicle (Fig. 4). Similarly, the tibial bone plug is passed through the femoral tunnel without twisting the graft about its axis, and the graft is made tense and anchored distally by tying the distal fixation sutures around a special bone screw with a constricted neck (Fig. 5).

Isometric graft position is tested by applying manual tension to the distally attached patellar tendon graft while the joint is moved between 90° flexion and full extension. If the graft is correctly positioned, it should undergo no more than 2–3 mm length change over the range of knee motion (Jakob 1985). Having "passed" this test, the graft is definitively attached under maximum tension with the knee flexed 45°. The reconstruction concludes with the intraoperative

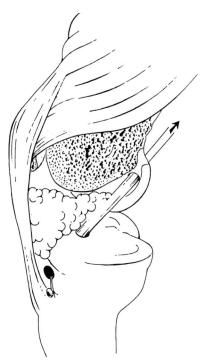

Fig. 5. Definitive placement of the graft within the joint. Fixation of the distal bone plug has been completed (from Jakob et al. 1988)

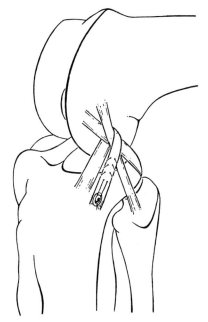

Fig. 6. Lateral extraarticular augmentation using a strip of iliotibial tract (from Jakob et al. 1988)

▷

Fig. 7. Medial extraarticular augmentation by semimembranosus tendon advancement

testing of anteroposterior drawer motion in 10°–15° flexion (Lachman test) and range-of-motion testing between full extension and 90° flexion.

Because chronic instabilities are invariably associated with deficiency of the secondary restraints, especially the posterolateral capsule (Butler et al. 1980), it is recommended that the cruciate reconstruction be augmented by an extraarticular "lateral repair" (Clancy et al. 1982; McIntosh and Darby 1976; We. Müller 1982). A distally based strip of iliotibial tract 10–12 cm long is dissected free and passed beneath the lateral collateral ligament and popliteus tendon (Jakob technique). With the knee flexed 45° and the tibia in neutral rotation, the mobilized strip is sutured to the popliteus tendon with absorbable material, and its free end is looped back and reattached behind Gerdy's tubercle with a screw or subperiosteal suture. Besides reinforcing the ACL reconstruction, this transfer also contributes to posterolateral stability by tightening the arcuate ligament complex (Fig. 6).

If posteromedial instability exists, the operation to this point can be further supplemented by advancing the horizontal slip of the semimembranosus tendon on a piece of bone (Noesberger et al. 1981) (Fig. 7). This procedure, which restores tension to the posteromedial capsule, was necessary in 19 of the 50 cases that we followed.

The orientation of the bone tunnels and the position of the bone plugs are documented by postoperative radiographs in 2 planes (Fig. 8).

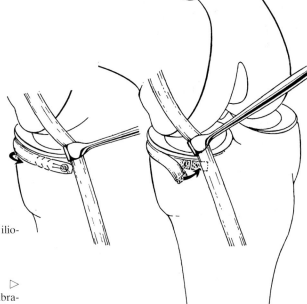

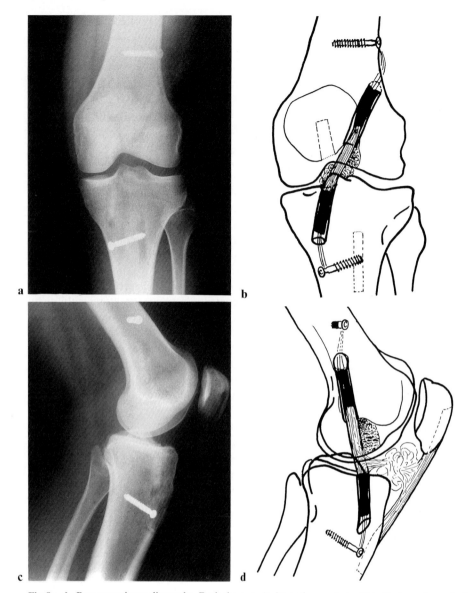

Fig.8a–d. Postoperative radiographs. Both the a.p. (a, b) and lateral projections (c, d) demonstrate the bone plugs of the graft seated within the bone tunnels. The location and orientation of the tunnels define the intraarticular position of the graft

Postoperative Treatment

The average length of postoperative immobilization was 7 weeks, with 24 patients wearing a long cylinder cast holding the knee in 30°–40° flexion, and 26 patients wearing a cast brace permitting motion between 20° and 60°. (In recent years we have come to favor early postoperative passive mobilization from a protective posterior plaster splint.) After several weeks' immobilization, all the patients were placed on an individualized rehabilitation program under the direction of a qualified physical therapist. The supervised rehabilitation was continued for more than 6 months in 35 patients; 2 underwent less than 6 weeks' rehabilitation. Thirty-nine patients confirmed at follow-up that they had faithfully complied with the designated rehabilitation program; only one patient considered the physical therapy to be unnecessary.

A Lenox-Hill knee brace was prescribed in 20 cases; 13 were still in use at follow-up, with 11 patients wearing them only during sports activities. The operated knees resumed full weight-bearing an average of 16 weeks after surgery, and flexion past 120° was achieved by 20 weeks. Extension deficits greater than 10° lasted an average of 21 weeks.

Table 7. Reoperations (n = 12)

Arthroscopy	Diagnostic	1
	Operative	3
Arthrotomy		4
Hardware removal	With	4
	Additional measures	
	Without	4

Table 8. Reoperations (n = 12)

Partial meniscectomy	2
Resection of scar tissue (infrapatellar fat pad)	4
Debulking of the reconstructed cruciate ligament	2
Projecting tibial bone plug	2
Widening of the intercondylar notch	1

Table 9. Residual complaints (n = 50)

Pain	
None	9
Slight/rare	36
Moderate/occasional	5
Severe/frequent	–
Swelling	
None	34
Slight/rare	15
Moderate/occasional	1
Severe/frequent	–
Giving way	
None	46
Rare	3
Occasional	1
Frequent	–

There were no serious *systemic complications. Local complications* consisted of 3 significant wound hematomas, which were cleared by percutaneous aspiration. One knee had to be manipulated under general anesthesia at 5 months to restore motion, and a total of 12 patients required further operative measures (Table 7). Three patients required a partial meniscectomy combined with debulking of the substitute ligament. Two patients had an extension loss necessitating arthroscopic surgery for the removal of scar tissue, and 2 other patients required ablation of a projecting tibial bone plug, supplemented in 1 case by widening of the intercondylar notch. No patients required further reconstruction of the ACL due to graft failure (Table 8), and none of the 50 patients sustained an injury that affected knee stability prior to follow-up.

Follow-Up

Follow-up was conducted according to a standard protocol designed expressly for documentation purposes, based on the evaluative criteria recommended by Marshall et al. (1977), Noyes et al. (1983), Daniel (1981), and Lysholm and Gillquist (1982).
At the start of the examination, the patient was asked to compare the function of the affected joint with that of the unaffected or normal knee and express the difference as a percentage. After this spontaneous subjective assessment, the patient's symptoms and clinical findings were documented, following the sequence of the protocol. Joint stability was always tested by 2 examiners, including the senior author (R.P.J.), and the results were graded according to the criteria of Hughston et al. (1976) and Torg et al.

(1976). The method of Jakob et al. (1981, 1987) was used to grade the pivot shift and reversed pivot shift tests.

Results

Subjective Evaluation and Residual Complaints

Three years after the ligament reconstruction, 46 patients were subjectively pleased with the result, and 6 considered the operated knee equivalent to the unaffected knee. Four patients were disappointed with the result because they had expected more. No result was rated unsatisfactory, which would have meant that the knee was worse than before the operation. Five patients reported frequent pain during normal daily activities, but only 9 patients were completely pain-free. Sixteen patients experienced exertion-dependent joint swelling, 3 mentioned problems with stair climbing, and 1 patient described a troublesome feeling of instability with frequent giving-way episodes. Forty-six no longer experienced giving-way episodes after the reconstruction (Table 9).

Work

The patients returned to work an average of 24 weeks postoperatively at the same level of performance, with a range from 3 weeks (student) to 60 weeks (factory worker). At follow-up all the patients had resumed full occupational activity except for one, a carpenter, who is drawing a partial pension for disability relating to the operated knee. One patient had to be

Table 10. Return to work and sports

Return to work		
Complete	49	
Partial due to knee	1	
Unable to resume work	–	
Change of occupation due to knee	1	
Return to sports activities		
Full/same types of sport	11	
Limited/same types of sport	16	43
Limited/lower-demand sport	16	
Disabled for sports due to knee	2	
Not athletically active	5	

Table 11. Range of motion compared with the unaffected knee, with allowance for hyperextensibility of the joints

Extension	
Equivalent to opposite knee	19
Limitation of 10° or less	20
Limitation greater than 10°	11
Flexion	
Equivalent to opposite knee	18
Limitation less than 10°	16
Limitation 10°–20°	13
Limitation greater than 20°	3
Symmetrical range of motion	8
Limitation of flexion *and* extension	21

retrained for work less strenuous to the knee and has done well in his new job (Table 10).

Sports

Twenty-seven patients were able to resume sports they participated in before their injury, but only 20% at the preinjury level. More than half the patients who had injured their knee in a particular sports activity returned to that type of sport. Two felt unable to participate in sports due to the affected knee, and 5 had never been active in sports (see Table 10).

Clinical Examination

Three patients exhibited pronounced atrophy of the thigh muscles with a 3-cm difference in thigh girth between the sides. Most patients showed no significant disparity. Capsular thickening was noted in 5 knees, and 3 had palpable effusion. The rectus femoris muscle was shortened in 28 patients and painful to stretch. Twenty-seven patients had femoropatellar crepitation, painful in only 13. Patellar motion was restricted in 13 patients, and in 2 cases patellar subluxation was noted in intermediate flexion.

Range of Motion

Range of motion in the operated knee was assessed by both active and passive testing and compared with the opposite side. In 8 patients we found no right-left differences in range of knee motion. An extension deficit was found in 31 knees; in 11 it exceeded 10°. A flexion deficit was noted in 32 of the operated joints, amounting to 10°–20° in 13 knees and more than 20° in 3. There was combined limitation of flexion and extension in 21 patients, and in 6 the total limitation of motion exceeded 30° (Table 11).

Stability

Sagittal displacement near extension, evaluated by the Lachman test, was negative in 18 patients, and 30 patients showed a slightly increased translation of 3–5 mm. All the operated joints had a palpable anterior end point, but in some cases it felt altered in relation to the uninvolved knee. With the knee flexed 70°–90° and the tibia in neutral rotation, only 1 patient displayed more than 5 mm of anterior drawer (2 +); in 22 patients it was slightly increased. Testing in external rotation elicited 0 anterior drawer in 12 patients, 3–5 mm in 32 patients, and > 5 mm in 6 patients (see Table 4). Valgus stress in extension elicited slight medial opening in only 2 cases, but the same test in 30° flexion was positive in 11 cases, and joint-space opening in 2 of those was pronounced. Varus stress elicited lateral opening in 23 joints in 30° flexion.

Forty-five patients had a negative pivot shift test, and the remaining 5 had a positive test only in forced internal rotation, which we call a trace pivot shift (see Table 5). A positive reverse pivot shift was elicited in 2/3 of our patients, but about 1/2 showed a lesser grade of reversed pivot shift in the unaffected knee as well.

Functional Capacity

As an adjunct to the clinical examination, the patients were told to perform 4 functional tests (standing and hopping on the affected leg, squatting, and kneeling). One-legged standing and hopping presented the fewest difficulties, but about half the patients had difficulty squatting, and 3 felt unable to bring the affected joint to a kneeling position (Table 12).

Table 12. Functional tests (n = 48[a])

One-legged stance	1	44
	2	4
Hopping on one leg	1	43
	2	3
	3	2
Squatting (> 90°)	1	22
	2	24
	3	2
Kneeling	1	11
	2	23
	3	11
	4	3

1 = No difficulty	3 = Great difficulty
2 = Slight difficulty	4 = Unable to perform test

[a] Two patients could not be tested due to problems unrelated to the knee.

Table 13. Overall evaluation by the Noyes score (n = 50)

Score	Number of patients	
50	5	⎫
48	5	⎪
46	7	⎬ 32
44	15	⎭
42	9	
32–40	6	
24–30	3	

Overall Evaluation (Noyes Score)

Using the scoring system of Noyes et al. (1983), based on pain, giving way, swelling, and activity restriction during daily living activities and sports, we can summarize our results as follows: Five patients scored the maximum of 50 points. These patients are the ones who rated their operated knee as being equivalent in every respect to the healthy side. Twenty-seven patients with mild complaints, such as slight pain during strenuous exertion, scored 44–48 points, and 15 patients with significant disability scored from 32 to 42 points. Three patients with scores of 24, 28, and 30 points were well outside the average range. The scoring system, designed chiefly for an athletic population, had to be adapted to our demographically mixed population that included housewives and non-athletes, and this tended to skew the results toward higher scores. Thus, 32 patients in our series (64%) scored between 44 and 50 points, with an average of 43 points (Table 13).

Discussion

The evaluation of knee ligament reconstructions is justifiably based on long-term results at 5 or more years, a requirement that our study does not fulfill. Moreover, our study covers only a relatively small series of 50 operated knees.

Against these limitations, we can point to criteria indicating that we were working with a representative population:

– No arbitrary patient selection
– All the patients had *chronic anterior knee instability*.
– The *same method* was employed in all patients.
– All the patients were operated on by the same surgeon (R. P. J.) or under his supervision.

These framing conditions enable us to compare our results with those previously published by other authors (Clancy 1983; Clancy et al. 1982; Hefti et al. 1982; Johnson et al. 1984; Jones 1970; Kieffer et al. 1984; Paterson and Trickey 1986).

The antecedent histories of these 50 patients were marked by painful, recurrent giving-way episodes at work, during daily activities, and during sports in the wake of a ligamentous knee injury sustained months or years before. Clinically, all the patients manifested anterior knee instability due to absence or insufficiency of the ACL.

Three years after ACL reconstruction with the central one-third of the patellar tendon, we found that more than 90% of our patients who presented for follow-up showed good or excellent knee stability by subjective and objective standards, even though 2/3 demonstrated a 2- to 3-mm increase of anterior drawer motion relative to the opposite knee in the Lachman test. We agree with Torg et al. (1976), Rosenberg and Rasmussen (1984), and Noesberger (1981) that the Lachman test is a simple and reliable clinical examination, provided it is performed correctly in the fully relaxed patient. The test permits a subtle assessment of two essential aspects of the ACL. The degree of anterior displacement – palpable medially between the anterior border of the tibial plateau and femoral condyle – characterizes the function of the ACL, while the softness or hardness of the anterior end point allows for the assessment of ligament quality (Johnson et al. 1984; Rosenberg and Rasmussen 1984).

Similar results are demonstrated by anterior drawer testing in 70°–90° of knee flexion, which we always performed in neutral, external, and internal tibial rotation. This examination mainly tests the secondary restraints (joint capsule, collateral ligaments), since it does not place maximum tension on the cruciate ligament (Rosenberg and Rasmussen 1984). It is of limited usefulness for evaluating the ACL, therefore.

The pivot shift test, an indispensable knee stability test that we have used for years, was negative in 90% of our population. In the remaining 10% the test was positive only while the tibia was in internal rotation ("trace pivot shift"; Jakob et al. 1987). Subjectively, this finding usually corresponds to a mild feeling of instability with occasional giving way during vigorous activities or while walking on uneven ground. It should be recalled that the pivot shift test, much like the Lachman test, is a specific examination for the ACL and that it was positive preoperatively in more than 90% of the patients (Galway and McIntosh 1980).

Considering the fact that Clancy (1983) and Clancy et al. (1982) found no significant loss of motion in their series of 50 patients, we were surprised to find that only 8 of our patients (16%) had equal ranges of motion in both knees, while 21 (42%) had limitation of motion in both flexion and extension (see Table 11). The substantial right-left disparities in our series can be explained by the fact that numerous patients had hyperextensible joints due to morphotype or constitutional ligament laxity. This can lead to an absolute right-left discrepancy of 10°–15° even though the patient has full extension in the operated knee. Thus, extension deficits of 5°–10° can be compensated without significant disability, but most patients with a loss of flexion feel hampered in their everyday activities. This is true even when the deficit is only a few degrees, as our experience with the squatting and kneeling tests confirms.

Three causal factors appear to have particular relevance to a clinically significant extension deficit (Jakob 1985; We. Müller 1982): impairment of isometry due to (1) faulty placement of the graft attachment sites, (2) insufficient graft length, and (3) graft impingement within a narrow intercondylar notch. We found that impingement can result from narrowing of the notch by osteophytes or scar tissue, excessive graft bulk, mechanical interference from a scarred vascular pedicle, or placing the distal insertion of the reconstructed ligament too far anteriorly or laterally. Analogous observations were made by Paterson and Trickey (1986), who stressed the importance of isometry and isotonicity of the graft during joint motion. Accordingly, we have adopted several measures, as needed, in an effort to forestall these complications: widening the intercondylar notch, adjusting the graft tension near extension (20°

flexion), and isometric graft fixation on the tibial plateau. Also, since 1985 we have used a free patellar tendon graft to eliminate the vascular connection with the fat pad, due largely to evidence in experimental animal studies (Drobny et al. 1984; Shino et al. 1984) that there are no significant differences between free and pedicled grafts in terms of revascularization and mechanical properties. The free, devascularized graft offers 2 crucial mechanical advantages: It is always long enough and occupies less space owing to the absence of the bulky fat pad pedicle. Besides these modifications of operative technique, we have also modified early postoperative rehabilitation by permitting forced extension exercises at only 6 weeks. Johnson et al. (1984) and Hefti et al. (1982) found comparable limitations of motion after ACL reconstructions using the Erikson technique (1976) or modified Jones procedure. In both techniques the patellar tendon strip is left attached distally. By contrast, Clancy (1983) and Clancy et al. (1982) noted an extension deficit in only 6 of their patients, and a flexion deficit in 14, which was less than 15° in all but 1 case.

Several patients suffered from femoropatellar crepitus and retropatellar pain, mainly during active extension against a resistance, but only 1 patient had significant disability. We repeatedly observed that patients tended to perceive femoropatellar symptoms as a feeling of instability. Clancy et al. (1982) described only 1 patient in their series who had severe femoropatellar pain, while Noyes et al. (1983) and Hefti et al. (1982) stressed the importance of patellar problems, whose etiology is obscure but presumably relates to a disturbance of femoropatellar alignment. Hefti et al. (1982) attributed the low incidence of retropatellar symptoms after knee operations by the Eriksson technique to the fact that that procedure involves incision of the lateral retinaculum. But chronic instabilities also may be associated with femoropatellar problems.

In this regard, Noyes et al. (1983) caution against overly intensive, active strengthening exercises of the extensor apparatus, as this can incite retropatellar symptoms that can lead to functional disability regardless of the type of operation performed. This problem is not observed with passive extension exercises.

There was 1 patient in our series who had an immediate postoperative herniation of the intrapatellar fat pad due to dehiscence of the patellar tendon, which was more a cosmetic problem than a source of pain. There was no instance of secondary rupture of the patellar tendon following removal of the central strip. Bonamo et al. (1984) reported on 2 cases of avulsion from the lower pole of the patella caused by significant trauma.

We were struck by the seemingly high incidence of irreparable meniscal lesions found at operation (82%), but when we compare our data with those of Clancy (1983) and Clancy et al. (1982), we find a comparable incidence of 86% in their series. McDaniel and Dameron (1980) found similar results in their follow-up study of 53 knees with an untreated rupture of the ACL.

During the past 10 years, reconstruction of the ACL with a strip of patellar tendon has evolved into a generally accepted and widely practiced technique, as the study of Bilko et al. (1986) confirms.

To date, our experience with this technique and the follow-up results in our first 50 cases at an average of 3 years postoperatively indicate that this method can satisfy the essential requirements in terms of knee joint stability. The results in these 50 patients are entirely comparable to those of Clancy (1983) and Clancy et al. (1982) and other authors (Hefti et al. 1982; Johnson et al. 1984; Paterson and Trickey 1986). Aside from the relatively pronounced limitations of motion in our series, we encountered no significant differences.

It remains to be determined whether the results presented are due to the hypothetically preserved vascular supply, as a comparative series using a free patellar tendon graft is still in progress.

Although cruciate ligament surgery has advanced considerably in recent years, owing largely to the impetus provided by numerous research studies, the technical aspects of the reconstruction still present a variety of problems. In this sense we agree with Noyes et al. (1984), who summarize the problems as follows:

An intraarticular cruciate substitution is a rather complex operative procedure, with many factors still to be studied. It requires selection of a graft with appropriate mechanical properties, meticulous surgical technique, correct fixation sites, correct adjustment of graft tension, postoperative protection allowing time for remodeling, and a careful and detailed rehabilitation program. A succession of biological remodeling events, out of the control of the surgeon, is ultimately required to achieve a successful result. This includes revascularization, collagen formation and fiber alignment, and remodeling of tissue fiber microgeometry. To what extent all of this occurs is presently unknown. The appropriate risks and benefits of biological ligament substitution must be weighed on this basis (Noyes et al. 1984, p. 352).

The authors thank Mr. J. Grünig for the excellent illustrations.

References

Alm A, Strömberg B (1974) Vascular anatomy of the patellar and cruciate ligaments. Acta Chir Scand [Suppl] 445: 25–35

Arnoczky SP (1983) Anatomy of the anterior cruciate ligament. Clin Orthop 172: 19–25

Arnoczky SP, Tarvin GB, Marshall JL (1982) Anterior cruciate ligament replacement using patellar tendon. An evaluation of graft revascularization in the dog. J Bone Joint Surg [Am] 64: 217–224

Bilko TE, Paulos LE, Feagin JA, Lambert KL, Cunningham HR (1986) Current trends in repair and rehabilitation of complete (acute) anterior cruciate ligament injuries. Analysis of 1984 questionnaire completed by ACL Study Group. Am J Sports Med 14: 143–147

Bonamo JJ, Krinick RM, Sporn AA (1984) Rupture of the patellar ligament after use of its central third for anterior cruciate reconstruction. Report of two cases. J Bone Joint Surg [Am] 66: 1294–1297

Brückner H (1966) Eine neue Methode der Kreuzbandplastik. Chirurg 9: 413–414

Butler DL, Noyes FR, Grood ES, Miller EH, Malek M (1979) Mechanical properties of transplants for the anterior cruciate ligament. Orthop Trans 3: 180–181

Butler DL, Noyes FR, Grood ES (1980) Ligamentous restraints to anterior-posterior drawer in the human knee. J Bone Joint Surg [Am] 62: 259–270

Clancy WG (1983) Anterior cruciate ligament functional instability: A static intra-articular and dynamic extra-articular procedure. Clin Orthop 172: 102–106

Clancy WG, Narechania RG, Rosenberg TD, Gmeiner JG, Wisnefske DD, Lange TA (1981) Anterior and posterior cruciate ligament reconstruction in rhesus monkeys. A histologic, microangiographic and biomechanical analysis. J Bone Joint Surg [Am] 63: 1270–1284

Clancy WG, Nelson DA, Reider B, Narechania RG (1982) Anterior cruciate ligament reconstruction using one-third of the patellar ligament, augmented by extra-articular tendon transfers. J Bone Joint Surg [Am] 64: 352–359

Daniel DM (1981) San Diego knee evaluation form. AAOS, Las Vegas, 1981

Drobny KT, Müller We, Wentzensen A, Perren SM (1984) Das Hoffagestielte Patellarsehnentransplantat beim vorderen Kreuzbandersatz. First European Congress of Knee Surgery and Arthroscopy, Berlin, 1984

Eriksson E (1976) Reconstruction of the anterior cruciate ligament. Orthop Clin North Am 7: 167–179

Galway RD, McIntosh DH (1980) The lateral pivot shift: A symptomatic sign of anterior cruciate insufficiency. Clin Orthop 147: 45–50

Hefti F, Gächter A, Jenny H, Morscher E (1982) Replacement of the anterior cruciate ligament. A comparative study of four different methods of reconstruction. Arch Orthop Trauma Surg 100: 83–94

Hughston JC, Andrews JR, Cross MJ, Moschi A (1976) Classification of knee ligament instabilities. Part I: The medial compartment and cruciate ligaments. Part II: The lateral compartment. J Bone Joint Surg [Am] 58: 159–179

Jakob RP (1985) Konzept der Isometrie. OAK-Workshop, Sept 1985

Jakob RP, Stäubli H-U, Hassler H (1981) Observations on rotatory instability of the lateral compartment of the knee. Acta Orthop Scand (Suppl 191) 52: 1–32

Jakob RP, Stäubli H-U, Deland JT (1987) Grading the pivot shift. J Bone Joint Surg [Br] 69: 294–299

Jakob RP, Kipfer W, Klaue K, Stäubli H-U, Gerber C (1988) Étude critique de la reconstitution du ligament croisé antérieur du genou par la plastie pédiculée sur le Hoffa à partir du tiers médian du tendon rotulien. 50 genoux opérés avec recul de 2 à 4 ans. Rev Chir Orthop 74: 44–51

Johnson RJ, Eriksson E, Haggmark T, Pope MH (1984) Five-to ten year follow-up evaluation after reconstruction of the anterior cruciate ligament. Clin Orthop 183: 122–140

Jones KG (1963) Reconstruction of the anterior cruciate ligament. J Bone Joint Surg [Am] 45: 925–932

Jones KG (1970) Reconstruction of the anterior cruciate ligament using the central one-third of the patellar ligament. J Bone Joint Surg [Am] 52: 1302–1308

Kieffer DA, Curnow RJ, Southwell RB, Tucker WF, Kendrick KK (1984) Anterior cruciate ligament arthroplasty. Am J Sports Med 12: 301–312

Lysholm J, Gillquist J (1982) Evaluation of knee ligament surgery results with special emphasis on use of a scoring scale. Am J Sports Med 10: 150–154

Marshall JL, Fetto JF, Botero PM (1977) Knee ligament injuries. A standardized evaluation method. Clin Orthop 123: 115–130

McDaniel WJ, Dameron TB (1980) Untreated ruptures of the anterior cruciate ligament. A follow-up study. J Bone Joint Surg [Am] 62: 696–705

McIntosh DL, Darby TA (1976) Lateral substitution reconstruction. J Bone Joint Surg [Br] 58: 142

Müller We (1982) Das Knie. Form, Funktion und ligamentäre Wiederherstellungschirurgie. Springer, Berlin Heidelberg New York

Noesberger B (1981) Grundlagen zur Diagnostik frischer und veralteter Kapselläsionen des Kniegelenkes. In: Jäger M, Hackenbroch MH, Refior HJ (Hrsg) Kapselbandläsionen des Kniegelenkes. Thieme, Stuttgart New York, S 78–87

Noesberger B, Jakob RP, Ganz R, Müller ME (1977) Reconstruction in cases of anteromedial instability of the knee. In: Chapchal G (ed) Injuries of the ligaments and their repair. Thieme, Stuttgart, pp 101–106

Noyes FR, Matthews DS, Mooar PA, Grood ES (1983) The symptomatic anterior cruciate-deficient knee. Part II: The results of rehabilitation, activity modification, and counseling on functional disability. J Bone Joint Surg [Am] 65: 163–174

Noyes FR, Butler DL, Grood ES, Zernicke RF, Hefzy MS (1984) Biomechanical analysis of human ligament grafts used in kneeligament repairs and reconstruction. J Bone Joint Surg [Am] 66: 344–352

Odensten M, Gillquist J (1985) Functional anatomy of the anterior cruciate ligament and a rationale for reconstruction. J Bone Joint Surg [Am] 67: 257–262

Palmer I (1938) On the injuries to the ligaments of the knee joint: A clinical study. Acta Chir Scand [Suppl 81] 53: 282

Paterson FWN, Trickey EL (1986) Anterior cruciate ligament reconstruction using part of the patellar tendon as a free graft. J Bone Joint Surg [Br] 68: 453–457

Paulos LE, Butler DL, Noyes FR, Grood ES (1983) Intra-articular cruciate reconstruction. II: Replacement with vascularized patellar tendon. Clin Orthop 172: 78–84

Rosenberg TD, Rasmussen GL (1984) The function of the anterior cruciate ligament during anterior drawer and Lachman's testing. An in vivo analysis in normal knees. Am J Sports Med 12: 318–322

Scapinelli R (1968) Studies on the vasculature of the human knee joint. Acta Anat 70: 305–331

Shino K, Kawasaki T, Hirose H, Gotoh I, Inoue M, Ono K (1984) Replacement of the anterior cruciate ligament by an allogeneic tendon graft. J Bone Joint Surg [Br] 66: 672–681

Torg JS, Conrad W, Kalen V (1976) Clinical diagnosis of anterior cruciate ligament instability in the athlete. Am J Sports Med 4: 84–93

Surgical Treatment of Anterior Cruciate Ligament Insufficiency: Comparison of Results of Repair, Primary Augmentation, and Reconstruction

R. Biedert, We. Müller, W. Hackenbruch, and R. Baumgartner

The results of operations on the anterior cruciate ligament (ACL) have improved substantially in recent years. To identify the precise factors involved in this positive development, we conducted a retrospective study in our own patients. It is hoped that our results will also pave the way for further advances in operating technique.

Materials and Methods

The patients selected for this study had undergone ACL surgery at the Bruderholz District Hospital, Switzerland, between 1981 and 1984. Out of the total pool of 600 patients, 200 were selected by lottery for review, and 163 of these could be evaluated.

The operations had been performed by a total of 10 physicians at the Orthopedic Department, using a standard operating technique.

Follow-up was conducted by the same orthopedist over a period of 3 months. Findings were documented on a special questionnaire covering the type and mechanism of injury, functional disability during everyday activities and sports, subjective complaints, overall subjective rating, etc. Stability relative to the opposite side (operated/nonoperated) and the objective results of the examiner were also documented.

A statistician assisted us in evaluating the results.

Time of follow-up. All operations had been performed between 12 and 48 months before. The average follow-up time was 29.4 months. The exact distribution is shown graphically in Fig. 1.

Age of patients. The youngest patient was 15 years of age, the oldest 64. The average age was 27.2 years.

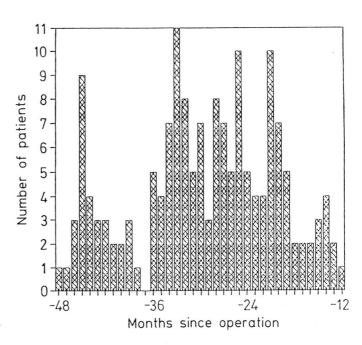

Fig. 1. Time of follow-up

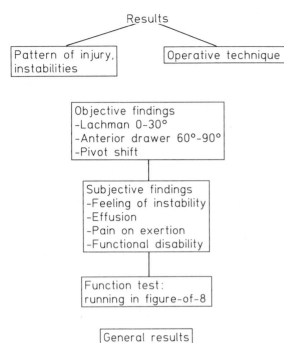

Results

Pattern of injury, instabilities

Operative technique

Objective findings
-Lachman 0-30°
-Anterior drawer 60°-90°
-Pivot shift

Subjective findings
-Feeling of instability
-Effusion
-Pain on exertion
-Functional disability

Function test:
running in figure-of-8

General results

Fig. 2. Overview of the evaluation

Table 1. Distribution by type of injury (n = 163)

Sports	139	(85.3%)
Motor vehicle	12	(7.3%)
Work	6	(3.7%)
Other	6	(3.7%)

Table 2. Distribution by type of sport (n = 139)

	Number	Percent (n = 139)	Total percent (n = 163)
Soccer	59	42	36.2
Skiing	50	36	30.7
Handball	7	5	4.3
Gymnastics	5	3.6	3.1
Tennis	4	2.9	2.5
Volleyball	3	2.2	1.8
Ice hockey, basketball, riding	2	1.4	1.2
Track and field, table tennis, squash, dancing; each:	1	0.7	0.6

Goal of Study

The results (more than 500 pages) were evaluated in order to address the following questions:

– What late result is likely to be associated with a certain pattern of injury and corresponding instability?
– What operative technique is best for achieving an optimum result?
– What is the impact of an ACL lesion on the patient's ability to perform in everyday tasks, extreme situations, and sports activities?

The focus of the evaluation, then, was on three major aspects relating to the injury, different operative techniques, and general results.

Our findings were subjected to a comparative analysis, and appropriate conclusions were drawn. Particular attention was given to the results of 8 specific examinations (Fig. 2).

Types of Injury

The great majority of ACL ruptures were sustained during sports activities (Table 1), followed by motor vehicle accidents; most patients in the latter group had been injured on motorcycles. Accidents at work and in various other settings accounted for the rest.

Distribution by Types of Sport (Table 2)

Soccer and skiing constituted the two highest risk groups, accounting for nearly 80% of all injuries. Other sports most commonly associated with ACL lesions were handball and gymnastics.

The causative mechanism of 73% of the injuries was valgus-flexion-external rotation. Only about 20% of injuries were caused by direct violence from an opponent.

Results by Patterns of Injury and Resulting Instabilities

Seven distinct combinations of knee injuries were noted at operation (Table 3). The corresponding instabilities were recorded in a diagram representing the 4 quadrants of the tibial plateau (Müller diagram, Fig. 3).

The results of the 8 findings that we consider most important are summarized in Table 4 for the 7 groups of injury combinations.

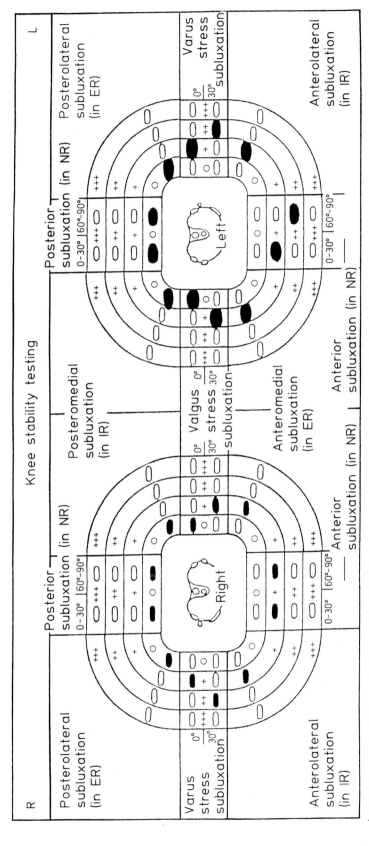

Fig. 3. Four-quadrant diagram for documenting instability

Table 3 see p. 405

Table 4. Results by injury and instability (data in percent)

Group		A	B	C	D	E	F	G
n=		32	22	19	36	23	20	11
Data in %								
Lachman 0-30°	0	32	32	21	36	33	17	9
	+	56	57	79	50	54	72	82
	+ +	9	11	0	14	13	11	9
	+ + +	3	0	0	0	0	0	0
Anterior drawer 60°-90°	0	6	3	6	3	9	0	0
	+	75	82	84	83	76	78	91
	+ +	19	15	10	14	15	22	9
	+ + +	0	0	0	0	0	0	0
Pivot shift	neg	60	57	58	64	59	39	45
	+	33	30	42	17	26	44	36
	+ +	7	13	0	19	15	11	19
Giving way	Preoperative	85	80	79	73	67	90	91
	Postoperative	9	13	11	14	11	22	9
Effusion	None	91	89	95	86	89	79	91
	Occasional	3	0	0	0	0	5	0
	Frequent	0	0	0	0	0	5	0
	On exertion	6	11	5	14	11	11	9
Exertional pain	None	67	59	53	58	59	78	91
	Occasional	33	38	47	40	39	17	9
	Constant	0	3	0	2	2	5	0
Functional disability	None	87	80	89	74	78	82	91
	Occasional	13	19	11	26	22	13	9
	Severe	0	1	0	0	0	5	0
Figure-of-8 running	Both sides	94	95	90	94	92	78	91
	Only 1 side	6	4	5	3	4	0	0
	Not possible	0	1	5	3	4	22	9

Table 3. Groups of injury combinations and number of patients affected

A: n = 32	ACL (isolated)
B: n = 22	ACL + POL
C: n = 19	ACL + POL + peripheral tear of medial meniscus
D: n = 36	ACL + MCL + POL
E: n = 23	ACL + MCL
F: n = 20	ACL + ALFTL + arcuate complex or popliteus corner
G: n = 11	ACL + ALFTL + arcuate complex or popliteus corner + POL

POL, Posterior oblique ligament (posterior medial collateral ligament); MCL, medial collateral ligament; ALFTL, antero-lateral femorotibial ligament

Significance of Injury Patterns and Instabilities

As a rule, the more structures are injured, the more difficult it is to achieve an optimum end result. The "most favorable" injury is an isolated tear of the ACL, which comprises the second largest of our 7 groups (group A, n = 32). However, because only 32% of this group showed complete stability on testing between 0° and 30°, and only 6% between 60° and 90°, it is reasonable to assume that the diagnosis was not always correct, and that there were concomitant injuries of the agonists (especially the posterior oblique ligament).

In group C, with a peripheral tear of the medial meniscus and posterior oblique ligament, the Lachman test was negative in only 21%. Group C was comparable to the other groups, however, in the range from 60° to 90°. This confirms that the semimembranosus corner and the posterior horn of the medial meniscus function as synergists for the ACL as the knee approaches extension.

The complex instabilities in groups F and G, with injury to the lateral structures, have the poorest prognosis and tend to have significantly poorer outcomes in most of the parameters tested. There were no significant differences in the pivot shift results, except in patients with complex lateral instabilities. Between 90% and 95% of the patients could run the figure-of-8 on both sides, 3%–6% on 1 side, and only 4 patients (excluding groups F and G) were unable to perform the test at all.

Results by Operative Technique

We divided the patients into 3 groups so that we could more meaningfully analyze and compare the operative results:

Table 5. Distribution of operations (the letters in parentheses designate the corresponding groups; ALFTL, Anterolateral femorotibial ligament)

Fresh (n = 91; 56%):	(H, I):	Isolated ACL: 12 repair = 5, augmentation = 7
	(K, L):	ACL + ALFTL: 19 repair = 8, augmentation = 11
	(M, N):	ACL + semimembranosus corner: 19 repair = 6, augmentation = 13
	(O, P):	ACL + ALFTL + semimembranosus corner: 28 repair = 14, augmentation = 14
	(Q, R):	ACL + arcuate complex/popliteus corner: 13 repair = 11, augmentation = 2
Chronic (n = 49; 30%):	(S):	Isolated ACL: 2
	(T):	ACL + ALFTL: 22
	(U):	ACL + semimembranosus corner: 12
	(V):	ACL + ALFTL + semimembranosus corner: 5
	(W):	ACL + arcuate complex/popliteus corner: 8
Previously operated (n = 23; 14%):	(X):	Isolated ACL: 1
	(Y):	ACL + ALFTL: 8
	(Z):	ACL + semimembranosus corner: 7
	(AA):	ACL + ALFTL + semimembranosus corner: 5
	(AB):	ACL + arcuate complex/popliteus corner: 2

– *Acute injuries*: Patients in this group had no previous history of knee problems and had their initial operation within 3 weeks after their injury.
– *Chronic instabilities*: These patients sustained their injury at least 4 weeks before, and they had had no previous knee surgery.
– *Previously operated instabilities*: Patients in this group had residual instability following 1–3 previous cruciate ligament operations.

The percentage distribution of the 3 main groups is shown in Table 5.

Group 1 (Acute Injuries)

Two major subgroups were identified:

– Patients who underwent simple suture *repair* or *reattachment* (N = repair, groups H, K, M, O, and Q)
– Patients who underwent *primary augmentation* of the ACL with a free or pedicled patellar tendon graft (central third, with proximal and distal bone blocks attached) (A = augmentation, groups I, L, N, P, and R)

The following additional procedures were employed to protect and relieve stress on the ACL during the healing period:

- Reconstruction of the ALFTL (anterolateral femorotibial ligament; Kaplan system), groups K and L
- Reconstruction of the semimembranosus corner (posterior oblique ligament, POL; posteromedial capsule, posterior horn of medial meniscus, capsular arm of semimembranosus muscle), groups M and N
- Combined reconstruction of the ALFTL and semimembranosus corner, groups O and P
- Reconstruction of the arcuate complex and popliteus corner (no popliteus bypass), groups Q and R

From the large volume of recorded data, Table 6 summarizes the results for the 8 parameters tested.

Evaluation and Discussion of Specific Results

Lachman Test

The best stability between 0° and 30° for fresh injuries was achieved by primary augmentation of the ACL with a patellar tendon graft combined with reconstruction of the ALFTL and semimembranosus corner (64% absolutely stable). Results were least favorable in the groups that underwent reconstruction of the arcuate complex or popliteus corner, but this is attributable to the complex instability itself and confirms the relationship of the results obtained to the existing pattern of injury.

Comparing repair and augmentation, we find that the results of primary augmentation are markedly better in the groups that had an isolated ACL repair or an isolated repair combined with reconstruction of the ALFTL and semimembranosus corner.

Pivot Shift

Primary augmentation yields significantly better results compared with repair or reattachment alone (maximum 82% negative versus maximum of 40%).

Reconstruction of the ALFTL appears to be an essential factor. It is not sufficient, however, to combine ALFTL reconstruction with ACL repair to achieve a good result. A significant reduction in pivot shift can be effected only by concomitant augmentation of the ACL. A similar percentage reduction in pivot shift can be achieved by reconstruction of the semimembranosus corner (compared with isolated surgery on the ACL). Adding semimembranosus reconstruction to ALFTL reconstruction does not provide further significant improvement, however. This means that at

least one of the adjunctive procedures for control of pivot shift must be performed.

Feeling of Instability

The patients with primary augmentation report significantly less subjective instability than those with primary repair (0%–9% vs. 12%–28%). The most marked improvement from 86% giving way preoperatively to 0% postoperatively was achieved by augmentation combined with reconstruction of the ALFTL and semimembranosus corner.

Pivot shift and giving way are directly interrelated not just clinically but also on the basis of the results obtained.

Figure-of-8 Running

All patients with an isolated operation on the ACL could run all legs of a figure-of-8 course without difficulty. This is surprising in view of the subjective postoperative instability in 20% and positive pivot shift in 43%–60%.

Patients who underwent reconstruction of the arcuate complex or popliteus corner had the greatest difficulty with this test.

Exertional Pain

On average, patients with a primary augmentation had less pain on exertion than the group that underwent repair. Again, the result can be improved by adding reconstruction of the ALFTL; this may relate to a reduction in giving way and the greater number of patients with a negative pivot shift.

Functional Disability

No patient was severely impaired in terms of functional capacity. Occasional functional disability occurred in an average of about 20% of the patients.

Effusion

Only 1 patient of 91 had chronic effusion. This case did not differ significantly from the others in terms of operative technique.

The groups that underwent surgery of the ACL (repair or augmentation) and reconstruction of the ALFTL alone did significantly poorer in terms of stability (0°–30° and 60°–90°) and postoperative giving way than the same groups in which reconstruction of the semimembranosus corner had been added. This has two implications:

Table 6. Results by operative technique: acute injuries (data in percent)

Group		H	I	K	L	M	N	O	P	Q	R
n=		5	7	14	14	11	2	6	13	8	11
		Data in %									
Lachman 0–30°	0	20	43	26	27	32	38	36	64	11	0
	+	20	57	62	54	60	54	50	36	72	50
	++	60	0	12	19	8	8	14	0	17	50
	+++	0	0	0	0	0	0	0	0.	0	0
Anterior drawer 60°–90°	0	20	28	12	9	16	8	14	22	0	0
	+	20	72	76	73	68	84	86	78	78	50
	++	60	0	12	18	16	8	0	0	22	50
	+++	0	0	0	0	0	0	0	0	0	0
Pivot shift	neg	40	57	26	82	32	69	36	78	17	50
	+	60	43	62	9	56	8	50	22	77	50
	++	0	0	12	9	12	23	14	0	6	0
Giving way	Preoperative	80	71	72	81	76	78	71	86	72	100
	Postoperative	20	0	12	9	28	8	14	0	22	0
Effusion	None	100	72	100	100	100	92	100	71	88	100
	Occasional	0	14	0	0	0	0	0	0	0	0
	Frequent	0	0	0	0	0	0	0	0	6	0
	On exertion	0	14	0	0	0	8	0	29	6	0
Exertional pain	None	40	57	62	72	68	54	36	57	67	100
	Occasional	60	43	38	28	32	38	64	43	33	0
	Constant	0	0	0	0	0	8	0	0	0	0
Functional disability	None	100	86	88	82	84	69	79	86	72	50
	Occasional	0	14	12	18	16	31	21	14	22	50
	Severe	0	0	0	0	0	0	0	0	0	0
Figure-of-8 running	Both sides	100	100	88	91	84	92	93	86	78	50
	Only 1 side	0	0	12	9	16	8	0	7	0	0
	Not possible	0	0	0	0	0	0	7	7	22	50

- A lesion of the semimembranosus corner is more common than statistically indicated, but undiagnosed.
- The importance of the structures in the semimembranosus corner has been underestimated. They serve not only to protect the intraarticular structures during the first postoperative year of healing but also perform a critically important synergistic role in general.

This realization calls for a more precise diagnostic evaluation, giving particular attention to the trauma history. It is known that an external rotation-flexion-valgus type of trauma ruptures the shortest posteromedial structures first, i.e., the POL before the ACL. Likewise, a pure hyperextension trauma leads to massive stretching in the posterior quadrants of the knee, probably causing significant lesions. Only hyperflexion or forced internal rotation in extension can rupture the ACL without also tearing the POL.

Chronic Instabilities

All operations for chronic instability included reconstruction of the ACL with a free or pedicled (fat pad) patellar tendon graft with attached proximal and distal bone blocks.
The individual results are listed in Table 7.

Discussion and Evaluation of Results

Stability

The stability in these patient groups, both in the ranges of 0°–30° and 60°–90°, is generally poorer up to a maximum of 5 mm (1 +). This is attributable to a progression of the existing instability with loosening of the secondary restraints. The end result could be markedly improved, however, by the selective reconstruction of these structures (semimembranosus corner, Kaplan system). This type of reconstruction was added in all but 2 patients with an isolated chronic tear of the ACL.
It is noteworthy that practically all groups displayed a 1 + to 2 + instability when testing was performed in 90° flexion.

Pivot Shift

No significant differences are apparent in the pivot shifts of knees with acute versus chronic instability. This clearly demonstrates the effect of reconstructing the ALFTL and/or the semimembranosus corner.

Giving Way

No patient in whom patellar tendon reconstruction of the ACL had been combined with reconstruction of the ALFTL and semimembranosus corner complained of subjective postoperative instability, even though this had been present in all patients prior to surgery. Again, results were poorest in the patients who underwent reconstruction of the arcuate complex or popliteus tendon.

Exertional Pain

The incidence of constant exertional pain was significantly higher than in the acutely operated patients. This is referable to the higher incidence of secondary chondropathies and degenerative meniscal lesions in the chronic group.

Effusion

No patient showed evidence of a chronic irritative effusion.

Figure-of-8 Running

A greater number of patients were unable to run both sides of the figure-of-8 course.

Previously Operated Patients

The previously operated patients constitute the smallest group, so the data in these patients represent tendencies rather than definitive results (Table 8).

Stability

Stability is worse compared with the acute and chronic instabilities. All patients had at least a 1 + instability in the range of 60°–90°.

Pivot Shift and Subjective Instability

Only 2 patients in this group had a 2 + pivot shift, and 1 complained of an unstable feeling after surgery. This again demonstrates the efficacy of ALFTL and semimembranosus reconstruction, even in previously operated patients.

Table 7. Results by operative technique: chronic instabilities (data in percent)

Group		S	T	U	V	W
	n=	2	22	12	5	8
		Data in %				
Lachman 0-30°	0	0	27	25	40	0
	+	100	69	67	60	100
	++	0	4	8	0	0
	+++	0	0	0	0	0
Anterior drawer 60°-90°	0	0	4	0	0	0
	+	100	87	83	100	88
	++	0	9	17	0	12
	+++	0	0	0	0	0
Pivot shift	neg	50	72	83	80	76
	+	50	24	17	20	24
	++	0	4	0	0	0
Giving way	Preoperative	0	96	92	100	100
	Postoperative	0	4	8	0	12
Effusion	None	100	92	84	100	64
	Occasional	0	4	8	0	12
	Frequent	0	0	0	0	0
	On exertion	0	4	8	0	24
Exertional pain	None	100	60	50	80	64
	Occasional	0	36	42	20	24
	Constant	0	4	8	0	12
Functional disability	None	100	72	83	80	76
	Occasional	0	28	17	20	24
	Severe	0	0	0	0	0
Figure-of-8 running	Both sides	100	86	83	80	76
	Only 1 side	0	14	17	0	24
	Not possible	0	0	0	20	0

General Results

Attitude Toward the Operation

A full 95.8% of the patients would consent to the operation again; 2.4% would not, and 1.8% might consent under certain conditions.

Use of the Knee

In 98% there was marked improvement in the activities of daily living, and 97% reported improvement in rigorous situations.

Condition of the Knee

The patients rated the condition of their knee as follows:

– 13% equivalent to the nonoperated side (completely normal)
– 75% greatly improved
– 11% improved
– 1% worse (1 patient)

Preoperative Athletic Disability

Before the operation 96% of the patients were severely disabled for athletic activities, and 4% were moderately disabled.

Table 8. Results by operative technique: previously operated instabilities (data in percent)

Group		X	Y	Z	AA	AB
	n=	1	8	7	5	2
		Data in %				
Lachman 0–30°	0	0	12	14	20	0
	+	100	64	72	60	100
	+ +	0	24	14	20	0
	+ + +	0	0	0	0	0
Anterior drawer 60°–90°	0	0	0	0	0	0
	+	100	76	72	80	100
	+ +	0	24	28	20	0
	+ + +	0	0	0	0	0
Pivot shift	neg	100	76	72	60	100
	+	0	24	14	20	0
	+ +	0	0	14	20	0
Giving way	Preoperative	100	88	86	80	100
	Postoperative	0	12	0	0	0
Effusion	None	100	88	72	80	50
	Occasional	0	0	14	0	50
	Frequent	0	0	0	0	0
	On exertion	0	12	14	20	0
Exertional pain	None	100	44	58	40	50
	Occasional	0	44	42	60	50
	Constant	0	12	0	0	0
Functional disability	None	100	50	86	80	100
	Occasional	0	50	14	20	0
	Severe	0	0	0	0	0
Figure-of-8 running	Both sides	100	76	86	80	50
	Only 1 side	0	24	14	20	50
	Not possible	0	0	0	0	0

Postoperative Athletic Disability

There was no athletic disability in 53% of the patients, mild disability in 39%, and severe disability in 8% (all with previous surgery).

Fibrosis of the Infrapatellar Fat Pad

In cases where a vascularized fat pad pedicle had been left attached to the patellar tendon graft, 9% of the patients complained of pain consistent with fat pad fibrosis. Of these, 4% had to be reoperated (arthroscopic shaving).

Complications

The following complications were documented postoperatively:

– Hematoma formation in 5%
– Infrapatellar nerve entrapment in 3%
– Infection in 1.2%

Social Status

None of the patients had to retire due to their injuries. A change of occupation was necessary in 2%, and 8% had to lighten their work load.

Range of Motion

The following ranges of motion were measured:

- Flexion deficit of 10° or less in 14 patients (9%)
- Flexion past 140° in 135 patients (83%)
- Extension deficit of 5° or less in 10 patients (6%)
- Recurvatum of 5° in 27 patients (16%)
- 10° recurvatum in 1 patient (0.6%)
- 20° recurvatum in 1 patient (0.6%)

No patient had an extension deficit of 10° or more at the time of follow-up.

There was clear evidence that as healing progresses, the range of extension and especially of flexion can continue to improve even after 1 year. In some cases almost 3 years passed before the patient was able to sit on his heels.

Conclusions

1. The more extensive the injury and associated instability, the more difficult it is to obtain a good late result. But the definitive outcome is not determined chiefly by the combination of injuries but by the type of operation that is performed.
2. Primary augmentation with a patellar tendon graft combined with reconstruction of the ALFTL and semimembranosus corner definitely yields the best results in acute ACL injuries.
3. Primary augmentation yields significantly better pivot-shift values than repair or reattachment.
4. Reconstruction of the ALFTL and, to a somewhat lesser degree, of the semimembranosus corner significantly reduces the incidence of pivot shift, but only when combined with ACL augmentation.
5. Giving-way symptoms are significantly less pronounced after primary augmentation than after repair or reattachment.
6. No patient with augmentation or replacement of the ACL with a patellar tendon graft combined with ALFTL and semimembranosus reconstruction complained of an unstable feeling after surgery.
7. Stability is significantly better in acutely operated patients than in the group with chronic instabilities. This does not apply to the pivot shift, however.
8. In all 3 operated groups (acute, chronic, previously operated), the results were poorest in patients who had a reconstruction of the arcuate complex or popliteus corner.
9. Stability is better in acutely operated patients than in patients with chronic instabilities, and it is better in the latter group than in patients who have had one or more previous operations.

Late Results after ACL Reconstruction with an Autologous Free Patellar Tendon Graft

W. Hackenbruch, W. Hey, and H. R. Henche

Replacement of the anterior cruciate ligament (ACL) with an autologous graft has become an established procedure in the management of chronic anterior knee instability. While clinical follow-up studies have confirmed good subjective and objective early results, little has been published to date on long-term results. It remains to be determined whether a good short-term result in a given patient also implies a good long-term outcome. In theory, there are 2 reasons why a primarily stable joint may become secondarily unstable:

- Excessive loading of the graft due to decompensation of the peripheral restraints
- Graft insufficiency based on a deficient blood supply or lack of collagen restructuring

To examine this question, we compared the operative results in a homogeneous clinical population for the years 1982 and 1988. The population consisted of 96 patients with an average age of 26 years (17–39) who underwent surgery for anterior cruciate insufficiency with disabling instability between 1978 and 1982. The operation was performed an average of 23 months (5–84) after the causal injury. Practically all cases were diagnosed by clinical examination, with tests eliciting a classic pivot shift sign in 92%. Only a few cases had been previously diagnosed by outpatient diagnostic arthroscopy under local anesthesia.

All patients underwent a standard operative procedure in which the ACL was replaced with a free autologous graft from the central third of the patellar tendon with attached proximal and distal bone blocks, using a modification of the techniques of Jones (1970) and Brückner and Brückner (1972). The trapezoidal distal bone block was wedged into the upper tibia, and the proximal end of the graft was fixed with a staple at the rim of the femoral tunnel (Fig. 1). In all cases the reconstruction was reinforced by the extraarticular anterolateral transfer of James and Slocum (1975), in which a distally based strip from the midportion of the iliotibial tract is routed beneath the lateral collateral ligament and lateral gastrocnemius head, looped back, and sutured to Gerdy's tubercle (Fig. 2).

Additional operative measures were not standardized and depended on the intraoperative findings and type of instability. A medial stabilizing procedure was performed in 54% of all patients (medial collateral ligament, semimembranosus corner), and repair of a peripheral meniscal tear was performed in 1/3 of all patients. Any meniscal and cartilage fragments causing mechanical interference were excised in the same sitting.

Postoperative treatment likewise followed a standard regimen and consisted basically of 6 weeks' immobilization in a plastic cast (Bycast), which was then changed for a modified Iowa brace in which partial weight bearing was allowed and finally complete weight bearing by the 16th week. Physical therapy was continued for at least 6 months, and strenuous sports activities were not permitted until 1 year postoperatively. Precise details on operative technique and aftercare have been fully described elsewhere (Hackenbruch and Henche 1981).

Of the 96 patients who gave responses on a written questionnaire, 73 could be evaluated. The 1982 respondents had had their operation an average of 23 months before follow-up (8–47). The final follow-up examination in 1988 was conducted an average of 7 1/2 years (6–9) after the operation.

From the large volume of information obtained, only identical questions could be meaningfully compared with each other (Table 1). Some 85% of the patients reported significant postperative improvement in 1982, while 95% reported significant improvement in 1988. All conditions being equal, 90% of the 1982 respondents and 97% of the 1988 respondents said they

Table 1. Patient responses to questionnaires (operation between 1978 and 1982); n = 73

	1982	1988
Significant improvement	85%	95%
Would consent to surgery again under the same conditions	90%	97%
Report complete relief of pain	63%	48%

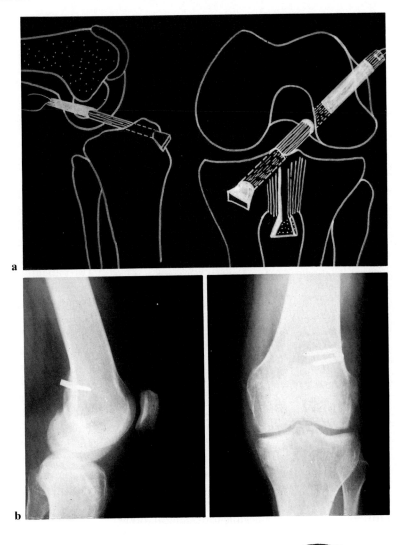

Fig. 1. a Schematic drawing of the placement of the graft for ACL reconstruction. **b** Corresponding radiographs

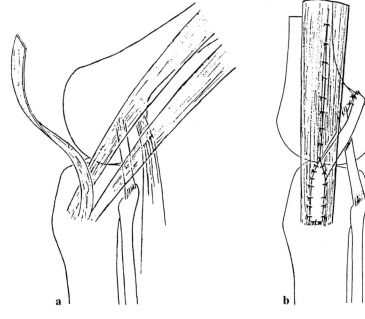

Fig. 2. a Graft mobilization for anterolateral stabilization. **b** Schematic appearance following fixation of the graft. Rerouting the iliotibial tract beneath the lateral collateral ligament and gastrocnemius tendon stabilizes against anterior tibial translation near extension (pivot shift)

Table 2. Clinical follow-up examination at 7 1/2 (6–9) years postoperatively; n = 56

Lachman test	Pivot shift	
Negative	Negative	23%
1 +	Negative	61%
1 + to 2 +	1 +	16%

Table 3. Evaluation of the result at 7 1/2 (6–9) years, using the scoring system of the New York Hospital for Special Surgery; n = 56

Score > 90	42.9%
Score 80–90	21.4%
Score < 80	35.7%

Table 4. Reoperations 6–9 years after ACL reconstruction; n = 73

Stabilizing procedure:	
ACL	1
Semimembranosus corner	1
Proximal tibial osteotomy	1
Resection of infrapatellar fat pad	2
Advancement of tibial tuberosity	1
Repair of muscle hernia	1
Scar revision	2
Removal of internal fixation material	5

would consent to the operation again, even though 63% of the 1982 respondents were completely pain-free as opposed to only 48% in 1988.

Fifty-six patients were available for a clinical follow-up examination with special emphasis on stability testing. In 23% of the patients, the stability of the operated knee was equivalent to that of the opposite knee. The pivot shift test was negative in 61%, but the Lachman test was positive (1 +). Sixteen percent of the patients showed significant residual instability with a positive pivot shift sign and positive Lachman test (1 + to 2 +). About half of these patients with a markedly poor result had undergone 1 or more previous operations (Table 2).

When the results were graded using the scoring system of the New York Hospital for Special Surgery, approximately two-thirds of all the patients scored higher than 80 points (Table 3).

Looking at the reoperation rate 6–9 years after the original surgery, we find that an additional stabilizing procedure was required in 2 patients who were assigned to the "poor result" group. In 1 patient the graft had been attached too far anteriorly on the femur in a nonisometric position. A second reconstruction was performed 3 years after the first, sup-

plemented by reuse of the old graft. Another patient underwent a stabilizing procedure on the semimembranosus corner combined with a modified pes anserinus transfer (Slocum and Larson 1968) to correct a disabling medial residual instability. One previously operated patient (total medial meniscectomy) underwent a proximal tibial osteotomy for incipient osteoarthritis. Advancement of the tibial tuberosity was performed in another patient with intractable retropatellar pain associated with preexisting patellar chondropathy. The rest of the reoperations were minor procedures and were more symptomatic in nature. Two scar revisions were performed medially in the area of the saphenous nerve, and 1 troublesome muscle hernia in the iliotibial band was repaired at the time the metallic fixation material was removed. Two patients required a partial arthroscopic resection of the infrapatellar fat pad for anterior knee pain, and 5 underwent removal of metallic fixation material (Table 4).

During analysis of the data obtained from the 1982 and 1988 examinations in the same homogeneous population, only responses to identical questions could be precisely compared, although additional information from the questionnaires and clinical examination do permit certain inferences to be drawn. The findings clearly indicate that the stability of the operated knee did not deteriorate from 1982 to 1988. It is also apparent that there was an increase in range of motion, with a corresponding improvement in athletic fitness and general knee use. This trend is clearly reflected in the responses to the first two questions (see Table 1). The increase in pain reported in the long-term result of 15% of the patients is obviously a result of meniscal and cartilage pathology, with most pain arising from the femoropatellar joint.

Analysis of the reoperations also confirms the generally good stability and range of motion in the long-term course. Only 2 patients required a stabilizing procedure on the knee (see Table 4). The fact that no patients required arthrolysis or manipulation under general anesthesia underscores the satisfactory long-term result in terms of motion range. Given the relatively large number of meniscus repairs, it is particularly noteworthy that no meniscectomies had to be performed during the long follow-up period.

The following conclusions can be drawn on the basis of our investigations: Good to excellent long-term stability is obtained in 84% of patients who undergo ACL reconstruction with the autologous free patellar tendon graft.

A good early result also implies a good long-term result, weakening the concept that a primarily stable joint is prone to secondary loosening. Based on the comparative results, it must be assumed that the long-term outcome is even more favorable than the early result.

Despite the stability achieved, only half the patients are completely free of pain; this can be attributed to associated meniscal and cartilage pathology. Even so, more than 90% of the patients questioned indicated that, with benefit of hindsight, they would consent to the same operation if the conditions were the same.

References

Brückner H, Brückner H (1972) Bandplastiken im Kniebereich nach dem Baukastenprinzip. Zentralbl Chir 3: 65–77

Hackenbruch W, Henche HR (1981) Diagnostik und Therapie von Kapselbandläsionen am Kniegelenk. Eular, Basel

Hackenbruch W, Henche HR, Müller We (1982) Operationsergebnisse bei chronischer vorderer Knieinstabilität. Vortrag, 3. Münchner Symposium für Sporttraumatologie, 13. 11. 1982

James SL, Slocum DB (1975) Sports medicine of the year. Sports Med 3: 260–271

Jones KK (1970) Reconstruction of the anterior cruciate ligament using the central one-third of the patellar ligament. J Bone Joint Surg [Am] 52: 1302–1308

Slocum DB, Larson RL (1968) The pes anserinus transplant. A surgical procedure for control of rotatory instability of the knee. J Bone Joint Surg [Am] 5: 226–242

Extraarticular Lateral Reconstructions

D. Fritschy and C. Freuler

Extraarticular ligament reconstructions on the lateral side of the knee joint are designed to stabilize the lateral tibial plateau beneath the femur. This is accomplished by constructing a lateral femorotibial ligament that functions as a checkrein against internal rotation of the tibia. In principle, then, these procedures are indicated for the control of lateral pivot shift, usually in patients with chronic ligamentous injury.

The medial ligament reconstructions, such as Slocum's pes anserinus transfer, are not discussed here as they do not affect anterolateral instabilty.

Two names are closely associated with the origin of extraarticular lateral transfers: Lemaire and MacIntosh. Interestingly, both authors described their extraarticular lateral transfer in papers in which they also described the "lateral pivot shift" for the first time. It is likely that Lemaire's 1967 publication would have been received across the Atlantic, and its concepts adopted, had it not been for the language barrier between the English- and French-speaking authors. The publications of Galway et al. (1972) are essentially English-language versions of Lemaire's papers that appeared 5 years before.

Lemaire (1980) has associated the lateral pivot shift phenomenon with anterior cruciate insufficiency since 1961. He describes the phenomenon in this way: "A sign, unfortunately not present in every case, appears to be pathognomonic for injury to the anterior cruciate ligament. It involves an anteromedial subluxation that is elicited as the knee approaches full extension. We place the foot in internal rotation while the knee is extended. If the muscles are completely relaxed, an anterior and medial subluxation can sometimes be elicited by exerting gentle pressure on the head of the fibula, accompanied by small excursions of the knee in flexion and extension. As these very gentle movements are carried out, an anterior jump ("ressaut") occurs at the start of flexion. The patient recognizes this shift at once as the subluxation he has been experiencing. Unfortunately, this sign is difficult to observe because perfect muscular relaxation is very difficult to achieve" (Lemaire 1980, p. 523).

Lemaire recognized this sign while he was investigating the mediocre results of meniscectomies. During this time he noted a frequent association of meniscal injuries with tears of the anterior cruciate ligament (ACL). For Lemaire, it was self-evident that both injuries required treatment. But since the repair of a long-standing ACL rupture was not feasible, and an anatomic reconstruction of the ACL was practically impossible, he opted for an extraarticular reconstruction, which he has practiced from 1961 until today, with ongoing refinements.

Meanwhile, MacIntosh and Darby (1976), who also described the pivot shift, proposed a lateral reconstruction procedure for the purpose of stabilizing the lateral tibial plateau beneath the femoral condyle in extension. We shall discuss their procedure and its results later in this article.

Several authors have described the role of the iliotibial tract in the lateral stabilization of the knee. The use of a portion of the tract to enhance anterolateral rotatory stability and decrease varus instability also has been reported. Recently Lobenhoffer et al. (1987), in a study of 100 knees, proved the existence of a fiber complex extending from the posterior portion of the iliotibial tract to the intermuscular septum. This anatomic structure corresponds to the "anterolateral femorotibial ligament" previously described by Müller. These retrograde fibers establish a solid, isometric connection between their femoral attachment and Gerdy's tubercle. All lateral tractopexies that respect the biomechanics of the knee joint must include these retrograde fibers.

Tenodesis of the iliotibial band (tractopexy) is intended to check anterolateral rotatory instability without lessening the active role of the tensor fascia latae. Andrews and Carson (1987), Hughston, and We. Müller (1983) described the best-known procedures.

Several American authors – most notably Ellison (1975), Losee et al. (1978), and James (1983) – have proposed their own modifications of the original MacIntosh procedure. These 3 authors represent the second mainstream in the Angloamerican literature. According to them, other surgeons have modified the

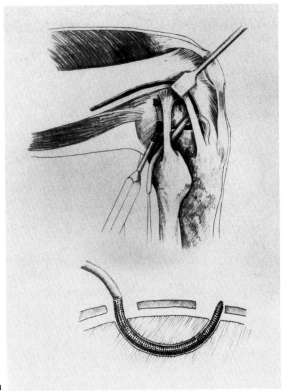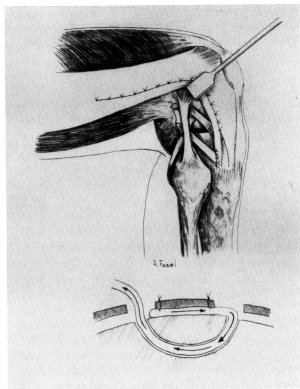

Fig. 1 a, b. Technique of Lemaire (1980)

technique without introducing significant changes or achieving spectacular improvement in results.

Here we shall focus on the techniques of Lemaire (1967) and MacIntosh and Darby (1976) and the modifications of Ellison (1975) and Losee et al. (1978).

Lemaire Technique (Fig. 1)

We shall describe the most recent modification, published by Lemaire in 1980.

The patient is positioned supine with a pneumatic tourniquet on the thigh. The knee is positioned on a holder in 40°–60° flexion so that the limb falls spontaneously into maximum external rotation. This position is very important and should be checked throughout the operation to see that it is maintained.

The lateral approach is made at the level of the condyle through an incision about 15 cm long, starting at Gerdy's tubercle and passing over the proximal attachment of the lateral collateral ligament to the central portion of the fascia lata of the iliotibial band. The fascial strip should be approximately 12–15 cm long and at least 1.5 cm wide. It is left attached distally to Gerdy's tubercle. The exact strip length varies with the size of the patient, but it must be long enough to produce a solid transfer. The proximal part of the strip should be cut from the posterior portion of the fascia lata, where the fibers are especially thick and strong. The more distal part of the strip includes the anterior portion of the band and passes tangential to the delicate anterior capsule.

The deep surface of the strip is cleanly dissected and freed of extraneous tissue.

Meticulous preparation of the fascial strip is essential to produce a solid transfer that will pass easily through the osseous tunnel. The next step is exposure of the lateral condyle. The synovial recess is retracted upward, and the proximal attachment of the lateral collateral ligament is freed and the proximal 2 cm of the ligament exposed. Its anterior and posterior margins and deep surface are carefully dissected free. The ligament is extrasynovial and well demarcated from the capsule, so its full circumference can be exposed without difficulty while protecting the underlying synovium, which must not be harmed.

The periosteum along the posterior edge of the lateral collateral ligament is elevated about 2–3 cm distally from the upper attachment of the ligament using a small, straight periosteal elevator. This zone is easily freed by retracting the synovial recess to one side and the suprapatellar quadriceps pouch to the other. The distal opening for the bone tunnel is located on the lower aspect of Gerdy's tubercle, the proximal opening at the upper limit of the elevated periosteum. The bone tunnel is cut with 2 reamers that are advanced from the entrances until they touch. The tunnel is smoothed with a short, round rasp. A staple is placed tangentially at the lower edge of the proximal tunnel entrance to prevent the tight fascial strip from sawing into the bone, which would lead to laxity of the repair.

The strip is pulled through the tunnel with the aid of a guide suture at its end. The suture should be carefully attached so that it does not pull out and keeps the end of the strip from flaring, which would hamper its passage through the bone tunnel. The strip is first pulled through beneath the lateral ligament and then beneath the elevated periosteum toward the upper tunnel entrance. It is now pulled very tight while the tibia is in neutral rotation. While still taut, the strip is fixed to the periosteum with several sutures; it is then routed down through the bone tunnel before it is pulled tight again. The reconstruction is completed by looping the strip back beneath the lateral ligament and fixing it to the distal iliotibial band with 3–5 nonabsorbable interrupted sutures. Together with the periosteal suture, this second suture provides fixation of the strip on both the anterior and posterior sides of the osseous tunnel. Finally the fascial defect is closed while the knee is in extension.

Postoperative Treatment

Crutch ambulation without weight bearing is started on the 2nd postoperative day, and weight bearing is resumed on day 15. Further rehabilitation is brief, and running exercises can be started after only 2 weeks, i.e., 1 month after the operation. Sports activities can be resumed at 6 weeks.

MacIntosh Technique

The procedure of MacIntosh and Darby (1976) is technically less demanding than the Lemaire procedure. The approach is made through a lateral incision approximately 20 cm long, and a strip of fascia lata 16 cm long and 1.5 cm wide, attached distally to Gerdy's tubercle, is mobilized from the iliotibial band. The strip is routed deep to the lateral collateral ligament and then toward the intermuscular septum on the posterior side of the femoral condyle, where it is secured. A hiatus is created in the septum, and the strip is passed through this opening from lateral to medial, looped downward and back beneath the lateral ligament, and secured just distal to its insertion into Gerdy's tubercle. It is attached there with a staple or suture while the knee is flexed and the tibia externally rotated, and the fascial defect is closed.

Postoperative Treatment

The extremity is immobilized in a long leg cast with the knee flexed 60° and the tibia externally rotated. The cast is changed at 2-week intervals and worn for a total of 6–8 weeks. Isometric quadriceps training is started the day after surgery, and non-weight-bearing crutch ambulation is permitted. After cast removal, the knee is protected in a brace for several months. Physical therapy is the same as that for an acute ligament repair. The patient is not permitted strenuous sports activities for 1 year.

Ellison Technique

The modification of Ellison (1975) aims at achieving a dynamic stabilizing effect. The knee is flexed 90° with a pneumatic tourniquet about the thigh. The skin incision starts just proximal to the lateral femoral condyle in the midline of the iliotibial band and ends distally between the tibial tuberosity and Gerdy's tubercle. First a 1.8-cm button of bone is cut from Gerdy's tubercle, then a strip of iliotibial band approximately 1.5 cm wide is cut, starting distally and proceeding proximally, gradually widening the strip so that the base is 3–4 times as wide as the distal end. This shape is designed to ensure an optimum blood supply and achieve a dynamic stabilizing efect. The foot is placed across the opposite thigh to tighten the lateral collateral ligament, and a blunt hemostat is passed beneath the dissected ligament to create a tunnel for passage of the fascial strip and attached bone fragment. A staple is used to anchor the bone fragment within a prepared tibial trough near the lateral edge of the patellar tendon. During attachment of the fragment, the lateral tibial condyle is held in a posteriorly reduced position while the knee is flexed 90° and the tibia is held in external rotation. When the transferred fascial strip is correctly positioned and tightened, the knee cannot be fully extended be-

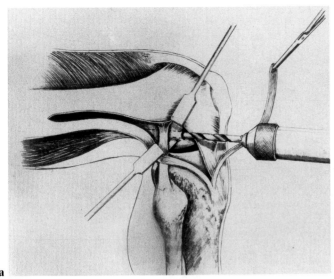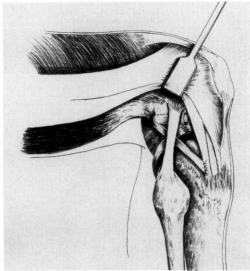

a   b

Fig. 2 a, b. Technique of Losee et al. (1978)

cause, as the knee extends, the proximal insertion of the lateral collateral ligament acts as a checkrein on the iliotibial strip to prevent full extension. During wound closure the iliotibial tract envelopes the transplant except for its wide proximal base. This creates a sleeve within which the transplant is free to glide. Care is taken to avoid placing sutures into the transferred strip as they would interfere with its excursion.

Postoperative Treatment

The limb is immobilized in a long leg cast with the knee flexed 60° and the tibia externally rotated. Further treatment is like that described for the procedure of MacIntosh and Darby (1976).

Losee Technique (Fig. 2)

The limb position and lateral incision are the same as in the Ellison procedure. A strip of iliotibial band 18 cm long and 1.5 cm wide is fashioned from the midportion of the tract and is left attached distally to Gerdy's tubercle. A superficial bone tunnel is created which starts on the anterolateral aspect of the femoral condyle, passes deep to the femoral attachment of the lateral collateral ligament and popliteus tendon, and emerges posterolaterally where the superior part of the posterior capsule, the lateral gastrocnemius head, and the iliotibial tract converge. The strip is pulled through the bone tunnel from anterior to pos-

terior and pulled tight with the knee flexed 90° and the tibia externally rotated. From there the strip passes through the femoral attachment of the intermuscular septum and the lateral gastrocnemius head, is woven through the lateral portion of the arcuate ligament complex, and is fixed at the posterolateral corner of the knee. The strip is again pulled taut inferiorly and anteriorly, which also tenses the posterior capsular structures and arcuate ligament, and is passed forward deep to the lateral ligament, approximately at the level of the joint line, and secured with interrupted sutures or a staple near Gerdy's tubercle while the knee is flexed 90° and the tibia is in maximum external rotation. The transferred strip checks anterior translation and internal rotation of the tibia while simultaneously reinforcing the anterolateral capsule and arcuate ligament. Several sutures may be added between the biceps femoris muscle and the posterior edge of the iliotibial tract.

Postoperative treatment is like that following the procedures of MacIntosh and Darby (1976) and Ellison (1975).

Tenodesis of the Iliotibial Band

Andrews and Carson (1987) (Fig. 3). With the knee flexed 90°, the iliotibial band is exposed through a lateral incision approximately 10 cm long. A longitudinal incision 10 cm long is made through the iliotibial band 4 cm from its posterior border. The distal and lateral portions of the femur are exposed, especially

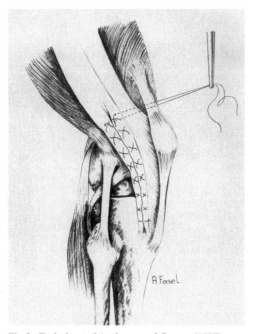

Fig. 3. Technique of Andrews and Carson (1987)

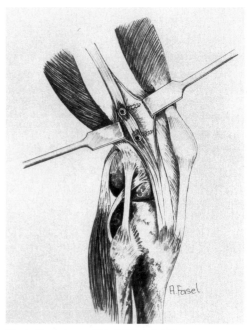

Fig. 4. Technique of We. Müller (1983)

the linea aspera by distal incision of the intermuscular septum. This area is freshened with an osteotome to promote adhesion of the "ligament" prepared by weaving sutures through 2 strips of iliotibial band.

An initial hole is drilled from lateral to medial through the femur at the distal attachment of the intermuscular septum on the linear aspera, as close as possible to the posterior cortex. A 2nd hole is drilled 1 cm anterior and 0.5 cm distal to the first. Exposure of the medial distal metaphysis permits localization of the drill holes and the osseous bridge over which the sutures will be tied. Two nonabsorbable, heavy-gauge sutures are woven through the posterior part of the iliotibial tract using the Bunnel technique, each suture encompassing a strip 1.5 cm in width. The 1st strip is prepared from Gerdy's tubercle, proceeding proximally 4–5 cm to the level of the posterior drill hole. An identical 2nd strip is prepared just anterior to the first, the criss-cross suture terminating at the level of the anterior drill hole. The 2 sutures are then pulled through the transfemoral drill holes and pulled taut on the medial side. With isometric placement of the sutures, the knee can move freely through a full range of motion, the anterior strip becoming taut in flexion, the posterior strip in extension. Finally the 2 sutures are tied together with the knee flexed 45° and the tibia externally rotated. The joint is immobilized in plaster for 4 weeks with the knee flexed 30°–45°.

W. Müller (1983) (Fig. 4). Two incisions are made in

the iliotibial tract parallel to its fibers, and a 1.5-cm-wide strip is dissected from the posterior portion of the tract. The lateral aspect of the femur is then freshened at the level of this strip. Isometry is first tested by fixing the strip with a Kirschner wire 2 mm long. Anterior instability must be eliminated in all positions of flexion and extension. Definitive fixation of the strip is performed with 2 AO/ASIF small-fragment screws 28 mm long, inserted over toothed washers. The strip is additionally sutured to the intermuscular septum before the iliotibial tract is closed over it with simple interrupted sutures. The limb is immobilized on a removable splint that permits early postoperative exercises.

Technique of Fritschy and Freuler (Fig. 5)

We likewise use the iliotibial tract to construct a lateral femorotibial ligament. We mobilize a 10–15 mm wide and 20 cm long strip from the posterior portion of the tract, preserving its attachment to Gerdy's tubercle. An osseous tunnel is reamed perpendicular to the axis of the linea aspera, just posterior to the attachment of the lateral collateral ligament. The strip is pulled through the tunnel from anterior to posterior and routed toward Gerdy's tubercle, where it is fixed to the tract with simple interrupted sutures.

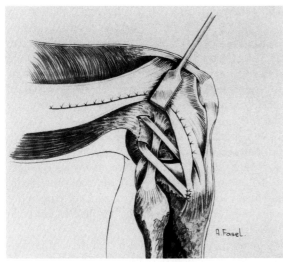

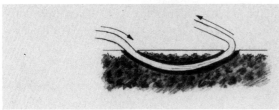

Fig. 5. Technique of Fritschy and Freuler

This technique avoids 3 difficulties inherent in other procedures:

- It is difficult to place the longitudinally oriented tunnel in the Losee technique (Losee et al. 1978) entirely within the bone because it runs parallel to the lateral femoral condyle.
- The proximal attachment in solid bone is more secure than the attachment to the intermuscular septum in the MacIntosh procedure (MacIntosh and Darby 1976).
- It is unnecessary to pass the strip deep to the lateral collateral ligament. Often this leads to laxness of the collateral ligament, which is not desirable. The transfer is just as solid when routed superficial to the lateral ligament.

Like Lemaire (1983), we advocate early mobilization under the protection of non-weight-bearing for 2 weeks, followed by a progressive resumption of normal function at 4–6 weeks.

Results

In his first series published in 1967, Lemaire found good results in 28 of the 30 patients. In a 1980 paper on operating technique, he noted that he had acquired experience in more than 2000 operations, but unfortunately the results were not published. In 1983 he reported on 156 patients who had been followed for 4 years (Lemaire 1983); these represented half the patients who had been operated in 1977. He found that most patients still had an anterior drawer sign, but that anterior subluxation of the lateral tibial plateau in internal rotation (lateral pivot shift) had been eliminated. Lemaire reports a 76% rate of good results, adding that the functional results are somewhat less favorable in patients with patellar chondropathy and when the injury is older than 2 months.

Schmid and Bandi (1986) reviewed 65 cases (22 chronic injuries, 43 acute) of ACL lesions that had been treated by the Lemaire procedure. Follow-up at 2–7 years indicated a good result in 80%–90% (Lysholm score and Marshall scale). These authors, who recommend the procedure for young patients as well as older active patients, believe that control of the pivot shift plays a key role.

In 1972 MacIntosh reviewed a series of 18 patients who had been operated by his technique, but the length of follow-up was insufficient to permit an evaluation of the results.

In 1976 MacIntosh and Darby published a review of 90 patients who had been followed for a period of 6 months to 5 years. The results were characterized as encouraging (MacIntosh and Darby 1976).

In 1978 Kennedy et al. described their experience with the Ellison procedure in 52 knees. Of the 28 patients who were available for follow-up at 6 months, the authors found good or excellent results in approximately half. Based on their findings, the authors recommended that the Ellison transfer be used only as an adjunctive procedure in lateral reconstructions of the knee.

Fox et al. (1980) evaluated the results in 76 patients who underwent a modification of the Ellison procedure in which the osteotomized bone fragment, attached to the iliotibial strip, is looped around the lateral collateral ligament and brought back to Gerdy's tubercle and fixed to the osteotomy site. At 1 year the authors noted results similar to those reported by Kennedy et al. In conclusion, they recommend a direct reconstruction of the ACL in addition to the extraarticular transfer for knees with a 2 + or 3 + instability.

In 1978 Losee reviewed a series of 84 patients who had been treated by his "sling and reef" operation

(Losee et al. 1978). It should be noted that Losee, in 1969, described a variant of the lateral pivot shift test that bears his name. His extraarticular procedure was inspired by MacIntosh. Fifty of the 84 patients were evaluated at 1 to 6 1/2 years after the operation. The results were rated in terms of function, stability, ability to work, and osteoarthritis. Using these criteria, the results were good in 41 knees, fair in 6, and poor in 3. Losee noted that ligament reconstructions tend to stretch out over time, and that the long-term result at 10–15 years might be poor.

Andrews reported excellent results with the technique that he has used since 1977: 62 knees (31 acute, 31 chronic) with anterolateral instablity were evaluated at least 2 years after operation, and 94% exhibited good results (Andrews and Carson 1987). This enthusiasm is not shared by all, and it is remarkable that Andrews himself no longer practices his own tehnique.

this protective effect has not been definitively proven. O'Brien found surprising results in a randomized series of ACL reconstructions: The combined reconstructions (intra- and extraarticular) are not superior to intraarticular reconstructions alone (O'Brien 1987). The current policy at the Hospital for Special Surgery is to avoid the use of extraarticular transfers.

English-speaking authors are generally more pessimistic in the assessment of their results. Today it appears that the Ellison procedure (1975) is no longer used alone for the treatment of anterior cruciate insufficiency. The Losee procedure appears to be better in the hands of the author, but this has not yet been confirmed in large series.

The general impression today is that the extraarticular transfer is a good operation for reinforcing a repair or reconstruction of the ACL. When used alone, however, it is inadequate for the control of ligamentous insufficiency.

Summary

We feel that a lateral extraarticular transfer procedure alone may be appropriate for 2 types of patient with symptomatic anterolateral instability:

– For the occasional athlete who does not want a major intraarticular operation with the attendant need for prolonged rehabilitation
– For patients 50 years of age or older who desire an improvement of knee function. Several authors have pointed out the hazards of intraarticular ligament surgery in this age group. The control of pivot shift is often sufficient for these patients.

Twenty-five years after his description of the lateral pivot shift and his extraarticular reconstruction, Lemaire has remained true to his philosophy. He still uses his transfer as an isolated operation, believing that it is both beneficial and does no harm. Lemaire's experience as an operator is impressive: His surgical patients number in the thousands. One objection that may be raised is that Lemaire has shown little concern for results. The 156 patients who have been followed to date are only a fraction of the thousands that have been operated on. In the orthopedic departments that employ the Lemaire transfer, either alone or as an adjunct to other procedures, surgeons acknowledge its efficacy as a lateral tenodesis while also noting, with Losee et al. (1978), that there is a tendency for the transfer to loosen over time.

Many authors use the extraarticular transfer to protect a repair or reconstruction of the ACL, although

References

Andrews JR, Carson WG Jr (1987) The role of extra-articular anterior cruciate ligament stabilization. In: Jackson DW, Drez D (eds) The anterior cruciale deficient knee. New concepts in ligament repair. Mosby, St. Louis
Campbell's Operative Orthopaedics (1980) Traumatic affections of joints, 6th edn, vol 1. Mosby, St. Louis, pp 967–972
Ellison AE (1975) A modified procedure for extra-articular replacement of the anterior cruciate ligament. Presented at Annual Meeting of American Orthopaedic Society for Sports Medicine. New Orleans/LA, July 1975
Fox JM, Blazina ME, Del Pizzo W, Ivey FM, Broukhim B (1980) Extra-articular stabilization of the knee joint for anterior instability. Clin Orthop 147: 56–61
Galway RO, Beaupré A, Mac Intosh DL (1972) Pivot shift: a clinical sign of symptomatic anterior cruciate insufficiency. J Bone Joint Surg [Br] 54: 763
James SL (1983) Knee ligament reconstruction. In: Evarts CM (ed) Surgery of the musculoskeletal system. Churchill Livingstone, New York, pp 31–104
Kennedy JC, Stewart R, Walker DM (1978) Anterolateral rotatory instability of the knee joint. J Bone Joint Surg [Am] 60: 1031–1039
Lemaire M (1967) Ruptures anciennes du ligament croisé antérieur du genou. J Chir 93: 311–320
Lemaire M (1980) Technique actuelle de plastie ligamentaire pour rupture ancienne du ligament croisé antérieur. Rev Chir Orthop 66: 523–525
Lemaire M (1983) Résultats de la plastie extra-articulaire palliative de la rupture du ligament croisé antérieur. Rev Chir Orthop 69: 278–282
Lobenhoffer P, Posel P, Witt F, Piehler J, Wirth CJ (1987) Distal femoral fixation of the iliotibial tract. Arch Orthop Trauma Surg 106: 285–290

Losee RE, Johnson TR, Southwick WO (1978) Anterior sub-luxation of the lateral tibial plateau. A diagnostic test and operative repair. J Bone Joint Surg [Am] 60: 1015–1030

Mac Intosh DL, Darby TA (1976) Lateral substitution recon-struction. J Bone Joint Surg [Br] 58: 142

Müller We (1983) The knee. Springer, Berlin Heidelberg, New York Tokyo

O'Brien SJ (1987) Results of ACL reconstruction using the in-frapatellar tendon. AOSSM Traveling Fellow Instructional Course, New York

Schmid F, Bandi W (1986) The operative-functional treat-ment of recent and old ligamentous lesions of the knee joint according to Lemaire. Abstract Book 2nd ESKA Congress, Basel, pp 53, 182–183

Arthroscopic Techniques of Anterior Cruciate Ligament Reconstruction

Kenneth Jones Technique of Arthroscopic Cruciate Reconstruction

J. D. Demottaz

Transarthroscopic reconstruction of the anterior cruciate ligament (ACL) by the Jones technique is still somewhat controversial. The results of arthroscopic cruciate ligament reconstructions are not yet as convincing as those of arthroscopic meniscectomy. Transarthroscopic reconstructions require a meticulous working technique and the ability to visualize anatomy in 3 dimensions, as in other orthopedic procedures. Nevertheless, the technical difficulties of arthroscopic reconstruction are no greater than those of arthroscopic meniscectomy. Although the anatomic sites of attachment of the ACL can be directly visualized, errors of judgment are possible. Generally the definitive drilling of the tibial and femoral bone tunnels constitutes the "point of no return." With the arthroscopic technique described here, definitive drilling is deferred until a precise analysis has been made of the anatomic insertion sites, possibly supplemented by a radiographic assessment of isometry.

The following instruments are required for the transarthroscopic reconstruction:

- 30° telescope
- Motorized shaver with cutting head, Dyovac forceps, curette
- 2 Kirschner wires of 1 mm diameter, 1 Kirschner wire of 2.5 mm diameter (same as the guidewire for the dynamic hip screw)
- 8-mm cannulated reamer (same as that for the dynamic hip screw)
- 4- and 4.5-mm drill bits
- Bone staples or screws with corresponding fixation instruments
- Straight needle
- If available, the small Storz aiming device for ACL reconstruction

The length of the operation is generally 1.5–2 h. Use of a tourniquet is rarely necessary.

Operative Technique

With the patient supine on the operating table, a tourniquet is placed about the thigh but not inflated. The knee is flexed 90°, the foot resting on a bolster; a lateral thigh support at the level of the tourniquet stabilizes the limb (Fig. 1) while permitting intraoperative knee flexion past 120°.

To shorten the duration of the arthroscopy and avoid possible edema due to fluid extravasation into perisynovial tissues, the patellar tendon graft is harvested through a 7-cm parapatellar incision before the arthroscope is introduced. The graft consists of the central one-third of the patellar tendon with an attached bone block from the tibial tuberosity at the distal end, and a bone block from the lower pole of the patella at the proximal end. A lateral supracondylar incision about 4 cm long is required for exposure of the transfemoral tunnel (Fig. 2).

The harvested patellar tendon graft is defatted, and a wire suture 0.8 mm in diameter is placed through each of the attached bone blocks. The arthroscope is introduced through an anterolateral portal as close to the patellar tendon as possible, without causing tendon damage. The knee joint is distended with Ringer's solution. All concomitant transarthroscopic

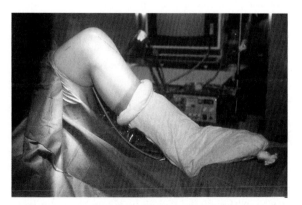

Fig. 1. The knee is positioned in 90° flexion with the foot on a padded rest and the thigh stabilized by a lateral support. The skin incision lines have been drawn

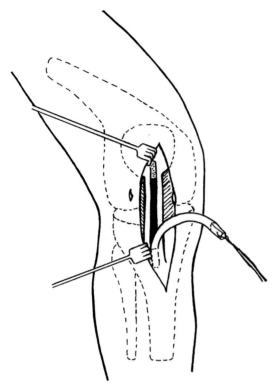

Fig. 2. Through a parapatellar approach, the central one-third of the patellar tendon is removed with attached bone blocks from the tibial tuberosity and distal patellar pole. Arthrotomy is not required

procedures such as partial meniscectomy or meniscal repair or reattachment are carried out first. The residual cruciate ligament stumps are removed and aspirated using the shaver or Dyovac forceps. Debridement of the cruciate stumps and adequate widening of the intercondylar notch (notch plasty) permit the surgeon to identify the attachment sites of the ACL on the femur and the anterior intercondylar area of the tibia. The extent of the notch plasty is difficult to estimate, and use of a graduated probe can be helpful. Odensten and Gillquist (1985) measured an average intercondylar notch width of 21 mm. It is difficult to gauge the depth of the intercondylar notch by the arthroscopic route.

Bone Tunnels

The technique described here is derived from the "one-tunnel" technique of Odensten and Gillquist (1985). Although the technique is much simpler with the Storz aiming device, it can be performed without any special aids.

Technique Without an Aiming Device

A Kirschner wire 1 mm in diameter is drilled into the tibia at a point approximately 2 cm distal to the joint line and 1 cm from the medial border of the distal patellar tendon. The direction of the wire forms a 30° angle with the femur on the sagittal plane (30° is easier to estimate than the 28° angle stated by Odensten and Gillquist). This angle measurement is accurate only if the knee is flexed exactly 90°.

We use arthroscopic triangulation to reach the tibial attachment of the ACL in the anterior intercondylar area. That point can be defined with 2 percutaneously inserted Kirschner wires, but an easier method is to touch the point with the converging tips of the shaver and arthroscope (Fig. 3). While an assistant keeps both instruments centered on the tibial attachment site, the operator drills a 1-mm Kirschner wire toward their insertion (the tibial insertion of the ACL). The wire is introduced at a 30° angle to the femur so that it will reach the correct proximal femoral attachment site. Once the wire has been drilled into the tibia to a sufficient depth, the arthroscope and shaver tips are retracted slightly from the tibial attachment so that the operator can more clearly see the emerging wire tip and check its position relative to the center of the attachment site. If the ideal attachment site is not located right away, a second 1-mm Kirschner wire is inserted from a slightly different entry point, leaving the first wire in place as a guide for positioning the second wire. Once a good wire placement has been achieved at the tibial attachment site, the wire is advanced farther through the intercondylar notch, sparing the synovial covering of the posterior cruciate ligament. The wire is advanced under arthroscopic guidance until it impales the anatomic attachment site on the femur. If the isometric femoral attachment is not found initially, another Kirschner wire is inserted in the proper direction until its position at the tibial and femoral attachment sites is anatomic. Generally the correct anatomic sites are found very quickly. If identification of the femoral attachment site proves difficult, it can be helpful to take a lateral radiograph of the knee (Fig. 4). The use of X-rays to check the Kirschner wire placement is recommended for beginners, because there is a tendency to place the Kirschner wire too far anteriorly on the roof of the intercondylar notch and on the tibial plateau. It is important to position the tibial site far enough medially to avoid graft impingement against the lateral femoral condyle. Once accurate placement of the 1-mm Kirschner wire has been achieved in both bones, the wire is replaced by a de-

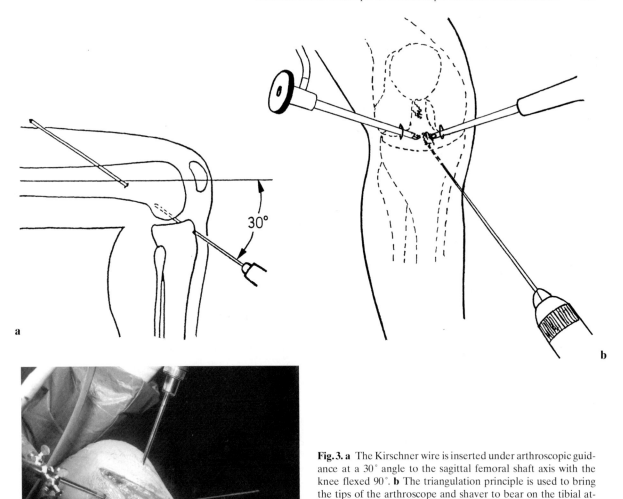

Fig. 3. a The Kirschner wire is inserted under arthroscopic guidance at a 30° angle to the sagittal femoral shaft axis with the knee flexed 90°. **b** The triangulation principle is used to bring the tips of the arthroscope and shaver to bear on the tibial attachment of the ACL. **c** In this operation the 2 Kirschner wires bear on the targeted point, but only the top wire is correctly oriented at a 30° angle to the sagittal femoral axis. The 2.5-mm Kirschner wire is then introduced along the correctly oriented guidewire

finitive 2.5-mm Kirschner wire inserted parallel to the first wire.

Technique Using the Storz Aiming Device

The aiming device is introduced into the knee through the anteromedial portal (Fig. 5). The tip A of the device engages against the femoral attachment F of the ACL, the curved portion B against the tibial attachment T. Part E of the device should then be parallel to the femur (Fig. 6).

A 2.5-mm Kirschner wire is drilled into the tibia through guide sleeve CD (Fig. 7) under arthroscopic control. The wire is advanced on through the femur until it emerges in the anterolateral supracondylar area. The aiming device can then easily be removed from the joint. Figure 8 shows the position of the Kirschner wire, which forms a 30° angle to the femoral shaft axis. If precise placement of the wire is in doubt, it can be checked by taking a lateral radiograph, and necessary adjustments can be made.

Testing Isometry

The 2.5-mm Kirschner wire is advanced until it emerges above the lateral femoral condyle, then it is carefully withdrawn. A No. 1/0 suture is passed upward through the 2.5-mm drill hole on a straight wire passer or long needle. Its upper end is grasped and

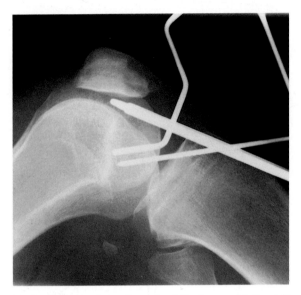

Fig. 4. Intraoperative radiograph of the knee, with the drill guide still in place

fixed with a clamp at the outlet of the femoral hole, and its lower end is held with the fingers (or with the Stryker isometric tension gauge) at the inlet of the tibial hole (Fig. 9). Now the knee is moved through a range from 0 to 110°, and the distal end of the thread is observed: Retraction of the suture into the joint during flexion means that the mouth of the femoral hole is placed too far anteriorly. If the suture retracts during extension, this generally means that the femoral attachment site is too posterior. If there is an abrupt inward excursion of the suture that occurs only in the last degrees of extension, the tibial attachment site is too anterior. Isometricity must be adjusted until there is no more than 2 mm of suture excursion in any position. This having been accomplished, the knee joint is returned to the original flexion angle, and the 2.5-mm Kirschner wire is reintroduced through the same hole (Fig. 10). Normally the wire will pass through without difficulty. Otherwise the rotational position of the knee must be adjusted while maintaining the same flexion angle. The latter is controlled by the position of the bolster beneath the foot.

Now the 2.5-mm Kirschner wire (e.g., the guidewire in the instrument set for the dynamic hip screw) is overdrilled with a 9- or 10-mm cannulated reamer. Power reaming is discontinued as soon as the bit emerges from the tibial plateau, and further insertion

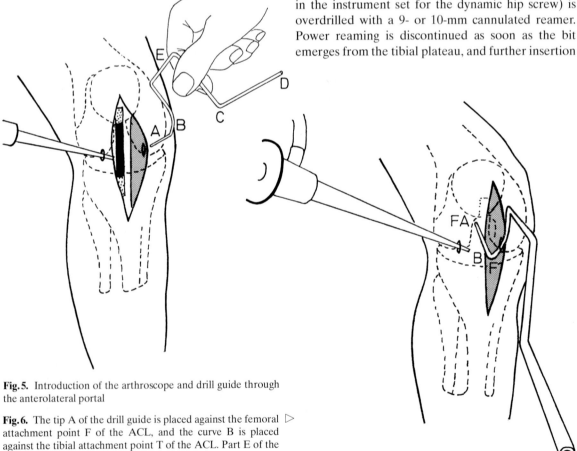

Fig. 5. Introduction of the arthroscope and drill guide through the anterolateral portal

Fig. 6. The tip A of the drill guide is placed against the femoral ▷ attachment point F of the ACL, and the curve B is placed against the tibial attachment point T of the ACL. Part E of the device should be parallel to the femoral shaft

Fig. 7. The 2.5-mm Kirschner wire is drilled into the tibia ▷ through part CD of the guide. Its passage through the joint is observed with the arthroscope. The wire is advanced on through the femur until it emerges from the bone in the antero-lateral supracondylar portion of the femoral metaphysis

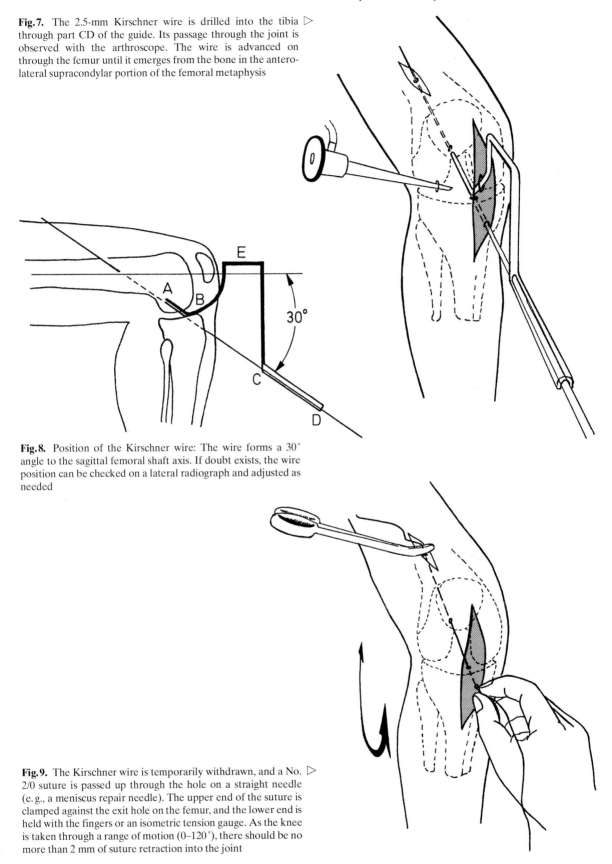

Fig. 8. Position of the Kirschner wire: The wire forms a 30° angle to the sagittal femoral shaft axis. If doubt exists, the wire position can be checked on a lateral radiograph and adjusted as needed

Fig. 9. The Kirschner wire is temporarily withdrawn, and a No. ▷ 2/0 suture is passed up through the hole on a straight needle (e. g., a meniscus repair needle). The upper end of the suture is clamped against the exit hole on the femur, and the lower end is held with the fingers or an isometric tension gauge. As the knee is taken through a range of motion (0–120°), there should be no more than 2 mm of suture retraction into the joint

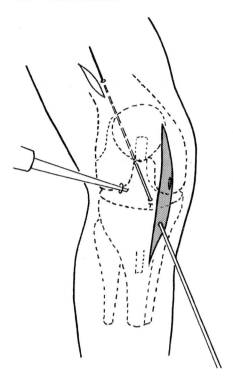

Fig. 10. Next the knee joint is returned to the same flexion angle as before (90°), and the 2.5-mm Kirschner wire is reintroduced

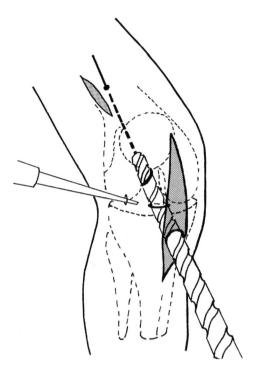

Fig. 11. The Kirschner wire is overdrilled with a 9- to 10-mm cannulated reamer

is done by manual rotation of the bit to avoid injury to the posterior cruciate ligament and its synovial covering.

The cannulated reamer is driven about 2 cm into the femur, creating a recess deep enough to accommodate the patellar bone plug of the ligament graft (Fig. 11). Then the reamer and Kirschner wire are withdrawn, and a 4-mm or 4.5-mm drill bit is inserted to complete the transfemoral tunnel with a channel of smaller diameter than the first 2 cm (which was reamed to 9–10 mm). The edges of the tunnel openings are rounded with a curette passed up through the tibial tunnel, and the soft tissues are debrided and smoothed with the shaver. Throughout the drilling and reaming process, one instrument (e. g., the Dynovac forceps), passed through an anteromedial portal, is kept within the joint to maintain soft-tissue retraction in the anterior part of the knee. The joint is carefully irrigated to remove the otherwise concealed debris.

Placement of the Graft

A Mersilene suture is pulled upward by the passer through both tunnels, followed by the wire previously tied to the patellar end of the graft (Fig. 12). This is done very easily if the following 3 conditions are satisfied:

– All soft tissues are removed from around the openings of the femoral and tibial tunnels.
– The proximal end of the bone block is rounded off.
– The diameter of the bone block and graft closely matches that of the tibial and femoral tunnels.

The medullary nail template has proven helpful for the accurate measurement of diameters. If necessary, a larger reamer may be selected and/or the size of the bone block may be reduced.

Fixation in the Femoral Tunnel

Before the proximal bone block is pulled into the femur, the upper end of the graft is given a 180° twist to achieve better isometry of the graft fibers in all po-

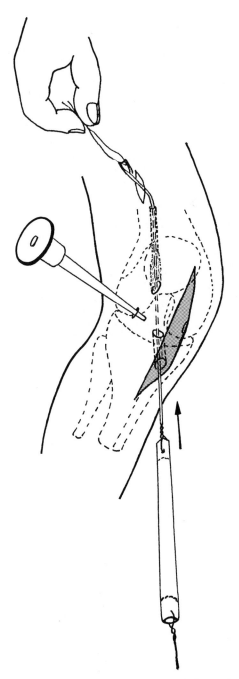

Fig. 12. The graft is introduced from below and pulled upward into the joint

and a notch plasty is performed to adequately widen the notch. Finally the wound is closed in layers over lateral subfascial and medial subcutaneous suction drains.

The postoperative rehabilitation program will be discussed later.

Comparative Results Over a 6-Month Period

Materials and Methods

We reviewed the postoperative results in our first 20 arthroscopically operated cases and compared them with the results of our last 20 conventional ACL reconstructions using the Jones technique. The indication for ACL replacement was the same in both groups: a chronic or acute rupture of the ACL with exertional pain and recurrent giving-way episodes with a feeling of instability.

Clinically we required a positive pivot shift test and a positive Lachman sign.

With regard to operating technique, the patellar tendon graft was harvested at the start of the operation, as described above, and the one-tunnel technique of Odensten and Gillquist (1985) was employed in all cases. Postoperative treatment consisted of immediate motion in an arc of 0–60°, non-weight-bearing for the first 6 weeks, no cast immobilization, and no motion splintage. Careful quadriceps exercises with simultaneous hamstring contraction are recommended for the first 2 months. Swimming is allowed in the 3rd month, bicycling in the 4th month, and jogging in the 6th month. Data on age, sex, interval from injury to operation, and concomitant procedures are listed in Table 1.

An isometric graft placement is considered the sine qua non for a good result (MacIntosh et al. 1977). Applying the criteria of Jackson and Reimann (1987), we considered the reconstruction isometric if the graft showed less than 2 mm of excursion during postoperative flexion of the knee from 0 to 110°. As the graft had been fixed with a wire loop, graft position could be assessed as good or poor on the basis of postoperative X-rays. The determination of postoperative isometry and the analysis of the femoral and tibial attachment sites were performed by an independent orthopedist, and radiographic isometry was assessed in accordance with previously published guidelines (Arnoczky 1983; Girgis et al. 1975; Jackson and Reimann 1987). The patients' histories were reviewed for analgesic use and length of hospital stay. Each patient was followed at monthly intervals, and

sitions of flexion. The graft is then fixed in place by tying the suture wires around screws or staples in the bone. We have found that it is unnecessary to place a large amount of tension on the graft. The knee is taken through a range of motion to test graft function. If the graft impinges against osteophytes in the intercondylar notch, the osteophytes are removed

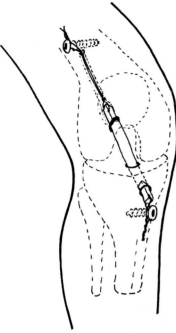

Fig. 13. The wire sutures in the graft are anchored to bone screws or staples

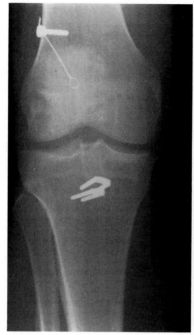
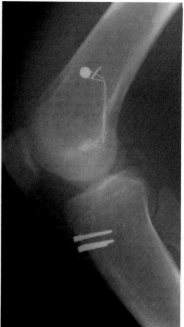

Fig. 14. Postoperative radiographs

Table 1. Reconstruction of the ACL with the central third of the patellar tendon

	Arthroscopic technique	Conventional open technique
Age		
Average age	30 years	29 years
Range	19–41 years	17–42 years
Sex		
Distribution	14 male, 6 female	11 male, 9 female
Interval from injury to operation		
Average	3.2 years	2.3 years
Range	0–7 years	0–6 years
Concomitant procedures		
Meniscectomy	4	5
Upper tibial valgus osteotomy	1	2
Other ligament reconstructions	2	1

complications such as pain and effusion were recorded. The range of motion and stability of the reconstructed knees were documented. We did not use a special knee scoring system to evaluate the results because we felt that the follow-up interval was too short.

Results

The perioperative isometry of the ACL substitute during flexion and extension was declared good in 19 of the 20 knees in the open reconstruction group and in 18 of the 20 knees in the arthroscopic group. Radiographic assessment of the tibial and femoral attachments by an independent observer yielded identical results. Only 4 of the patients in the arthroscopic group took narcotic medication for postoperative pain, as opposed to 14 of the 20 patients who had an open reconstruction. Seven patients in the arthroscopic group required no analgesic medication of any kind, whereas all patients in the open reconstruction group required at least Novamin for pain.

Effusion: By the 3rd postoperative day, intraarticular effusion was no longer detectable in 18 of the 20 arthroscopic patients, versus only 2 patients in the open group. The length of hospitalization was equal in both groups, averaging 5 days (4–7 days).

Postoperative complications: Early postoperative complications consisted of 1 deep vein thrombosis in the arthroscopic group, and 1 gastric ulcer and 1 massive local hematoma in the open reconstruction group. There were no postoperative infections. Reflex sympathetic dystrophy developed as a late complication in 3 female patients in the arthroscopic group (all had an acute ACL rupture). Follow-up in the 4th postoperative month revealed an extension loss of 10° or more in 8 patients of each group. One patient in each group required manipulation of the joint under general anesthesia, one required removal of a bone staple, and one required transarthroscopic debridement of the graft.

By the 6th postoperative month, the results in the open reconstruction group were somewhat better than in the arthroscopic group. Only 10 of the 20 arthroscopic patients were subjectively satisfied with their result, compared with 15 in the conventionally reconstructed group. Eight of the 20 arthroscopic patients complained of pain and effusion on exertion, as opposed to only 5 in the open reconstruction group. Eight of the 20 arthroscopic patients were able to jog by the 6th month, as opposed to 14 in the open group. An extension loss of 5°–10° was noted in 8 patients of the arthroscopic group and in 6 patients of the open reconstruction group. The pivot shift test was negative in all patients of both groups. One patient in the arthroscopic group had a positive residual Lachman sign. He was 1 of the 2 patients found to have poor graft isometry; the other had a painless knee with a negative Lachman sign.

Discussion

In this study we present a preliminary report comparing the results of 20 arthroscopic ACL reconstructions using the central third of the patellar tendon and 20 open ACL reconstructions using the Kenneth Jones technique. We did not begin testing isometry before reaming the bone tunnels until the 10th patient in the arthroscopic series. This could account for the 2 unfavorable cases relating to anisometry of the graft attachment. The transarthroscopic technique is widely used for the implantation of prosthetic ACL substitutes (Bousquet 1984; Hendler 1987; Jackson and Reimann 1987). To date there have been few reports on transarthroscopic ACL reconstruction using an autologous graft, although this technique corresponds to the conventional open cruciate substitution or augmentation. Imbert (1986) transplants the quadriceps and patellar tendon using the over-the-top McIntosh technique under arthroscopic control.
Gillquist (1987) found that the arthroscopic implantation of a Dacron graft offers no advantages over the conventional technique. He attributed this in part to the difficulty of using the drill guide during arthroscopy and partly to the imprecision of transarthros-

copic notch plasty. For this reason we recently developed an aiming device, patterned after the Stryker device, that enables us to identify the femoral and tibial attachment sites with precision. The size of this new device has been modified for arthroscopic use. The most important innovation is a guide sleeve instead of a tunnel for the insertion of Kirschner guidewires (see Fig. 6). As a general rule, drill guides are designed for use with drill bits rather than Kirschner wires for the preoperative determination of isometry, and they force the surgeon to drill the tunnels before he can test isometry. The Storz device eliminates this drawback. The arthroscopic reconstruction can also be performed without an aiming device. This technique seems somewhat crude and requires a good 3-dimensional spatial sense, but it is relatively safe. The transarthroscopic technique is reasonably safe as long as a constant, designated angle of knee flexion is maintained during Kirschner wire insertion. A surgeon well versed in arthroscopic surgical technique may find the transarthroscopic reconstruction simpler and more convenient than the conventional open technique, although the arthroscopic technique takes just as much operating time. We feel that the arthroscopic technique is advantageous in that it provides better visualization of the joint interior, allows for better evaluation of the menisci by visual inspection and probing, and permits an accurate assessment of cartilage pathology. Continuous perioperative irrigation facilitates the clearing of debris from the bone, cartilage, and ligaments. Because arthrotomy is omitted, damage to proprioceptive elements also can be reduced, resulting in a significant reduction of postoperative pain. It remains to be tested whether the transarthroscopic technique will help to avoid late sequelae such as secondary osteoarthritis, femoropatellar pain, and secondary graft deficiency. The transarthroscopic technique inflicts small surgical wounds and allows for more rapid rehabilitation. If there are drawbacks to the technique, they relate to insufficient arthroscopic experience. Transarthroscopic visual estimation can be very deceptive, and the dependence of the procedure on the technical environment is absolute, although this dependence becomes less critical as operator experience increases. Despite progress in the transarthroscopic reconstruction technique, concomitant extraarticular reconstruction or augmentation procedures should not be overlooked. The extraarticular procedures that we currently perform are repair of the medial or lateral capsule and ligaments, biceps tendon augmentation of the lateral collateral ligament, or transposition of the femoral attachment of the collateral ligaments and popliteus tendon. In cases where we add a posterolateral reconstruction to the ACL replacement, we also generally perform a slight valgus osteotomy of the proximal tibia using the technique of Bousquet (1984). We feel that this realigning osteotomy is critical to the success of the lateral reconstruction procedures in patients with coexisting genu varum. Although these measures are extraarticular, we have found that they do not pose an obstacle to the transarthroscopic cruciate reconstruction, which is performed immediately following the extraarticular procedure.

References

Arnoczky SP (1983) Anatomy of the anterior cruciate ligament. Clin Orthop 172: 19-25

Bousquet G (1984) Les indications thérapeutiques dans les laxités chroniques du genou. Cinquièmes Journées Lyonnaises de Chirurgie du Genou, Lyon

Gillquist J (1987) Arthroscopic reconstruction of the anterior cruciate ligament. International Arthroscopy Association, Triennial Scientific Meeting, Sidney, April 1987

Girgis FG, Marshall JL, Al Monajem ARS (1975) The cruciate ligaments of the knee joint. Clin Orthop 106: 216-231

Hendler RC (1987) A uni-tunnel technique for arthroscopic anterior cruciate ligament reconstruction. International Arthroscopy Assocciation, Triennial Scientific Meeting, Sidney, April 1987

Imbert JC (1986) Ligamentoplastie mixte intra et extra articulaire sous controlle endoscopique. Réunion du G. E. R. F., Lyon, 11-12 April 1986

Jackson DW, Reiman PR (1987) Principles of arthroscopic anterior cruciate reconstruction. In: Jackson DW, Drez D jr (eds) The anterior cruciate deficient knee. Mosby, St. Louis, pp 273-285

McIntosh DL, Tregonning RJA (1977) A follow-up study and evaluation of the „over the top" repair of acute tears of the anterior cruciate ligament. J Bone Joint Surg [Br] 59: 511

Müller We (1983) The Knee. Springer, Berlin Heidelberg New York Tokyo

Odensten M, Gillquist J (1985) Functional anatomy of the anterior cruciate ligament and a rationale for reconstruction. J Bone Joint Surg [Am] 67: 257-262

Rosenberg TD (1984) Arthroscopic technique for anterior cruciate ligament surgery. Technical Bulletin, Acufex Microsurgical Inc

Rosenberg TD (1986) Technique for rear entry ACL guide. Technical Bulletin, Acufex Microsurgical Inc

Arthroscopically Assisted Cruciate Ligament Reconstruction Using a Free Patellar Tendon Graft

P. M. Ballmer and R. P. Jakob

The undisputed advantages of arthroscopic surgery over arthrotomy, together with increasing surgical experience and refined techniques, have caused operations on the cruciate ligaments to move increasingly into the arthroscopic realm.

The favorable results of transplanting the central one-third of the patellar tendon to reconstruct the anterior cruciate ligament (ACL) in knees with chronic anterior instablity (Clancy et al. 1982; Jakob et al. 1988), compared with the disappointing results of direct repairs of the acutely torn ACL (see article by Ballmer et al., p.293ff.; Feagin and Curl 1976; Lysholm et al. 1982), had caused us to favor a primary patellar tendon reconstruction even for acute ACL injuries. We performed the reconstruction as a free graft due to evidence refuting the theoretical superiority of grafts vascularized through the infrapatellar fat pad (Clancy 1988; Paulos et al. 1983). This also enabled us to perform the reconstruction by the transligamentous route, i.e., without a medial arthrotomy. These cases were distinguished by a marked reduction in postoperative morbidity. However, the limited exposure increased the technical difficulty of the procedure, and the interior of the knee joint was difficult to explore, so we often had to precede the operation by diagnostic arthroscopy. It was a natural step, then, to proceed to an arthroscopically assisted ACL reconstruction. In this chapter we shall describe the technique that we have used since 1987.

Technique

Examination under Anesthesia

With benefit of epidural or general anesthesia, the injured knee is examined and compared with the healthy opposite side, and stability data are recorded. If findings are complex or unclear, a comparative radiographic evaluation is performed by obtaining stress X-rays in the frontal and sagittal planes (Stäubli et al. 1985).

Preoperative Preparation

The operation is performed in the supine position with a pneumatic tourniquet. The distal thigh is supported on a knee rest whose angle can be freely adjusted during the operation. The operative field (midthigh to calf) is draped with plastic film, and the distal lower leg and foot are wrapped in a sterile plastic sack. The tourniquet is not inflated until all instruments have been installed.

Graft Removal

If preoperative findings are unclear, the cruciate reconstruction is preceded by diagnostic arthroscopy. When cruciate insufficiency has been confirmed, we begin the operation by harvesting the graft. The patellar tendon is approached through an anterior skin incision approximately 10 cm long that starts 2 cm proximal to the distal pole of the patella and extends to the tibial tuberosity; the tendon is exposed by longitudinal incision of the paratenon. The central one-third (9–12 mm) of the patellar tendon and the adjacent bone blocks are outlined with a scalpel (Fig. 1). Two drill holes are made in each bone block with a 2.0-mm bit. First the distal bone block is removed from the tibial tuberosity (length 20 mm, width 10 mm, depth 10 mm) with an oscillating saw and chisel. After separation of the infrapatellar fat pad from the patellar tendon, the proximal bone block is removed from the patella. The patellar bone plug has a conical shape (distal width 10 mm, proximal width 15 mm, length 20 mm, depth 10 mm). To avoid fracturing the patellar apex and opening the joint cavity, the block is removed with the saw or chisel by a frontal osteotomy directed parallel to the retropatellar joint surface (Fig. 2).

A second incision 5 cm long is made proximal to the lateral femoral epicondyle. The iliotibial tract is split longitudinally, the vastus lateralis is reflected forward, and the metadiaphyseal region of the femur is exposed.

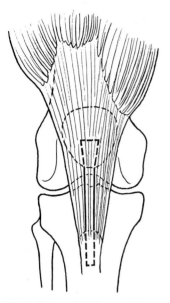

Fig. 1. Removal of the central one-third of the patellar tendon

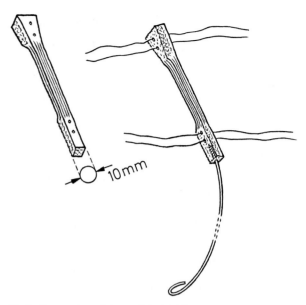

Fig. 3. Preparation of the graft (axial Kirschner wire in the distal bone block)

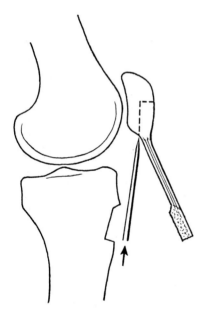

Fig. 2. The proximal bone block is removed by a frontal osteotomy directed parallel to the retropatellar joint surface

Graft Preparation

To save time, an assistant usually prepares the graft during the subsequent arthroscopic examination. The tibial bone block is trimmed to a diameter of 10 mm, which is checked with a calibration sleeve. The distal half of the patellar bone block is also trimmed to a 10-mm diameter. The proximal half is left cone-shaped so that later it can be wedged into the femoral tunnel. Both blocks are armed with 2 heavy-gauge nonabsorbable sutures (No. 3) passed through the predrilled 2.0-mm holes. To facilitate handling of the distal tibial block, a threaded 1.6-mm Kirschner wire is twisted axially into the distal end through a pre-drilled 1.5-mm pilot hole placed to avoid splitting the bone. The Kirschner wire is given a slight curve, and the end is looped to form an eyelet (Fig. 3).

Diagnostic Arthroscopy

Ordinarily we use 3 portals for the arthroscopic phase the arthroscope anterolaterally, the instruments anteromedially, and the inflow channel supero-medially. The parapatellar anterolateral and ante-romedial portals are established through the existing skin incision. Diagnostic arthroscopy is performed with the knee in 20°–30° flexion. Cartilage lesions and meniscal injuries are managed according to standard criteria. If a meniscus repair is indicated, the sutures are preplaced, but not yet tied, using standard arthroscopic technique (Jakob et al. 1988).

Arthroscopic ACL Reconstruction

With an acute midsubstance tear of the ACL, the ligament remnants are removed with a shaver passed through the anteromedial portal. The junction with the over-the-top region must be clearly visible. The

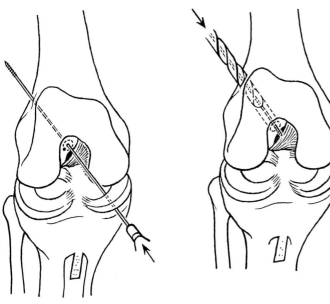

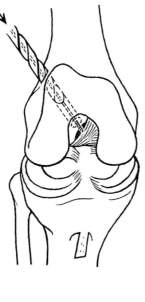

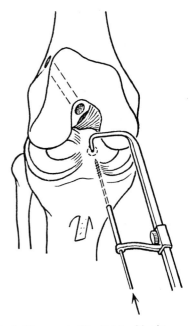

Fig. 4. Placement of the femoral guide-wire (5 mm posterolateral to the isometric point)

Fig. 5. Reaming the femoral bone tunnel

Fig. 6. Placement of the tibial guidewire (5 mm anteromedial to the isometric point) using the drill guide

shoulder of the shaver should be directed toward the posterior cruciate ligament (PCL) to avoid iatrogenic injury. In chronically unstable knees with a stenotic intercondylar notch, we perform a widening notch plasty with a spherical burr. The junction with the over-the-top region is identified with a probe, and the isometric point on the femur is verified. Through a small inferomedial stab incision just above the tibial plateau, a 1.6-mm Kirschner wire is manually inserted beneath the medial meniscus and advanced past the medial condyle toward the femoral attachment of the ACL. A 2.5-mm threaded Kirschner wire is then introduced through the same approach using a power drill, aiming for a point approximately 5 mm posterolateral to the isometric point (Fig. 4). The tip of the wire is embedded by turning it through several rotations. As the position of the Kirschner wire is monitored arthroscopically, the knee is flexed to 90°–120°, and the wire is drilled out through the lateral side of the femur; its emergence is verified by palpation through the lateral incision. The wire is then withdrawn from the lateral side until its end is still just within the joint space, and the knee is returned to its original position of 30° flexion. The femoral tunnel is created by overdrilling the wire from the outside in with the 10.0-mm cannulated reamer, and the intra-articular rim of the tunnel is smoothed with a round burr (Fig. 5). To avoid fluid loss, the outlet of the bone tunnel is sealed with a plastic plug.

To construct the tibial tunnel, we insert the tip of the AO/ASIF drill guide through the anteromedial portal, approximately 5 mm anteromedial to the isometric ligament attachment. A 2.5-mm threaded Kirschner wire is introduced through the drill guide, and its position is checked (Fig. 6). It is then over-drilled from the outside in with the 10.0-mm cannu-lated reamer. Again, the intraarticular opening of the tunnel is smoothed with the round burr, and any pro-jecting cruciate ligament remnants are debrided with the shaver (Fig. 7).

In preparation for intraarticular graft placement, 2 guide sutures are passed up through the tunnels with an arthroscopic forceps and brought out the femoral side under arthroscopic guidance. The tibial bone block is snared, 1 guide suture engaging the 1.6-mm Kirschner wire, the other engaging the 2 nonabsorb-able threads. The sutures and wire having been passed through the joint and brought out of the tibial tunnel, the tibial bone block is pulled through the femoral tunnel into the joint. By manipulation of the Kirschner wire, it is a simple matter to center the bone block in the tibial tunnel and give the graft a slight twist to simulate the helicoid course of the nor-mal ACL (Fig. 8). An impactor is used to wedge the proximal bone block down into the opening of the femoral tunnel. Next we pull the distal threads taut to test graft isometry and lack of impingement in the in-tercondylar notch. With the knee in full extension,

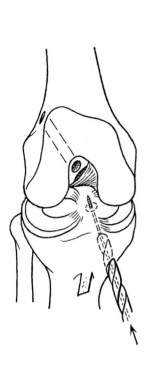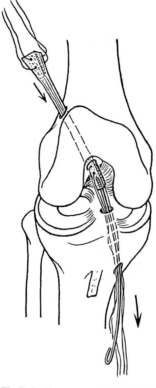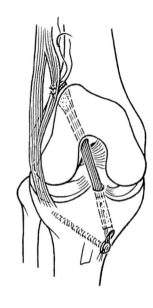

Fig. 9. The proximal bone block is wedged into the femoral tunnel (with a tractopexy), and the tibial bone block is anchored to a bone screw

Fig. 7. Reaming the tibial bone tunnel   **Fig. 8.** Pulling the graft into the joint

the taut distal sutures are tied over a 3.5-mm cortical bone screw with metal washer. If the lateral opening of the femoral tunnel has been isometrically placed (Krachow and Brooks 1983) and extraarticular reinforcement is desired, the proximal nonabsorbable sutures can be utilized for an extraarticular repair. This is done by passing the sutures through the previously exposed deep layer of the iliotibial tract and reinforcing its attachment to the isometric insertion point of the tract on the femur: a deep tractopexy. With a good interference-fit fixation of the bone block, however, the sutures may be removed (Fig. 9).

If a meniscal repair was done, the preplaced sutures are now tightened and tied. The wound is closed over multiple suction drains. The defect in the patellar tendon is not closed, but the paratenon is reapproximated to prevent patella baja.

Postoperative Treatment

Postoperatively the knee is placed in a simple rubber knee immobilizer. After the suction drains are removed, the knee is mobilized on an electric passive motion splint. The physiotherapist instructs the patient in quadriceps strengthening exercises with sim-

ultaneous hamstring contraction in a 40°–70° arc. Isolated quadriceps contraction in a 0–30° arc is not permitted until 3 months. The patient ambulates on crutches for 6 weeks with partial weight bearing of 15 kg and progresses to full weight bearing in the 7th week, at which time the immobilizer is discarded.

Discussion

Initial reports on arthroscopic cruciate ligament procedures are not convincing (Bartlett 1983; Brade 1986; Fox et al. 1985). However, the disappointing short-term results are due less to the arthroscopic technique itself than to the methods used for repairing or reconstructing the ligament, and they are comparable to the similarly poor results of open operations.

In recent years, however, increasing attention has been paid to applying the experience and insights gained in open cruciate ligament operations to arthroscopic procedures (Brown 1988; Chandler 1988; Clancy 1988; Friedman 1988; Jackson and Reiman 1987; Wilcox and Jackson 1987). All these studies pertain to ACL reconstructions using autologous tissue. Besides fascia lata (Chandler 1988), authors have used quadriceps tendon (Stäubli, personal communication) and especially patellar tendon grafts (Brown 1988; Clancy 1988) in acutely and chronically ACL-deficient knees. Basically the techniques are comparable to arthroscopic cruciate ligament reconstructions. While some authors place the arthroscope in an anterolateral portal (Friedman 1988; Jackson and Reiman 1987), others prefer the anteromedial approach, especially for the femoral preparation (Brown 1988; Chandler 1988; Clancy 1988), as this provides better visualization of the over-the-top region. Most authors remove the cruciate ligament remnants prior to reconstruction (Brown 1988; Clancy 1988; Friedman 1988; Jackson and Reiman 1987; Wilcox and Jackson 1987). Some routinely perform a notch plasty (Brown 1988; Chandler 1988; Friedman 1988), while others reserve it for selected cases (Jackson and Reiman 1987; Wilcox and Jackson 1987). Most authors (Brown 1988; Chandler 1988; Clancy 1988; Jackson and Reiman 1987; Wilcox and Jackson 1987) use a special instrument (Graf 1987) to test the isometry of the selected femoral and tibial insertion points. In reconstructions with the patellar tendon, however, the definitive Kirschner wire should be placed in a slightly anisometric position (posterolateral on the femur and anteromedial on the tibia) because the patellar tendon graft occupies an eccentric position in the bone tunnels (Clancy et al. 1982; Graf 1987).

Inserting the femoral Kirschner guidewire from the inside out is advantageous in that the entry point can be selected with greater accuracy than with an "over the top" drill guide, in which the Kirschner wire is inserted from the outside in. But the disadvantages of the inside-out technique are a less precise control of the exit site on the lateral femur and possible damage to the medial condyle and PCL. Outside-in placement of the tibial Kirschner wire with the aid of a drill guide and the use of a cannulated reamer to drill the femoral and tibial tunnels have become established as the techniques of choice (Brown 1988; Clancy 1988; Friedman 1988; Jackson and Reiman 1987; Wilxoc and Jackson 1987).

Unlike other authors (Chandler 1988; Clancy 1988; Friedman 1988; Jackson and Reiman 1987), we harvest the graft before inserting the arthroscope whenever possible, because this avoids edematous swelling of the subcutaneous fat and softening of the tendon tissue by the irrigation fluid, the arthroscopic portals can be established through the existing skin incision, and the infrapatellar fat pad prolapses into the patellar tendon defect during the arthroscopy, providing a clearer view of the joint interior.

In our experience and that of other authors (Brown 1988; Chandler 1988; Clancy 1988; Friedman 1988; Jackson and Reimann 1987; Wilxoc and Jackson 1987), arthroscopically assisted reconstruction of the ACL offers the following advantages:

– Better anatomic (isometric) placement of the bone tunnels
– Easier joint inspection and meniscus repair
– No division of the extensor apparatus with impaired patellar tracking and no compromise of proprioception by arthrotomy
– No cartilage dehydration
– No wound problems due to undermining of soft tissues
– Less postoperative pain
– Faster rehabilitation (better mobility, less muscle atrophy)
– Shorter hospital stay

Against these significant advantages, we may cite several less important disadvantages. The arthroscopic technique demands a skilled, experienced surgeon to minimize the duration of the procedure. After an initial learning curve, the average operating time for an arthroscopically assisted ACL reconstruction alone at our center is 1 1/2 h. An arthroscopy set is needed, so the equipment requirements are somewhat greater than for an open reconstruction. Finally, additional incisions are necessary in chronically unstable joints with deficient secondary restraints and in acutely unstable joints with associated ligament injuries.

In summary, the arthroscopically assisted ACL reconstruction has proven effective in our hands. We are impressed by the short-term results, which are marked by good stability and, in most cases, symmetrical ranges of knee motion. We realize, of course, that longer follow-up periods are needed before definitive conclusions can be drawn.

References

Bartlett EC (1983) Arthroscopic repair and augmentation of the anterior cruciate ligament in cadaver knees. Clin Orthop 172: 107–111

Brade A (1986) Mittelfristige Ergebnisse nach arthroskopischer Kreuzbandersatzplastik mit Dacron-Bändern. Mitteilung 3. Kongreß der Arbeitsgemeinschaft für Arthroskopie Basel

Brown CH (1988) Rationale and technique of arthroscopically assisted anterior cruciate reconstruction. Third Congress of the European Society of Knee Surgery and Arthroscopy, Amsterdam

Chandler EJ (1988) Arthroscopic-aided anterior cruciate ligament reconstruction using autogenous fascia lata graft both intra and extra-articularly. American Academy of Orthopaedic Surgeons, Atlanta, USA

Clancy WG, Nelson DA, Reider B, Narecharia RG (1982) Anterior cruciate ligament reconstruction using one-third of the patellar ligament, augmented by extra-articular tendon transfer. J Bone Joint Surg [Am] 64: 352-359

Clancy WG (1988) Arthroscopic anterior cruciate ligament reconstruction with patellar tendon. Techniques Orthop 2/4: 13-22

Feagin JA, Curl WW (1976) Isolated tear of the anterior cruciate ligament: 5-year follow-up study. Am J Sports Med 4: 95-100

Fox JM, Shermann OH, Mardolf K (1985) Arthroscopic anterior cruciate ligament repair: Preliminary results and instrumented testing for anterior stability. Arthroscopy 1: 175-181

Friedman MJ (1988) Arthroscopic semitendinosus (gracilis) reconstruction for anterior cruciate ligament deficiency. Techniques Orthop 2: 74-80

Graf B (1987) Isometric placement of substitutes for the anterior cruciate ligament. In: Jackson DW (ed) The anterior cruciate deficient knee. Mosby, St. Louis Washington/DC Toronto, pp 102-113

Jackson DW, Reiman PR (1987) Principles of arthroscopic anterior cruciate reconstruction. In: Jackson DW (ed) The anterior cruciate deficient knee. Mosby, St. Louis Washington/DC Toronto, pp 273-285

Jakob RP, Kipfer W, Klaue K, Stäubli H-U, Gerber C (1988) Étude critique de la reconstruction du ligament croisé antérieur du genou par la plastie pédiculée sur le Hoffa à partir du tiers médian du tendon rotulien. Rev Chir Orthop 74: 44-51

Jakob RP, Stäubli H-U, Zuber K, Esser M (1988) The arthroscopic meniscal repair. Am J Sports Med 16: 137-142

Krachow KA, Brooks RL (1983) Optimization of knee ligament position for lateral extraarticular reconstruction. Am J Sports Med 11: 293-301

Lysholm J, Gillquist J, Liljedahl SO (1982) Long term results after early treatment of the knee injuries. Acta Orthop Scand 53: 109-118

Noyes FR, Butler DL, Paulos LE (1983) Intra-articular cruciate reconstruction I: Perspectives on graft strengths, vascularization and immediate motion after replacement. Clin Orthop 172: 71-77

Paulos LE, Butler DL, Noyes FR (1983) Intra-articular cruciate reconstruction II: Replacement with vascularized patellar tendon. Clin Orthop 172: 78-84

Stäubli H-U, Jakob RP, Noesberger B (1985) Anterior-posterior knee instability and stress radiography. A prospective biomechanical analysis with the knee in extension. In: Perren SM, Schneider E (eds) Biomechanics: Current Interdisciplinary Research. Nijhoff, Dordrecht Boston Lancaster

Wilcox PG, Jackson DW (1987) Arthroscopic anterior cruciate ligament reconstruction. Arthroscopy 6/3: 513-524

Arthroscopically Assisted ACL Reconstruction Using Autologous Quadriceps Tendon

H.-U. Stäubli

In this study we present an arthroscopically assisted technique for replacing the anterior cruciate ligament (ACL) with autologous tissue from the quadriceps tendon. This procedure is based on the following principles:

1. Duplication of the natural course of the ACL based on 3-dimensional preoperative planning (Stäubli 1988)
2. Imitation of the natural tension of the ACL (Hassenpflug et al. 1985)
3. Restoration of physiologic joint kinematics (Müller 1988) and physiologic tensile forces in the cruciate ligament (Engebretsen et al. 1988)
4. Preservation of proprioception and of functionally important nerve endings in the tibial stump of the ACL (Kennedy et al. 1982; Schultz et al. 1984)
5. Arthroscopic and radiographic functional tests of guidewire position before definitive reaming of the tibial and femoral tunnels (Stäubli 1990)
6. Adequate widening of the intercondylar notch under arthroscopic control before and after intra-articular graft placement (Rosenberg et al. 1988)
7. Use of a strong substitute material composed of autologous quadriceps tendon for the technique as modified by Blauth (1984)
8. Stable graft fixation (Lambert and Cunningham 1988)
9. Early postoperative rehabilitation (Arvidson and Eriksson 1988)

Indications for Transarthroscopic Reconstruction (Table 1)

Arthroscopically assisted substitution or augmentation is indicated in young patients with subjectively disabling, clinically significant anterior subluxation of the tibia. Marked anterior subluxation of the tibia with respect to the femur should be confirmed in candidates by stressradiography (Stäubli 1990). This 1st group is distinguished clinically by a functionally disabling insufficiency of the ACL with a markedly posi-

Table 1. Indications for transarthroscopic ACL reconstruction

Subjectively disabling, clinically significant, radiographically documented anterior subluxation of the tibia

ACL insufficiency and reparable peripheral meniscus tear

Significant ACL insufficiency with negative general selection criteria (age > 45 years, obesity, lack of cooperation, etc.)

Patients with significant anterior residual laxity following deficient primary repair or reconstruction

ACL insufficiency in a young, active individual with postmeniscectomy varus osteoarthritis of the knee

Ruptured prosthetic cruciate ligament or significant anterior residual laxity following a prosthetic reconstruction

tive Lachman sign (anterior subluxation near extension), an absent anterior end point, and a positive grade II or grade III pivot shift (Jakob et al. 1987).

The 2nd group of candidates for arthroscopic reconstruction consists of patients with documented ACL insufficiency and reparable peripheral meniscal tears.

A relative indication for arthroscopic reconstruction exists in a 3rd group of patients with significant ACL deficiency who are poor candidates for an open reconstruction on general grounds (advanced age, obesity, lack of cooperation, low motivation) and who would otherwise require treatment with a knee brace.

The 4th group comprises patients with significantly disabling residual laxity following a deficient primary repair or primary reconstruction of the ACL.

The 5th group consists of patients with an unstable osteoarthritic knee whose age and activity level contraindicate a prosthetic ACL replacement.

The 6th group comprises patients with a ruptured prosthetic ACL and an unstable knee. In these patients, anisometric bone tunnels must be filled with autologous bone tissue to ensure an anatomic placement of the autologous graft before the new reconstruction is performed.

In patients with unstable postmeniscectomy varus osteoarthritis of the knee, transarthroscopic ACL reconstruction can be combined with a valgus osteotomy of the upper tibia. Postoperative rehabilitation time, time away from work, and associated secondary costs can be significantly reduced by the combined procedure.

Clinical Examination

Localized tenderness, quantity of effusion, active and passive subluxation signs, and varus/valgus opening are tested before the induction of anesthesia. Standard X-ray films supplement the initial examination. Under epidural anesthesia, joint stability is systematically tested according to OAK guidelines (Müller et al. 1988).

Stressradiography under Anesthesia

Stressradiographs taken with 178 N (20 kp) of anterior and posterior drawer stress applied to the slightly flexed knee joint serve to document the objective limits of knee instability (Stäubli 1990).

Patient Preparation and Position

The patient is positioned supine, and the whole lower extremity is prepped from the iliac crest to the toes. Following adequate aseptic preparation, the operative field is draped with sterile towels. A self-adhering drape and a sterile, waterproof plastic bag cover the region from the toes to the calf. An incise drape is applied about the knee, and a sterile Esmarch thigh tourniquet is applied with the knee flexed 90°. The tourniquet is not inflated until instrument functions have been tested. A sterile leg holder makes it easier to adjust the knee position between 0 and 130° flexion. Unobstructed knee motion is important, since the area of isometry diminishes with increasing flexion and forms a small band-shaped area when the knee is flexed 120° (Hefzy et al. 1988).

Arthroscopic Equipment and Instrumentation

The necessary arthroscopic equipment and instruments are listed in Table 2. The instruments required for the arthroscopically controlled ACL reconstruction are listed in Table 3. The instruments needed for graft removal, intraarticular graft placement, and graft fixation are listed in Table 4.

Table 2. Arthroscopic equipment and instrumentation

Fluid bag and Y-tubing
Arthroscope (30° and 70° oblique telescopes)
Obturator (sheath)
Probing hook
Light source
Light cable
Arthroscopic camera
Camera drape
Rotary instruments (shavers)
Shaver heads and cannulas
Meniscus repair needles
AO/ASIF distractor (optional for meniscus repairs)
Sterile-draped image intensifier with cross-table beam

Table 3. Instruments for transarthroscopic reconstruction

Kirschner wires of 2.5 mm diameter (assorted lengths)
Cannulated reamers of 6 mm, 8 mm, 10 mm, and 12 mm diameter
Cannulated cutters of 8 mm, 10 mm, and 12 mm diameter
Drilling template for Kirschner wires
Polyethylene plugs for sealing the bone tunnels (6, 8, 10 mm diameter)
Burr and rasps for rounding the tunnel edges
Set of curettes

Table 4. Instruments for removal, placement and fixation of the graft

Simal chisels, 5 and 10 mm
2.0-mm drill bit and drill sleeve
Small AO/ASIF drill
AO/ASIF vibrating saw with small blade
Straight needles for fixation of the graft ends and nonabsorbable sutures
Small Johnson grasping forceps for the pull-through suture
AO/ASIF 2.5-mm screws with smooth shank
Trial ACL prosthesis

Technique of Arthroscopically Assisted ACL Replacement with the Quadriceps Tendon and a Patellar Bone Block (Modification of Blauth 1984)

Organization of the Operative Field, Equipment Setup and Function Tests

A sterile tubing system is connected by a Y-piece to two 3-liter fluid bags, and the desired length of tubing is brought in through prefabricated openings in the waterproof limb drape. The fiberoptic light cable is connected to the light source. A suction tube is installed. The endoscopic camera is covered with a sterile plastic sleeve whose distal end is secured with a clamp. Rotary instruments (shaver with power cord), 2 separate suction tubing systems, and an electrocautery are installed and their function tested.

The leg is exsanguinated with a sterile rubber bandage, and the Esmarch thigh tourniquet is inflated to 300–400 mmHg. The knee is positioned in 45° flexion on a sterile leg holder that permits adjustment of the knee position up to 130° for testing isometry (q. v.).

Diagnostic Knee Arthroscopy and Functional Probing

The skin incision for the inflow cannula is placed superomedially. The incision for the arthroscope portal is placed anterolaterally, adjacent to the patellar tendon and cranial to the infrapatellar fat pad. The skin incision for the probing hook, shaver, and meniscus repair needles is placed anteromedially. After distention of the joint cavity with irrigating fluid through the inflow portal by the medial condyle, the arthroscopic sheath with blunt obturator is introduced with the knee flexed 45°; then the knee is extended and the sheath is directed into the suprapatellar pouch. The suction tubing is connected to the arthroscope sheath, the 30° telescope is exchanged for the obturator, and the light cable is attached. The sterile-draped endoscopic camera is connected to the scope.

ACL Insufficiency and Meniscal Lesions

Reparable vertical or oblique tears in the peripheral vascular portion of the meniscus are repaired transarthroscopically by using meniscal repair needles with various radii of curvature after preliminary submeniscal abrasion and freshening of the tear site and the creation of vascular channels. In tight joints, use of the AO/ASIF distractor (applied in the distraction mode) can improve access for submeniscal abrasion, placement of mattress sutures in the upper and lower edges of the meniscus, and tying the sutures (compression mode) (Jakob et al. 1988).

Irreparable meniscal lesions are managed by a partial meniscectomy that preserves a maximum amount of undamaged functional residual meniscus tissue.

Preparation of the Intercondylar Notch

Splayed, incarcerated, functionally useless remnants of the ACL stump are sparingly resected with the synovial shaver while preserving as much intact residual tissue as possible. The femoral ACL stump is generally resected in its entirety until the femoral attachment site is completely exposed. Anterior osteophytes on the intercondylar roof ("guillotine" osteophytes) in a chronically ACL-deficient joint and osteophytes on the lateral femoral condyle that narrow the lateral half of the intercondylar notch are resected to the extent necessary to avoid graft impingement. The synovial covering of the PCL is spared. Generally the osteophytes are resected after definitive placement of the Kirschner guidewires (Caution: hemorrhage and red-out of the arthroscopic field may occur).

Three-Dimensional Orientation of the Transtibial Guidewire and Reaming of the Tibial Tunnel

The 3-cm anteromedial skin incision starts about 3–5 cm distal to the anterosuperior border of the medial tibial plateau and ends above the cranial margin of the pes anserinus next to the tibial tuberosity. The shaver with obturator is passed through the anteromedial portal into the lateral half of the intercondylar notch under arthroscopic guidance. The obturator simulates the later course of the substitute ligament and simultaneously measures the width of the lateral half of the intercondylar space (clearance between the PCL and the intercondylar surface of the lateral femoral condyle). The tip of the shaver cannula points toward the femoral attachment of the ACL. The shaft of the cannula is above the center of the tibial attachment site. A drill guide is useful for defining the orientation of the ligament on the transverse plane (15° anteromedial), which in turn defines the placement of the skin incision (Fig. 1).

A small amount of periosteum is stripped from the anteromedial surface of the tibia, and a 2.5-mm threaded Kirschner guidewire is carefully drilled toward the center of the tibial attachment site. If this wire is off-center, another 2.5-mm Kirschner guidewire is inserted in a corrected position until the wire pierces the center of the attachment area. The placement of this wire is checked arthroscopically, and it is observed as the knee is extended to check for impingement against the anterior rim of the intercondylar roof. In the fully extended knee, the guidewire should assume a position 3–5 mm posterior to the distal edge of the anterior intercondylar roof after ade-

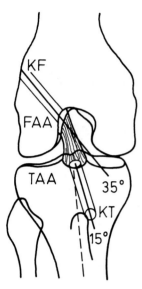

Fig. 1. The Kirschner guidewire for the tibial tunnel (KT), inserted anteromedially at a 15° angle, is centered on the anteromedial border of the tibial area of attachment (TAA). The Kirschner guidewire for the femoral tunnel (KF), inserted inside-out at a 35° angle, is centered on the anteromedial portion of the femoral area of attachment (FAA). It is overdrilled from the outside in

quate widening of Grant's notch. If the guidewire is located too far anteriorly or medially, its position is adjusted using a drill template to avoid later graft impingement. If the exact position of the Kirschner wire is in doubt, it should be checked by image intensification fluoroscopy with a cross-table beam, giving attention to the relationship between the edge of the intercondylar roof and the tibial attachment site in the extended knee. When definitive guidewire placement has been confirmed, the transtibial tunnel is reamed and sealed with a plug. Under arthroscopic guidance, the tibial guidewire is first overdrilled with the 6-mm cannulated reamer, then with the 8-mm reamer. The 10-mm reamer is advanced only to the subchondral zone, preserving the peripheral remnants of the distal cruciate stump if at all possible. The tunnel opening is smoothed with a curette and round burr and sealed with a polyethylene plug. Now the projected function of the graft is tested by passing an abrader through the tibial tunnel and checking its course in the lateral half of the intercondylar notch. If the instrument impinges against the lateral condyle, projecting osteophytes are removed with the abrader tip. If there is impingement against the anterior roof of the intercondylar notch, the tunnel must be widened posteriorly, or additional osteophytes at the anterior edge of the roof must be removed.

Placement of the Transfemoral Kirschner Wire in the Inside-Out Two-Tunnel Technique

The 2.5-mm threaded Kirschner guidewire is introduced through the medial portal directly adjacent to the medial border of the patellar tendon and directly above the anterior horn of the medial meniscus or transverse knee ligament and is passed through the center of the lateral half of the intercondylar notch under arthroscopic control. Sparing the PCL, the tip of the Kirschner wire is advanced manually toward the lateral posterosuperior border of the intercondylar notch to the femoral attachment of the ACL (see Fig. 1). At this point the arthroscope and irrigation cannula are withdrawn. The knee is flexed to 125°, and the exact position of the Kirschner wire tip on the sagittal plane is checked against the preoperative plan by using the image intensifier and fluoroscopic control (Fig. 2).

To check the position of the transfemoral Kirschner wire at the femoral attachment of the anteromedial bundle of the ACL, the cross-table image intensifier is moved in a proximal direction over the knee joint, which is oriented for an orthograde lateral projection. The calculated center of the femoral attachment site is located anteroinferior to the intersection of 2 reference lines: a tangent to the caudal border of the intercondylar roof and a line corresponding to the anterior femoropopliteal metaphyseal boundary.

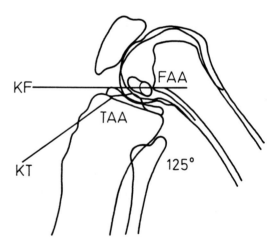

Fig. 2. Relative position of the tibial Kirschner wire (KT) and femoral Kirschner wire (KF) with respect to the tibial area of attachment (TAA) and femoral area of attachment (FAA), shown on the sagittal plane with the knee flexed 125°. In this position the femoral Kirschner wire is perpendicular to the intercondylar roof and rests against its border. In accordance with the "most isometric" zone, this wire should not be shifted *anteriorly* along the boundary of the intercondylar roof tangent but should be placed *distally* corresponding to the posterior metaphyseal boundary line

This point is located by first advancing the guidewire to the "over the top" position. This is done carefully to avoid damage to popliteal vessels. Under image intensifier control, the threaded tip of the Kirschner guidewire is retracted slightly and drilled about 1 mm deep into the attachment site of the anteromedial bundle of the ACL, 4–5 mm caudal to the point of intersection of the reference lines.

Before the Kirschner wire is definitively inserted through the femur, its position is checked again by image intensification fluoroscopy. The transfemoral Kirschner wire is oriented toward the lateral metaphyseal-shaft boundary of the femur with the knee in maximum flexion. There should be minimal tunnel divergence with respect to the anatomic alignment of the ACL. The Kirschner guidewire is now drilled through the femur from the inside out.

Lateral Skin Incision

A lateral skin incision 6–8 cm long is made on the line connecting the greater trochanter and lateral femoral epicondyle. The fascia lata is incised at a relatively anterior site, cranial to the incoming iliotibial tract fibers, while preserving the lateral femorotibial ligamentous attachments. The vastus lateralis muscle is detached from the lateral intermuscular septum, sparing the Kaplan fiber system. The periosteum at the metaphyseal-shaft boundary is incised around the tip of the Kirschner wire; the lateral intermuscular septum is not released as far as the over-the-top position. From the time the transfemoral Kirschner wire is inserted, the knee is maintained at a constant 125° flexion to avoid bending of the guidewire, which would complicate reaming of the condylar tunnel.

The transfemoral Kirschner wire is withdrawn upward until its tip is still just visible in the intercondylar notch. The tip position is checked arthroscopically in relation to the femoral attachment site and the remnants of the femoral ACL stump. If the Kirschner wire is too far posterior or anterior, a corrected Kirschner wire is inserted from the outside in. Its position is again checked by image intensification before definitive reaming is performed. The tip position is checked arthroscopically as it relates to the lateral border of the PCL and to the intercondylar surface of the lateral femoral condyle before overreaming.

Reaming the Femoral Tunnel by the Outside-In Technique

The shortened transfemoral guidewire is overdrilled with the 6-mm, 8-mm, or 10-mm cannulated reamer (depending on limb morphotype, constitutional laxity, and intercondylar notch width) from the superolateral aspect of the femur. A tissue protector sleeve shields the vastus lateralis muscle fibers from harm. Under arthroscopic guidance, the reamer is directed toward the center of the femoral attachment site. When diminished resistance is felt, the reamer is withdrawn and the Kirschner wire removed. This avoids damage to the synovial investment of the PCL.

The internal aperture of the femoral tunnel is smoothed with a round burr, curved file, and abrader under arthroscopic vision. With the arthroscope in the anterolateral portal and the shaver in the anteromedial portal, the reaming debris is aspirated under arthroscopic control.

Graft Selection, Removal, and Preparation

A skin incision 6–7 cm long is made on the midline over the proximal border of the patella in preparation for harvesting the free autologous quadriceps tendon graft on a trapezoidal bone block from the patellar base. The muscle fascia is incised longitudinally, and the tendinous layer of the quadriceps between the muscle bellies of the vastus medialis and vastual lateralis is exposed for a length of 6 cm. The galea aponeurotica of the extensor apparatus is incised longitudinally with a scalpel. A trapezoidal bone block that measures 10 mm at the proximal border of the patellar base and widens distally is outlined with a Simal chisel. The ends of the bone block are marked with the 2.0-mm drill bit to avoid stress concentration at the end of the graft bed. The trapezoidal bone block is excised with the vibrating saw at a depth of 6–8 mm. The cut is made from the proximal side, holding the blade perpendicular to the anterior patellar surface so that the cut does not go too deep. A transverse distal saw cut completes excision of the 10- to 12-mm-long bone block. A strip of quadriceps tendon 6–8 cm long, 10–12 mm wide, and 6–8 mm thick is then excised proximally in continuity with the patellar bone block. Care is taken not to enter the suprapatellar pouch if at all possible. If this should occur, the synovium is repaired with an absorbable watertight suture line. In contrast to the Blauth technique for a two-slip quadriceps tendon reconstruction of the ACL, the rectus femoris is not detached, and the skin incision for harvesting the graft is significantly smaller. The donor defect is closed transversely with absorbable coapting sutures. At times it is preferable to harvest the graft before the arthroscopic procedure is performed.

Snaring the Graft Ends

The quadriceps tendon strip is snared proximally and dissected distally to an adequate thickness. The proximal border of the patellar base is osteotomized at the desired depth, parallel to the anterior patellar surface, using the saw or Simal chisel. The bone block is carefully separated from the patellar base. Wedge-shaped chisels should not be used as they are apt to fissure or fracture the bone. The bone block from the patellar base is perforated transversely with two 2.0-mm drill holes, and 2 nonabsorbable sutures are passed through these fixation holes with a straight needle in a figure-of-8 pattern and tied over the end of the bone block. The proximal tendinous end of the graft is snared with 4 nonabsorbable inverting sutures.

Trial Insertion of a Prosthesis

With the knee flexed 45°–60°, a small grasping forceps is passed into the tibial tunnel from below and directed through the lateral half of the intercondylar notch into the femoral tunnel. A U-shaped loop of thread is brought down through the femoral tunnel and out the tibial tunnel while the proximal end of the thread is secured with a clamp. The arthroscopic passing device is pulled into the joint to check the course of the new ligament, and joint play and graft behavior are observed arthroscopically through a range of knee motion. Projecting osteophytes or ACL remnants are removed with the synovial shaver or bone abrader until the graft can function without impingement.

Testing Isometry

The distal end of the passing device is secured with a clamp, and the knee is placed through a range of motion from full extension to 130° flexion while the trial graft is observed for change of length at different flexion angles. Less than 2–3 mm of excursion is considered to indicate acceptable isometry, and the passing device may be replaced with the cruciate ligament graft. If there is doubt as to the position of the graft and its course, this can be checked with the image intensifier by inserting a sterile, distally cuffed pediatric endotracheal tube that has been filled with radiographic contrast medium. Engebretsen et al. (1988a, b) and Hassenpflug et al. (1985) note that tightening of the graft in the last 10° before full extension is a physiologic phenomenon reflecting the increasing tension on the cruciate ligament as the knee approaches extension and the recruitment of all the graft fibers.

Pulling the Graft into the Joint

The proximally tapering quadriceps tendon strip is fastened to the distal end of the passing device and pulled into the joint through the tibial tunnel, through the tibial remnant of the ACL stump, and through the lateral half of the intercondylar notch into the smoothed intraarticular opening of the femoral tunnel under arthroscopic guidance. As the graft is pulled into place, the distally widening bone block is impacted vertically into the tibial tunnel until it is firmly anchored there at the subchondral level. The junction of the bone block with the quadriceps tendon (where the Sharpey fibers enter the tendon) is placed so that it is flush with the superior osseous boundary of the anterior intercondylar area. This ensures that the physiologic junctional zone between the quadriceps tendon and patellar base, a zone with structural transitional elements, is placed in the region where shearing and bending forces will be transmitted to the tibial insertion site.

Graft Tension and Graft Fixation

First the graft is fixed on the distal side by tying the impacted bone block to a transverse bicortical tibial screw with nonabsorbable sutures.

Adjustment of graft tension: With the knee flexed 20°, 2 of the 4 nonabsorbable looped threads placed in the tendinous proximal end of the graft are tentatively fixed to a bicortical screw with smooth shank and washer driven transversely into the femur. Now the knee is extended to the neutral position, avoiding any recurvatum or hyperextension. The 2 remaining looped graft sutures are fixed to the bicortical screw under moderate tension. Before tying the threads definitively, the surgeon tests residual anterior laxity near extension, which should equal 2–3 mm. If an extension deficit of 5° or more is noted, or if there is a complete lack of physiologic residual anterior displacement near extension, the graft is loosened slightly until its tension is as close to physiologic as possible. Following the adjustment of graft tension (which is flexion-dependent and increases near full extension), the sutures are definitively tied around the smooth shank of the transverse bicortical screw with the knee extended. Finally the fixation screw is driven home in extension. In patients with lax ligaments, the sutures are tightened with the knee flexed 20°.

Arthroscopic Check of Graft Placement

Under arthroscopic control, the knee is placed through several ranges of motion between 130° flexion and full extension. The graft is again checked for impingement against the anteroinferior rim of the intercondylar roof while the knee is fully extended. Any residual projecting osteophytes are removed with the abrader under vision with the knee flexed 90° while the graft is protected. Any graft irregularities or graft fibers that were mechanically damaged when pulled through the joint are sparingly removed with the synovial shaver under arthroscopic guidance. The knee joint is irrigated until it is completely cleared of synovial villi, bone particles, and drilling debris. Finally graft tension is tested with the probing hook.

Wound Closure and Drainage

After copious intraarticular irrigation, a suction drain is passed into the joint through the superomedial irrigation portal under visual control. Another drain is placed at the quadriceps tendon donor site, a third is placed subfascially beneath the vastus lateralis, and a fourth is placed inferomedially in the region of the tibial bone tunnel.

Postoperative Positioning and Treatment

The knee is elevated in 60° flexion until the drains are removed 24–48 h postoperatively. The epidural catheter is left in place for 2–3 days, as Arvidson and Eriksson recommend (1988). The patient then starts flexion-extension exercises and intermittent passive motion therapy in the range from 0° to 90°. The flexion arc is gradually increased. An extension deficit of 5° is left in lax individuals for the first 4 weeks, at which time the range is manually increased to 0°. Flexion to 100° is allowed for the first 4 weeks, and to 120° in weeks 5 and 6. Optionally, a plastic knee immobilizer may be worn at night that maintains the joint in a position of near extension. Hydrotherapy in a walking pool and "duck standing" with the knees flexed 70° while bearing 50% of the body weight are permitted by the 5th postoperative day. "Duck walking" is allowed by the 3rd week. The patient is instructed and supervised daily in isometric quadriceps setting exercises and quadriceps-hamstring co-contractions. The patient is encouraged to mobilize the patella by grasping it with the fingers and moving it mediolaterally and craniocaudally several times daily. The load on the knee is increased weekly in 10-kg increments, starting with 15–20 kg on the 3rd postoperative day. If the active extension loss is less than 10°, an effort is made to achieve full weight bearing. A knee brace is worn to limit terminal extension. An elevated heel is indicated for 3 months in patients with lax ligaments to prevent hyperextension.

Discussion

Open techniques have proven effective for autologous reconstruction of the ACL. With accurate placement of sufficiently strong autologous graft material, current reconstructive procedures yield satisfactory knee stability in approximately 80% of patients.

An arthroscopically controlled reconstruction with autologous graft material of adequate strength offers the following advantages:

1. The 3 arthroscopic portals, which measure only 5 mm in diameter, prevent drying of the cartilage surfaces like that occurring in open reconstructions. The articular cartilage is not exposed to the air, and there is less chance of damage to the chondrocytes.
2. Joint distention by the irrigating fluid improves visualization of the knee interior. Mechanical damage by conventional retractors is avoided.
3. The arthroscopic technique eliminates the parapatellar medial or lateral arthrotomy, incision of the medial or lateral retinaculum, and detachment of the vastus medialis or lateralis, thus preserving the integrity of the extensor mechanism and retinacula. Partial resection of the infrapatellar fat pad as in the transligamentous approach is avoided, so that proprioceptive control mechanisms are spared (Kennedy et al. 1982; Schultz et al. 1984).
4. Accurate placement of the transtibial and transfemoral Kirschner guidewires under arthroscopic

control and functional testing of the position and orientation of the wires *before definitive reaming* of the bone tunnels permit an anatomically precise placement of the ACL substitute (Stäubli 1990).

5. The magnification effect of the video camera provides a "microsurgical" view of the operative field that enables the surgeon to work with enhanced precision.

6. The continuous joint irrigation and selective use of the synovial shaver allow for thorough perioperative clearing of tendinous, synovial and osseous debris from the joint.

7. Arthroscopy, supplemented by intraoperative image intensification and radiographs, permits the tibial and femoral Kirschner guidewires to be placed with greater accuracy before reaming is commenced. This can improve the isometry of the reconstruction (Hefzy et al. 1989; Stäubli 1988).

8. Chamfering of the intraarticular tunnel openings can be done more precisely under arthroscopic guidance.

9. Function testing of the proposed graft with a trial prosthesis reveals impingement problems before definitive intraarticular graft placement, so that the definitive graft orientation or intercondylar notch width can be corrected accordingly.

10. Following graft placement, any adjustments of the intercondylar notch configuration can be carried out under arthroscopic vision while protecting the graft.

The disadvantages of transarthroscopic reconstruction are as follows:

1. The equipment and personnel requirements of the procedure are formidable. All installed equipment and instruments must be function-tested before the tourniquet is applied, and it is essential to have an efficiently organized and structured operating environment.

2. The duration of the transarthroscopic reconstruction presently averages 1 1/2 to 1 3/4 h (after the initial learning period).

3. The center of the femoral attachment site can be difficult to see in a narrow intercondylar notch, so the position and orientation of the transfemoral Kirschner wire can be difficult to assess visually. The use of image intensification fluoroscopy to check the exact placement and orientation of the 2 Kirschner guidewires has become routine. If the transfemoral Kirschner guidewire is inserted from the inside out using arthroscopic control alone, we have found that the femoral tunnel will be placed 5–6 mm too far anteriorly. The same error can

occur in the single-tunnel technique (Good et al. 1987; Rosenberg et al. 1988).

4. Graft donor defect and donor pathology: With practice, a quadriceps tendon strip 6–8 cm long, 10–12 mm wide, and 6–8 mm thick can be removed without opening the suprapatellar pouch. The residual quadriceps tendon thickness over the pouch can be assessed by diaphanoscopy. We have not experienced vastus medialis/lateralis innervation problems in the postoperative period. Complaints in the area of the donor defect past 120° of flexion are occasionally reported 6–8 weeks after surgery, but these pass without treatment. Kneeling is not painful because there are no incisions in the weight-bearing portion of the tibial tuberosity. No cases of patella baja have been observed with this technique (51 arthroscopic reconstructions in 1 1/2 years from September 1987 to March 1989). When the bone block is excised from the center of the patellar base, care must be taken that the vibrating saw does not cut too deeply. A tangential radiograph of both knees in 30° flexion provides useful preoperative information on the patellar configuration and helps to avoid iatrogenic fissuring or fracturing of the patella (2 fissures in our series). Stress concentration at the ends of the bone block can be avoided by predrilling the block with a 2.0-mm bit. This will reduce stress concentration at the end of the graft bed.

5. A possible disadvantage of the arthroscopic technique is the absence of pain and large range of knee motion that is possible within a relatively short time compared with conventional open surgery. This means that patients will require continual guidance and supervision. Graft protection during the remodeling period, which generally lasts for 12 months or more, requires constant, motivational patient guidance to avoid excessive loading of the reconstructed ligament during that period.

6. Reconstruction under arthroscopic guidance calls for experience in performing a variety of interventional arthroscopic procedures. Before applying the technique clinically, the surgeon should first practice it in cadaveric knees under the personal instruction and supervision of an experienced operator. The long-term results of arthroscopic ACL reconstructions are not yet known, although it is reasonable to speculate that the graft, which is 2–3 mm thicker and 2–3 mm wider than the free central third of the patellar tendon, will provide similarly good long-term results (W. Blauth, personal communication).

7. Transarthroscopic reconstruction performed under image intensifier control is a "high-tech" reconstructive procedure. Necessary biological remodeling processes such as *neoenthesis* (restoration of the ligament-bone attachment) and *"neoligamentization"* (restructuring of the collagen fiber bundles) are not directly affected by this method.

8. Associated injuries of the popliteus tendon and its fascicles and significant posteromedial lesions of the secondary restraints should not go untreated despite arthroscopically controlled reconstruction of the central pivot.

References

Arvidson I, Eriksson E (1988) Counteracting muscle atrophy after ACL injury. Scientific bases for a rehabilitation program. In: Feagin J jr (ed) The crucial ligaments. Churchill Livingstone, New York Edinburgh London Melbourne, pp 451–464

Blauth W (1984) Die zweizügelige Ersatzplastik des vorderen Kreuzbandes aus der Quadricepssehne. Unfallheilkunde 87: 45–51

Engebretsen L, Lew WD, Lewis JL, Hunter RE (1988a) Knee joint motion and ligament force before and after primary repair of acute anterior cruciate ligament rupture. Acta Orthop Scand

Engebretsen L, Lew WD, Lewis JL, Hunter RE (1988b) Knee joint motion and ligament force before and after primary augmented repair of the acute anterior cruciate ligament. Acta Orthop Scand

Good L, Odensten M, Gillquist J (1987) Precision in reconstruction of the anterior cruciate ligament. A new positioning device compared with hand drilling. Acta Orthop Scand 58: 658–661

Hassenpflug J, Blauth W, Rose D (1985) Zum Spannungsverhalten von Transplantaten zum Ersatz des vorderen Kreuzbandes. Unfallchirurg 1988: 151–158

Hefzy MS, Grood ES, Hoyes FR (1988) Factors affecting the region of most isometric femoral attachments. Part II: The anterior cruciate ligament. Am J Sports Med 17: 208–216

Jakob RP, Stäubli H-U, Deland JT (1987) Grading the pivot shift. Objective tests with implications for treatment. J Bone Joint Surg [Br] 69: 294–299

Jakob RP, Stäubli H-U, Zuber K, Esser M (1988) The arthroscopic meniscal repair. Techniques and clinical experience. Am J Sports Med 16: 137–142

Kennedy JL, Alexander IJ, Hayes KC (1982) Nerve supply of the human knee and its functional importance. Am J Sports Med 10: 329–335

Lambert KL, Cunningham RR (1988) Anatomic substitution of the anterior cruciate ligament using a vascularized patellar tendon graft with interference fixation. In: Feagin J jr (ed) The crucial ligaments. Churchill Livingstone, New York Edinburgh London Melbourne, pp 401–408

Müller We (1988) Kinematics of the cruciate ligaments. In: Feagin J jr (ed) The crucial ligaments. Churchill Livingstone, New York Edinburgh London Melbourne, pp 217–233

Müller We, Biedert R, Hefti F, Jakob RP, Munzinger U, Stäubli H-U (1988) OAK Knee evaluation. A new way to assess knee ligament injuries. Clin Orthop 232: 37–50

Rosenberg TD, Paulos LE, Abbott PJ (1988) Arthroscopic cruciate repair and reconstruction: An overview and descriptions of technique. In: Feagin J jr (ed) The crucial ligaments. Churchill Livingstone, New York Edinburgh London Melbourne, pp 409–423

Schultz RA, Miller DL, Kerr CS, Micheli L (1984) Mechanoreceptors in human cruciate ligaments. A histological study. J Bone Joint Surg [Am] 66: 1072–1076

Stäubli H-U (1988) Preoperative planning to determine anatomic attachment areas in anterior cruciate ligament reconstruction. ACL study group conference. March 19–26th, Snowmass, Aspen/CO

Stäubli H-U (1990a) Preoperative planning for anterior cruciate ligament reconstruction. Technique based on radiographic views reflecting individual patient morphology. (In preparation)

Stäubli H-U, (1990b) Limits of compartmental knee motion. Acta Orthop Scand [Suppl] (submitted for publication)

Cruciate Reconstruction under Arthroscopic Control: Technique and Preliminary Results

P. Chambat and E. Pradat

Since 1979 we have used the free central one-third of the patellar tendon with proximal and distal bone blocks for reconstruction of the anterior cruciate ligament (ACL). We used to reinforce the intraarticular substitution by harvesting part of the quadriceps tendon in continuity with the patellar bone block. The tibial-tuberosity bone block was introduced into the tibial tunnel and anchored to a tibial cortex screw with a metal wire. The patellar bone block was fixed within a deep supracondylar slot whose base was in the anteromedial portion of the ACL attachment on the intercondylar aspect of the lateral femoral condyle. The quadriceps tendon emerging from the lateral femoral condyle was passed forward beneath the lateral collateral ligament and anchored in a tunnel in Gerdy's tubercle with the tibia held in slight external rotation. The knee was mobilized early after surgery.

The advantages of this operation were confirmed by various studies, which showed the following:

- The central one-third of the patellar tendon is the strongest autologous replacement material currently available that does not cause significant weakening of the residual patellar ligament (Butler et al. 1979).
- Complete mobilization of the distal bone fragment, necessary to ensure correct placement of the patellar bone block on the intercondylar surface of the lateral femoral condyle, does not adversely affect graft revascularization compared with a graft left attached to a distal pedicle (Ginsberg et al. 1980; Scapinelli 1968).
- The bone block method of graft fixation is superior to all other fixation methods, especially when a screw is driven into the tunnel to strengthen the interference fit (Lambert 1983; Kurosaka et al. 1983).
- One result of this mechanical advantage is that bony consolidation of the bone block within the tunnel occurs within 3 months after surgery by a progressive ingrowth of osteoid from the transplanted bone block (Cabaud et al. 1974; Chambat et al. 1984; Clancy et al. 1981).

- The good mechanical fixation of the graft permits the early institution of rehabilitation, which is beneficial for graft remodeling (Burks et al. 1984; Noyes et al. 1983; Rigal et al. 1982).
- By 1 year, the remodeling of a graft with an initial width of 14 mm has produced a rupture strength comparable to that of the normal ACL (Arnoczky et al. 1982; Cabaud et al. 1974; Fayard et al. 1982; Clancy et al. 1981; Noyes et al. 1983).

Considering all of these reconstructive principles, it seems logical to attempt this procedure under arthroscopic control as a means of avoiding anterior arthrotomy and reducing iatrogenic morbidity.

Arthroscopic Technique

Since September 1985, we have performed this operation under arthroscopic guidance. *We no longer augment the procedure with an extraarticular transfer of quadriceps tendon.*

Arthroscopic Search for Intraarticular Lesions

The procedure begins with an arthroscopic examination of the knee (Fig. 1). If meniscal lesions are found, the following options are available:

- Arthroscopic resection of a meniscal flap, leaving the remaining half of the meniscus intact
- Repair of vertical tears in the vascular zone, using a retroligamentous approach for posterior tears, and a double anteromedial and posterior approach for a long tear extending into the anterior horn (in this case we abandon the arthroscopic technique in favor of an open reconstruction)

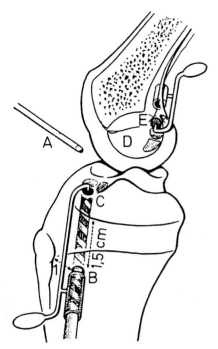

Fig. 1. The arthroscope *(A)* is in the anterolateral portal. The inlet of the tibial tunnel *(B)* is 1.5 cm distal to the joint line and 1 cm medial to the medial border of the patellar tendon; the outlet is at the attachment site of the anteromedial bundle *(C)* (confirmed arthroscopically). Though it opens within the joint, the tunnel takes a nearly horizontal course. Soft tissues are stripped from the intercondylar surface of the lateral femoral condyle. Obstructing osteophytes are removed by a notch plasty. The femoral tunnel is tangential to the posterosuperior cartilage boundary and is centered on the intercondylar portion of the lateral femoral condyle

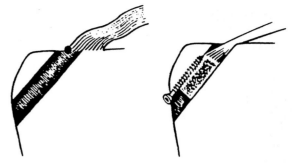

Fig. 2. Position and interference-fit fixation of the bone block in the tibial tunnel. Placement of the tibial tunnel on the sagittal plane in relation to the anteromedial bundle of the ACL. The tibial tunnel should exit in the anterior portion of the original ACL attachment so that the substitute, which occupies the posterior part of the tunnel, will have an anatomic course

outlet (Fig. 2). The intraarticular tunnel opening is carefully cleaned of bone, cartilage and tendon debris with the shaver to eliminate the risk of soft-tissue invagination when the graft is pulled through. Arthroscopically, the surgeon clears the intercondylar surface of the lateral femoral condyle of soft tissues with a periosteal elevator by pushing aside the remnants of the ACL stump and adherent synovial tissue. This will facilitate passage of the graft. Obstructing osteophytes are removed with a motorized cutter, and a narrowed intercondylar notch is widened by an adequate notch plasty. This condyloplasty is especially indicated for stenotic changes but should not be too extensive as it might jeopardize the already precarious bony congruity of the joint.

Tibial Bone Tunnel and Preparation of the Intercondylar Surface of the Lateral Femoral Condyle

Access for drilling the tibial bone tunnel is gained through a 3-cm skin incision centered over the tibial tuberosity. The periosteum is stripped from the site of the proposed tunnel inlet, 1.5 cm distal to the tibial plateau and 1 cm medial to the patellar tendon (see Fig. 1). This results in a very low-angle ("horizontal") tibial bone tunnel, which facilitates pull-through of the graft by decreasing the angulation at the internal opening of the tibial tunnel. The 9-mm tibial tunnel is drilled under arthroscopic control using a drill guide. The intraarticular tunnel opening is located at the attachment site of the anteromedial bundle of the ACL (see Fig. 1). To achieve the most isometric placement, the tunnel opening should be centered on the most distal anteromedial fibers of the ACL, because the 3- to 4-mm-wide tendinous portion of the new ligament will emerge through the posterior half of the tunnel

Graft Removal and Preparation

The graft is harvested through 2 skin incisions, one centered on the tibial tuberosity, the other over the distal pole of the patella (Fig. 3). The new ligament is taken from the central third of the patellar tendon. The bone block from the tibial tuberosity measures $1 \times 1 \times 1.5$ cm and is perforated in its proximal portion with a 2.0-mm drill bit. The tendinous part of the graft is 10–12 mm wide and is dissected subcutaneously up to the lower pole of the patella. The tibial bone block with attached patellar tendon is delivered through the proximal skin incision, where a trapezoidal bone block (15 mm wide proximally, 10 mm wide distally) is excised with an oscillating saw.

This block is likewise perforated with the 2.0-mm bit. The graft is prepared for transplantation by trimming the tibial bone block to a size that can be pulled through a 9-mm bone tunnel with a loop of metal

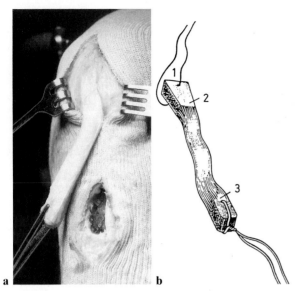

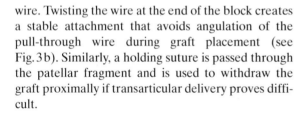

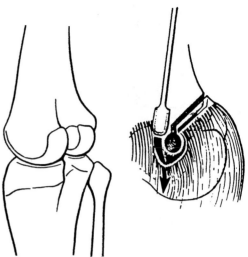

Fig. 3a, b. Two 3-cm skin incisions are centered on the tibial tuberosity and patella **(a)**, and the graft is removed **(b)**. *1* Full-thickness patellar bone block (measures 1.5×1.0 cm proximally and 1.0×1.0 cm distally) armed with pull-through suture. *2* Tendinous graft width is 1.0 to 1.4 cm, according to patellar tendon volume; should always be less than half the anatomic width. *3* Tibial bone block measures $1.0 \times 1.0 \times 1.5$ cm, armed with 8–10 mm metal wire

Fig. 4. A lateral skin incision 3 cm proximal to the lateral femoral epicondyle gives access to the intercondylar notch without damaging the posterolateral capsule and ligaments. A 9-mm tunnel is drilled through the femur above the lateral intermuscular septum, aiming for the attachment of the anteromedial bundle of the ACL on the intercondylar surface of the lateral condyle. The tunnel is unroofed with 2 parallel saw cuts spaced 3 mm apart. This U-shaped channel runs parallel to the femoral diaphysis, so it emerges outside the posterior joint capsule

wire. Twisting the wire at the end of the block creates a stable attachment that avoids angulation of the pull-through wire during graft placement (see Fig. 3b). Similarly, a holding suture is passed through the patellar fragment and is used to withdraw the graft proximally if transarticular delivery proves difficult.

Drilling the Femoral Tunnel

Access for drilling the femoral tunnel is gained through a 3–4 cm skin incision above the lateral condyle. The fascia lata is incised longitudinally through its middle fibers. The periosteum is then incised anterior to the lateral intermuscular septum and is stripped from the posterior femoral metaphysis with a periosteal elevator. This instrument is then directed obliquely downward to give access to the posterior portion of the intercondylar notch (Fig. 4). This permits exposure of the lateral supracondylar metaphysis without causing trauma to posterolateral capsuloligamentous structures. A drill guide is placed posterior to the lateral femoral condyle, and a 9-mm transfemoral tunnel is drilled from the outside in, starting from above the posterolateral capsular insertion and aiming for the attachment of the antero-

medial bundle of the ACL on the intercondylar surface of the lateral condyle (see Fig. 1). The correct position of the intraarticular tunnel mouth is verified by arthroscopy.

Next the femoral tunnel is partially unroofed with 2 saw cuts parallel to the femoral diaphysis, sparing the capsular insertion. With a width of 2–3 mm, this notchlike opening is narrower than the femoral tunnel. Its purpose is explained below (see Fig. 4).

Graft Placement and Fixation

A looped pull-through suture is grasped with a slightly curved and flexible suture passer introduced through the tibial bone tunnel (Fig. 5). Passage of the instrument is facilitated by extending the knee (*A* in Fig. 5) so that the instrument will be parallel to the intercondylar roof (*A* and *B* in Fig. 5). By then flexing the knee, the instrument tip is brought to rest against the posterior femoral metaphysis in such a way that the pull-through suture is easier to retrieve (*C* in Fig. 5). The metal wire on the graft is threaded through the loop of the pull-through suture, and the new ligament is pulled down through the joint so that the tibial bone block is anterior.

The new ligament is first aligned axially in the U-

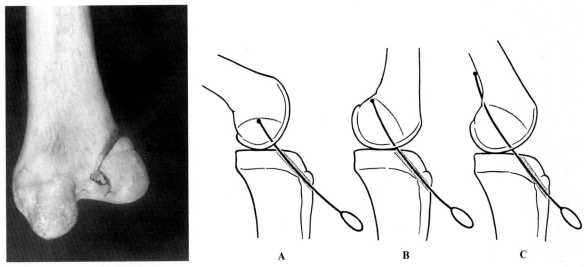

Fig. 5. A looped suture is carried up through the joint on a flexible passer and is used to pull the graft into place. The instrument is introduced through the tibial tunnel *(A)*; the knee is extended *(B)* and then flexed again to direct the tip of the passer posterolaterally to the femoral metaphysis *(C)*. The end of the suture is retrieved in the lateral skin incision

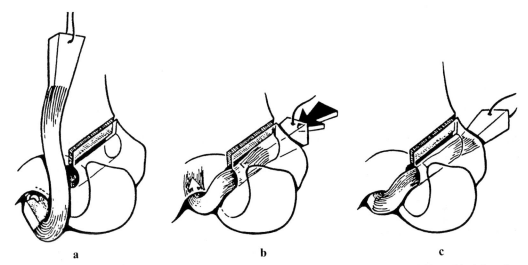

Fig. 6 a–c. Femoral fixation of the graft; replacement of the pull-through suture with a metal wire. **a** Initially the substitute is outside the U-shaped channel and is aligned parallel to it. As there is no angulation, forward and downward traction on the graft draws it through the posterior capsule. Once the tibial bone block is inside the joint, the proximal tendinous portion of the graft is slipped into the prepared femoral slot. **b** Continued anterior and distal traction pulls the tibial bone block into the tibial tunnel while the patellar block wedges into the femoral tunnel owing to its trapezoidal shape **(c)**. The drawings illustrate the U-shaped profile of the femoral channel. The pull-through suture is passed at the first attempt, and there is no angulation at the mouth of the tibial tunnel, which therefore can be made somewhat larger

shaped femoral channel (Fig. 6a). Previous stripping of the soft tissues from the posterior femoral metaphysis prevents angulation and facilitates access through the joint capsule.

The patellar tendon strip is slipped into the U-shaped slot, which is just wide enough to accommodate the graft (Fig. 6b). The graft is then pulled forward and downward to draw the trapezoidal patellar bone block into the opening of the femoral tunnel. The traction is continued until the trapezoidal block wedges into place (*C* in Fig. 5). Once the distal end of the block is flush with the intercondylar surface of the lateral femoral condyle, the block can enter no farther. The tibial bone block enters the transtibial tunnel with resistance, although passage is aided by the relatively horizontal course of the tunnel and by the

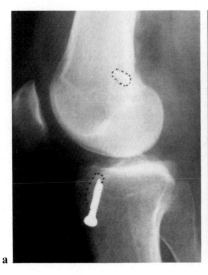 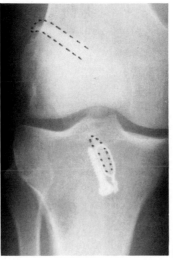

a   b

Fig. 7 a, b. Postoperative radiographs of the tibial and femoral bone tunnels (marked). **a** Sagittal plane, **b** frontal plane

rigid attachment of the metal guidewire to the bone block, which avoids angulation. Definitive interference-fit fixation of the distal bone block is achieved by driving a screw between the block and the tunnel wall (see Figs. 2, 7).

Postoperative Course and Rehabilitation

The knee, which does not bear weight for the first 45 days, is immediately mobilized through a 10°–90° range of motion. A slightly flexed knee position is maintained for 90 days postoperatively by having the patient wear an elevated heel. After 90 days, an effort is made to achieve full extension while avoiding hyperextension (accepting a relative extension deficit). Meanwhile an intensive hamstring strengthening program is begun, while quadriceps strengthening is controlled so that the graft is not damaged.

Results

From September 1985 to July 1986, 72 patients underwent surgery at our center for ACL insufficiency with varying degrees of accompanying deficiency of the posteromedial and posterolateral structures. All cases were managed by an intraarticular reconstruction with no extraarticular augmentation. Because of certain problems that will be explained below, we had to use a conventional arthrotomy for the repair. This permitted us to analyze the 2 groups separately and compare the results.

Case Material

Isolated ACL Reconstruction

Of the 72 patients who had the reconstruction, 56 were followed for an average of 17 months (12–23 months). We shall report results only for the 56 patients whom we personally examined at follow-up.

The operation was arthroscopically controlled in 36 patients, 3 of whom underwent a concomitant partial meniscectomy. In 3 cases a posterior vertical meniscal tear was repaired through a conventional retroligamentous aproach. Arthrotomy was performed in 20 cases. Three of these involved second operations in which scarring made it difficult to harvest the graft. Ten patients required an arthrotomy for meniscal repair; the indication for this procedure was extended to include chronic bucket-handle tears. In 7 cases technical difficulties necessitated conversion to an open operation (5 of 7 in the initial phase).

ACL Reconstruction
Plus Extraarticular Augmentation

Fifty patients operated before September 1985 for the same indication were reexamined an average of 21 months after reconstruction. We compared the results based on:

– The postoperative course
– The anatomic, functional, and esthetic results after more than 1 year

Comparison of Results

Postoperative Sequelae

It is difficult to compare the intensity of postoperative pain in both groups because pain sensation is purely subjective. We can, however, objectively evaluate postoperative swelling and joint effusion by measuring the joint circumference at the level of the patella with the knee flexed 20°. At 48 h, joint circumference relative to the nonoperated side was increased in 5% of the group that only had arthroscopic surgery, versus 12% in the arthrotomized group and 18% in patients who had an extraarticular augmentation. This girth discrepancy was still apparent at 14 days, though to a lesser degree.

Differences in joint circumference do not correlate precisely with subjective pain. Two patients developed a subcutaneous hematoma at the graft donor site following arthroscopic surgery due to inadequate hemostasis.

Anatomic Results: Dynamic Lachman Test

A positive Lachman test was not elicited in any of the patients who had an ACL reconstruction without extraarticular augmentation. Dynamic radiographic documentation of the Lachman test (lateral projection in 5° knee flexion with quadriceps contraction against a 7-kg ankle weight) confirmed these good results. To an accuracy of 2 mm, the value was equal to or less than that of the opposite side in 46% of patients.

All the patients exhibited a firm anterior end point on translation testing, but in 15% there was an increase relative to the opposite healthy knee, implying that the graft was functioning (intact end point) in a slightly elongated condition. This change in the Lachman test was noted in equal percentages of the cases with and without arthrotomy. Of the patients who had an extraarticular augmentation, 2% showed a positive Lachman test while 20% had increased anterior translation with an intact ACL end point. Lachman testing with unconstrained tibial rotation quite often demonstrates a relative increase in anterior translation of the lateral tibial plateau. In the non augmented series (ACL reconstruction without extra articular augmentation), we attribute this phenomenon to a slight loss of control of the lateral compartment caused by the anteromedial placement of the tibial ACL attachment. This insignificant loss of restraint in the anterolateral compartment was not demonstrable in the augmented series, although half of those patients did exhibit in-

Table 1. Dynamic Lachman test (data in mm)

	Pre-operative	Post-operative	Healthy knee
Without extraarticular augmentation			
Total (n = 56)	9.8	5.1	4.2
Arthrotomy (n = 22)	10.1	5.3	4.3
Arthroscopy (n = 34)	9.7	5.1	4.2
With extraarticular augmentation			
Total (n = 50)	10.4	5.4	4.2

creased passive external rotation of the knee in 90° flexion, representing an increased posterior translation of the lateral tibial plateau caused by the extraarticular procedure (Table 1).

The equally good results in both series are explained by a reestablishment of restraint to recurvatum, which stabilizes the knee in extension. In both series (8 without and 10 with extraarticular augmentation), we noted a slight decrease in physiologic anterior joint play relative to the nonoperated side.

Dynamic Subluxation Tests

Two knees in the nonaugmented series showed mildly positive dynamic subluxation tests in medial rotation. Both had been operated arthroscopically, and in both the femoral attachment of the substitute ACL had been placed too far anteriorly. Twelve percent of the knees showed unphysiologic displacement of the lateral tibial plateau caused by loss of anterolateral restraint, but it was too slight to represent a true pivot shift (in the French nomenclature, a "ressaut bâtard"). The incidence of dynamic subluxation phenomena was the same regardless of whether or not the construction had been performed arthroscopically. In the augmented series, 4% of the dynamic subluxation tests in internal rotation were positive, and 20% were unphysiologic, tending to show a posterior subluxation (reversed pivot shift) more than anterior subluxation.

Functional Results

We used the Arpège evaluation system based on activity level (competitive sports, recreational sports, athletically active, athletically inactive), stability, pain, fatiguability, and range of knee motion (scored on a 0–9 scale).

Activity Level

Among patients who were athletically active, we found equal percentages who dropped from competitive to recreational sports and from recreational sports to athletic inactivity. Arthroscopic reconstruction cannot prevent the decline to a lower level of sports activity.

Stability

Nonaugmented series: The total knee score increased from 5.8/g to 8.4/g regardless of the technique employed. The number of arthrotomies at the start of the series was due to the high incidence of associated meniscal injuries, which lowered scores (Table 2).
Augmented series: The knee score increased from 4.5/g to 8.6/g (see Table 2).

Table 2. Knee score

	Preoperative	Postoperative
Without extraarticular augmentation		
Total (n = 56)	5.1/9	8.4/9
Arthrotomy (n = 22)	3.7/9	8.5/9
Arthroscopy (n = 34)	6/9	8.2/9
With extraarticular augmentation		
Total (n = 50)	4.5/9	8.6/9

Pain and Stress Tolerance

The final score in the nonaugmented series was 7.8/9. There was no significant difference between scores with (7.9/9) and without arthrotomy (7.7/9). The results were somewhat lower in the augmented series (7.3/9).

Range of Motion

There was no difference in range of motion between the augmented and nonaugmented series. Generally, 79% were in category 9 (flexion > 130°, no extension loss), 18% in category 8 (flexion < 130°, extension loss < 5°), and 3% in category 7 (marked loss of flexion or extension or both).
We paid particular attention to preventing complete extension during rehabilitation. The object of avoiding hyperextension is to avoid stretching of the new ligament at the anterior rim of the intercondylar roof. This relative extension deficit, though desired, can

Table 3. Range of knee motion (data in %)

	Without extraarticular augmentation Arthrotomy	With extraarticular augmentation Arthroscopy	
Extension loss < 5°	26	14	25
Extension or recurvatum < opposite side	31	39	35
Equal amounts of recurvatum	43	47	40

mask residual anterior laxity near extension and thus distort the result of the radiographically documented Lachman test in 10° flexion. None of the knees examined had reached a degree of recurvatum exceeding that of the opposite side. Complete extension is more difficult to regain following an extraarticular augmentation.
The arthroscopic technique does not necessarily facilitate rehabilitation, as illustrated by 2 patients in this series who had an arduous rehabilitation and did not achieve an acceptable range of motion until 5 months postoperatively.

Analysis of Tunnel Placement

Taking the attachment of the anteromedial bundle as a reference point, we observed no error of tunnel placement on AP radiographs. On lateral views, the tunnel was placed too far anteriorly in 5 knees with arthroscopic reconstructions and in 2 knees with arthrotomies (nonaugmented series).

Skin Incisions

An important advantage of the arthroscopic technique is that it requires only 2 anterior skin incisions and one 3-cm lateral incision, as opposed to the 15-cm anterior incision and 3-cm lateral incision required in an open reconstruction. If an extraarticular procedure is added, the skin incision is 20–25 cm long.
The following conclusions may be drawn:

– Reconstruction of the ACL with the central one-third of the patellar tendon (graft width 11–12 mm) is sufficient to stabilize the knee without extraarticular augmentation (even in joints with associated anterolateral subluxation), provided the medial meniscus can be preserved.

- An anatomically precise reconstruction can be carried out under arthroscopic control from an anterolateral portal.
- The arthroscopic technique reduces the incidence of postoperative hematoma.
- Smaller incisions are cosmetically more appealing and do not alter the anatomic or functional results after a follow-up period of 17 months.

References

Arnoczky SP, Tarvin GB, Marshall JL (1982) Anterior cruciate ligament replacement using patellar tendon. An evaluation of graft revascularisation in the dog. J Bone Joint Surg [Am] 64: 217–224

Burks R, Daniel D, Losse G (1984) The effect of continuous passive motion on anterior cruciale ligament reconstruction stability. Am J Sports Med 12: 323–327

Butler D, Noyes F, Grood E, Miller E, Malek M (1979) Mechanical properties of transplants for anterior cruciate ligament. Orthop Trans 3: 180

Cabaud HE, Rodkey WG, Feagin JA (1974) Experimental studies of acute anterior cruciate ligament injury and repair. Am J Sports Med 7: 18

Chambat P, Walch G, Deschamps G (1984) Les lésions aiguës du LCA du genou à proposer de 71 malades revus. Rev Chir Orthop [Suppl 2]: 70

Clancy WG jr, Narechania RG, Rosember TD et al. (1981) Anterior and posterior cruciate ligament reconstruction in Rhesus monkeys. A histological, microangiographic, and biomechanical analysis. J Bone Joint Surg [Am] 63: 1270–1284

Clancy WG jr, Nelson DA, Reider B et al. (1982) Anterior cruciate ligament reconstruction using one-third of the patellar ligament, augmented by extra-articular tendon transfers. J Bone Joint Surg [Am] 64: 352–359

Fayard JP, Chambat P, Dejour H (1982) Etude expérimentale chez le chien du remplacement du LCA par un transplant libre du tendon rotulien. Rev Chir Orthop [Suppl 2]: 90–60

Ginsburg JH, Whiteside LA, Piper TL (1980) Nutrient pathways in transfered patellar tendon used for ACL reconstruction. Am J Sports Med 8: 15

Hoogland T, Hillen B (1984) Intra-articular reconstruction of the anterior cruciate ligament: an experimental study of length changes in different ligament reconstruction. Clin Orthop 185: 197–202

Jones KG (1963) Reconstruction of the anterior cruciate ligament. A technique using the central one-third of the patellar ligament. J Bone Joint Surg [Am] 45: 925–932

Kurosaka M, Yoshiya S, Andrish JT (1987) A biomechanical comparison of different surgical techniques of graft fixation in anterior cruciate ligament reconstruction. Am J Sports Med 15: 225

Lambert KL (1983) Vascularized patellar tendon graft with rigid internal fixation for anterior cruciate ligament insufficiency. Clin Orthop 172: 85–89

Norwood LA, Cross MJ (1979) Anterior cruciate ligament: Functional anatomy of its bundles in rotatory instabilities. Am J Sports Med 7: 23–26

Noyes FR, Delucus JL, Torvik PJ (1974) Biomechanics of anterior cruciate ligament failure: Analysis of strain rate sensitivity and mechanisms of failure in primates. J Bone Joint Surg [Am] 56: 236–253

Noyes FR, Butler DL, Paulos LE, Grood ES (1983) Intra-articular cruciate reconstruction, Part I: perspective on graft strength, vascularisation and immediate motion after replacement. Clin Orthop 172: 71

Noyes FR, Butler DL, Grood ES (1984) Biomechanical analysis of human ligament grafts used in knee-ligament repairs and reconstructions. J Bone Joint Surg [Am] 66: 344–352

Rigal F, Chambat P, Fayard JP, Dejour H (1982) La rééducation des plasties ligamentaires du genou selon la technique de Kenneth Jones. Ann Kinesither 4

Scapinelli R (1968) Studies of the vascularisation of the human knee joint. Acta Anat 70: 305

Torg JS, Conrad W, Kalen V (1976) Clinical diagnosis of anterior cruciate ligament instability in the athlete. Am J Sports Med 4: 84–93

Injuries of Posterolateral Structures and the Posterior Cruciate Ligament

Lateral and Posterolateral Rotatory Instability of the Knee

R. P. Jakob and J. P. Warner

Injuries of the lateral and posterolateral structures of the knee joint are uncommon and have received relatively little attention compared with the extensive body of literature on ligamentous knee injuries in general (Abbot et al. 1941; Brantigan and Voshell 1941; DeLee et al. 1983 a,b; Galleazzi 1927; Galway 1972; Helfet 1974; Hughston 1962; Hughston et al. 1976 a,b; Järvisen and Kannas 1985; Larson 1975; MacIntosh 1974; MacIntosh and Darby 1976; Marshall and Rubin 1977; Nicholas 1978; O'Donoghue 1950, 1955; Palmer 1938; Slocum et al. 1973; Smillie 1959). O'Donoghue (1950, 1955) and Abbot et al. (1941), who added greatly to our knowledge of knee ligament injuries, formulated a new concept favoring the aggressive surgical treatment of these lesions. But the clinical series published to date have included only isolated reports of lateral ligament injuries, and authors in general have tended to ascribe relatively little clinical importance to them (Baker et al. 1983; DeLee et al. 1983 a,b; Hughston and Jacobson 1985; Hughston and Norwood 1980; Hughston et al. 1976 b; Jobe 1980; Kannus 1989; Kennedy 1983; Kennedy and Swan 1972; Naver and Aalberg 1985; Nicholas 1978; Novich and Newark 1960; Towne et al. 1971). The literature on the functional anatomy and pathomechanics of the lateral compartment is likewise modest (Bruser 1960; Cohn and Mains 1979; Fukubayashi et al. 1982; Fulkerson and Gonling 1980; Gollehon et al. 1987; Gould et al. 1984; Grood et al. 1981, 1988; Jakob et al. 1981; Johnson 1979; Kaplan 1961; Marshall et al. 1972; Noyes et al. 1980, 1983; Terry et al. 1986; Wang and Marshall 1977; Wang and Walker 1973).

Hughston et al. (1976 b) were the first to underscore the combined, complex nature of instabilities involving the lateral compartment of the knee.

They recognized 6 types of acute and chronic lateral instability:

- Anterolateral rotatory instability (ALRI)
- Posterolateral rotatory instability (PLRI)
- Combined ALRI and PLRI
- Combined anteromedial rotatory instability (AMRI) and ALRI
- Combined ALRI, PLRI and AMRI
- Acute straight (one-plane) lateral instability (SLI)

Of these 6 types, PLRI and SLI have been given the least attention. ALRI is defined as a forward rotatory subluxation of the lateral tibial plateau with respect to the lateral femoral condyle, the tibia rotating internally about the axis of the intact posterior cruciate ligament (PCL). This type of instability is consistently associated with a tear of the anterior cruciate ligament (ACL) and is the most common isolated ligamentous injury in the knee (Cabaud and Slocum 1977; Ellison 1975; Fetto and Marshall 1979; Jakob et al. 1981; Kennedy et al. 1978; Losee et al. 1978).

PLRI has been defined as a posterior rotatory subluxation of the lateral tibial plateau with respect to the lateral femoral condyle in which the tibia rotates externally about the axis of the intact PCL (Bousquet 1972; DeHaven 1978; Hughston et al. 1976b; Jakob et al. 1981; Kennedy et al. 1977; Trillat 1977; Trillat et al. 1972). It soon became clear, however, that the presumed integrity of the PCL often was not confirmed, and the concept of rotatory instability with an intact central pivot had to be discarded (Gollehon 1987; Jakob et al. 1981; Müller et al. 1988).

SLI is a severe one-plane instability caused by the disruption of all lateral structures combined with a rupture of the PCL and possibly of the ACL (DeLee et al. 1983 b; Hughston et al. 1976b). In the present article, SLI and PLRI are treated both as isolated injuries and as injuries combined with other instabilities. Though given relatively little attention in the past, SLI and PLRI are important in connection with the new OAK concept of ligament instabilities (OAK = Swiss Orthopedic Study Group for the Knee).

There is much confusion in the literature regarding the pathomechanics and accompanying pathoanatomy of lateral ligamentous knee injuries. A spectrum of lesions have been described in articles dealing with the surgical treatment of lateral ligament instabilities (Table 1). In contrast to earlier observations, it is now generally recognized that lateral ligament injuries are very frequently combined with in-

Table 1. Lateral structural lesions in the knee, excluding combined rotatory instabilities

Study (diagnosis no.)	Anatomic lesions (%)											
	ACL	PCL	LCL	Arcuate ligament	Popliteus	Central third of lateral capsule	ITT	Lateral gastrocnemius	Biceps femoris	Lateral meniscus	Medial meniscus	Peroneal nerve
Baker et al. (1983) (acute PLRI-17)	65%	0%	59%	100%	94%	–	12%	35%	47%	24%	6%	12%
DeLee et al. (1983a) (acute PLRI-12)[a]	0%	0%	100%	100%	100%	67%	17%	0%	75%	25%	0%	0%
Hughston et al. (1976b)												
(acute PLRI-6)	17%	–	–	100%	–	–	–	17%	33%	17%	–	0%
(acute PLRI-6)	33%	0%	–	–	–	83%	–	–	–	50%	33%	0%
(chronic PLRI-8)	25%	–	–	100%	50%	–	–	25%	–	50%	25%	0%
(chronic PLRI-20)	75%	–	–	–	–	100%	–	–	–	65%	75%	0%
Hughston and Jacobson (1985) (chronic PLRI-18)	–	–	37%	100%	58%	–	–	–	–	–	–	–
DeLee et al. (1983b) (acute lateral one-plane-10)	100%	100%'	100%	100%	100%	100%	50%	20%	80%	70%	0%	30%
Towne et al. (1971) (acute one-plane-17)	56%	17%	94%	–	6%	44%	34%	11%	61%	34%	11%	56%

PLRI, Posterolateral rotary instability; *ALRI*, anterolateral rotary instability; *LCL*, lateral collateral ligament; *ITT*, iliotibial tract; *LM*, lateral meniscus; *MM*, medial meniscus; *ACL*, anterior cruciate ligament; *PCL*, posterior cruciate ligament

[a] In this study the arcuate ligament, LCL, and popliteus were listed together and treated as a combined injury of the arcuate complex

juries of the ACL and PCL (Gollehon et al. 1987; Hughston and Jacobson 1985l; Hughston et al. 1976b; Trickey 1980). This clinical observation is supported by sequential ligament sectioning experiments in cadavers, which have shown that lesions of the popliteus tendon and lateral ligament complex often give rise to complicated instability patterns that are not adequately described by the traditional classification system of Hughston et al. (1976b) (Fabbricciani et al. 1982; Gollehon et al. 1987; Hertel 1980; Jakob et al. 1981; Kennedy 1983; Noesberger and Paillot 1976; Noyes et al. 1983; Trickey 1984a,b; Trillat et al. 1978). A true alternative to the Hughston system has not yet been devised.

Straight Lateral Instability (SLI)

Knee injuries resulting in SLI are relatively uncommon and are comparable in severity to the lateral "pentade" or even a dislocation of the knee. Very little has been published about this type of instability, its surgical features, and its prognosis (DeLee et la. 1983b; Highet and Homes 1982; Hughston et al. 1976b; Loos et al. 1981; Morre and Larsen 1980; Novich and Newark 1960; Platt 1924, 1940; Towne et al. 1971; Watson-James 1931). Typically it is caused by a violent, high-energy impact trauma sustained in a motor vehicle accident, although recent series from North America indicate a rising incidence of SLI in conjunction with contact sports (DeLee et al. 1983b; Kannus 1989). True SLI, which would be a relatively mild condition caused by an isolated tear of the lateral collateral ligament, is probably rare. This mechanism is typically described as a sudden, violent varus stress induced by a blow to the medial side of the extended knee (DeLee et al. 1983b; Towne et al. 1971). Indeed, a number of these injuries actually represent extended knee dislocations that reduce spontaneously before they are seen by a physician (Abbot et al. 1941; DeLee et al. 1983b; Moore and Larson 1980); concomitant medial tibial plateau fractures are described in some studies (DeLee et al. 1983b; Towne et al. 1971). A variety of lesions have been observed during surgical intervention (see Table 1). Although Hughston et al. describe 3 cases of SLI in a series of 89 lateral ligament instabilities, they do not report on late results. DeLee et al. (1983b), in a review of 735 surgically treated acute ligamentous knee injuries, report on 10 patients with severe SLI. Forty percent of these injuries were caused by a varus trauma sustained during football, and all the patients had a 3 + varus laxity in full extension with no associ-

ated rotatory instability. Numerous other studies describe lateral ligament injuries coexisting with a tear of the PCL. Moore and Larson (1980) observed 3 such lesions in 18 cases, Hughston et al. (1980) 2 in 29, and Loos et al. (1981) 18 in 59. Only Moore and Larson (1980) distinguish patients with a combined injury of the PCL and lateral collateral ligament from patients with an isolated tear of the PCL.

Platt, in 1924 and 1940, wrote on 6 cases of peroneal nerve lesions coexisting with a severe lateral ligament injury. Later, Watson-Jones (1931) and others (DeLee et al. 1983a; Highet and Holmes 1942; Novich and Newark 1960; Platt 1924) drew attention to this important associated injury. Recently Towne et al. (1971) and DeLee et al. (1983b) observed associated traction injuries of the peroneal nerve in 56% and 30%, respectively, of their SLI patients.

Most authors express reservations about the prognosis of these injuries (DeLee 1983b; Kannus 1989; Towne et al. 1971). De Lee et al. (1983b) report that only 1 of 7 patients with severe SLI returned to competitive sports following surgical treatment. After a 7-year follow-up and despite the fact that 6 of 7 patients had only a 1 + varus laxity in full extension and 30° flexion, only 4 of the patients were satisfied with the result. Recently, Kannus (1989) reported on the nonoperative treatment of grade 2 and grade 3 injuries of the lateral compartment. A grade 3 lesion was defined as a 3 + varus laxity in 30° flexion and a 1–2 + laxity in extension. This is interpreted as evidence of a severe SLI, although the degree of associated rotatory instability was not defined. At final follow-up examination, 75% of the patients exhibited significant athletic disability. Objective evaluation showed signs of a more complex instability with a rotatory component. Fifty percent of the patients showed radiographic signs of osteoarthritis.

Posterolateral Rotatory Instability (PLRI)

Hughston et al. (1976b; Hughston and Jacobsen 1985) and DeLee et al. (1983a) defined PLRI as a type of instability caused by injury to the arcuate complex of the knee (arcuate ligament, lateral collateral ligament, popliteus tendon and aponeurosis, lateral head of gastrocnemius) (DeLee 1983a; Grood et al. 1981; Hughston et al. 1976b; Hughston and Norwood 1980; Nicholas 1978; Noyes et al. 1980). There is excessive external rotation of the lateral tibial plateau, which subluxates about the intact axis of the PCL with respect to the lateral femoral condyle. This concept is supported by clinical studies on posterolateral instability by Baker et al. (1983) and

DeLee et al. (1983a) in which no PCL lesions were found in a series of 29 cases. Recent findings, however, have cast doubt on the notion of the PCL as the rotational center of the knee. A series of clinical studies have demonstrated the frequent coexistence of PCL lesions with lateral and posterolateral injuries (Gollehon et al. 1987; Jakob et al. 1981; Müller et al. 1988), and sequential ligament sectioning studies (Gollehon et al. 1987; Fabricciani et al. 1982; Hertel 1980; Jakob et al. 1981; Kennedy and Towler 1971; Noesberger and Paillot 1976; Noyes et al. 1983; Trickey 1984a,b; Trillat et al. 1978) suggest that a close relationship exists between the lateral structures and the cruciate ligaments. Indeed, PLRI becomes significant only when an injury of the arcuate complex is combined with a lesion of the PCL. Recently Müller et al. (1988) and Jakob et al. (1981) stressed the need for a more comprehensive classification of ligamentous instabilities.

PLRI is considerably less common than ALRI (Hughston et al. 1976b; Nicholas 1978). Frequently it is overlooked in examinations of acute knee injuries and is diagnosed only in chronic cases where PLRI is accompanied by other instabilities (Baker et al. 1983; Hughston et al. 1976b; Hughston and Jacobson 1985). Most authors agree that the clinical signs of both the acute and chronic forms are subtle and frequently misleading (Hughston and Jacobson 1985; Hughston and Norwood 1980; Hughston et al. 1976b; Jakob et al. 1981).

In acute ligamentous injuries that progress to a chronic form of ALRI with secondary deficiency of the static and dynamic restraints on the lateral side, it is common for ALRI and PLRI to coexist (Jakob et al. 1981; Nicholas 1978). Indeed, most forms of PLRI occur in a setting of combined rotatory instabilities (Baker et al. 1983; DeLee et al. 1983a; Hughston and Jacobson 1985; Hughston et al. 1976b). In a series of 89 consecutively operated lateral collateral ligament injuries, Hughston et al. (1976b) found that 6 patients had ALRI combined with PLRI and AMRL, 10 had ALRI plus PLRI, and 12 had isolated forms of PLRI. In 140 patients operated for chronic posterolateral knee instability, Hughston and Jacobson (1985) noted 30 patients with coexisting ALRI, 11 with AMRI plus PLRI, 36 with AMRI plus PLRI plus ALRI, and 18 with isolated PLRI. In a series of 31 cases of acute PLRI, Baker et al. (1983) reported on 17 cases operated for severe PLRI; 10 of these showed associated rotatory instabilities, ALRI being the most common. DeLee et al. (1983a,b), reviewing 735 surgically treated acute ligament injuries, found that 22 had a combination of ALRI and PLRI while only 12 had acute PLRI.

The conclusions that may be drawn from the natural history of PLRI with regard to prognosis and indications for treatment are controversial and based on scant objective documentation. Funk (1983) stated that the true incidence of these injuries is underestimated in the literature, because he frequently observed mild PLRI in professional athletes that was successfully managed by nonoperative treatment. Baker et al. (1983) and other authors (Kannus 1989; Nicholas 1978) likewise observed patients with mild PLRI who returned fully to their preinjury level of sports activity following a period of cast immobilization and formal physiotherapy. Naver and Aalberg (1985) recently described a case of isolated avulsion of the femoral attachment of the popliteus tendon in a soccer player caused by an external rotation-deceleration mechanism in the flexed knee. Reportedly, this patient did well following excision of the small bone fragment from the popliteus tendon. These observations, however, should not draw attention from the fact that significant chronic posterolateral instabilities are commonly observed in association with insufficiency of the PCL.

Functional Anatomy of the Lateral Compartment of the Knee

DeLee et al. (1983a,b) defined lateral ligament lesions as involving a region bounded anteriorly by the lateral patellar border and posteriorly by the PCL. A number of in vitro dissections have supplied a detailed description of the complex ligamentous structures in this region (Gollehon et al. 1987; Johnson 1979; Kaplan 1957a, 1962; Last 1950; Marshall et al. 1972; Wang and Marshall 1977). Seebacher et al. (1982) described the lateral structures of the knee as consisting of 3 distinct layers and characterized 3 major variations of the posterolateral ligamentous structures. DeLee et al. (1983b) described the structures of this region by subdividing the lateral compartment into 3 parts from an anatomical and functional standpoint. A number of authors have investigated the specific anatomic relationships of the iliotibial tract (Bruser 1960; Colonna 1930; Fulkerson and Gonling 1980; Gill 1931; Heyman 1924; Isnar 1947; Irwin 1949; Jakob et al. 1981; Johnson 1979; Kaplan 1988; Kennedy et al. 1978; MacIntosh 1974; Mayer 1930; Soudar et al. 1939; Terry et al. 1986), the popliteal hiatus (Cohn and Mains 1979), the popliteus muscle (Barnett and Richardson 1953; Basmajian and Lovejoy 1971; Fabricciani et al. 1982; Last 1950; Naver and Aalberg 1985; Southmayd and Quig-

ley 1982; Wang and Marshall 1977), the arcuate ligament (Kaplan 1961), and the biceps femoris tendon
(Marshall et al. 1972). DeLee et al. (1983 a,b), Wang
and Marshall (1977), and Gollehon et al. (1987)
noted that the close relationship among the ligamentous structures in the posterolateral corner would
make an isolated ligament injury extremely unlikely.
Thus, most surgeons view the posterolateral corner
as a functional tendoligamentous unit referred to as
the "arcuate ligament complex" or simply the "arcuate complex" (DeLee et al. 1983 a; Hughston et al.
1976 b; Nicholas 1973; Sisk 1987). This complex encompasses the arcuate ligament, the lateral collateral
ligament, the aponeurotic and tendinous portions of
the popliteus muscle, and the lateral head of the
gastrocnemius muscle. The arcuate ligament is
formed by the multiple insertions of the popliteus
tendon together with the condensation of the fascia
over the posterior surface of the muscle (DeLee et al.
1983 a). The mechanical and kinematic demands on
the anatomy and function of the lateral compartment
of the knee must be understood in terms of clinical
observations and in vitro observations from sequential ligament sectioning studies on cadaver knees.

The posterolateral corner of the knee is comprised of
a "loop" of capsuloligamentous and tendinous structures that are statically and dynamically interdepen-
dent and which control tibiofemoral external rotation
and femorotibial coaptation (DeLee et al. 1983 a;
Fürst 1903; Hughston et al. 1976 b; Kaplan 1961;
Larsson 1975; Last 1950; Nicholas 1978). This group
of structures makes up the arcuate complex (Baker
et al. 1983; DeLee et al. 1983 a,b; Hughston et al.
1976 b).

The posterior third of the lateral capsular ligament is
reinforced by the popliteus muscle (Fig. 1), which
arises at the posterior tibial margin, runs obliquely
upward and forward, and inserts on the lateral femoral condyle deep to the lateral collateral ligament
(Basmajian and Lovejoy 1971; Fürst 1903; Jobe 1980;
Kaplan 1957 b; Last 1950). The most important component of this muscle is the peroneal-popliteal fibers
that attach to the lateral meniscus (Cohn and Mains
1979; Fürst 1903; Kaplan 1957 b; Last 1950; Wang and
Marshall 1977). The popliteus tendon and muscle
form an active-passive posterolateral checkrein that
limits posterolateral rotation of the tibia on the femur
and whose tension powerfully coapts the femorotibial articular surfaces (Figs. 2, 3). Other important
functions are the passive restraint of tibiofemoral external rotation in flexion and extension (Southmayd
and Quigley 1982), active internal rotation of the
tibia on the femur (Last 1950), and retraction of the
lateral meniscus (Hughston 1962). Basmajian and

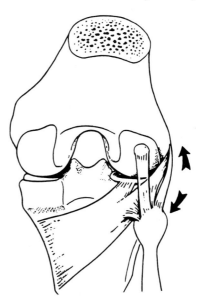

Fig. 1. "Coaptation" of the lateral compartment, after Bousquet et al. (1986)

Lovejoy (1971) and Barnett and Richardson (1953)
state that the popliteus is the only muscle that restrains active translation of the femur on the tibia
when the knee is flexed. Additionally, this muscle in-
teracts functionally with the iliotibial tract and biceps
femoris to provide dynamic stabilization of the lateral
compartment (see Fig. 3).

The *middle third of the lateral capsular ligament* arises
near Gerdy's tubercle and expands backward and upward to blend with the capsule above the lateral collateral ligament (Jobe 1980). Functionally, the meniscotibial fibers form the strongest component of this
ligament (Hughston et al. 1976 b; Johnson 1979). Although Grood et al. (1981), Noyes et al. (1981), and
Hughston et al. (1976 b) believe that the middle third
of the capsule is a secondary restraint of minimal
importance to varus stability, DeLee et al. (1983 a)
noted damage to this structure in 33% of patients
with acute PLRI.

The *lateral collateral ligament* has been characterized
as a relatively unimportant restraint (Brantigan and
Voshell 1941; Kaplan 1957 a, 1962; Segond 1879; Sisk
1987). This component of the arcuate complex descends from the lateral femoral condyle to its insertion on the head of the fibula (Jobe 1980). Along its
course, it reinforces the posterior third of the capsule
(Grood et al. 1981; Kaplan 1957 a; Noyes et al. 1980).
Although Grood et al. (1981) and Noyes et al. (1981)
contend that the lateral collateral ligament is the
principal checkrein against varus opening, clinical
observations have rarely demonstrated an isolated

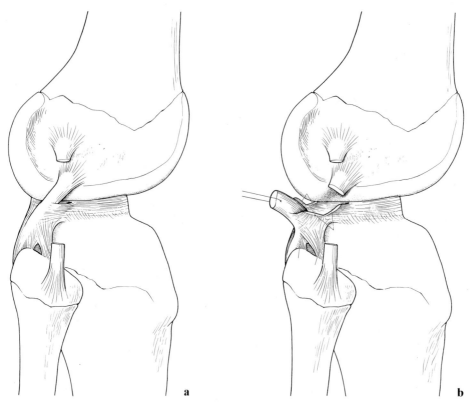

Fig. 2a, b. Popliteus muscle. **a** Femoral attachment, lateral collateral ligament resected. **b** Course of the popliteus tendon, sectioned and retracted to show its site of attachment to the lateral meniscus. (From Stäubli and Birrer 1990)

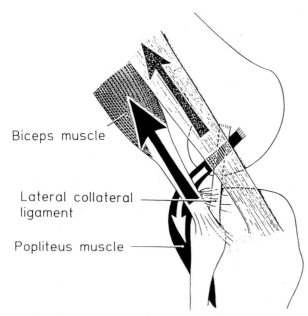

Fig. 3. Dynamic stabilizing actions of the iliotibial tract, biceps femoris muscle, and popliteus muscle. (From Müller 1983)

lesion of this component of the arcuate complex (DeLee 1983 a,b).

Larsson (1975) and Kaplan (1957b, 1961) described the "fabellofibular ligament" or "short collateral ligament" as a variable and poorly defined component of the arcuate complex, in which sutures can be anchored to reinforce a posterolateral repair (Kaplan 1957b, 1961; Larsson 1975). Seebacher et al. (1982) described 3 different anatomic variants of the arcuate complex that are important in the surgical treatment of posterolateral ligament injuries (Fig. 4).

The lateral meniscus is stabilized by the capsule and the peroneal-popliteal (medial) portion of the popliteus tendon (Cohn and Mains 1979). Though more mobile than the medial meniscus, it contributes significantly to the stability of the lateral compartment by creating a concave articular surface on the anatomically convex or saddle-shaped lateral tibial plateau (Galway et al. 1972; Jobe 1980) (Fig. 5).

The *biceps femoris muscle* descends posterior to the iliotibial tract, inserts on the fibular head along the lateral collateral ligament, and also sends strong attachments to the iliotibial tract, Gerdy's tubercle, lateral collateral ligament, the posterior third of the cap-

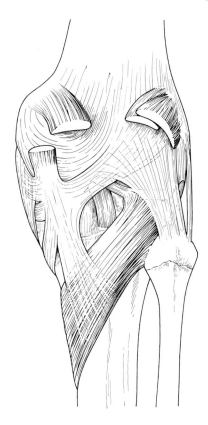

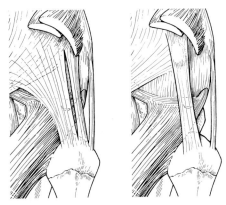

Fig. 4. Variants of the arcuate complex (see text and chapter by Hunziker et al., p. 31 ff.)

sule, and the lateral tibia (DeLee et al. 1983 a). With the popliteus muscle and iliotibial tract, the biceps functions as a strong dynamic lateral stabilizer and a powerful external rotator of the tibia (DeLee et al. 1983 a; Ellison 1975) (see Fig. 3).

The *lateral head of the gastrocnemius muscle* makes a variable contribution to the arcuate complex. In cadaveric dissections, Jakob et al. (1981) noted several instances where this structure was strongly developed and blended with the arcuate ligament.

The *iliotibial tract* has been described as the most important stabilizer of the lateral compartment (DeLee et al. 1983 a), but until recently only Kaplan (1957 b, 1988) described the nature of this stabilizing action. The region called the "Kaplan fibers" is one of the most important parts of this structure in terms of lateral stabilization. This portion of the iliotibial tract blends with the insertion of the intermuscular septum at the supracondylar and femoral tubercle. It runs distally to the tubercle of Gerdy on the tibia (Jakob et al. 1981). Kaplan (1957 b, 1981) assumes that this structure functions as an accessory anterolateral ligament. In more recent reports, Terry et al. (1986) described this region as the "deep capsulo-osseous layer," Müller (1983) as the "femorotibial ligament," and Lobenhoffer et al. (1987) as the "retrograde fiber

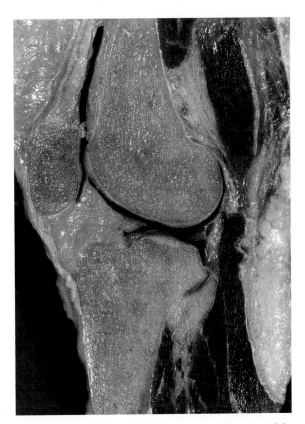

Fig. 5. A sagittal section through the lateral compartment of the knee shows how the lateral meniscus imparts a functional concavity to the anatomically convex lateral tibial plateau, enhancing stability

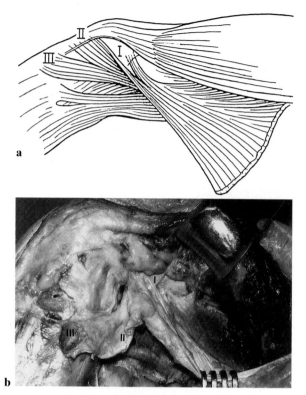

Fig. 6. The 3 insertions of the iliotibial tract. *I* Part of the ITT that blends with the intermuscular septum and inserts on the supracondylar tubercle (Kaplan fibers). The attachments of the ITT to the patellar tendon (*II*) and Gerdy's tubercle (*III*) have been removed to show that there is no attachment on the lateral aspect of the femoral condyle. (From Jakob et al. 1981)

tract." Each of these descriptions confirms Kaplan's own description and underscores the functional importance of this ITT structure that runs between the distal femur and tibia to create, in effect, an accessory anterolateral ligament (Fig. 6). During flexion the ITT tightens and moves backward while exerting a force vector that tends to cause external rotation and posterior translation of the lateral tibia (Jakob et al. 1981; Kaplan 1988; Terry et al. 1986). In extension, the entire ITT glides forward and generally is protected from varus and posterolateral injuries (DeLee et al. 1983a; Hughston et al. 1976b).

Relevant Biomechanics of the Lateral Side of the Knee

The lateral ligament complex differs markedly from the medial structures in its morphology and function (Hughston et al. 1976b). The ligamentous structures on the lateral side of the knee joint are substantially more robust than on the medial side and are subjected to greater forces during gait (Jakob et al. 1981; Müller et al. 1988; Nicholas 1978). When the knee reaches or approaches full extension during the stance phase of gait, the medial compartment is compressed while the lateral compartment is under tension (Müller et al. 1988; Nicholas 1978). A net distracting force acts upon the posterolateral corner. This is an expression of the biomechanics of the lower extremity, which places the mechanical limb axis slightly medial to the center of the knee (Charmion 1984) (Fig. 7). Bousquet (1972), Bousquet et al. (1986), and Charmion (1984) introduced the concept of morphotype and noted that a tendency toward varus and recurvatum angulation in the one-legged stance due to medial deviation of the mechanical limb axis is responsible for distraction and de-coaptation of the lateral compartment.

In 1976 Hughston et al. (1976b) devised a classification that deepened our awareness of the compartmental aspects of lateral knee injuries (Table 2), although the distinction between translational and rotational instabilities was somewhat arbitrary. In this scheme the PCL represents the anatomic axis about

Table 2. Six types of lateral knee instability (from Hughston et al. 1976)

	Pathomechanics	Anatomic lesion
PCL intact	1. ALRI	Middle third of lateral capsule ACL
	2. PLRI	Arcuate complex
	3. Combined ALRI + PLRI	ACL Arcuate complex + / − iliotibial tract
	4. Combined ALRI + AMRI	Middle third of medial capsule Middle third of lateral capsule ACL
	5. Combined ALRI + AMRI + PLRI	Middle third of medial capsule Middle third of lateral capsule Arcuate complex ACL
PCL not intact	6. Acute straight lateral instability	Arcuate complex PCL ACL

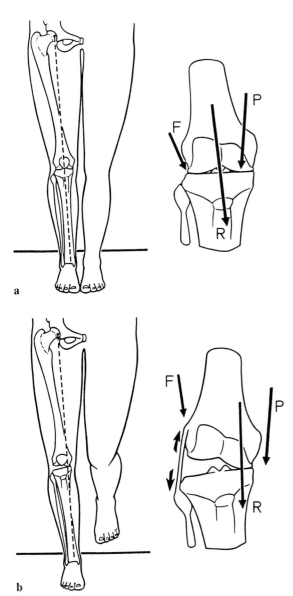

which the lateral tibial plateau rotates externally and subluxates relative to the femoral condyle when posterolateral instability is present (DeLee et al. 1983a,b; Hughston et al. 1976b; Hughston and Norwood 1980). Disruption of the PCL combined with injuries of the arcuate complex would by definition lead to SLI (Hughston et al. 1976b). Kennedy (1983) and DeLee et al. (1983b) took issue with this concept by noting that the distinction between true SLI and PLRI was a simplification of clinical reality. Moreover, cadaver experiments by Hertel (1980), Jakob et al. (1981), Gollehon et al. (1987), and others (Fabbricciani et al. 1982; Kennedy and Towler 1971; Noesberger and Paillet 1976; Noyes et al. 1983; Trickey 1984a,b; Trillat et al. 1978) clearly showed that the rotational axis of a knee with damaged lateral ligaments does not correspond to the PCL, and that the pathomechanical situation resulting from the injuries always represents a combination of rotation and translation. The complexity of the capsuloligamentous apparatus led Noyes et al. (1983) to propose the concept of the "envelope of motion" (in which joint components are free to move) as a means of describing clinical pathomechanics more precisely. Recently Müller et al. (1988) presented the OAK scheme for clinical evaluation of the functional significance of a given instability (see chapter by Müller et al., p. 123 ff.). This approach is based on the concept that rotational and translational knee motions never occur in isolation but are invariably combined with each other, and that clinical tests should be performed using an "unconstrained" technique. Also, factors such as constitution, inherent ligamentous laxity, and morphytype should be taken into account. Within the framework of this new concept, SLI and PLRI are viewed as examples of coupled translational and rotational motions.

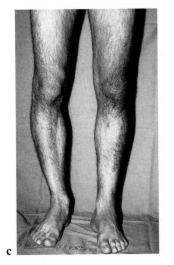

◁ **Fig. 7. a** In the normal knee the mechanical axis of the limb runs slightly medial to the center of the joint. With a varus morphotype or with injury to the arcuate complex, the axis is shifted medially. **b** Standing on one leg increases the loss of coaptation in the lateral compartment, with resultant stretching of the lateral capsule and ligaments and excessive loading of the medial compartment. **c** With chronic posterolateral instability, the morphotypic varus overload is increased. (From Charmion 1984)

Table 3. Clinical signs of lateral and posterolateral instability

Diagnosis	Lesion	Clinical signs
SLI (mild)	Isolated LCL (rare)	1 + Varus opening in 20° flexion
SLI (severe)	LCL Arcuate complex PCL + / − ACL	2–3 + Varus opening in full extension 1 + ERR 1 + PD in neutral rotation 1 + AD in internal rotation True hyperextension only with tear of ACL
PLRI (mild)	LCL Arcuate complex + / − Lateral meniscus (PCL intact)	1 + ERR 1 + PLD 2 + RPST 2–3 + Varus opening in 20° flexion Slightly increased external rotation in 30° and 90° flexion PD greater at 30° than at 90°
PLRI (severe)	LCL Arcuate complex + / − Lateral meniscus + PCL	1 + ERR 1 + PD in neutral rotation 2–3 + Varus opening in full extension Markedly increased external rotation in 30° and 90° flexion
ALRI	ACL Middle third of lateral capsule	1 + True pivot shift sign 1 + Lachman (AD in 20° flexion) 1 + AD in 90° flexion (passive)
Isolated PCL	+ PCL + / − Ligs of Wrisberg and Humphrey	1 + Active AD (false-positive reduced from position of posterior subluxation) + / − PD in neutral rotation and 90° flexion
Combined ALRI and PLRI	+ ACL + Arcuate complex + / − PCL + Middle third of lateral capsule	1 + True pivot shift sign 1 + RPST 1 + Lachman 1 + ERR 1 + PLD or PD in neutral rotation 1 + Passive external rotation icrease in 20° flexion

ERR, External rotation-recurvatum test; *PLD*, posterolateral drawer; *RPST*, reversed pivot shift test; *PD*, posterior drawer; *AD*, anterior drawer; *SLI*, straight lateral instability; *PCL*, posterior cruciate ligament; *ACL*, anterior cruciate ligament; *LCL*, lateral collateral ligament

Clinical Evaluation of Straight Lateral Instability and of Acute and Chronic Posterolateral Rotatory Instability in the Knee

Acute (Severe) Straight Lateral Instability

History and Clinical Examination

Because severe SLI is associated with extensive disruption of the lateral compartment and cruciate ligaments, these injuries are all diagnosable in the acute stage. Indeed, dislocation of the knee must be excluded in these cases, and assessment of neurovascular status is an integral part of the workup (DeLee et al. 1983b). A significant number of patients exhibit common peroneal nerve injury (DeLee et al. 1983a; Platt 1924; Towne et al. 1971; Watson-Jones 1931), and the finding of a neurologic deficit is helpful in as-

sessing the severity of the trauma. Posttraumatic hemarthrosis often resolves spontaneously as a result of capsular disruption. The clinical signs are summarized in Table 3. It is particularly noteworthy that the pronounced 3 + varus laxity in extension is a reliable indicator of associated PCL injury (DeLee 1983b).

Conventional and Stress Radiography, Examination under Anesthesia, and Arthroscopy

Conventional radiographs may demonstrate associated injuries such as an avulsion fracture of the fibular head, an avulsion of Gerdy's tubercle, or a nondisplaced fracture of the medial tibial plateau. We routinely obtain stressradiographs to establish the direction and degree of the ligamentous instability, although in severe cases one must consider the risk of causing additional peroneal damage by stressing open the lateral compartment (Towne et al. 1971). Examination under anesthesia is also helpful as it eliminates protective muscular contractions due to pain. The clinical stress tests must be performed carefully to avoid neurovascular damage. Although DeLee et al. (1983 a,b) feel that arthroscopy is contraindicated in these acute cases due to the risk of fluid extravasation, we have used it successfully and uneventfully to exclude or confirm intraarticular pathology.

Acute Posterolateral Rotatory Instability

History and Clinical Examination

The history of this injury is frequently marked by a collision between a pedestrian and motor vehicle or a violent blow sustained during contact sports (Baker et al. 1983; DeLee et al. 1983 a; Hughston and Jacobson 1985; Hughston and Norwood 1980; Hughston et al. 1976 b). The most common mechanism of injury is an anteromedial blow to the proximal tibia in the extended knee, driving the tibia backward into varus hyperextension and external rotation. Typically this blow is sustained from an automobile bumper or from the shoulder of a tackler in football (Baker et al. 1983; Hughston and Norwood 1980; Hughston et al. 1976 b).

Symptoms are often mild in the acute stage (DeLee et al. 1983 a; Hughston and Jacobson 1985; Hughston and Norwood 1980). Typically there are mild lateral complaints associated with posterolateral tenderness or a contusion over the medial upper tibia (DeLee et al. 1983 a; Hughston and Jacobson 1985; Hughston and Norwood 1980). Examination without anesthesia can be hampered by muscle spasm, apprehension, and pain (DeLee et al. 1983 a; Hughston and Norwood 1980), so we examine all of our patients under anesthesia and by stressradiography. The diagnosis of PLRI as an isolated condition or combined with other rotatory instabilities can be difficult and requires a thorough knowledge of the appropriate stability tests and a meticulous technique (Hughston and Norwood 1980). Besides the pivot shift sign, Lachman test, and standard anterior drawer test used to diagnose anterior instability, we favor 3 special tests (Jakob et al. 1981) that are specific for posterolateral instability: the external rotation-recurvatum test and posterolateral drawer test of Hughston and Norwood (1980) and the reversed pivot shift test of Jakob et al. (1981).

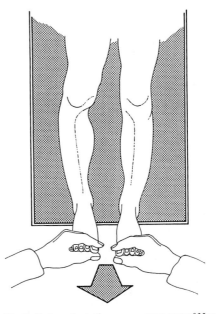

Fig. 8. External rotation-recurvatum test of Hughston. With the patient relaxed and supine, both legs are lifted up by the toes. When posterolateral instability is present, the leg will assume a position of hyperextension and varus angulation, with simultaneous external rotation of the tibia. (From Jakob et al. 1981)

External Rotation-Recurvatum Test (Hughston and Norwood 1980; Hughston et al. 1976 a,b)

This test demonstrates the abnormal relationship between the tibia and femur near extension (Fig. 8). Falling of the leg into hyperextension and varus bowing in this test should be distinguished from true hyperextension occurring in association with a concomitant rupture of the ACL (Hughston and Norwood 1980; Jakob et al. 1981; Nicholas 1978).

Posterolateral Drawer Test

Bousquet (1972), Bousquet et al. (1986), and Hughston and Norwood (1980) are the authors of this sign (Figs. 9, 10). The test demonstrates the abnormal relationship between the tibia and femur in flexion. When the sign is elicited, it is necessary to differentiate an isolated peripheral lesion from an injury that also involves the PCL. Hughston and Norwood (1980) state that a positive posterior drawer sign in neutral tibial rotation signifies a tear of the PCL. Jakob et al. (1981) state that an isolated posterolateral lesion is expressed as a posterolateral translation of the tibia in external rotation that reduces in neutral rotation, measurable by the posterior sag of the

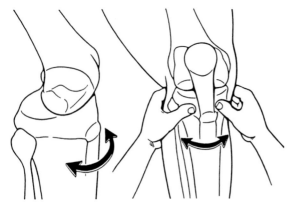

Fig. 9. Hypermotility of the lateral compartment ("posterolateral syndrome"). (From Charmion 1984)

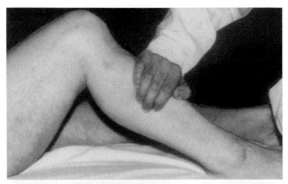

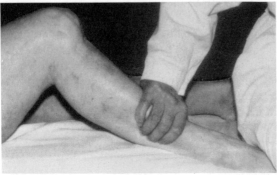

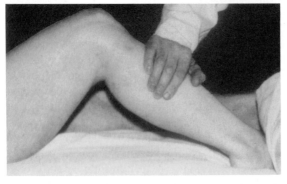

Fig. 10. A posterior drawer sign of 2 + in neutral rotation, 3 + in external rotation, and 0 in internal rotation is typical of severe posterolateral instability. (From Jakob et al. 1981)

proximal tibia or loss of the normal "step" in the proximal tibial border relative to the femur. In internal rotation, tightening of the medial collateral ligament and posterior capsule prevent the posterior translation, or make it difficult to elicit, even in the absence of the PCL. Clancy et al. (1983) claim that abolition of the posterior drawer sign in a PCL-deficient knee implies that both meniscofemoral ligaments (Wrisberg and Humphrey) are sufficient. Grood et al. (1988) and Gallehon et al. (1987) observed that a posterior drawer sign that is more prominent in 30° of knee flexion that at 90° signifies an isolated injury of the arcuate complex. It is clear that a lesion of the PCL allows greater posterior translation in flexion than near extension, creating a situation precisely opposite to that in the Lachman test for ACL insufficiency. Nevertheless, the posterior translation can also be demonstrated in the form of a posterior drawer sign near extension. Shelbourne (1988) recently described a dynamic posterior tibial subluxation test that gives an impressive clinical demonstration of the posterior drawer sign but unfortunately cannot differentiate between pure posterolateral instability and a combined instability (PCL-associated type) or even anterior instability. In this sense the sign expresses nothing more than the difficulty of determining the direction of displacement and the neutral positions when the drawer sign is elicited. The evaluation is further complicated by the fact that this sign can also be positive in knees with anterior instability (true pivot shift).

Reversed Pivot Shift Test (Jakob et al. 1981)

The reversed pivot shift test is a dynamic test in which motions occur so rapidly that the true extent of translation and rotation is difficult to assess (Müller et al. 1988). Even so, the sign can furnish useful information on the functional instability that is present in a given patient (Fig. 11). Like the true pivot shift sign of anterior instability, the reversed pivot shift phenomenon expresses the dynamic functional instability that is subjectively perceived by the patient. Characteristic of posterolateral instability, this sign is distinct from that associated with isolated injuries of the PCL or posteromedial instability. The examination is best performed under anesthesia in acutely injured patients.

The pathomechanics of the clinically elicited sign are best described in terms of abnormal tibial motion upon the relatively immobile femur. In the actual situation the phenomenon probably involves a reciprocal sequence of events in which the femur exhibits

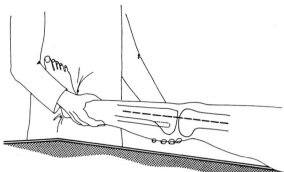

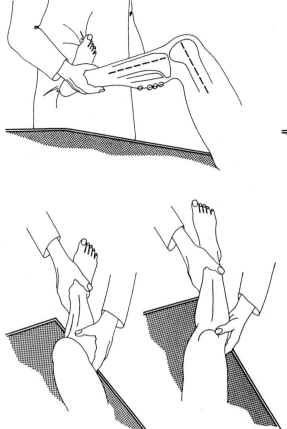

Fig. 11. Demonstration of the reversed pivot shift sign. The patient is placed supine on the examining table. To test the right knee, the examiner lifts the foot and ankle with his right hand, resting it against the right side of his pelvis. The left hand supports the lateral side of the calf with the palm on the proximal fibula. The examiner now flexes the knee to 70°–80°. In the presence of posterolateral instability, external rotation of the foot in this position will cause the lateral tibia to subluxate posteriorly in relation to the lateral femoral condyle. This is evidenced by a posterior sag of the lateral tibial plateau. The examiner now extends the knee and leans slightly against the foot to transmit an axial load through the leg and a valgus stress to the knee. When the knee reaches 20° flexion, the lateral tibial plateau reduces from its position of posterior subluxation with a reverse pivot-shift-like motion. If the test is initiated with the tibia in the reduced position of full extension and neutral rotation, and the knee is flexed rapidly while the foot is allowed to rotate externally, a similar shift will occur at about 10° of flexion as the tibia falls into posterior subluxation. (From Jakob et al. 1981)

abnormal motion on the tibia, which is fixed by contact of the foot with the ground. As we see in Fig. 12, the test can be performed in a way that demonstrates both the subluxation phase and the reduction phase of the phenomenon. The sign should be judged clinically significant only if it affects one side exclusively or predominantly and if other signs of posterolateral instability are present (Jakob et al. 1981), because many patients, especially females, with constitutional ligamentous laxity will exhibit physiologic translations of the lateral compartment that may be interpreted as a 1 + reversed pivot shift. Based on their experience in cadaver studies, the authors (Jakob et al. 1981) suggest that a reversed pivot shift sign of 2 + signifies an isolated lesion of the arcuate complex while a 3 + sign implies that a PCL injury is also present.

Varus Stress Test

Many authors believe that 2 + to 3 + lateral joint opening in 30° flexion reflects a lesion of the arcuate complex, while 2 + to 3 + opening in extension im-

plies a concomitant lesion of the PCL (DeLee et al. 1983a; Hughston and Jacobson 1985; Hughston et al. 1976b). It is difficult, however, to interpret varus opening of the fully extended knee due to the possibility of simultaneous external rotation of the tibia on the femur (DeLee et al. 1983a; Hughston et al. 1976b).

Conventional and Stressradiography, Examination under Anesthesia, and Arthroscopy

Besides avulsion of the fibular head and the rare fracture of the medial tibial plateau, radiographs frequently demonstrate a Segond fracture (Segond 1879) of the lateral tibial plateau. Woods et al. (1979) call this the "lateral capsular sign" and claim that it is commonly associated with lesions of the ACL, though other studies have been unable to confirm this (Baker et al. 1983; DeLee et al. 1983a; Johnson 1979). Examination under anesthesia is extremely important for identifying the neutral point between anterior and posterior translation. Stressradiography is very useful in this situation to establish the direc-

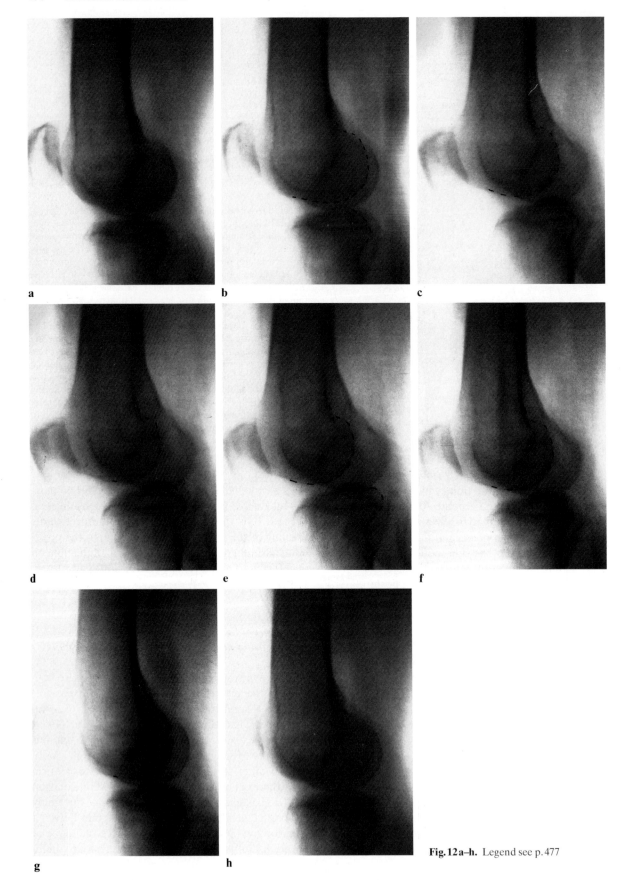

Fig. 12a–h. Legend see p. 477

tion and degree of instability on the frontal and sagittal planes (Stäubli and Jakob 1990; Järvisen and Kannas 1985) (Fig. 13). Arthroscopy provides a valuable adjunct for detecting concomitant meniscal lesions and associated injuries of the central pivot.

Chronic Posterolateral Rotatory Instability

History and Physical Examination

Chronic PLRI often presents more conspicuous signs than an acute injury, and it is commonly accompanied by other instabilities (Hughston and Jacobson 1985; Hughston et al. 1976b). Typical complaints are a feeling of the knee "giving way backward" into hyperextension and inability to lock the knee in full extension during walking and standing (Hughston and Jacobson 1985; Hughston and Norwood 1980; Hughston et al. 1976a,b; Nicholas 1978). When we observe these patients during gait, we find that they keep the knee flexed to avoid excessive internal rotation and posterior subluxation of the lateral tibial plateau relative to the lateral femoral condyle (Hughston and Norwood 1980; Jakob et al. 1981). They do better when they wear a shoe with a raised heel, as this keeps the knee flexed throughout the gait cycle. In one-legged stance, slight to pronounced varus angulation is noted due to lateral separation of the articular surfaces (see Fig. 7). Most patients are easily examined without anesthesia since there is little muscle spasm. The OAK approach to the examination of this condition includes a quantitative description of the degree of compartmental displacement in relation to factors of constitutional laxity and morphotype. This method attempts to expand the traditional Hughston classification by these factors so that isolated and combined instabilities can be discriminated in terms of translation and rotation (Noyes et al. 1983). The morphotype is assessed on the frontal plane in the one-legged stance for varus or valgus, on the sagittal plane for recurvatum and ante-

curvatum, and on the transverse plane for internal and external rotation. The degree of varus angulation has important implications for the therapeutic management of chronic symptomatic PLRI.

Combined Instabilities

The differentiation between the true and reversed pivot shift signs is extremely important, because anterolateral instability is frequently combined with posterolateral instability (Bousquet 1982; Hughston et al. 1976b; Kennedy et al. 1977). The true pivot shift, reflecting anterolateral instability, is an expression of abnormal internal tibial rotation with anterior subluxation of the lateral tibial plateau (Jakob et al. 1981). The vertical axis is shifted medially and anteriorly. The 2 dynamic signs are compared schematically in Fig. 14. The position of the foot significantly influences the test. If the 2 signs are equivocal, a shift that is more prominent in internal rotation is likely to be a true pivot shift, whereas the reversed pivot shift becomes weaker or disappears in internal rotation. If both instabilities are pronounced, a double or "two-phase" pivot shift can be elicited. A positive anterior drawer sign, Lachman sign, and posterolateral drawer sign also will be present, and there will be a 1+ to 2+ varus stress test in 30° of flexion, provided the PCL is intact.

Conventional Radiography and Arthroscopy

Radiographs commonly demonstrate osteoarthritic changes in knees with chronic PLRI. This relates causally to the excessive loading of the medial compartment due to the acquired varus morphotype, and the X-ray findings may include subchondral sclerosis, cysts, joint-space narrowing, and marginal osteophytes.

As in acute injuries, arthroscopy is essential for defining the associated intraarticular pathology and assisting the planning of reconstructive measures on the central pivot.

◁ **Fig. 12a–h.** Sequential frames from a cineradiogram (frequency 24 frames/s) taken during the reverse pivot shift maneuver, elicited from a position of extension to slight flexion and then back to extension. For technical reasons the tibia is held in neutral rotation, so the rotational phenomenon occurs at the level of the femur, which is probably the case when the patient feels his knee "give way." The lateral femoral condyle and lateral tibial plateau are marked with *dashed lines*. Within 1/3 of a second the lateral femoral condyle shifts forward on the lateral tibial plateau in 10°–20° of flexion (**d, e**) and reduces in extension (**a, h**). (From Jakob et al. 1981)

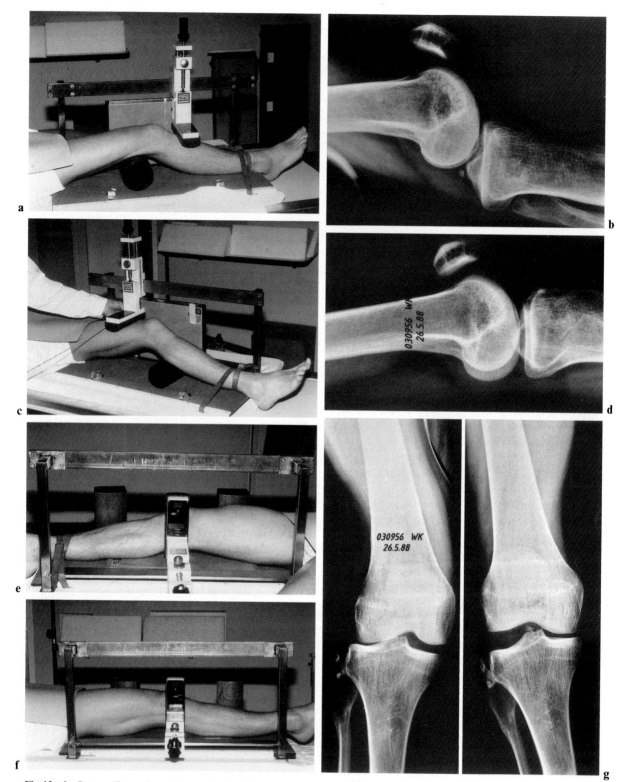

Fig. 13a–h. Stressradiography under anesthesia using a stress of 20 kp. **a, b** Posterior drawer. **c, d** Anterior translation (Lachman). **e–g** Varus, valgus stress. **h** see p. 479

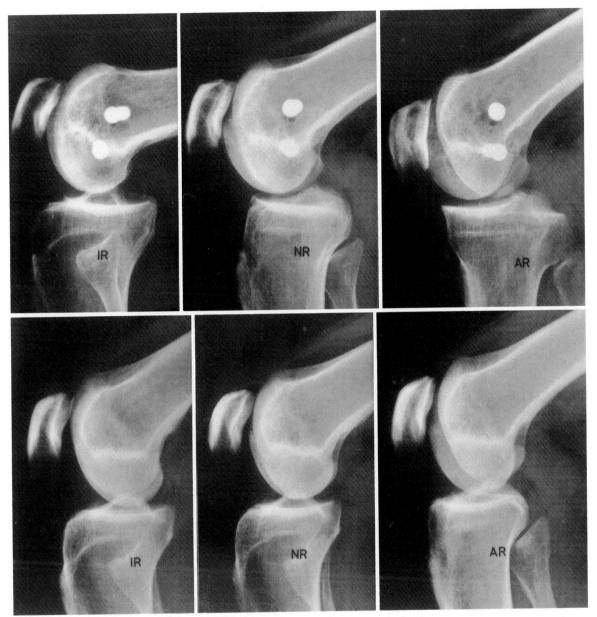

Fig. 13h. Posterior translation is more pronounced in 90° flexion than near extension (significant posterior or posterolateral instability, compared with the opposite knee)

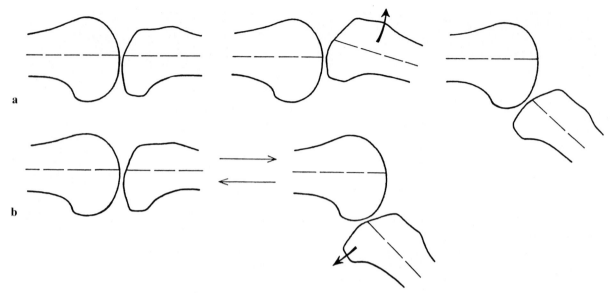

Fig. 14a, b. Comparison of the true and reversed pivot shift. **a** In the true pivot shift, the lateral tibial plateau shifts from a reduced position in extension into anterior subluxation in slight flexion and reduces again at 30° flexion. **b** In the reversed pivot shift, the lateral tibial plateau falls from a reduced position in extension into posterior subluxation and flexion. (From Jakob et al. 1981)

Therapeutic Options

Surgical Treatment of Acute SLI and PLRI

"Mild" instability cases have been variously described in the literature. Baker et al. (1983), Kannus (1989), and DeLee et al. (1983a) all emphasized the mild "1 + form" during clinical testing. The patients were able to resume all previous sports activities after cast immobilization followed by a supervised program of physiotherapy. Our treatment follows the recommendations of these authors for the conservative management of patients who show a 1 + varus instability on clinical and radiographic stress testing with the knee flexed 30° and show no varus instability in full extension. The reversed pivot shift sign should be 2 + or less. The external rotation-recurvatum test should show minimal instability, and there should be only a trace posterolateral drawer. As mentioned above, these injuries are difficult to evaluate and, we feel, require a comprehensive workup that includes examination under anesthesia, stressradiographs, and arthroscopic inspection. Stressradiography is the only quantitative procedure available for determining the direction and degree of instability in combined forms (see Fig. 13). In acute cases with moderately severe instability, we tend to favor operative treatment. This is because residual varus laxity following a lateral ligament injury tends to incite a pro-

gressive de-coaptation of the lateral articular surfaces. The conservative treatment of these injuries is less likely to yield a favorable outcome than in analogous medial injuries. As Bousquet et al. (1986) explain, this is a result of the progressive varus deformity and unphysiologic compression of the medial compartment (see Fig. 7). In cases where stress-radiography demonstrates lateral opening of 10 mm or more relative to the opposite side, it is likely that there is an associated injury of the central pivot accompanying the lesion of the arcuate complex (see Fig. 13).

Acute repairs should be performed within 2 weeks of the injury, for otherwise scarring and induration will hamper separation of the tissue layers (DeLee et al. 1983a; Hughston and Jacobson 1985). First the intraarticular pathology is assessed arthroscopically. The extraarticular approach is made through a lateral parapatellar incsion, and secondary incisions are added as findings require (Baker et al. 1983; DeLee

▷

Fig. 15a–h. Woman 49 years of age who sustained a varus injury of the right knee in a train accident. Acute anterolateral instability with bony avulsion of Gerdy's tubercle (**a, b**). Marked varus opening on the 20-kp stress films (**c** valgus, **d** varus). Marked anterior translation of 18 mm with no posterior instability (**e, f**). Avulsion fracture managed by screw fixation, with semitendinosus-augmented repair of the ACL (**g, h**)

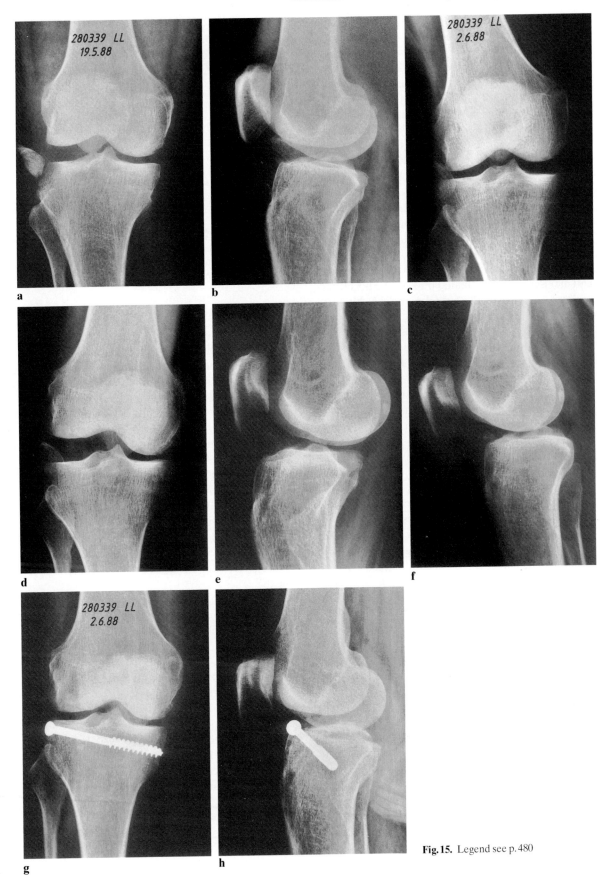

Fig. 15. Legend see p. 480

et al. 1983a,b; Fukubayashi et al. 1982). The examiner is guided by the hematoma in his initial evaluation of the pathology. The common peroneal nerve is inspected behind the biceps tendon. If it is completely severed, it may be amenable to direct repair (Novich and Newark 1960; Towne et al. 1971), or the torn ends may simply be reapproximated as a prelude to later definitive repair (Sisk 1987). If continuity is preserved (neurapraxia, axonotmesis), it is acceptable to wait for up to 18 months owing to reports of favorable spontaneous healing rates up to 69% (Kennedy 1983).

The biceps femoris tendon may be ruptured at its fibular insertion or avulsed on a piece of bone. Lesions of the iliotibial tract are rare and partial in nature (Baker et al. 1983) (Fig. 15).

Arthroscopically detected lesions of the central pivot and menisci should be treated prior to the posterolateral repair. Tears of the lateral meniscus should be tended to, as its structure contributes significantly to the stability of the lateral compartment (DeLee et al. 1983a). At sites where ACL repair is required, it is performed through the same anterolateral arthrotomy for distal lesions or through a separate anteromedial arthrotomy for femoral lesions. The sutures are passed through osseous channels, brought out and tied at the end of the operation following repair of the posterolateral lesion. A bony tibial PCL avulsion should be repaired by screw fixation through a posterior approach using the technique of Trickey (1980), Novich and Newark (1960), or O'Donoghue (1950). A femoral avulsion is reattached with nonabsorbable transosseous sutures passed through the femur. This repair is often reinforced by a patellar tendon graft and synthetic augmentation. The same applies to the more common distal tibial ligament avulsion, which we repair under arthroscopic guidance by drilling a tibial bone tunnel from the anterior side, passing a 70° scope through the intercondylar notch, and placing an accessory posteromedial incision. The drill guide may be passed through the intercondylar notch or introduced separately through the posteromedial incision, depending on the technique.

Often the severity of the trauma will dissect the popliteus tendon from the rest of the arcuate complex, usually in a muscular avulsion type of injury (Fig. 16). Unfortunately, distinction of the individual tissue planes can prove quite difficult at operation (Hughston and Jacobson 1985). Ruptures of the popliteus most commonly occur at its musculotendinous junction or at the popliteal hiatus (Fig. 17). The visualization of this region can be difficult and requires mobilization and release of the lateral head of the

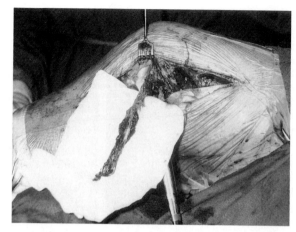

Fig. 16. Avulsion of the popliteus muscle. In this acute injury, the popliteus tendon is intact proximally at its femoral attachment but has been avulsed from the muscle

gastrocnemius (Sisk 1987). If the popliteus tendon has been avulsed distally from the muscle, the free tendon end can be used to reinforce the lateral collateral ligament, or it can be routed forward through a tibial bone tunnel using the "popliteus bypass" technique of Müller (1983). Avulsions of the popliteus tendon from its femoral attachment are repaired with transosseous sutures and a fixation screw. The peroneal-popliteal segment of this muscle and the popliteal hiatus must be inspected and repaired.

Following the popliteal repair, attention is turned to identifying the lateral collateral ligament and the arcuate ligament with its variations (fabellofibular ligament). The torn lateral collateral ligament is repaired and if necessary reinforced with a distally based strip of biceps tendon, as described by Müller (1983) (Fig. 18).

The anterolateral capsule may be avulsed from the tibia on a small flake of bone (Johnson 1979; Segond 1879; Woods et al. 1979). This lesion is repaired with transosseous sutures or screws. Interstitial tears are repaired with reefing sutures (Cabaud and Slocum 1977). Tension is restored to the arcuate complex by advancing the lateral border anteriorly and the posterior border toward the PCL (Sisk 1987). Additionally, the lateral head of the gastrocnemius can be "tacked" forward (Hughston and Norwood 1980; Fukubayashi et al. 1982). Careful inspection of the deep portion of the iliotibial tract is important; the Kaplan fiber region must be accurately repaired as it functions as the origin of the accessory lateral ligament (Lobenhoffer et al. 1987; Müller 1983; Terry et al. 1986).

This reconstruction should be performed with the knee flexed and the tibia internally rotated with re-

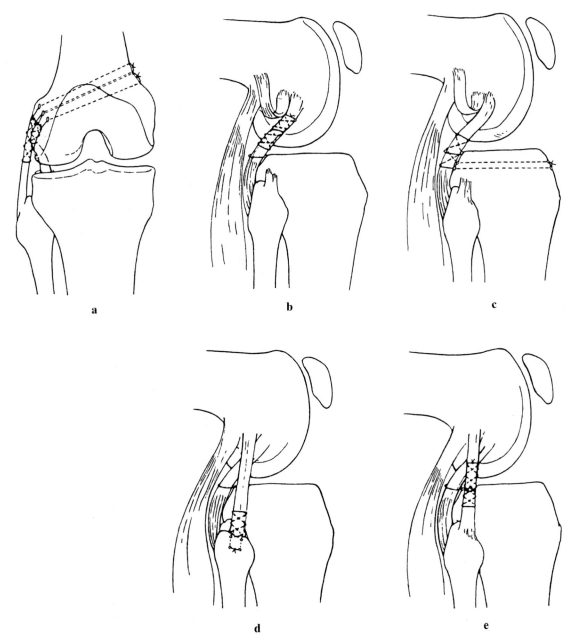

Fig. 17 a–e. Reconstruction techniques for acute ruptures of the lateral collateral ligament (LCL) and popliteus tendon. **a** Repair of a femoral avulsion of the LCL and popliteus tendon using transosseous sutures. **b** Repair of a ruptured popliteus tendon by the Bunnell technique. **c** Repair of a musculotendinous avulsion of the popliteus by tenodesis to the posterior tibia with transosseous Bunnell pullout sutures. **d** Repair of a distal osseous avulsion of the LCL. **e** Repair of a midsubstance rupture of the LCL. (From Sisk 1987)

spect to the lateral femoral condyle. The incision is closed over a suction drain, and the leg is immobilized in a long cast with the knee flexed 60° and the tibia in slight internal rotation. A pelvic support can be incorporated into the cast to prevent external rotation (Baker et al. 1983), but we have had no experience with this technique.

Chronic Posterolateral and Lateral Instability

In cases of chronic instability, the degree and direction of the instability must be accurately determined. The clinical workup for identifying accompanying instabilities must be conducted with great precision (Hughston and Jacobson 1985; Hughston et al.

1976 b; Jakob et al. 1981; Müller et al. 1988; Sisk 1987; Stäubli and Jakob 1990). In most cases we have observed that chronic symptomatic PLRI is particularly disabling when accompanied by cruciate ligament insufficiency (Bousquet et al. 1986; Jakob et al. 1981; Müller et al. 1988; Sisk 1987). It is not uncommon for ALRI to coexist with PLRI in patients with chronic anterior cruciate insufficiency. In some of these cases, initial examination fails to disclose a lesion of the ACL, which then is expressed chronically as combined ALRI and PLRI. This underscores the importance of differentiating between a true and reversed pivot shift sign (see Fig. 14). In most patients with symptomatic PLRI, we find an accompanying lesion and insufficiency of the PCL. We use stress radiography in these cases to establish the degree and direction of the instability (see Fig. 13). Sagittal and frontal stressradiographs that demonstrate translation or varus opening of more than 10 mm compared with the uninjured side indicate significant laxity of the central pivot and the arcuate complex. Chronic PLRI requiring operative treatment is frequently marked

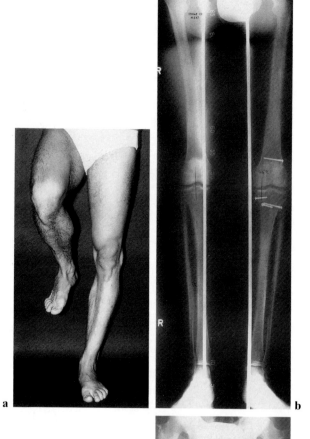

a

b

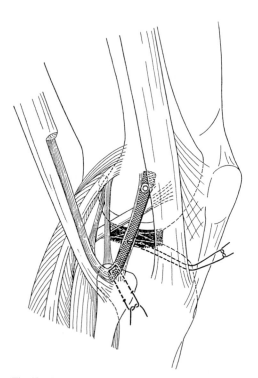

Fig. 18. Reconstruction of the LCL using the distally based anterior third of the biceps tendon. (From Müller 1983)

▷

Fig. 19. In patients with marked genu varum, the treatment of posterolateral instability must start with a realigning osteotomy. An open-wedge type of osteotomy was performed in this patient, a 39-year-old man

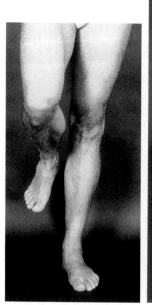

c

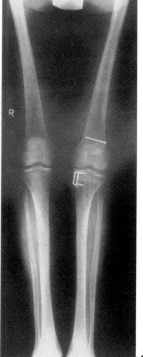

d

by pain, apprehension, instability, and clinical findings with a 3 + posterolateral drawer, a 3 + reversed pivot shift, and varus angulation on loading. We divide chronic PLRI into a form with pure posterior translation and a form with concomitant varus instability.

Generally, a combined extra- and intraarticular reconstruction is necessary for the management of chronic PLRI. The intraarticular part usually requires replacement with a patellar tendon graft and synthetic augmentation, performed under arthroscopic guidance. The intraarticular reconstruction usually precedes the posterolateral repair.

Hughston and Jacobson (1985), Trillat (1978), Bousquet et al. (1986), Müller (1983), and others (Charmion 1984; Jaeger 1984; Lerat 1977; MacIntosh and Darby 1976; Slocum et al. 1973) deserve mention in connection with reconstructions for chronic PLRI. We generally use the techniques recommended by Bousquet et al. (1986) and Müller (1983), as they are appropriate for the severe form of lateral ligament lesions. Basically we advocate the necessity of soft-tissue reconstruction including the central pivot and the integration of Bousquet's morphotype concept. We evaluate the limb morphotype by taking a full-length standing radiograph of each lower extremity (Fig. 19). In cases of significant varus angulation associated with chronic PLRI, a corrective open-wedge osteotomy of 5°–6° is sufficient to restore correct mechanical alignment. The advantage of the open-wedge osteotomy over a closed-wedge osteotomy is that it adds tension to the medial and posterolateral soft tissues. This is especially important in patients with global laxity. Owing to the connections between the oblique popliteal ligament and arcuate ligament,

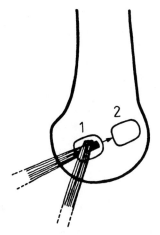

Fig. 20. In the technique of Trillat, later adopted by Hughston, the common femoral osseous attachment of the popliteus tendon and LCL is advanced proximally and anteriorly. The lateral meniscus and popliteal hiatus can be inspected prior to fixation of the bone flap

the medial open-wedge osteotomy tightens the oblique popliteal fibers, which at least in theory imparts tension to lateral structures as well. In some cases we have found that the osteotomy in itself provides sufficient stabilization, which is why we always begin with that procedure.

The critical first phase of the soft-tissue reconstructions begins by identifying and mobilizing the common peroneal nerve to protect it from direct injury or excessive traction by improperly placed reef sutures (Hughston and Jacobson 1985; Sisk 1987). The popliteus tendon and lateral collateral ligament are exposed and inspected. Since we respect the importance of isometricity of the lateral and medial

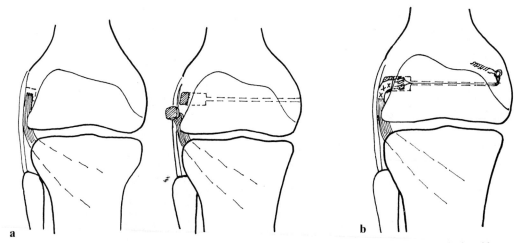

a   b

Fig. 21 a, b. Recession or "countersinking" of the popliteus tendon in the femur. This technique, which we described in 1982, restores tension to the loose tendon at its anatomic site of femoral attachment

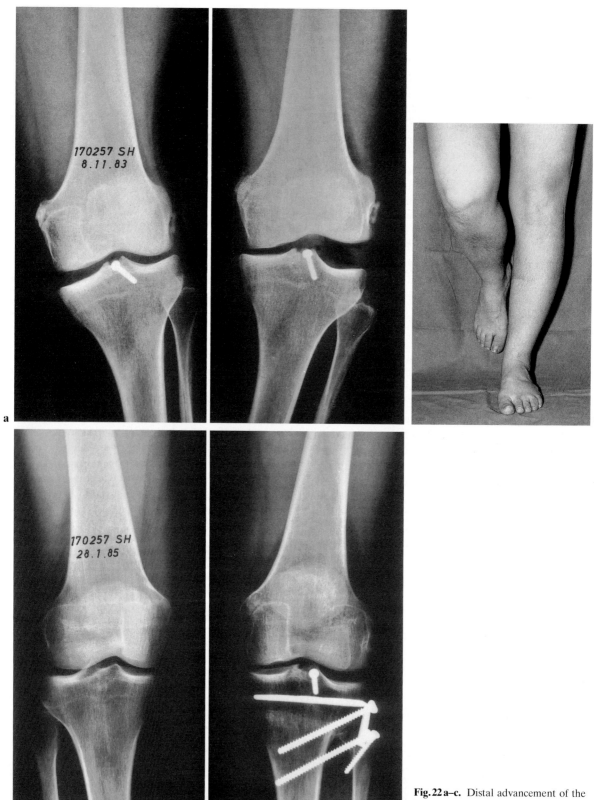

Fig. 22 a–c. Distal advancement of the LCL with a concomitant valgus osteotomy of the proximal tibia and screw fixation of the distally transposed fibular head, which tightens the LCL

collateral ligament structures according to the rules of Burmester (Menschik 1974, 1977), we do not recommend anterosuperior advancement of the common osseous origin of the popliteus tendon and collateral ligament as advocated by Trillat (1978) and Hughston and Jacobson (1985). We believe that the resulting tensile stress on the lateral collateral ligament interferes with normal kinematics and will eventually stretch the ligament and render it deficient. In these cases of a presumed proximal lesion with good quality of the popliteus tendon, we excise the femoral attachment of the popliteus tendon on a bone fragment measuring 10×10 mm. We then "countersink" this bone plug by drilling a hole of matching size in the lateral femoral condyle precisely at the original attachment site, inlaying the bone plug with attached tendon, and fixing the plug with a screw and washer. This restores tension to the tendon while preserving isometry (Fig. 21). Proximal lesions of the collateral ligament are treated separately in a similar fashion. The popliteal hiatus should be carefully inspected and repaired.

In some cases tension should be restored by advancing the insertion of the collateral ligament distally. This is done by osteotomizing the neck of the fibula, resecting a bone segment, and reapproximating the fibula with bone screws (Fig. 22). Due to the sometimes disappointing results of this technique, however, we have employed the "countersink" method since 1982.

If the quality of the popliteus tendon is inadequate for a proximal transfer, replacement becomes necessary. Bousquet has recommended 2 soft-tissue procedures. For his *"petit poplité"* reconstruction, he uses the central one-third of the biceps tendon to replace the popliteus tendon (Fig. 23); for his *"grand poplité"* he originally used fascia late, changing later to the central third of the patellar tendon to improve the quality of the reconstruction. In 1983, Müller recommended a soft-tissue operation similar to that of Bousquet (Fig. 24). Like Bousquet, Müller believes that the popliteus tendon is the most important component of the arcuate complex. He proposes (1983) that advancement and repair of the popliteus tendon

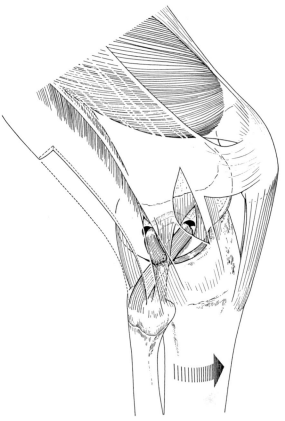

Fig. 23. "Small" popliteus reconstruction, modified from Bousquet. We use a 10- to 12-cm-long strip of biceps tendon (1/2 thickness) based distally on the fibular head to reconstruct the peroneal insertion of the popliteus. We pass the tendon beneath the LCL to the popliteus insertion and loop it back through a U-shaped tunnel in the lateral femoral condyle, where it emerges between the attachments of the LCL and lateral gastrocnemius tendon. The strip is sutured to the LCL and overlying capsule. This reconstruction can be reinforced with an augmentation band

▷

Fig. 24. "Grand poplité" reconstruction of Bousquet. The central one-third of the iliotibial tract, distally based and about 15–20 cm long, is routed posteriorly through a lateral bone tunnel in the proximal tibia, passed obliquely up along the course of the popliteus tendon to the femoral attachment of the tendon, passed back through a short femoral bone tunnel (as in the *petit poplité*), and finally sutured distally to the arcuate ligament above the fibular head. (From Bousquet et al. 1986)

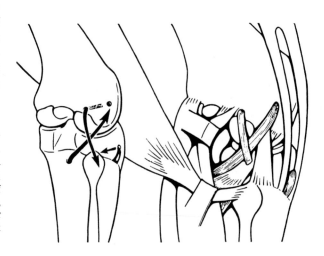

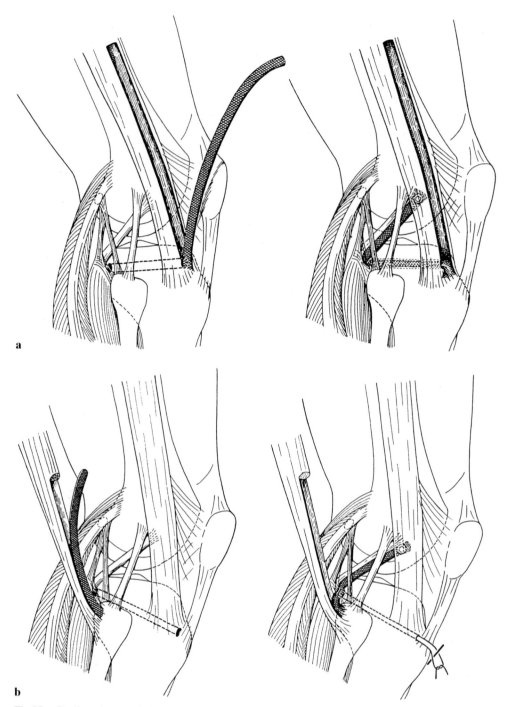

Fig. 25. a Popliteus bypass of Müller using a strip from the anterior iliotibial tract 1.5 cm wide and 16–20 cm long. The distally based strip is passed backward through a 4.5-mm tunnel in the tibial plateau (as in the *grand poplité*) and emerges directly below the cartilage surface in the region of the popliteus tendon groove. The strip is then pulled obliquely upward and forward, sutured to the posterolateral capsule, brought forward along the popliteus tendon, and fixed to the bone with a screw and plastic washer, staple, or transosseous sutures. **b** The popliteus bypass can be performed using 1/3 of the biceps tendon. The graft, based distally on the fibular head, is passed to the posterolateral corner through a soft-tissue tunnel. It is then anchored to the posterolateral tibia with transosseous sutures, brought upward and fixed along the course of the popliteus tendon as in **a**. (From Müller 1983)

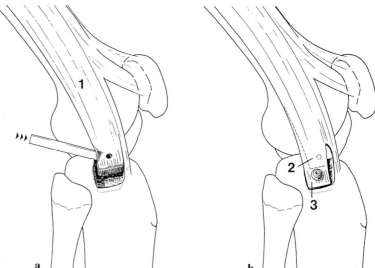

Fig. 26 a, b. Posterior and distal advancement of Gerdy's tubercle (see text)

and collateral ligament be done separately, since common advancement of these structures places than in an orientation too different from their natural anatomy. In cases where the popliteus tendon is stretched and irreparable, Müller recommends his bypass technique using a strip from the iliotibial tract or biceps tendon (Fig. 25).

We have come to believe that the transfer of large portions of the iliotibial tract predisposes to loss of lateral coaptation. There is also a risk that this relatively weak structure will become stretched over time. Moreover, the transfers are routed in part through a tibial bone tunnel that only roughly approximates the isometry of the popliteus tendon. Because the popliteus tendon is basically a nonisometric structure, it must be dynamically stabilized by muscular tension. Any static reconstruction, then, will probably become deficient over time. Like Bousquet (1986), we have observed this failure even when stronger materials such as patellar tendon were used. At the same time, there is a danger that a patellar tendon graft fixed to the bone, like that used in Bousquet's *grand poplité* reconstruction, will cause limitation of motion. Currently we perform a "small" popliteus reconstruction using a biceps tendon strip 1.5 cm wide and 10–12 cm long, which is passed directly beneath the scar of the lateral collateral ligament and routed backward through a transosseous femoral tunnel. Emerging behind the collateral ligament, the end of the strip is brought down and attached to the fibular head. This part can be reinforced by other reconstructions, and we do not hesitate to use prosthetic augmentation (Kennedy's LAD, PRO-LAD). So far we have not found a direct,

efficient technique for reinforcing the lateral collateral ligament, although we do advance Gerdy's tubercle distally and slightly posteriorly by 1–1.5 cm (Fig. 26) to tighten the deep portions of the iliotibial tract with the collateral ligament and reinforce the accessory femorotibial lateral ligament.

In patients exhibiting posterolateral and anterolateral instability with increased varus opening, we recommend the following peripheral reconstruction, which we have found to be the best combination:

- A small popliteus reconstruction using the biceps tendon to relieve posterolateral hyperrotation
- Correct anterolateral hyperrotation with a lateral repair using the Lemaire technique, in which the tunnel in the femoral condyle receives the biceps graft from the front and the strip of iliotibial tract from the rear
- If necessary, reinforce the reconstruction with a synthetic augmentation strip 18–20 cm long.

The successful treatment of posterolateral instability requires attention to the central pivot, especially the PCL. Operations that involve only a peripheral posterolateral reconstruction without restoring the central pivot are rarely performed today. Increasingly, there is a tendency to treat the central pivot, the arcuate complex, and occasionally even posteromedial instability in patients with severe posterior and posterolateral instabilities. The reconstructions in such a case would be as follows:

- Arthroscopically assisted reconstruction of the PCL using the patellar tendon, reinforced by a synthetic augmentation band, with concomitant in-

spection of the meniscus and cartilage and necessary meniscal repair (Fig. 27 a–c)
– "Small" posterolateral reconstruction of the popliteus tendon, possibly with a concomitant anterolateral Lemaire plasty, both reinforced by synthetic
augmentation (Fig. 27 c)

– Posteromedial reconstruction using a strip of semimembranosus tendon, also augmented, for coexisting posteromedial instability (Fig. 27 d)

In summary, our concept involves a step-by-step surgical reconstruction dictated by the severity of the ligamentous injury (Table 4). Because the combination of soft-tissue and bony reconstructions is a very

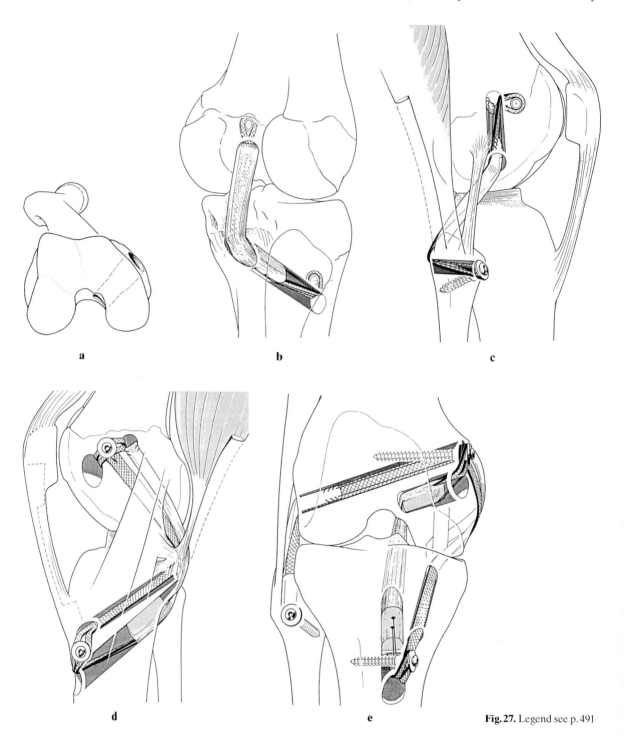

Fig. 27. Legend see p. 491

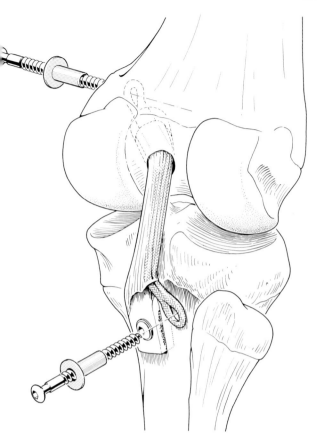

Fig. 28. Two-stage PCL reconstruction using patellar ligament augmented by a Prolad fixed with anchorage sleeves and screws. (Prolad – Protek ligament augmentation device – Protek, Bern, Switzerland)

Table 4. Recommended procedures for chronic posterolateral instability

Lesion	Surgical procedure
1. Pronounced varus morphotype	Open-wedge osteotomy
2. Torn PCL	Reconstruction with central third of patellar tendon, reinforced by synthetic augmentation (semiarthroscopic)
3. Proximal tear of popliteus tendon	Recession of popliteus insertion
4. Midthird or distal popliteus tear	Small popliteus reconstruction using the biceps tendon (may be augmented)
5. Proximal tear of lateral collateral ligament	Recession of lateral collateral ligament insertion
6. Midsubstance tear of lateral collateral ligament	Distal or posterior advancement of Gerdy's tubercle
7. Laxity of arcuate complex and posterior capsule	Reefing of arcuate ligament
8. Combined anterolateral and posterolateral lesions plus varus instability	Peripheral lateral extraarticular reconstruction of Lemaire plus small popliteus reconstruction of Bousquet, augmented with a synthetic strip; augmented reconstruction of the PCL
9. Posteromedial instability	Semimembranosus transfer with augmentation

extensive operation, we recommend a staged approach beginning with a corrective osteotomy followed by the ligament reconstruction 3–6 months later.

More recently we have adopted a PCL reconstruction technique which splits the surgery into anterior and a posterior approaches. The problem was that we had difficulty placing the tibial attachment anatomically from in front without kinking the graft around the corner of the tibia. We perform the anterior part with fixation of the bone plug wedged into the medial femoral condyle, keeping the bone tendon junction at the inner wall of the notch (Fig. 28). We fix the Prolad solidly with a grummet at the medial femoral cortex

◁ **Fig. 27 a–e.** All instability components should be taken into account in the treatment of posterolateral instability. With acute or chronic instability, coexisting instability of the PCL also must be treated, along with any posterolateral laxity that is present. **a, b** Reconstruction of the PCL using a 14-mm-wide strip from the central third of the patellar tendon with attached bone blocks (trapezoidal patellar block), reinforced with a synthetic augmentation band. The graft is pulled upward into the joint, wedging the proximal bone plug in the femoral condyle. The synthetic band and autologous graft are each fixed with a screw. The synthetic strip is inserted by closed technique beneath the most anterior layer of the patellar tendon graft. **c** Small lateral popliteus reconstruction using one-half the biceps tendon, reinforced by augmentation with a thin, narrow synthetic band passed obliquely through the fibular head and brought out me-

dially through the femoral tunnel, where it is anchored at the fixaton site of the PCL. **d** Reconstruction to relieve posteromedial instability. A strip of semimembranosus tendon based on the tibia is passed beneath the posterior oblique ligament to the medial epicondyle or adductor tubercle, where it is attached by intraosseous fixation. If a small popliteus reconstruction has been done on the lateral side in the same patient, the semimembranosus strip can be pulled into the femoral tunnel, which has been anatomically positioned using a drill guide. A synthetic augmentation strip passes from the anterolateral aspect of the upper tibia to the semimembranosus attachment (drill guide!). In this way 1 femoral screw can anchor 2 or 3 augmentations. **e** Central, lateral, and medial reconstructions with corresponding augmentations

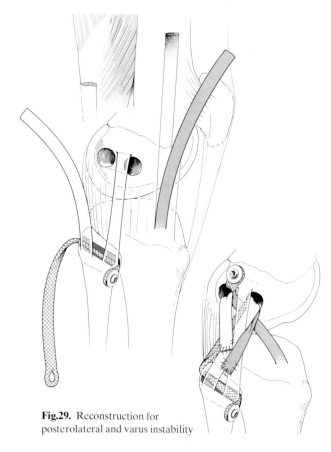

Fig. 29. Reconstruction for posterolateral and varus instability

and tie the bone plug sutures around at an appropriate distance to allow distal fixation. We then close the wound anteriorly and turn the patient to the prone position and redrape him. This can either be done immediately or a week later.

Posteriorly we enter through a straight midline incision lateral or medial to the neurovascular bundle, above and below the branches to the lateral gastrocnemius muscle (Fig. 29). The bone plug is then retrieved through a longitudinal incision of the posterior capsule dividing the oblique popliteal ligament. A bony bed is prepared with the chisel to receive the flat tibial plug, which is fixed with a screw and metal washer under appropriate tension. The Prolad is then fixed with the anchorage sleeve to the tibia, beside the bone plug. This technique is obviously more extensive; however, it is worth the effort and the early results are more gratifying. With posterolateral hyperrotation this is combined with a small Prolad augmented popliteus plasty. With varus instability we add a Lemaire-type plasty (Fig. 29).

The authors thank Mr. H. Holzherr, Department of Instructional Media, University of Bern and Inselspital Bern, for providing the illustrations (Figs. 2, 4, 23, 26, 27).

References

Abbot LC, Saunders BM, Bost FC, Anderson CE (1941) Injuries to the knee joint. J Bone Joint Surg 26: 503–521

Baker CL, Norwood LA, Hughston JC (1983) Acute posterolateral rotatory instability of the knee. J Bone Joint Surg [Am] 65: 614–618

Barnett CH, Richardson AT (1953) The postural function of the popliteus muscle. Am Phys Med 1: 177–179

Basmajian JU, Lovejoy JF (1971) Functions of the popliteus muscle in man. A multifactorial electromyographic study. J Bone Joint Surg [Am] 53: 557–562

Bousquet (1972) Les lésions graves récentes, classification et principe du traitement. Rev Chir Orthop 58 [Suppl 1]: 49–56

Bousquet G, Charmion L, Passot JP, Girardin P, Relave M, Gazielly D (1986) Stabilisation du condyle externe du genou dans les laxités antérieures chroniques. Importance du muscle poplité. Rev Chir Orthop 72: 427–434

Brantigan OC, Voshell AF (1941) The mechanics of the ligaments and menisci of the knee joint. J Bone Joint Surg 23: 44–66

Bruser DM (1960) A direct lateral approach to the lateral compartment of the knee joint. J Bone Joint Surg [Br] 42: 348–351

Cabaud HE, Slocum DB (1977) The diagnosis of chronic anterolateral rotatory instability of the knee. Am J Sports Med 5: 99–105

Charmion L (1984) Conception de la stabilisation du condyle externe du genou dans les laxités antérieures chroniques ou intégration du muscle poplité dans la chirurgie ligamentaire du genou. Thèse présentée à l'Université de Saint-Etienne

Cohn AK, Mains DB (1979) Popliteal hiatus of the lateral meniscus. Anatomy and measurement at dissection of 10 specimen. Am J Sports Med 7: 221–226

Colonna PC (1930) A fascia check-bank for relief of paralytic genu recurvatum. Am Surg 91: 624–626

Clancy WG, Shelbourne KD, Zoellner GB, Keene JS, Reider B, Rosenberg TD (1983) Treatment of knee joint instability secondary to rupture of the posterior cruciate ligament, J Bone Joint Surg [Am] 65: 310–322

DeHaven KE (1978) Classification and diagnosis of knee instabilities. Symposium on reconstructive surgery of the knee. Mosby, St. Louis

DeLee JC, Riley MB, Rockwood CA (1983a) Acute posterolateral rotatory instability of the knee. Am J Sports Med 11: 199–207

DeLee JD, Riley MB, Rockwood CA (1983b) Acute straight lateral instability of the knee. Am J Sports Med 11: 404–411

Ellison AE (1975) Anterolateral rotatory instability. The knee in sports, continuing education course. The American Academy of Orthopaedic Surgeons, Ann Arbor/MI

Fabbriciani C, Oransky M, Zoppi U (1982) Il muscolo popliteo: Studio anatomico. Arch Ital Anat Embriol 87: 203–217

Fetto JF, Marshall R (1979) Injury to the anterior cruciate ligament producing the pivot-shift sign. An experimental study in cadaver specimens. J Bone Joint Surg [Am] 61: 710–714

Fukubayashi T, Torzilli PA, Sherman MF, Warren RF (1982) An in vitro biomechanical evaluation of anterior-posterior motion of the knee. Tibial replacement, rotation, and torque. J Bone Joint Surg [Am] 64: 258–264

Fulkerson JP, Gonling HB (1980) Anatomy of the knee joint lateral retinaculum. Clin Orthop 153: 183–188

Fürst CM (1903) Der Musculus Popliteus und seine Sehne. Acta Regiae Societatis Physiographicae Lundensis. E. Malmström Lund

Funk FJ (1983) Discussion. In: DeLee JC, Riley MB, Rockwood CA (eds) Acute posterolateral rotatory instability of the knee. Am J Sports Med. 11: 199–207

Galeazzi R (1927) Clinical and experimental study of lesions of the semi-lunar cartilages of the knee joint. J Bone Joint Surg 9: 515–523

Galway RD (1972) Pivot-shift syndrome. J Bone Joint Surg [Br] 54: 558

Galway RD, Beaupre A, MacIntosh DL (1972) Pivot shift: a clinical sign of symptomatic anterior cruciate insufficiency. J Bone Joint Surg [Br] 54: 763

Gill AB (1931) Operation for correction of paralytic genu recurvatum. J Bone Joint Surg [Br]: 44–53

Gollehon DL, Torzilli PA, Warren RF (1987) The role of the posterolateral und cruciate ligament in stability of the human knee. J Bone Surg [Am] 69: 233–242

Gould JD, Torzilli PA, Adams TC, Warren RF, Levy M (1984) The effect of lateral meniscectomy on knee motion. Trans Orthop Res Soc 9: 25

Grood ES, Noyes FR, Butler DL, Suntay WJ (1981) Ligamentous and capsular restraints preventing medial and lateral laxity in intact human cadaver knees. J Bone Joint Surg [Am] 63: 1257–1269

Grood ES, Stowers SF, Noyes FR (1988) Limits of movement in the human knee. Effect of sectioning the posterior cruciate ligament and posterolateral structures. J Bone Joint Surg [Am] 70: 88–97

Helfet AJ (1974) Disorders of the knee. In: Nicholas JA (ed) Rehabilitation of the knee. Lippincott, Philadelphia

Hertel P (1980) Verletzungen und Spannung von Kniebändern. Hefte Unfallheilkd 142: 1–94

Heyman C (1924) A method for the correction of paralytic genu recurvatum. J Bone Joint Surg 6: 689–695

Highet WB, Holmes W (1942) Traction injuries to the lateral popliteal nerve and traction injuries to peripheral nerves after suture. Br J Surg 30: 212–233

Hughston JC (1962) Acute knee injuries in athletes. Clin Orthop 23: 114–133

Hughston JC, Jacobson KE (1985) Chronic posterolateral rotatory instability of the knee. J Bone Joint Surg [Am] 67: 351–359

Hughston JC, Norwood LA (1980) The posterolateral drawer text and external rotational recurvatum test for posterolateral rotatory instability. Clin Orthop 147: 82–87

Hughston JC, Andrews JR, Cross MJ, Moschi A (1976a) Classification of knee ligament instabilities, Part I. The medial compartment and cruciate ligaments. J Bone Joint Surg [Am] 58: 159–172

Hughston JC, Andrews JR, Cross MJ, Moschi A (1976b) Classification of knee ligament instabilities, Part II. The lateral compartment. J Bone Joint Surg [Am] 58: 173–179

Hughston JC, Bowden JA, Andrews JR et al. (1980) Acute tears of the posterior cruciate ligament. J Bone Joint Surg [Am] 62: 438–450

Isnar VT (1947) Functional aspects of the abductor muscles of the hip. J Bone Joint Surg 29: 607–619

Irwin CE (1949) The iliotibial band. Its role in producing deformity in poliomyelitis. J Bone Joint Surg [Am] 31: 141–146

Jaeger JH (1984) Techniques chirurgicales pour une lésion du compartiment externe. In: Bonnel F, Jaeger JH, Mansat C (éds) Les laxités chroniques du genu. Masson, Paris, pp 148–153

Jakob RP, Hassler H, Stäubli H-U (1981) Observations on rotatory instability of the lateral compartment of the knee. Acta Orthop Scand 191: 6–27

Järvisen M, Kannas P (1985) Clinical and radiological long-term results after primary knee ligament surgery. Arch Orthop Trauma Surg 104: 1–6

Jobe FW (1980) Acute tears of the lateral complex. In: Funk FJ (ed) AAOS. Symposium on the athlete's knee. Surgical Repair and reconstruction. Mosby, St. Louis Toronto London, pp 164–172

Johnson LL (1979) Lateral capsular ligament complex: anatomical and surgical considerations. Am J Sports Med 7: 156–160

Kannus P (1989) Non-operative treatment of grade II and III sprains of the lateral ligament compartment of the knee. Am J Sports Med 17: 83–88

Kaplan EB (1957a) Factors responsible for the static stability of the knee joint. Bull Hosp Jt Dis 18: 51–59

Kaplan EB (1957b) Surgical approach to the lateral (peroneal) side of the knee joint. Surg Gynecol Obstet 104: 346–356

Kaplan EB (1961) The fabellofibular and short lateral ligament of the knee joint. J Bone Joint Surg [Am] 43: 169–179

Kaplan EB (1962) Some aspects of functional anatomy of the human knee joint. Clin Orthop 23: 18–29

Kaplan EB (1988) The iliotibial tract. J Bone Joint Surg [Am] 40: 817–832

Kennedy JC (1983) Discussion. In: DeLee JC, Riley MB, Rockwood CA (eds) Acute straight lateral instability of the knee. Am J Sports Med 11: 404–411

Kennedy JC, Swan WJ (1972) Lateral instability of the knee following lateral compartment injury. J Bone Joint Surg [Br] 54: 763

Kennedy J, Towler RJ (1971) Medial and anterior instability of the knee. J Bone Joint Surg [Am] 53: 1257

Kennedy JC, Roth JH, Walker DM (1974) Posterior cruciate ligament injuries. Orthop Digest 7: 19–31

Kennedy JC, Nicholas JA, Allen WC, James SL (1977) Classification of knee joint instability resulting from ligamentous damage. Vortrag, Knee Workshop Heidelberg

Kennedy JC, Stewart R, Walker DM (1978) Anterolateral rotatory instability of the knee joint, an early analysis of the Ellison procedure. J Bone Joint Surg [Am] 60: 1031–1034

Larson RL (1975) Part 2: Dislocation and ligamentous injuries of the knee. In: Rockwood CA, Green DP (eds) Fractures. Lippincott, New York, pp 1182–1245

Last RJ (1950) The popliteus muscle and the lateral meniscus. J Bone Joint Surg [Br] 32: 93–99

Lerat JL (1977) Les laxités chroniques du compartiment externe. In: Trillat A, Dejour H, Bousquet G (éds) Chirurgie du genou. 3èmes Journées Lyon, Simép, pp 107–112

Lobenhoffer P, Posel P, Witt S, Piehler J, Wirth CJ (1987) Distal femoral fixation of the iliotibial tract. Archiv Orthop Trauma Surg 106: 285–290

Loos WC, Fox JM, Blazina ME et al. (1981) Acute posterior cruciate ligament injuries. Am J Sports Med 9: 86–92

Losee RE, Johnson E Tho, Southwick WO (1978) Anterior subluxation of the lateral tibial plateau. J Bone Joint Surg [Am] 60: 1015–1030

MacIntosh DL (1974) The anterior cruciate ligament: the over-the-top repair. Annual Meeting of the American Academy of Orthopaedic Surgeons, Dallas/TX

494   R.P. Jakob and J.P. Warner

MacIntosh DL, Darby TA (1976) Lateral substitution reconstruction. J Bone Joint Surg [Br] 58: 142

Marshall JL, Rubin RM (1977) Knee ligament injuries. Orthop Clin North Am 8: 641–668

Marshall JL, Girgis FG, Zelko R (1972) The biceps femoris tendon and its functional significance. J Bone Joint Surg [Am] 54: 1444–1450

Mayer L (1930) An operation for the cure of paralytic genu recurvatum. J Bone Joint Surg 12: 845–852

Menschik A (1974) Mechanik des Kniegelenks, Teil 1. Z Orthop 112: 481–495

Menschik A (1977) The basic kinematic principle of the collateral ligaments, demonstrated on the knee joint. In: Chapchal G (ed) Injuries of the ligaments and their repair. Thieme, Stuttgart, pp 9–16

Moore HA, Larson RL (1980) Posterior cruciate ligament injuries. Am J Sports Med 8: 68–78

Müller We (1983) The knee: Form, function and ligamentous reconstruction. Springer, Berlin Heidelberg New York

Müller We, Biedert R, Hefti F, Jakob RP, Munzinger U, Stäubli H-U (1988) OAK knee evaluation. A new way to assess knee ligament injuries. Clin Orthop 232: 37–50

Naver L, Aalberg JR (1985) Avulsion of the popliteus tendon. A rare case of chondral fracture and hemarthrosis. Am J Sports Med 13: 423–424

Nicholas JA (1973) The five-one reconstruction for anteromedial instability of the knee. J Bone Joint Surg [Am] 55: 899–922

Nicholas JA (1978) Acute and chronic lateral instabilities of the knee: diagnosis, characteristics and treatment. In: Evarts CM (ed) AAOS Symposium on reconstructive surgery of the knee. Mosby, St. Louis, pp 187–206

Noesberger B, Paillot JM (1976) Biomécanique du genou. Springer, Berlin Heidelberg New York

Novich NM, Newark NJ (1960) Adduction injury of the knee with rupture of the common peroneal nerve. J Bone Joint Surg [Am] 42: 1372–1376

Noyes FR, Grood ES, Butler DL, Paulos LE (1980) Clinical biomechanics of the knee-ligament. Restraints and functional stability. American Academy of Orthopaedic Surgeons, Symposium on the Athletic Knee. Mosby, St. Louis, pp 1–35

Noyes FR, Grood ES, Suntay WJ, Butler DL (1983) The three dimensional laxity of the anterior cruciate deficient knee as determined by clinical laxity tests. Iowa Orthop J 3: 32–44

O'Donoghue DH (1950) Surgical treatment of fresh injuries to the major ligaments of the knee. J Bone Joint Surg [Am] 32: 721–738

O'Donoghue DH (1955) An analysis of end results of surgical treatment of major injuries to the ligaments of the knee. J Bone Joint Surg [Am] 37: 1–54

Palmer I (1938) On the injuries to the ligaments of the knee joint. Act Chir Scand 81 [Suppl 53]

Platt H (1924) On the peripheral nerve complication of certain fractures. J Bone Joint Surg 10: 403–414

Platt H (1940) Traction lesions of the external popliteal nerve. Lancet II: 612–614

Seebacher JR, Inglez AE, Marshall JL, Warren RF (1982) The structure of the posterolateral aspect of the knee. J Bone Joint Surg [Am] 64: 536–541

Segond P (1879) Recherches cliniques et experimentales sur les épanchements sanguins du genou par entorse. Le Progrés Médical: 297, 319, 340, 379, 400, 419

Shelbourne RD, Benedict F, McCarroll JR, Rettig AC (1988) Dynamic posterior shift test. Am J Sports Med 17: 275–277

Sisk TD (1987) Knee injuries. In: Crenshaw AH (ed) Campbell's operative orthopaedics. Mosby, St. Louis, 2283–2496

Slocum DB, Larson RL, James LS (1973) Late reconstruction procedures used to stabilize the knee. Orthop Clin North Am 4: 679

Smillie IS (1950) Injuries of the knee joint, 2nd edn. Livingstone, Edinburgh

Soudar K, Audekercke R, Murtens M (1939) Methods, difficulties, and inaccuracies in the study of the human joint kinematics and pathokinematics by the instant axis concept. Example: The knee joint. J Biochem 12: 27–33

Southmayd W, Quigley TB (1982) The forgotten popliteus muscle. Its usefulness in correction of anteromedial rotatory instability of the knee. A preliminary report. Clin Orthop 164: 9–12

Stäubli H-U, Birrer S (1990) The popliteus tendon and its fascicles at the popliteal hiatus: Gross anatomy and functional arthroscopic evaluation with and without anterior cruciate ligament deficiency. J Arthroscopy Vol 6 Nr. 3 209–220. 1990

Stäubli H-U, Jakob RP (1990) Posterior instability of the knee near extension. A clinical and stress radiographic analysis of acute injuries of the posterior cruciate ligament. J Bone Joint Surg [Br] 72: 225–230

Terry GC, Hughston JC, Norwood LA (1986) The anatomy of the iliopatellar band and iliotibial tract. Am J Sports Med 14: 39–45

Towne LC, Blazina ME, Marmor L, Lawrence JF (1971) Lateral compartment syndrome of the knee. Clin Orthop 76: 160–168

Trickey EL (1980) Injuries to the posterior cruciate ligament. Diagnosis and treatment of early injuries and reconstruction of late instability. Clin Orthop 147: 76–81

Trickey EL (1984a) Acute ligamentous injuries. In: Jackson JP, Waugh W (eds) Surgery of the knee-joint. Chapman & Hall, London

Trickey EL (1984b) Chronic ligamentous injuries. In: Jackson JP, Waugh W (eds) Surgery of the knee joint. Chapman & Hall, London, pp 172–191

Trillat A (1977) Les laxités postéroexternes du genou. Vortrag Knee Workshop Heidelberg

Trillat A (1978) Posterolateral instability. In: Schulitz KP, Krahl H, Stein WH (1978) Late reconstruction of injured ligaments of the knee. Springer, Berlin Heidelberg New York, pp 99–105

Trillat A, Ficat P, Bousquet G et al. (1972) Symposium sur les laxités traumatiques du genou. Rev Chir Orthop 58 [Suppl 1]: 31–116

Trillat A, Dejour H, Bousquet G (éds) (1978) Chirurgie du genou. 2èmes Journées Lyon, Septembre 77. Simép, Villeurbanne

Wang JB, Marshall JL (1977) The popliteus as a static stabilizer of the knee. Orthop Res Soc Proc

Wang CJ, Walker PS (1973) The effects of flexion and rotation on the length patterns of the ligaments of the knee. J Biomech 6: 587–596

Watson-Jones R (1931) Styloid process of fibula in the knee joint with peroneal palsy. J Bone Joint Surg 13: 258–260

Woods GW, Stanley RF, Tullos HS (1979) Lateral capsular sign: x-ray due to a significant knee instability. Am J Sports Med 7: 27–33

The Popliteus Tendon and Its Fascicles in the Popliteal Hiatus: Arthroscopic Functional Anatomy with and without ACL Insufficiency

H.-U. Stäubli and St. Birrer

Based on anatomic investigations of the structure (Bousquet 1977; Fabbriciani et al. 1982a,b; Fürst 1903; Last 1948; Tabutin 1977) and function of the popliteus system (Basmajian and Lovejoy 1971; Bousquet 1977; Jakob et al. 1981; Stäubli and Birrer 1989; Stäubli and Jakob 1988; Stäubli et al. 1981), the arthroscopically visible structures of the popliteal hiatus (Patel 1981) were functionally analyzed. The normal functional anatomy was compared with arthroscopically detectable lesions of the popliteus system in acute ruptures of the anterior cruciate ligament (ACL) and chronic ACL-deficient knees (Stäubli and Birrer 1989, 1990).

Anatomy

The popliteus system is integrated into the arcuate ligament complex. The musculotendinous-aponeurotic connections of the popliteus system are composed of the following structural elements (Figs. 1–4):

– Popliteus muscle
– Posterosuperior popliteomeniscal fascicle
– Arcuate popliteal ligament
– Popliteofibular fascicle
– Anteroinferior popliteomeniscal fascicle
– Popliteus tendon
– Femoral attachment of the popliteus tendon

The *popliteus muscle* passes laterally upward from the posteromedial aspect of the proximal tibial metaphysis above the soleal line. The medial portion of the popliteus muscle inserts broadly on the posterior segment of the lateral meniscus (posterosuperior popliteomeniscal fascicle), while the lateral portion passes beneath the arcuate popliteal ligament, to which it is adherent (Fabbriciani et al. 1982a). The popliteus tendon attaches to the posterosuperior and anterosuperior fibular apex by a broad slip, the popliteofibular fascicle. The popliteus tendon inserts on the posterior and middle segments of the lateral meniscus by 2 fascicles, the superior and inferior popliteomeniscal fascicles (Figs. 2–5). The tendon, the

popliteomeniscal fascicles, and the lateral wall of the lateral meniscus together define the popliteal hiatus (Cohn and Mains 1979; Patel 1981; Stäubli and Birrer 1989a,b). The popliteus tendon is covered by synovium within the hiatus. It inserts on the lateral femoral condyle at the end of the popliteal groove, i.e., the popliteal sulcus (Basmajian and Lovejoy 1971; Fürst 1903). In extension the popliteus tendon passes beyond the lateral border of the lateral femoral condyle, and in flexion it lies within the "popliteal

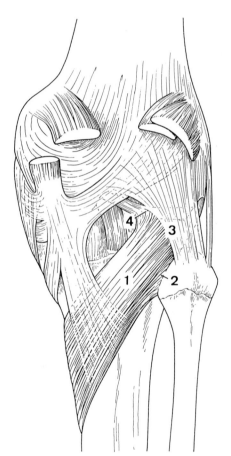

Fig. 1. Right knee, posterior aspect. *1*, Popliteus muscle; *2*, popliteofibular fascicle; *3*, arcuate popliteal ligament; *4*, posterosuperior popliteomeniscal fascicle. (From Stäubli and Birrer 1990)

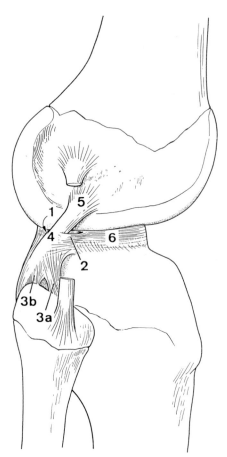

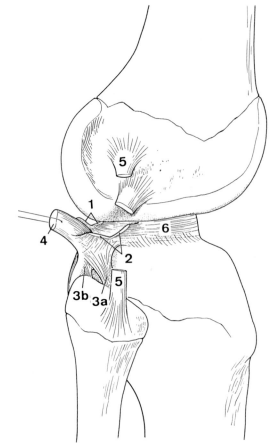

Fig. 2. Right knee, lateral aspect (lateral collateral ligament resected). *1*, Posterosuperior popliteomeniscal fascicle; *2*, inferior popliteomeniscal fascicle; *3a*, popliteofibular fascicle, anterior portion; *3b*, popliteofibular fascicle, posterior portion; *4*, popliteus tendon; *5*, femoral attachment of popliteus tendon; *6*, lateral meniscus. (From Stäubli and Birrer 1990)

Fig. 3. Popliteus tendon and popliteomeniscal fascicle. Right knee, lateral aspect (popliteus tendon divided and retracted). *1*, Posterosuperior popliteomeniscal fascicle; *2*, inferior popliteomeniscal fascicle; *3a*, popliteofibular fascicle, anterior portion; *3b*, popliteofibular fascicle, posterior portion; *4*, popliteus tendon; *5*, lateral collateral ligament (resected); *6*, lateral meniscus. (From Stäubli and Birrer 1990)

sulcus," a recess located below the lateral femoral epicondyle (Fürst 1903).

Arthroscopic Anatomy

From the standard anterolateral portal, part of the popliteus system can be inspected and functionally evaluated in the popliteal hiatus using a 30° wide-angle arthroscope (Patel 1981; Stäubli and Birrer 1989 a,b). An understanding of the functional anatomy of the popliteal hiatus presupposes a knowledge of the 3-dimensional anatomy of the popliteus system (see Fig. 5). The entrance of the popliteal hiatus is bounded superomedially by the lateral femoral condyle, superolaterally by the popliteus tendon, infero-

laterally and inferomedially by the inferior fascicle of the popliteomeniscal fiber attachments, and medially by the vertical wall of the middle segment of the lateral meniscus (Fig. 6).

Right Popliteal Hiatus

Anterolateral Approach

The 30° wide-angle arthroscope is introduced from the anterolateral portal. After inspection of the suprapatellar pouch and femoropatellar compartment with the knee extended and the scope inverted, the arthroscope is advanced into the lateral recess alongside the lateral femoral condyle and retracted under arthroscopic vision.

Fig.4. Right knee, posterolateral aspect from above. The biceps tendon, iliotibial tract, arcuate popliteal ligament, lateral collateral ligament, and posterolateral capsule have been resected to show the deep structures. *1*, Lateral meniscus; *2*, inferior popliteomeniscal fascicle; *3*, popliteus tendon (divided and retracted); *4a*, popliteofibular fascicle, anterior portion; *4b*, popliteofibular fascicle, posterior portion; *5*, superior popliteomeniscal fascicle; *6*, popliteus muscle; *7*, posterior meniscofemoral ligament (of Wrisberg); *8*, posterior cruciate ligament; *9* anterior meniscofemoral ligament (of Humphry); *10*, anterior cruciate ligament; *11*, head of fibula. (From Stäubli and Birrer 1990)   ▷

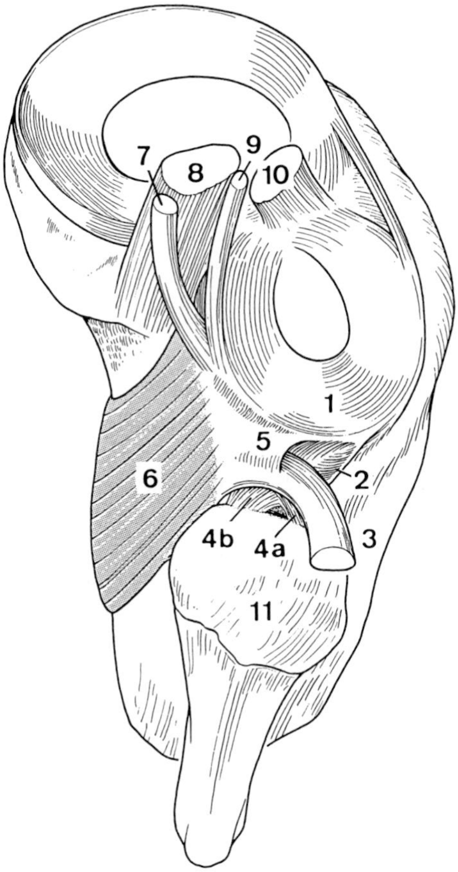

Fig.5a, b. Anatomy of the structures of the popliteal hiatus. Right knee, anterolateral aspect. *1*, Lateral collateral ligament; *2*, popliteus tendon; *3*, cartilage of lateral femoral condyle; *4*, lateral meniscus; *5*, inferior popliteomeniscal fascicle; *6*, anterior portion of popliteofibular fascicle; *7*, posterior portion of popliteofibular fascicle; *8*, head of fibula. (From Stäubli and Birrer 1990)

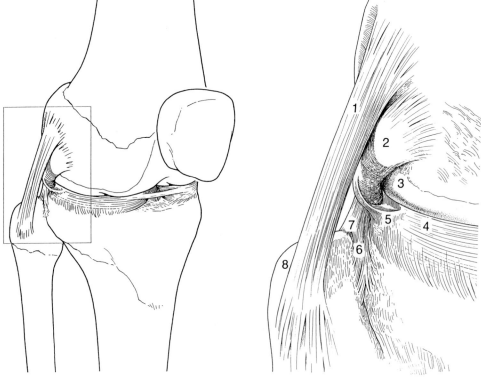

a   b

The knee is flexed to 20° with the tibia in neutral rotation, and the arthroscopic field is oriented by the vertical wall of the lateral meniscus.

Inlet of the Popliteal Hiatus (see Fig. 6)

With the tibia in neutral rotation, the femoral attachment of the popliteus tendon is evaluated. The anteroinferior popliteomeniscal fascicle, the fibers connecting the popliteus tendon to the meniscus (popliteomeniscal part), and the fibers connecting the meniscus to the popliteus tendon (meniscopopliteal part) bound the entrance of the popliteal hiatus inferolaterally and inferomedially. It is bounded medially by the vertical wall of the middle segment of the lateral meniscus (Cohn and Mains 1979) (see Fig. 6).

To obtain a deeper view into the popliteal hiatus, the tibia is internally rotated. When the cruciate ligaments are intact, this maneuver causes the lateral tibial plateau to shift slightly forward while the popliteofibular fibers act like a checkrein to hold the popliteus tendon laterally and inferiorly. The popliteus tendon runs vertically to its femoral attachment site. Through the coupled anterior translation and internal rotation of the tibia, the lateral meniscus shifts medially while the popliteus tendon remains fixed at the femur and fibula, thereby opening up the popliteal hiatus (Stäubli and Birrer 1989 a, b).

Middle Segment of the Popliteal Hiatus (Fig. 7)

The middle segment of the popliteal hiatus is bounded as follows: The cranial boundary (roof) is formed anteriorly by the lateral femoral condyle and posteriorly by the superior popliteomeniscal fascicle. The lateral boundary is formed by the popliteus tendon, whose intraarticular portion is covered by synovium. The middle segment of the hiatus is bounded inferolaterally by the popliteomeniscal part of the inferior fascicle, and inferomedially by the meniscopopliteal part. With the tibia in neutral rotation, the popliteus tendon occupies the center of the hiatus (Fig. 7). The tendon shifts anteroinferiorly in internal rotation (Fig. 8) and posterosuperiorly in external rotation (Fig. 9).

If the arthroscope is retracted slightly with the *tibia in external rotation*, the function of the popliteus tendon and its relation to the superior popliteomeniscal fascicle can be assessed. With external rotation the lateral tibial plateau undergoes a slight posterior shift about the intact central pivot. The popliteus tendon is

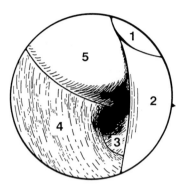

Fig. 6. Entrance of the popliteal hiatus, arthroscopic view from the anterolateral portal (right knee). *1*, Cartilage of lateral femoral condyle; *2*, lateral meniscus; *3*, inferior popliteomeniscal fascicle, meniscopopliteal part; *4*, inferior popliteomeniscal fascicle, popliteomeniscal part; *5*, popliteus tendon. (From Stäubli and Birrer 1990)

made tense by the geometry of its femoral attachment and by the restraining "pulley system" of the popliteofibular fibers and comes to occupy the posterior portion of the popliteal hiatus. The superior popliteomeniscal fascicle and the intact popliteofibular structures (which are not directly visible by arthroscopy) prevent further recession of the lateral tibial plateau. In a knee with an intact posterior cruciate ligament (PCL), the posterior translation of the lateral tibial plateau and the passive external rotation of the tibia are controlled by the popliteus tendon and its system of fibrous attachments (Patel 1981).

On internal rotation of the tibia, the lateral tibial plateau shifts forward until checked by the ACL, while the vertical popliteomeniscal portion of the anteroinferior fascicle tightens.

ACL Insufficiency

Following a violent knee injury with a subjective giving-way sensation and immediate effusion, systematic palpation will frequently disclose tenderness at the middle third of the lateral capsule, at the attachment of the popliteus tendon on the lateral femoral condyle, or in the posterior portion of the fibular head over the arcuate ligament complex. The clinical testing of sagittal stability in the ACL-deficient knee will reveal anterior subluxation of the tibia near extension with an absent end-point (positive Lachman sign). A coupled anterior translation and internal rotation of the tibia relative to the femur is clinically demonstrable. If the coupled anterior translation-internal rotation exceeds a value of 10–15 mm, there will generally be *associated injuries of the arcuate com-*

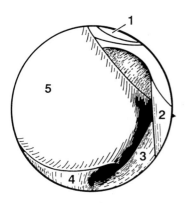

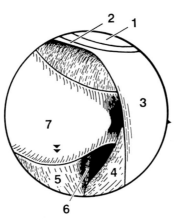

Fig. 7. Middle segment of the popliteal hiatus, arthroscopic view from the anterolateral portal (right knee). Tibia in neutral rotation, varus stress, normal anatomy. *1*, Lateral femoral condyle; *2*, vertical wall of lateral meniscus; *3*, meniscopopliteal part (inferior fascicle); *4*, popliteomeniscal part (inferior fascicle); *5*, popliteus tendon. In neutral tibial rotation the popliteus tendon is centered in the popliteal hiatus. (From Stäubli and Birrer 1990)

Fig. 8. Middle segment of the popliteal hiatus, arthroscopic view from the anterolateral portal (right knee). Tibia in internal rotation, varus stress, normal anatomy. *1*, Cartilage of lateral femoral condyle; *2*, superior popliteomeniscal fascicle; *3*, vertical wall of lateral meniscus; *4*, meniscopopliteal part of inferior fascicle; *5*, popliteomeniscal part of inferior fascicle; *6*, popliteofibular fascicle, part merging with inferior fascicle; *7*, popliteus tendon. With combined internal rotation and a varus stress, the checkrein function of the popliteofibular fascicle (*filled triangles*) becomes apparent. (From Stäubli and Birrer 1990)

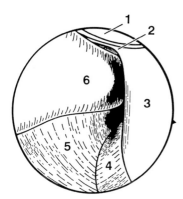

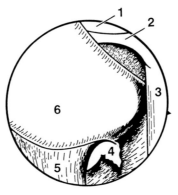

Fig. 9. Middle segment of the popliteal hiatus, arthroscopic view from the anterolateral portal (right knee). Tibia in external rotation, normal anatomy. *1*, Cartilage of lateral femoral condyle; *2*, superior popliteomeniscal fascicle; *3*, vertical wall of lateral meniscus; *4*, meniscopopliteal part of inferior fascicle; *5*, popliteomeniscal part of inferior fascicle; *6*, popliteus tendon. On external rotation of the tibia, the popliteus tendon engages against the superior fascicle. (From Stäubli and Birrer 1990)

Fig. 10. Middle segment of the popliteal hiatus, arthroscopic view from the anterolateral portal (right knee). Tibia in internal rotation, meniscopopliteal part of inferior fascicle is torn. *1*, Cartilage of lateral femoral condyle; *2*, superior fascicle; *3*, vertical wall of lateral meniscus; *4*, torn meniscopopliteal part of inferior fascicle; *5*, popliteomeniscal part of inferior fascicle; *6*, popliteus tendon. (From Stäubli and Birrer 1990)

plex, depending on constitutional ligamentous laxity and morphotype and the severity of the initial anterior subluxation.

The following lesions of the popliteus tendon and its fascicles have been diagnosed by a systematic, functional arthroscopic evaluation of the popliteal hiatus (Stäubli and Birrer 1989/1990):

– *Rupture of the anteroinferior popliteomeniscal fascicle.* One can distinguish lesions of the meniscopopliteal part of the inferior fascicle (Fig. 10) and the popliteomeniscal part (Fig. 11). Tears of the inferior fascicle may run parallel to the meniscal rim.
– *Rupture of the posterosuperior popliteomeniscal fascicle* (Fig. 12). This involves a tear in the fibers connecting the medial portion of the popliteus

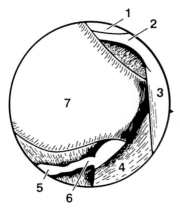

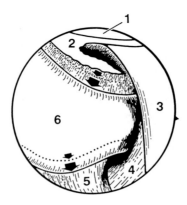

Fig. 11. Middle segment of the popliteal hiatus, arthroscopic view from the anterolateral portal (right knee). Tibia in internal rotation, tear of inferior fascial and popliteofibular fascicle. *1*, Cartilage of lateral femoral condyle; *2*, superior fascicle; *3*, vertical wall of lateral meniscus; *4*, meniscopopliteal part of inferior fascicle; *5*, popliteomeniscal part of inferior fascicle (torn); *6*, popliteofibular fascicle (torn); *7*, popliteus tendon. A combined injury of the inferior and popliteofibular fascicles removes restraint to combined external rotation-posterior translation and varus opening. The checkrein function of the popliteofibular fascicle is abolished. (From Stäubli and Birrer 1990)

Fig. 12. Middle segment of the popliteal hiatus, arthroscopic view from the anterolateral portal (right knee). Tibia in internal rotation, tear of superior fascicle. *1*, Cartilage of lateral femoral condyle; *2*, torn superior fascicle; *3*, vertical wall of lateral meniscus; *4*, meniscopopliteal part of inferior fascicle; *5*, popliteomeniscal part of inferior fascicle; *6*, popliteus tendon. When the superior fascicle is torn, the popliteus tendon is pulled inferolaterally by the restraining action of the popliteofibular fascicle (*arrows*). (From Stäubli and Birrer 1990)

Table 1. Structural lesions of the popliteus tendon and its fascicles in the popliteal hiatus

	Intact ACL + PCL control knees (n = 182)		Acute ACL disruptions (n = 104)		Chronic ACL deficiencies (n = 63)	
	n	%	n	%	n	%
Site of lesion(s)						
No of lesions	140	76.9	6	5.8	5	7.9
Popliteus tendom (isolated)	2	1.1	1	1.0	1	1.6
Lateral meniscus (isolated)	5	2.8	2	1.9	4	6.3
Superior popliteomeniscal fascicle	9	4.9	10	9.6	3	4.8
Inferior popliteomeniscal fascicle	21	11.5	22	21.1	12	19.0
Superior and inferior fascicle	0	0.0	28	26.9	20	31.7
Combination of more than two lesions	5	2.8	35	33.7	18	28.6

ACL, anterior cruciate ligament; PCL, posterior cruciate ligament.

muscle to the lateral meniscus, causing the popliteal hiatus to expand posterosuperiorly. Sites of bloody imbibition and variable fiber tears in the superior fascicle are accessible to arthroscopic detection.

– *Lesions at the attachment of the popliteus tendon.* Vertical fiber tears that run parallel to the anterior border of the popliteus tendon and extend to the popliteomeniscal part of the inferior fascicle can be verified by arthroscopy.

The incidence of lesions of the popliteus tendon and its fascicles blending into the posterior and middle segments of the lateral meniscus is shown in Table 1 (Stäubli and Birrer 1991). The incidence of structural lesions of the popliteus system was 23.1% in the control knees (n = 182), 94.2% in acute ACL ruptures (n = 104), and 92.1% in chronic ACL-deficient knees (n = 63) (Stäubli and Birrer 1991).

Discussion

D. Patel emphasized the functional importance of the popliteal hiatus and its fibrous attachments in his description of proximal approaches for knee arthroscopy (1981). Fabbriciani et al. (1982a,b) investigated the gross anatomy of the popliteus muscle and arcuate ligament. Jakob et al. (1981), Stäubli et al. (1981), Stäubli and Birrer (1989, 1990), and Stäubli and Jakob (1988) noted the importance of the posterolateral structures in the context of pathomechanical studies on the reversed pivot shift (Jakob et al. 1981). In the present study we have attempted to apply current knowledge on the gross anatomy of the popliteus system and its attachments to the structures of the popliteal hiatus that are accessible to arthroscopic functional evaluation. The following elements of the popliteus tendon and its fibrous attachments could be functionally evaluated in the popliteal hiatus:

- The anterolateral attachment of the popliteus tendon on the femoral condyle
- The entrance of the popliteal hiatus with the popliteus tendon and inferior popliteomeniscal fascicle (popliteomeniscal and meniscopopliteal parts)
- The superior popliteomeniscal fascicle (which bounds the popliteal hiatus posterosuperiorly)
- The vertical wall of the lateral meniscus (which bounds medially the middle segment of the popliteal hiatus)

The attachment of the popliteus tendon, the medial translation of the lateral meniscus under a varus stress, its lateral translation under a valgus stress, and the neutral position in neutral rotation can all be evaluated at the hiatal inlet. When a varus stress is applied while the tibia is internally rotated, the lateral checkrein function of the popliteus system can be arthroscopically assessed. With coupled anterior translation and internal rotation of the tibia, the superior popliteomeniscal fascicle (posterior) and the inferior popliteomeniscal fascicle can be functionally evaluated (Stäubli and Birrer 1989, 1990).

The function of the popliteofibular fibers can be tested indirectly by means of the "pulley effect," which holds the popliteus tendon in an inferolateral position during internal rotation when the popliteofibular fascicle is intact.

ACL Insufficiency

When there is significant ACL insufficiency with increased anterior translation and internal rotation of the tibia (anterolateral subluxation), tenderness over the arcuate complex, and signs of accompanying posterolateral rotatory instability, arthroscopy can demonstrate lesions involving the superior and inferior popliteomeniscal fascicles and the femoral attachment of the popliteus tendon. The lesions of the popliteus tendon and its fibrous attachments in the region of the popliteal hiatus are generally part of a more extensive associated injury of the arcuate complex. The severity and extent of the initial associated injuries of the popliteus system and the sites where these secondary restraints are deficient can be analyzed in the region accessible to arthroscopic inspection. We believe that a systematic search should be made for significant lesions of the popliteus system so that they can be repaired during reconstruction of the ACL. The severity of the initial associated injuries in the posterolateral portion of the popliteus system, limb morphotype, and constitutional ligamentous laxity can account for the phenomenon of primary posterolateral rotatory instability coexisting with acute rupture or chronic insufficiency of the ACL and for secondary varus coaptation loss in the chronically ACL-deficient knee.

References

Basmajian JV, Lovejoy JF (1971) Functions of the popliteus muscle in man. A multifactorial electromyographic study. J Bone Joint Surg [Am] 53: 557–562

Bousquet G (1977) Anatomophysiologie du genou. Chirurgie du Genou. Troisièmes Journées Lyon, Septembre 1977. Simép, Villeurbanne, pp 12–19

Cohn AK, Mains DB (1979) Popliteal hiatus of the lateral meniscus. Anatomy and measurement at dissection of 10 specimens. Am J Sports Med 7/4: 221–226

Fabbriciani C, Oransky M, Zoppi U (1982a) Il muscolo popliteo. Studio anatomico. Arch Ital Anat Embriol 87: 203–217

Fabbriciani C, Oransky M, Zoppi U (1982b) Il legamento popliteo arcuato e le sue varianti. Int J Sports Traumatol 4/3: 171–178

Fürst CM (1903) Der Muskulus Popliteus und seine Sehne. Lunds Universitets Arsserift, Bd 39. Lund, Malmström

Jakob RP, Hassler H, Stäubli H-U (1981) Observations on rotatory instability of the lateral compartment of the knee. Acta Orthop Scand [Suppl 191]: 1–32

Last RJ (1948) Some anatomical details of the knee joint. J Bone Joint Surg [Br] 30: 683–688

Patel D (1981) Proximal approaches to arthroscopic surgery of the knee. Am J Sports Med 9/5: 296–303

Stäubli H-U, Birrer S (1989) Functional arthroscopic evaluation of the popliteal hiatus: Normal anatomy – anterior cruciate ligament (ACL) deficiency. Abstract book, Congress of the International Arthroscopy Association Rome 6th–8th May 1989

Stäubli H-U, Birrer S (1990) The popliteus tendon and its fascicles at the popliteal hiatus: Gross anatomy and functional arthroscopic evaluation with and without anterior cruciate ligament deficiency. J. Arthroscopy Vol 6 Nr. 3: 209–220

Stäubli HU, Birrer S (1991) Läsion der Popliteussehne ind ihrer Faszikel im Hiatus popliteus. Makroskopie Anatomie und funktionelle videoarthroskopische Evaluation bei intakten Kreusbändern und bei vorderer Kreusbandinsiuffizienz. SFA (Stiftung zur Förderung der Arthroskopie, 7200 Tuttlingen, Deuschland). Arthroskopie Aktuell 4

Stäubli H-U, Jakob RP (1988) Posterolateral compartmental knee instability – an experimental study. Third congress of the European Society of Knee Surgery and Arthroscopy (ESKA), Amsterdam, 7 (abstract)

Stäubli H-U, Jakob RP, Noesberger B (1981) Experimentelle Grundlagen zur Diagnostik der postero-lateralen Knierotationsinstabilität. In: Jäger M, Hackenbroch MH, Refior HJ (Hrsg) Kapselbandläsionen des Kniegelenkes. Thieme, Stuttgart New York S 109–116

Stäubli HU, Rauschning W (1991) Popliteus tendon and lateral meniscus: gross and multiplaner cyrosectional anantomy of the knee. Am Knee Surg 4 (3): 110–121

Tabutin J (1977) Anatomie du compartiment externe. Chirurgie du Genou. Troisièmes Journées Lyon, Septembre 1977. Simep, Villeurbanne, pp 9–11

Synthetic Materials
for Ligament Reconstruction

Biomechanical Considerations

S. N. Freudiger

Autologous tissues have been taken from various sites for reconstruction of the anterior cruciate ligament (ACL) (Noyes et al. 1984). The patellar tendon finally emerged as the most utilized source of autograft material (Clancy and Ray 1987). But even patellar tendon replacements of the ACL have not proven perfect in all patients 5–10 years after the operation (Johnson et al. 1984; Roth et al. 1985). Extraarticular techniques also have been proposed for ACL reconstruction (e.g., the Lemaire procedure).

The ongoing controversies in ACL reconstruction have prompted interest in exploring the clinical usefulness of synthetic materials for ligament replacement. At present the development of artificial ligaments is still in its infancy, and clinical results are not yet available for postoperative periods of more than 5–10 years. Though the potential of synthetic materials is great, their long-term biological effects are not yet fully known.

Types of Artificial Ligaments

Prostheses are advantageous in that they provide a high degree of mechanical strength right away, permitting the patient to start rehabilitation shortly after surgery. Also (ethical considerations aside), artificial ligaments can be replaced in the event of recurring failure, an advantage that may be of particular benefit to professional athletes.

Augmentation generally refers to the mechanical support of an autologous tissue. The purpose of an augmentation device is to reduce stresses on the biological graft during revascularization and thereafter to protect the graft from excessive loading. Augmentation can therefore accelerate rehabilitation and improve long-term results.

A *scaffold* is a device designed to promote the apposition and ingrowth of new tissue in order to to create a new ligament. Because of their typically small cross section, scaffolds are normally much weaker than natural ligaments, so prolonged rehabilitation is required. Another concern is our limited knowledge about the mechanical quality of the newly formed tissue.

Biomechanical Boundary Conditions

The ACL and its Synergists

From a mechanical viewpoint, the knee may be considered a statically indeterminate system, with more than one structure available to carry the reactive loads. But if one considers the inherent stiffness and global orientation of the individual structures as well as the shapes of the articular surfaces (condyles and plateaus), the important structures may be found to respond to specific types of load. Thus, the ACL may be found primarily to restrain anterior tibial translation and internal rotation and to ensure that the rolling-gliding mechanism of the knee is maintained. In performing these functions, the ACL relies on synergistic structures, i. e., on the posterior oblique ligament to respond to internal rotation (Müller 1982) and on the posterior cruciate ligament (PCL) to control the rolling-gliding mechanism. This synergism is the main reason why the elasticity of an artificial ACL should closely match that of the human ligament (preservation of rotational axes, restoration of rolling-gliding, etc.).

Elasticity

Much has been published on the mechanical properties of the human ACL, yet few authors have taken into account the age of the donors in their evaluations. For this reason, we have selected Noyes and Grood (1976) as the principal reference.

It is not sufficient for an artificial ligament to have the same strain as a natural ligament. From a biomechanical standpoint, its elongation under a given load must be the same. An equivalent strain is sufficient only if the natural and artificial ligaments have the same initial lengths or functional lengths. This condi-

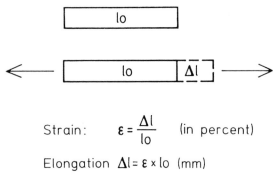

Fig. 1. Definition of strain (ε) and length change (δ). $l_0 =$ Initial length

tion is not satisfied in an over-the-top reconstruction, and the greater initial length of the implanted ligament must be taken into consideration. The definitions of strain and elongation are reflected in Fig. 1. Frequently the strain is multiplied by 100 and expressed as a percentage.

Strength

Data on the strength of the human ACL may be found in Noyes and Grood (1976). Here we shall note only that artificial ligaments should have greater mechanical strength to compensate for their lack of proprioceptive properties. The magnitude of this reserve factor is still unknown, but it must not be so great as to induce further cartilaginous, osseous, or synovial damage if a new trauma occurs following an artificial ligament reconstruction. One way to ensure this is to provide the artificial ligament with a predetermined breaking point. In any case, the strength of the attachment is usually less than that of the prosthesis itself.

Stress Level

There is still disagreement among biomechanical experts as to the physiologic loads that develop in the ACL (Workshop of the European Society of Biomechanics 1987). The following values have been reported in the literature (Chen and Black 1980; Morrison 1969):

- Level walking: 169 N,
- Descending a ramp: 445 N,
- Jogging (with friction): 630 N.

The following model offers another way to estimate the magnitude of the load:

A skier has adjusted the front clamps of his safety binding to the no. 5 setting, corresponding to a torque of 50 Nm (according to DIN 7881). If the skier wants his binding to release, this amount of torque must be transmitted through the knee. If this torque is produced by internal rotation that is restrained by the ACL together with the posterior oblique ligament, then the load acting on the ACL is 1400 N, as shown in Fig. 2. Ligament protection by muscular contraction is disregarded in this model. This situation could occur, for example, during a fall in which loads are imposed in less time than is required for the initiation of protective muscular reflexes. Perhaps this model can account for some of the many lesions of the ACL that are sustained while skiing.

Finally, the loads on the ACL resulting in a typical case of internal loads will be estimated: Close to full extension, the quadriceps becomes an antagonist to the ACL (Feagin et al. 1982). There have been several reports of ACL tears sustained by skiers who had not fallen (Figueras et al. 1987), where a faulty quad-

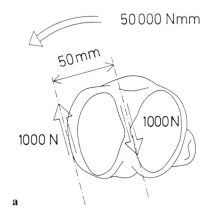

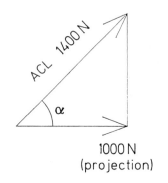

Fig. 2. a Coupled forces on the knee joint plane involved in the transmission of a torque in internal rotation. **b** Projection of an ACL force onto the plane of the tibial plateau

riceps reflex is assumed to have overloaded the ACL. Assuming that the patellar tendon is inclined forward 10° from the vertical while the ACL is inclined 45° backward, the load on the ACL can reach about 25% that on the patellar tendon. According to Noyes et al. (1984), the patellar tendon (medial and central thirds) has a strength of at least 5600 N. Thus, if the quadriceps generates a load of 5600 N in the patellar tendon, a load of 1400 N can develop in the ACL.

Load Cycles

A variety of models can also be derived for estimating load cycles, i.e., the frequency of occurrence of a given load over a certain period of time. Chen and Black (1980), for example, estimated the following load cycles:

- Level walking: 2,500,000/year,
- Descending a ramp: 3700/year,
- Jogging: 640,000/year.

For purposes of illustration, I will now present my own model. Assuming 1 hour of jogging per week at 15 km/h and a stride length of 75 cm, one finds:

- 15,000 m/week
- 20,000 strides/week
- 10,000 cycles/week and knee
- 500,000 cycles/year
- 1,000,000 cycles in 2 years
- 10,000,000 cycles in 20 years

Prosthesis

Proflex[1]

The Proflex prosthesis will be used for illustrative purposes. This device was designed by Mansat, developed by Sulzer, and tested clinically and mechanically by Protek. Its principal features are its elasticity and its functionally differentiated cross sections. It is made from textured polyethylene terephthalate (PET) fiber formed into multiple tubes that are braided together. The prosthesis is prestretched to match the elasticity of the human ligament (Fig.3), and its ultimate strength is approximately 4500 N (1 mm/s, Ringer solution, 37° C).

[1] Proflex = Tersuisse (polyethylene terephthalate) fiber; Protek AG Bern, Stadtbachstr. 64, CH-3001 Bern, Switzerland.

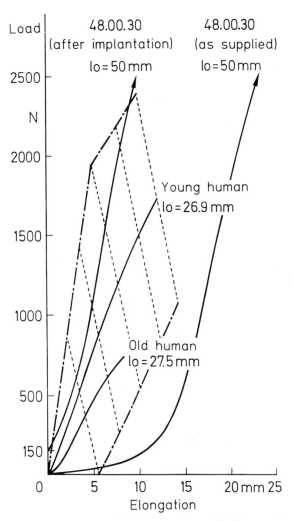

Fig.3. Comparison of the elasticity of an artificial ligament in various states with the elasticity of human ACLs. Linear and maximum points of mean and extreme values of human ligaments, after Noyes et al. (1976). l_0 = Initial length

Operating Technique

The operating technique continues to be a major concern in ACL reconstructions. There is still considerable contrast between the over-the-top and the transcondylar techniques. Despite numerous studies on the effects of varying the attachment sites (Gely et al. 1984; Grood et al. 1986; Hoogland and Hillen 1984; Odensten and Gillquist 1985), we are only beginning to understand the effects on the loading of the reconstructed ACL and on normal kinematics. Odensten and Gillquist (1985) and Hoogland and Hillen (1984), for example, report a length change of approximately 8–10 mm from flexion to extension with a graft routed over the top of the femur to the center of the

508   S. N. Freudiger

tibial insertion area. No force can be derived from this length change, however. Of course, elongation normally generates a force, but in this case the force also creates a reaction which is thought to be carried mainly by the PCL. This reaction itself elongates the PCL by a certain amount, which reduces the resultant elongation of the ACL, where a smaller force will develop. This situation establishes a *new state of equilibrium*, which in turn affects normal kinematics, resulting, for example, in posterior subluxation of the tibia in extension, an extension deficit, or even an increase in terminal external rotation. The results of 2 laboratory experiments are noteworthy in this context:

– In 5 intact knee specimens, the automatic (external) rotation was found to average 6.3°. With the ACL excised, the automatic rotation decreased to 1.2°. If isometry is understood to mean *no* length change from flexion to extension, then the joint would behave the same after an isometric ACL reconstruction as it would without an ACL, i.e., a significant portion of the automatic rotation would be lost.
– If a prestretched Proflex ligament prosthesis (model 48.01.30) is routed over the top of the femoral condyle and through the center of the tibial insertion area, and is attached in 30° flexion with a preload of 50 N, 126 N is required by the quadriceps to achieve full extension while 112 N is developed in the prosthesis. For attachment in 60° flexion, 123 N is required by the quadriceps, while 146 N is developed in the prosthesis.

Based on the second finding it may be concluded that, from a purely mechanical standpoint, the optimum preload and knee flexion angle for fixation of the prosthesis have been found if, at the end of rehabilitation, the patient can achieve full extension, signifying that the potential of the prosthesis is being utilized to its full extent.

There is also a significant difference between the over-the-top and transcondylar routes in terms of the torsion exerted on the ACL substitute when the knee moves from flexion to extension. Bending components are predominant in the first technique, and torsional components in the second. Thus, a prosthesis designed for transcondylar placement should have low torsion stiffness to avoid abrasion at the entrance of the condylar tunnel. Because the Proflex prosthesis has high torsion stiffness due to its diagonal braid, it is suitable only for the over-the-top route.

Finally, the tibial placement of the ACL replacement is also a matter of compromise in an over-the-top reconstruction. If the tibial tunnel is too far anterior, in-

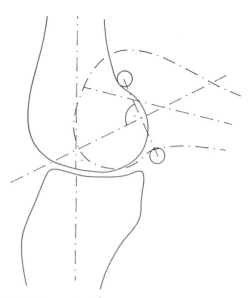

Fig. 4. Perpendicular bisector through 2 selected ligament positions

tercondylar notch impingement will occur in extension, causing potentially damaging shear loads on the prosthesis at the tunnel entrance. If the tibial tunnel is too far posterior, excessive length change from flexion to extension may result. This concept is easily visualized geometrically by connecting the 2 over-the-top positions (in flexion and extension) by a straight line and drawing a perpendicular bisector through the line. The farther the tibial entrance is from the intersection of the bisector and the tibial plateau, the greater the associated length change (Fig. 4).

Mechanical Testing

The mechanical testing of textile structures is an exacting task that begins with the clamping of the specimens and end with determining the effects of the viscoelastic properties, since their behavior changes from one load cycle to the next, even within the elastic range. Textile structures can therefore be regarded as a kind of "living" material.

Mounting the Specimen

Two different types of grip had to be designed for clamping Proflex specimens in an Instron test machine (Fig. 5). Figure 6 shows grips with a continuous clamp mechanism for determining ultimate breaking strength. The disadvantage of continuous

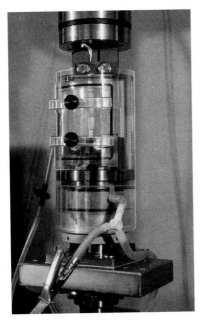

Fig. 5. Artificial ligament mounted for static testing in the Instron HE 1530/1270 test machine

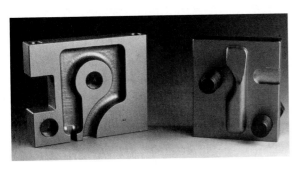

Fig. 6. Grip with continuous clamp mechanism

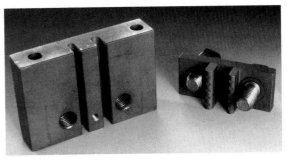

Fig. 7. Grip with concentrated clamp mechanism

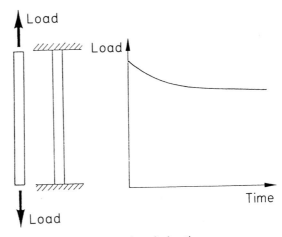

Fig. 8. Graphic representation of relaxation

clamping inside the grip is that the point of zero strain is unknown, so strain cannot be measured at the same time. Therefore a second type of grip (Fig. 7) was designed with a concentrated clamp mechanism that precisely defines the location of zero strain. However, these grips damage the ligament within the clamping groove, causing it to rupture below its ultimate strength.

Viscoelasticity

Viscoelasticity is a rheologic term denoting the flow properties of a given material. Viscoelasticity basically refers to time dependency, both in the loading phase and in the recovery phase following load release. Its significance in an artificial ligament is shown

graphically in Fig. 8 (relaxation) and Fig. 9 (creep). Testing relaxation involves applying a certain load to a specimen, holding it at the new length, and observing the decay of internal force (reaction) over time. Testing creep involves applying a constant load to a specimen and observing its elongation over time. Thus, relaxation is the decrease in force over time at a constant length, while creep is the increase in length over time at a constant force.

Control

A tensile testing machine is generally either stroke-controlled or load-controlled. In stroke control, the specimen is loaded by displacement from a lower to an upper stroke limit (Fig. 10); in load control, by dis-

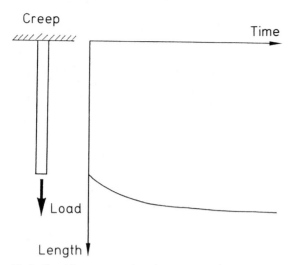

Fig. 9. Graphic representation of creep

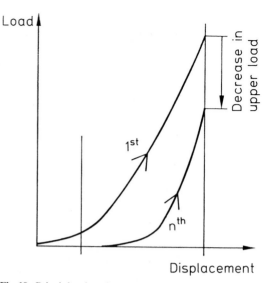

Fig. 10. Principle of stroke control

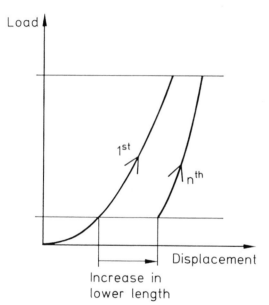

Fig. 11. Principle of load control

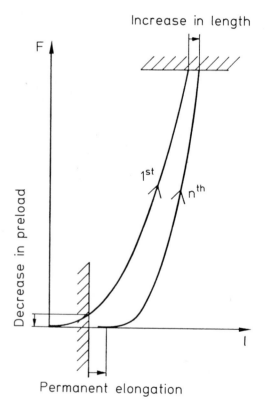

Fig. 12. Combined load-stroke control ▷

placement from a lower to an upper load limit (Fig. 11). The question arises as to which of these two types of control is better suited for testing an artificial ligament, and especially for cyclic loading. Clinically, the initial length of the substitute ligament is determined by the attachment of the second end. The liga-

ment therefore cannot shorten below this length when subjected to subsequent positive loading. The lower limit, then, should be stroke-controlled. At the same time, a knee is normally subjected to loading by external forces that, depending on the load case, may cause a reaction force to develop in the ACL. Therefore the upper limit should be load-controlled. In the fatigue testing of an artificial ligament, then, stroke control should be used for the lower limit and load control for the upper limit (Fig. 12). Such an experimental procedure can yield 4 types of information simultaneously:

– Decrease in preload
– Occurrence of permanent elongation
– Increase in elongation at the upper load
– Change of elasticity (slope of the curve).

Fatigue

The Proflex prosthesis was subjected to various fatigue tests using the combined load- and stroke-control system. Drawing on the results of Chen and Black (1980), the prosthesis was tested for 10 million cycles at a constant upper load of 650 N. The load spectra shown in Fig. 13 were also used to test the ability of the prosthesis to withstand the higher peak loads that may occur in young athletes. One hundred such spectra yield a total load of 1,010,100 cycles, broken down as follows:

– 1,000,000 × 500 N,
– 10,000 × 1000 N,
– 100 × 1500 N.

The permanant strain results were as follows:

	$10^7 \times 650$ N	100 Load spectra
– First-generation Proflex (48.00.30)	4.9%	4.0%
– Second-generation Proflex (48.01.30)	2.1%	1.7%

These tests were conducted at 3 Hz in Ringer's solution at 37° C.

An interesting observation was made in the load spectrum experiment (Fig. 14). After the first peak load of 1500 N, the ligament was able to recover by 0.5% during the subsequent 10,000 cycles at 500 N. This is a typical viscoelastic property, which could have been exploited to a much greater degree if recovery periods had been interpolated after each individual load cycle. Although such rest periods would more closely approximate reality, they would greatly prolong the fatigue tests. It must be considered that it takes 38.6 days to complete 10 million cycles at 3 Hz, and that the ultimate purpose of fatigue testing is to predict the future in a minimum amount of time.

Fatigue: Bending

Another type of fatigue test focuses on the bending properties of the artificial ligament. The actual bending behavior of an artificial ligament depends to a large degree on connective tissue formation, which in

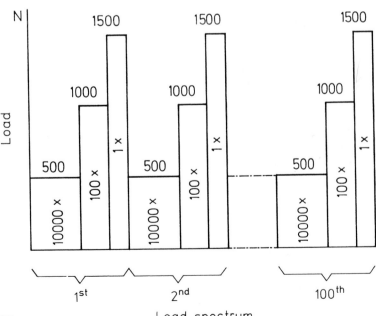

Fig. 13. Selected load spectra

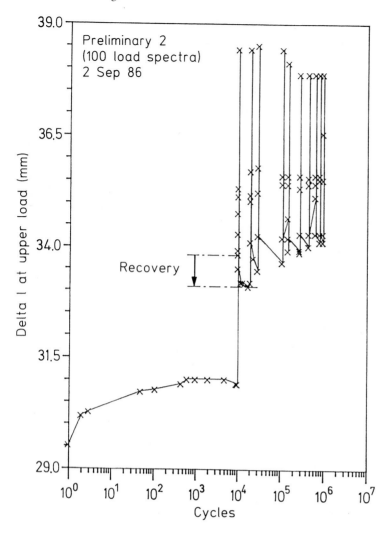

Fig. 14. Test protocol, including a recovery phase

favorable cases (fibrocartilage) can provide effective protection for the prosthesis. Bending behavior depends even more strongly on the operating technique, i.e., the angular deviation from a straight line and the radii at the edges of the bone tunnel openings. For example, the tibial tunnel can be placed so that the ligament substitute forms an approximately straight line when the knee is close to extension, thus avoiding additional bending during the loads that frequently occur at these flexion angles.

In an attempt to reflect the clinical worse-case situation, the test setup illustrated in Fig. 15 has been designed. It simulates the behavior of an artificial ligament at the edge of the tibial tunnel on the tibial plateau. The ligament is attached 30 mm below the rim, which means that the movement of the ligament around the edge of the sleeve duplicates the clinical situation. The amount of travel is thus a function of the applied load and the elasticity of the ligament being tested. Since the test is performed in Ringer's solution, the sleeve simulating the tibial tunnel is made of ceramic to avoid corrosion. The radius of the edge is 1.5 mm. The applied load is 150 N and the constant deviation angle 30°. After 10 million cycles, the ligament is tensile tested and the ultimate breaking loads before and after the bending test are compared. The results with the Proflex ligament are shown below; the Proflex IV is an experimental ligament made of a hybrid fiber system.

	Before	After
Proflex II	4500 N	1270 N
Proflex IV	6000 N	4485 N

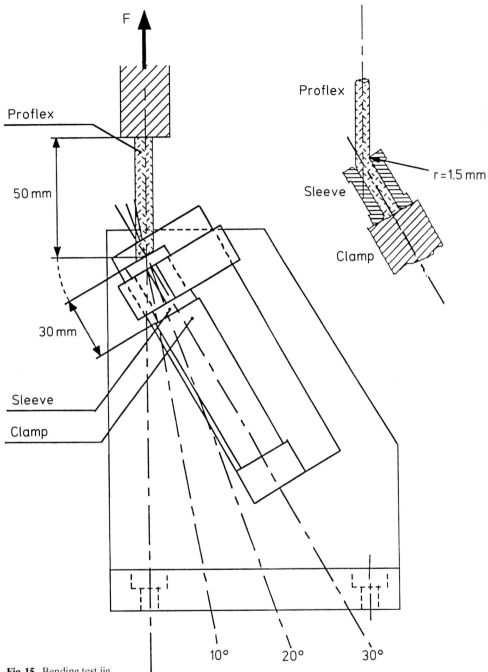

Fig. 15. Bending test jig

Long-Term Behavior of Prostheses

An important parameter in evaluating the long-term behavior of a prosthesis is permanent elongation. Practically all textile structures undergo permanent elongation when subjected to repetitive tensile loads. But what is the permissible amoung of permanent elongation in an ACL prosthesis? We shall assume a ligament with a functional length of 50 mm implanted by the over-the-top route and inclined 45° (Fig. 16). If this ligament elongates by the factor a, then the Lachman value, for example, increases approximately by the factor b, which is about 40% greater than a, because with an elongated ACL, the tibia does not separate from the femur, but rather the ligament assumes a new inclination and become more lax.

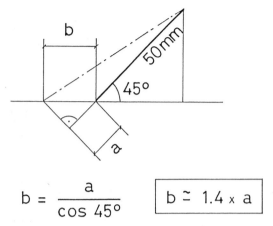

$$b = \frac{a}{\cos 45°}$$

$$\boxed{b \simeq 1.4 \times a}$$

Fig. 16. Effect of ligament inclination in the sagittal plane

Numerical data:

Permanent strain	Lachman increase
1%	0.7 mm
3%	2.1 mm
5%	3.5 mm

The amount of permanent strain that is permissible at the end of the specified life span of a prosthesis has not yet been described. Based on the foregoing assumptions, the permanent strain as measured in a load-stroke-controlled test should not exceed 3%.

Comparison of Clinical Laxity Measurements with Laboratory Results

The clinical documentation of the first-generation Proflex (48.00.30) consisted in the evaluation (July 1987) of 32 two-year results, which indicated a 2.4-mm difference between the operated and non-operated sides in the instrumented Lachman test.

The first-generation Proflex exhibits a permanent strain of 3.15% after 1 million cycles at 650 N, which would correspond to a Lachman increase of 2.2 mm based on the foregoing assumptions. At 650 N, typical for jogging, 2 years would equal approximately 1 million cycles, resulting in extremely good agreement between the 2.4-mm Lachman increase measured clinically and the 2.2-mm increase determined in the laboratory.

The author is aware that instrumented Lachman tests often yield data with a large scatter of values, and that assumptions had to be made regarding functional ligament lengths, ligament inclinations, load levels, and load cycles, and that consequently this agreement must be viewed with a critical attitude. Despite this, pursuing these measurements and assumptions

must be encouraged so that the gap between clinical and laboratory results can be narrowed.

It should be noted that 3.15% permanent strain after 1 million cycles is still not an optimum result. This fact, as well as clinical results, led to the development of a second-generation Proflex (48.01.30) that is prestretched during manufacture. This can reduce permanent elongation to approximately one-half.

Attachment

Perhaps the fastest and simplest way to attach artificial ligaments is by stapling. Since the Proflex ligament is attached with staples, pullout tests were performed on cadaveric bones. Because the tibial attachment is supported by friction owing to the angular deviation of the ligament at the tunnel openings, the femoral attachment was considered more critical than the tibial attachment and was selected for testing. The ligament was also passed around the lateral condyle (Fig. 17) but at a smaller angle of wrap (conservative). An important finding in these tests was: It is not meaningful to speak of maximum pullout force in reference to the staple fixation. In a bio-

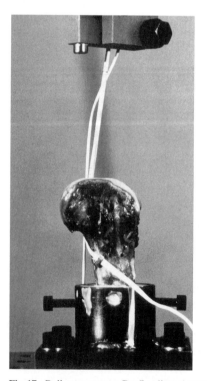

Fig. 17. Pullout test on a Proflex ligament stapled to a femoral stump

mechanical sense, it is more useful to determine the force at which the ligament starts to slip underneath the staple. This slippage has exactly the same consequences as permanent elongation of the ligament itself.

The following staples were tested in conjunction with the Proflex ligament: Union, Richards (small), and an original Protek design. The results in young bones averaged about 1600 N for the onset of slippage and about 1900 N for final pullout.

These values represent the situation immediately after implantation. In removing artificial ligaments implanted by the over-the-top technique, surgeons have frequently noted a marked adhesion of the ligament to the posterior capsule wall, which may considerably increase the load transfer capacity of the femoral attachment. The tibial part of the ligament also tends to resist removal, as the newly formed connective tissue adheres to the tunnel wall.

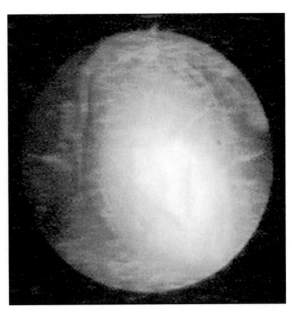

Fig. 18. Artificial ligament surrounded by connective tissue 2 1/2 months after implantation

Biocompatibility

Artificial ligaments incite a foreign body reaction that is expressed in connective tissue proliferation. Figure 18 shows an arthroscopic view of a Proflex ligament surrounded by connective tissue 2 1/2 months after implantation. The histologic examination of a Proflex implanted for 5 months shows the presence of richly vascularized connective tissue (Fig. 19). Another histologic evaluation of a Proflex implanted for 9 months shows fibrocartilage in the over-the-top region (Fig. 20). This fibrocartilage layer can effectively protect the ligament from abrasion against the bone and is a welcome development from a mechanical standpoint. Further studies are being done to elucidate the mechanism of fibrocartilage formation on artificial ligaments.

Augmentation

The mechanical requirements for an augmentation device are both stringent and contradictory: On the one hand, the device must protect the patellar tendon graft from excessive loads while the graft is undergoing revascularization; on the other, it should not cause undesired stress shielding. These time-varying requirements on load distribution call for finely adapted elasticities. Clancy et al. (1981) made a significant contribution to this problem, as shown graphically in Fig. 21. Unfortunately their data pertain to monkeys, and at present one can only speculate on the applicability of their findings to humans (Clancy and Ray 1987).

In theory, several desired properties of an augmentation device that meets the requirements illustrated in Fig. 21 can be proposed:

- The stiffness of the augmentation device declines between 6 and 12 months.
- The augmentation device undergoes a specified permanent elongation between 6 and 12 months and thereafter shares graft loads only beyond a certain amount of strain.
- The augmentation device is implanted in a differential way (with a certain initial laxness) so that, from the outset, graft loads are shared only beyond a certain amount of strain.

These suggestions are based on the assumption that both ends of the augmentation device are attached to bone. However, Van Kampen et al. (1987) recommend attaching only one end of the device to bone while suturing the other end to the biological graft to achieve a gradual transfer of load from the augmentation device to the graft. While this technique reduces strain in the patellar tendon graft and their associated effects, such as permanent elongation, it does not enhance the strength of the reconstruction (the weakest link remains).

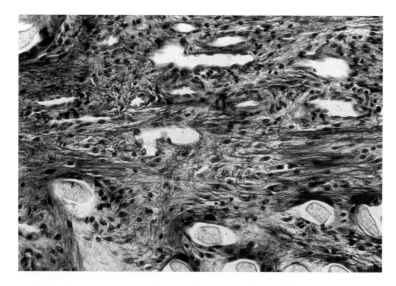

Fig. 19. Histologic section through newly formed connective tissue (after 5 months), showing numerous blood vessels

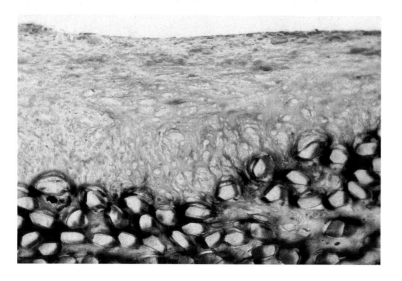

Fig. 20. Fibrocartilage on the over-the-top portion of an artificial ligament after 9 months

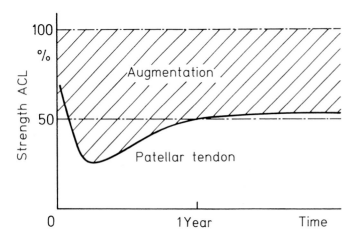

Fig. 21. Strength variation of a patellar tendon graft

Conclusion

The development of artificial ligaments is still in its initial stages, and the clinical and biomechanical requirements for these devices are not yet fully understood. There is still no testing procedure that can reliably predict the long-term performance of an artificial ligament. Operating techniques remain a major unknown. Stability can be restored in most cases using current reconstruction techniques, but will these techniques also restore kinematics in a way that will prevent long-term osteoarthritic change? We still know little about the biological effects of possible wear debris (e. g., synthetic synovitis). Ruptures of artificial ligaments can often be ascribed to incorrect placement of the insertion sites, or perhaps to impingement of the ligament against an intercondylar notch that was not adequately widened (notch plasty, osteophyte removal) before implantation. Has too little attention been given to the precision mechanics that underlie a cruciate ligament implantation? Does the cruciate reconstruction require pre- or intraoperative planning that will help the surgeon better evaluate geometric relationships? One device for this purpose may be the tensiometer, which should assist the surgeon in locating suitable isometric attachment sites. Finally, there is a need to encourage greater cooperation among different centers, since the complete, systematic documentation of clinical case material remains the only way to clarify the true behavior of artificial ligaments in the human body.

We are grateful to D. Wyder (MEM Institute for Biomechanics), D. Ulrich, Dr. U. Soltesz (FhG Institute for Material Engineering), and M. Eicher (Protek) for their work in the development of new testing procedures and for conducting the numerous tests.

References

Chen EH, Black J (1980) Materials design analysis of the prosthetic anterior cruciate ligament. J Biomed Mat Res 14: 567

Clancy WG, Ray JM (1987) Anterior cruciate ligament autografts. In: Jackson DW, Drez D (eds) The anterior cruciate deficient knee, new concepts in ligament repair. Mosby, St. Louis, P 193

Clancy WG, Narechania RG, Rosenberg TD, Gmeiner JG, Wisnefske DD, Lange TA (1981) Anterior and posterior cruciate ligament reconstruction in rhesus monkeys. J Bone Joint Surg [Am] 63: 1270

Feagin JA, Cabaud HE, Curl WW (1982) The anterior cruciate ligament: Radiographic and clinical signs of successful and unsuccessful repairs. Clin Orthop 164: 54

Figueras JM, Escalas F, Vidal A, Morgenstern R, Buló JM, Merino JA, Espadaler-Gamisans JM (1987) The anterior cruciate ligament injury in skiers. Skiing trauma and safety. In: Johnson RJ, Mote CD (eds) Sixth International Symposium, ASTM STP 938. ASTM Philadelphia, p 55

Gely P, Drouin G, Thiry PS, Tremblay GR (1984) Torsion and bending imposed on a new anterior cruciate ligament prosthesis during knee flexion: An evaluation method. Biomech Eng 106: 285

Grood ES, Hefzy MS, Butler DL, Noyes FR (1986) Intraarticular vs. over the top placement of anterior cruciate ligament substitute. 32nd Annual ORS, New Orleans, Feb. 1986, p 79

Hoogland T, Hillen B (1984) Intra-articular reconstruction of the anterior cruciate ligament. Clin Orthop 185: 197

Johnson RJ, Eriksson E, Haggmark T, Pope MH (1984) Five-to ten-year follow-up evaluation after the reconstruction of the anterior cruciate ligament. Clin Orthop 183: 122

Morrison JB (1969) Function of the knee joint in various activities. Biomed Eng December: 573

Müller We (1982) Das Knie: Form, Funktion und ligamentäre Wiederherstellungschirurgie. Springer, Berlin Heidelberg New York

Noyes FR, Grood ES (1976) The strength of the anterior cruciate ligament in humans and rhesus monkeys. J Bone Joint Surg [Am] 58: 1074

Noyes FR, Butler DL, Grood ES, Zernicke RF, Hefzy MS (1984) Biomechanical analysis of human ligament grafts used in knee-ligament repairs and reconstructions. J Bone Joint Surg [Am] 66: 344

Odensten M, Gillquist J (1985) Functional anatomy of the anterior cruciate ligament and a rationale for reconstruction. J Bone Joint Surg [Am] 67: 257

Roth JH, Kennedy JC, Lockstadt H, McCallum CL, Cunning LA (1985) Polypropylene braid augmented and non-augmented intraarticular anterior cruciate ligament reconstruction. Am J Sports Med 13/5: 321

Van Kampen CL, Mendenhall HV, McPherson GK (1987) Synthetic augmentation of biological anterior cruciate ligament substitutions. In: Jackson DW, Drez D (eds) The anterior cruciate deficient knee, new concepts in ligament repair. Mosby, St. Louis, p 226

Workshop of the European Society of Biomechanics (1987) Biomechanics of human knee ligaments. Reisensburg, Ulm

Current Status of Synthetic Ligament Reconstruction

U. Munzinger

Autologous reconstruction of the deficient anterior cruciate ligament (ACL) has a reported success rate of 75%–80% in the recent literature (Alm 1973; Arnoczky et al. 1982; Arvidsson et al. 1981; Clancy et al. 1982; Eriksson 1976; Henning 1979; Hughston and Barrett 1983; Johnson et al. 1984; Jones 1980; Lysholm et al. 1981; Nicholas 1973; Oretorp 1979; Poppon and Prudhon 1977; Wirth 1984). The observation periods on which these data are based are relatively short. In failed reconstructions or patients needing multiple reoperations, increased use has been made of alloplastic ligaments. This makes for a simpler operation, and the immediate strength of the ligament substitute allows for earlier and more rapid rehabilitation.

Extensive biomechanical and laboratory research has been conducted in this area. A series of clinical studies is in progress, and a number of these ligaments are already available commercially. The results of a comparative clinical study (Proflex, patellar tendon, Kennedy LAD, Stryker, Leeds-Keio, Gore-Tex, Telos) are summarized in Table 1.

The present article is concerned with the biomechanics of these artificial ligaments and the indications for their use. The advantages and disadvantages of the ligaments are presented along with the results of current clinical studies. The materials used for cruciate ligament reconstructions can be classified as follows:

Augmentation device:[1]
- Autologous
- Allogeneic (homologous)
- Biodegradable
- Nonbiodegradable

Prosthesis (alloplast):
- Polymers, polytetrafluoroethylene (PTFE) (Gore-Tex), polyethylene or terephthalate (dacron, Proflex, Trevira, etc.)
- Tendons (allogeneic, xenogeneic, e.g. Xenotech, etc.)

Scaffold:
- Carbon fibers
- Polymers
- Others

Properties of the Cruciate Ligaments Compared with Artificial Ligaments (Table 2)

A comparison of the material properties of artificial and natural ligaments must be based upon comparable terminologies, units, and test methods. The standard unit of force is the newton (N), and the standard unit of tensile and compressive stress is the pascal (Pa).

Force or Load (N)

The maximum force or maximum tensile load represents the value that a material can withstand before breaking or tearing. This value is between 475 and 1730 N for the ACL, and between 650 and 1710 for the PCL (Kennedy 1978, 1983; Kennedy and Fowler 1971; Kennedy and Willis 1976; Kennedy et al. 1954, 1976, 1978; Noyes 1977; Noyes and Grood 1977; Noyes et al. 1973, 1974, 1978, 1980 a,b, 1983 a,b).

Compressive and Tensile Stress (Pa)

The maximum tensile or compressive stress refers to the forces that a material can absorb per unit of cross-sectional area, i.e., force per unit area.

Strain (%)

The elasticity of a material can be represented by 2 different curves (Fig. 1): force versus length change, or stress versus strain. Strain equals the change in length divided by the original length and is expressed as a percentage. Both the curves are similar, showing

---

[1] Composite graft: a combination of autologous and allogeneic material.

Table 1. Compartive clinical study of artificial ligaments

Ligament		Proflex 48.00.30	Lig. patellae		Kennedy LAD	Stryker	Leeds-Keio	Gore-Tex	Telos
Femoral placement		Over the top	Anatomic	Over the top	Over the top	Over the top	Anatomic	Over the top	Anatomic
References		Mansat et al. (1984)	Johnson et al. (1984)	Roth et al. (1985)	Roth et al. (1985)	Orthopedic and Rehabilitation Devices Pauel 1986	Fujikawa (1986)	Gore-Tex	Mockwitz (1985) Contzen (1985) Mockwitz et al.
Number of patients		62	87	68	45	123	220	187	36
Follow-up (years)		2	7.9	5.5	4.1	2		3	4
Drawer at 70°/90° flexion	normal		– 1.0 – 1.0 mm 31%	8%	20%	85% (Stryker & Leeds-Keio)		26%	75%
	+		1.1 – 2.0 mm 19%	34%	42%			54%	19.4%
	+ +		2.1 – 4.0 mm 39%	34%	36%			15%	5.6%
	+ + +		4.1 – 6.0 mm 12%	24%	2%			5%	–
Pivot shift test	0	53%	72%	37%	51%	97% (Stryker)		69%	
	1	39%	18%	32%	38%			22%	
	2	8%	10%	18%	11%			7%	
	3	–	–	13%	–			2%	
Lachman test	normal	69%	– 1.0 – 1.0 mm 27%	21%	40%	98% (Stryker)	85%	38%	
	+	26%	1.1 – 2.0 mm 11%	45%	51%			45%	
	+ +	3%	2.1 – 4.0 mm 33%	24%	7%			11%	
	+ + +	2%	4.1 – 6.0 mm 15% 6.1 – + 14	10%	2%			6%	
Lysholm score		(pre 61)				93 (84% good to excellent)			
Stair climbing	easy	94%	86%					80%	83%
	difficult	6%	11%					17%	17%
	impossible	–	–					2%	–
Swelling	none	86%		79%	87%			59%	
	mild	12%		18%	11%			34%	
	marked	2%		3%	2%			7%	
Pain	none	89%	25%	55%	73%			44%	61%
	mild	11%	44%	31%	25%			30%	39%
	moderate	–	23%	11%	–			24%	–
	severe	–	8%	3%	2%			2%	–
Condition	much better	90%	7%	16%	67%	85% (Stryker & Leeds-Keio)		84%	52.7%
	better		64%	50%	15%			8%	30.6%
	same	10%	25%	16%	11%			8%	16.7%
	worse	–	4%	18%	6%			8%	–
Complications		6.4% "minor" 2.1% "major"	30%	42%	31%	9%		16% (1021 patients)	

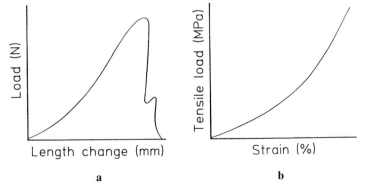

Fig. 1. a Load vs. elongation. The first part of the curve indicates the elasticity of the material. The increasing slope of the curve reflects increasing stiffness until failure occurs. **b** Percent material strain with increasing tensile load

Load (N)

Length change (mm)

a

Tensile load (MPa)

Strain (%)

b

Table 2. Biomechanical characteristics of the artificial ligaments

	Elongation (from initial length) (%/s)	Maximum load, breaking load (N)	Transition from elastic to plastic deformation (N)	Elongation (%) at transition from elastic to plastic deformation	Creep (%/δ)	Force to fatigue failure (N) and number of load cycles	Stiffness (KN/m)
ACL	100	1730 ± 660	1170 ± 750	25.5 ± 8			182 ± 56
Carbon	Data not available	2461 ± 238	F 300 N	1.14	NA	60 1 × 10⁶	–
Stryker Meadox	117	3045 ± 15	–	15	1% 1 × 10⁶	2850 1 × 10⁶	42 ± 1
Leeds-Keio	50	2000	–	–	3 – 5% 1400 N	830 30 × 10⁶	–
Proflex	20–100	4000	.....	.....	2% 650 N 10 × 10⁶	.....	.....
LAD (8 mm)	4	1730 ± 660	NA	20	3% 500 N 1 × 10⁶	1560 1 × 10⁶	330
Gore-Tex	2.6	4830 ± 280	1000	2 – 5	4% 285 N 300 × 10⁶	1495 10 × 10⁶	322
Xenograft	100	2210 ± 210	NA	4	0.2% 534 N 2 × 10⁴	2200 10 × 10⁶	56.9

an initially gradual upslope indicating a high elasticity at smaller loads (low stiffness, high elasticity). As more and more fibers become tense, the curve becomes steeper indicating less length change as the load increases.

Elongation (%) = Length Increase/Original Length

The elastic deformation of a material characterizes its ability to return to its original length following the release of a tensile force. Plastic deformation denotes permanent elongation. The ACL can elongate by 15%–20% before plastic deformation begins.

Stiffness (N/m^2)

Stiffness, expressed by the elastic modulus (N/m²), is the resistance of a material to deformation. It is represented graphically as the plot of force against length change. The elastic modulus is found by dividing tensile stress by strain and is expressed in N/m². A flat curve signifies low resistance to deformation, a steep curve high resistance to deformation:

$$\delta = E \cdot \varepsilon, \; E = \frac{\sigma}{\varepsilon}.$$

Creep

Artificial materials undergo plastic elongation when subjected to multiple cyclic loads. This phenomenon is known as "creep." Minimum elongation after load cycling under conditions comparable to physiologic loading is an essential property for an artificial ligament. Cruciate ligaments or artificial ligaments should be tested between 500 and 1400 N for 1 to 30×10^6 cycles. The plastic elongation induced by this test ranges from 1%–5% in synthetic materials.

Fatigue

Fatigue is associated with the phenomenon of creep. Biological materials have the ability to adapt and strengthen under loading. Artificial materials lack this property and eventually fail with plastic deformation and a decline in rupture strength, culminating in massive stretching or complete failure.

Biocompatibility

Biocompatibility is tested in the laboratory and in animal models. Artificial ligaments are tested in media similar to body fluids, and spectrophotometric analysis is used to determine whether any chemical substances are leached out. Tissue cultures are prepared, and finally laboratory animals are used to test histologic responses to the artificial substances, and mechanical tests are conducted under lifelike conditions. Olson (1988) tested currently used synthetic ligaments in rabbits by injecting wear particles from the various ligaments into the knee joint and then examining the tissues histologically. He also developed a protocol for analyzing failed reconstructions in human patients.

The following questions are still unresolved:

– What is the best animal model for investigating alloplastic ligament replacement?
– What clinical course is needed before an alloplastic ligament is approved for use (2, 3, or 5 years)?
– How large a population must be followed according to stringent criteria?
– How many different centers should participate in such a study?

Augmentation Devices

Nonbiodegradable LAD
(Ligament Augmentation Device)

Synthetic augmentation is intended for use in conjunction with a biological graft. The function of the synthetic band is to protect the biological graft from excessive loads during early healing, since the graft loses a significant portion of its original mechanical strength during this initial period. At the same time, the biological graft must carry some portion of the load in order to stimulate remodeling.

Two conditions must be satisfied:

– The augmentation device should not be attached to the bone at both ends, as this causes excessive stress protection of the biological graft.
– The attachment between the artificial and natural ligament must be such that the biological graft always carries a portion of the load ("load sharing").

Because of the gradually increasing load carried by the biological graft, the tissue eventually develops a ligamentous structure. In the long term, most the forces should be carried by the biological ligament.

In an *animal experiment* the ACL was excised in 54 goats and replaced by a patellar tendon graft. Half the reconstructions were augmented with an LAD (Roth 1985). The degeneration and regeneration of the autologous tissue was histologically evaluated in both groups (at 3, 6 and 12 months). The amount of regenerated and oriented collagen was significantly greater in the augmented group, especially at 6 and 12 months. Tissue ingrowth into the LAD was observed only at the periphery; there was no ingrowth of osseous tissue into the autologous graft or the LAD. When initial cast immobilization was dispensed with, significantly less chondromalacia was noted in the patellofemoral joint, and collagen regeneration was accelerated, initially in the augmented group. When the LAD was attached at both ends, the composite rupture strength of the augmentation device and autologous ligament was markedly reduced, and there were isolated instances of LAD failure.

Clinically, 43 unaugmented cases with a follow-up of 64 months were compared with 45 augmented cases followed for 50 months. The incidence of recurrent ACL insufficiency was 32% in the unaugmented group versus 11% in the augmented group. In the objective tests (KT 1000 arthrometer, Dybex, one-leg hop for distance), the augmented group was slightly better (both groups were cast-immobilized in 20°–30° flexion for the first 6 weeks).

Biodegradable Reinforcement
(Rehm and Schultheis 1985)

Compatibility is as important biologically as a proliferative stimulus for the formation of directionally oriented collagenous fiber network. The goal of biodegradable reinforcement is the formation of a biological substitute as an alternative to a permanently implanted ligament prosthesis.

Clinically a PDS (polydioxanone) degradable augmentation device was implanted in 10 patients using the Hey-Groves technique. The alloplastic band was inserted into the fascial strip, separately tightened, and fixed with a 3.5-mm small-fragment screw and washer. The patients were followed for 6–18 months; all were evaluated clinically, and 7 endoscopically and histologically.

The augmentated ACL reconstruction restored ligamentous stability in 9 of the 10 knee joints. Six of the endoscopic examinations showed a stiff regenerative structure. Excisional biopsies of the extraarticular portion of the ligament near the fixation screw revealed the desired longitudinally directed collagen fiber network and the PDS remnants.

Cabaud et al. (1982) transected the ACL proximally in 12 dogs, reapproximated it with sutures, and reinforced it with polyglycolic acid (PGA) composed of 30 braided 2/0 Dexon threads. At 2 weeks the ACL was well supported by the PGA band with no signs of synovitis. By 5 weeks the ACL had grown together, and the PGA band had been absorbed with no inflammatory or fibrotic reaction. Mechanical testing of the ligament at 4 months showed a maximum strength of approximately 54 kg, and histologic examination showed collagen-producing cells at the repair site. The PGA band functions as a splint and reinforcement. Some differences from human ligament injuries should be noted: The ligament was sharply divided in the experiment, whereas traumatic rupture of the ACL involves loss of substance with some degree of destruction and elongation. The synovium is generally torn and the blood supply compromised. In the experiment, the synovium was carefully preserved. When an absorbable ligament is used in humans, the absorption should proceed at a much slower rate since healing progresses more slowly than in dogs and the autologous tissue must be protected for 4–6 months.

Scaffolds

Carbon Fibers (see Table 2)

Jenkins first reported in 1980 on carbon fibers as a raw material for alloplastic ligament and tendon prostheses. Today, ligaments for use in human patients are made from 32 strands, each composed of 3000 individual filaments, braided together at a weave angle of 43°. Some of the disadvantages of carbon fibers, such as high sensitivity to shear forces and low elasticity, can be eliminated through new manufacturing techniques (Burri and Claes 1983; Claes et al. 1981; Wolter et al. 1978). The rationale for using carbon fibers for alloplastic tendon or ligament replacement is that the material does not lose its mechanical properties due to fiber breakage until endogenous ligament or tendon reparative tissue can assume this mechanical function as a result of fibrous tissue ingrowth into the implant (Jenkins and Jenkins 1977; Wolter et al. 1978). The histologic examination of carbon fiber ligaments after prolonged implantation in animals showed a hypocellular, tendon-like regenerative structure surrounding the individual carbon fibers (Forster 1976; Forster et al. 1978; Jenkins and Jenkins 1977; Wolter et al. 1978). Broken fibers can release carbon micro-particles that are phagocytized and collect in the lymphatic system or in parenchymatous organs (Burri 1980). Burri and Neugebauer (1981), Neugebauer et al. (1980), and Wolter et al. (1978) have described operative techniques for the implantation of carbon fiber ligaments in the knee. The implant is fixed to the bone by tucking the ends beneath proximally and distally based bone flaps on the femoral condyle and tibial plateau and compressing the flaps against the bone with fixation plates (Burri and Neugebauer 1981; Neugebauer et al. 1981; Wolter et al. 1979). Neugebauer and Burri (1981) reviewed 45 cases in which a carbon fiber implant was used for knee ligament reconstruction. Follow-ups were performed an average of 14.6 months postoperatively. Overall, the results were good in 88% of the cases and poor in 11%. Jenkins (1980) reported 43 good to satisfactory late results in 47 carbon fiber ligament reconstructions.

Hexel PLA Coated Carbon (Weiss 1985)

The usefulness of carbon fibers for cruciate ligament replacement is compromised by premature mechanical degradation. Coating the carbon with an absorbable copolymer (polylactic acid and polycapralactone) is believed to extend the intraarticular life of the carbon fibers until tissue ingrowth can occur. This material has been tested at 25 centers and used in approximately 1000 patients. From this multicentric study, the New Jersey Medical School has reviewed 110 knee ligament reconstructions with a follow-up of at least 1 year (including 36 with 2-year follow-ups). The patients had an average of 1.6 (0–13) previous operations. The coated carbon band was used along with autologous tissue for augmentation or by itself for reconstruction; the majority of cases were combined cruciate ligament and peripheral reconstructions. This study relied mainly on Cybex evaluations at 6-month intervals using a 100-point scoring system. Effusion was noted in 1/5 of the patients, and the KT 1000 arthrometer demonstrated good or excellent stability in a majority of the patients.

Leeds-Keio Ligament (Polyester) (Seedhom 1985)

The long-term success of an artificial cruciate ligament replacement depends on several factors:

– Isometric placement
– Mode of attachment
– Mechanical compatibility of the prosthetic ligament with the natural cruciate ligament
– The fatigue life of the artificial ligament

If errors are made, the first criterion will have immediate effects consisting of a restriction of joint motion or the persistence of instability. The remaining criteria are critical to the long-term success of the reconstruction.

The Leeds-Keio ligament is made of a polyester fiber (dacron in the U.S., Terylene in England) woven into a 2-part graft, 1 part tubular and the 2nd part flat.

Animal Experiments

The ACL was excised from 1 knee in each of 5 pigs and replaced with the prosthetic ligament. The animals were killed from 1 to 17 months after implantation. While only 1–2 fractures between the bone plug and tunnel were noted at 1 month, 4 such fractures were noted at 7 months. After that time the central portion of the bone plug was resorbed. At 9 months the boundary between the bone plug and tunnel was effaced, and there was extensive attachment of the bone plug to its surroundings.

Grossly, all the intraarticular fibers were covered by tissue after an average of 17.5 months. Histologically, the fibers were permeated by a granular necrotic material alternating with collagen and fibroblasts.

In summary, it was found that:

- The Leeds-Keio ligament has a maximum tensile strength of 2000 N.
- The stiffness of gas-sterilized ligaments is comparable to that of the natural ligament.
- The energy to failure is 18 Nm, versus 8–10 Nm for the natural ligament.

The prosthesis was implanted into 121 knees of human patients (104 ACL, 10 PCL, 7 ACL and PCL). Eighty-one patients were followed for more than 12 months, 43 of them for more than 24 months. The Lachman test and jerk test were satisfactory in 85% of the patients. Sixty percent achieved a full range of motion, and 15% had more than 21% loss of motion. Five of 8 active athletes were able to return to their original sport. Eighty-five percent of the patients were subjectively satisfied with the result, and 85% were objectively better than before the operation. Two patients required reoperation for instability. There was no reported evidence of joint effusion, synovitis, or infection. Arthroscopic biopsies taken in selected cases showed abundant longitudinally oriented collagen fibers. Histologic examination showed little inflammatory change in the synovial membranes about the ligament.

Cruciate Ligament Prostheses (Alloplasts)

Gore-Tex

The Gore-Tex ligament is made from a single fiber of expanded polytetrafluoroethylene (PTFE). The fiber is folded into bundles and braided in such a way that a eyelet for fixation is formed at each end of the prosthesis. For reconstruction of the ACL, the implant is passed through a tibial tunnel, routed over the top of the femur, inserted into a short proximal femoral tunnel, and its ends are initially fixed with screws. Definitive fixation must rely on bony and fibrous tissue ingrowth in the bone tunnels, made possible by the high porosity of the graft (the fibrils have a minimum size of 60 μm). The usual mechanical tests were performed, the bending fatigue tests using a load of only about 100 N.

Animal Experiments

The ACLs in 17 sheep were replaced with a Gore-Tex ligament for a maximum of 1 year. Maximum tensile strength was approximately 5000 N with an average elongation of 9%. Histologic examination confirmed tissue ingrowth into the prosthesis. The intraarticular portion of the graft was permeated by synovial and connective tissue, and imprecisely defined tissue lay in the around the graft inside the bone tunnels. Biocompatibility was good, with no demonstrable mutagenic or toxic effects.

Mechanical testing was designed to assess the potential life of the prosthesis, especially with regard to creep and bending strength (fatigue bending).

The "life span" of the prosthesis with respect to elongation is 6.0×10^8 cycles. It is assumed that an average individual will subject the ligament to 4.2×10^6 load cycles per year. One imprecision of the mechanical test procedure is that the ligament was cyclically tested at a constant load, which is unlike the very diverse loads occurring in daily life. The over-the-top positioning results in progressive laxity as flexion increases. The nonanatomic placement was chosen to extend the life of the prosthesis. Broken fibers found at the posterior rim of the tibial inlet on the intercondylar eminence were attributed to a peculiar knee geometry. The stiffness of the natural ligament is reported to be 129–183 N per mm (Noyes and Grood 1976).

The Gore-Tex ligament shows an average stiffness of 219 N per mm. The maximum tensile strength of the cruciate ligament in sheep averages 1912 N, and 1730 N in younger humans (52). The fixation or tearout strength is 1380 N.

Clinical Experience

A multicentric study (Gore-Tex 1988) covered 187 patients (68% male, 32% female) averaging 27.5 years of age who were followed for a minimum of 3 years. While 84% had a 2 + to 3 + Lachman test before operation, 38% had a negative Lachman test at about 3 years postoperatively, and 50% had a negative test at 1–2 years; 17% exhibited a 2 + to 3 + Lachman displacement. Ten percent of the patients experienced significant giving way postoperatively, and another 17% reported a vague "giving way sensation"; 30% of patients reported mild pain, 24% moderate pain. Mild swelling was noted in about 34% of the patients and marked swelling in about 7%. Stair climbing was the only function test evaluated, with approximately 25% of patients experiencing difficulties. About 10% of patients reported disability in daily living activities after 1 year or more. About 5% rated their condition as worse than before the operation. Rupture of the ligament was recorded in 6% of the patients, and the infection rate was 2.7%.

Proflex (48.00.30)

The Proflex ligament consists of 28 tubular layers of the polyester polyethylene terephthalate (PT, Tersuisse). The central (intraarticular) portion of the ligament is elastic, with fiber directions and diameters changing in response to tensile stresses. The knee stiffness approximates that of the natural ACL. In vitro experiments have failed to demonstrate cytotoxic effects. The PT material is compatible with cell growth. The device is implanted using a tibial tunnel and an over-the-top femoral placement. After the ligament is stapled to the femur, it is tightened to a force of 150 N and fixed medially to the tibia with a second staple, then the ends are buried in the femoral and tibial bone. The rupture strength is approximately 4500 N at a stress of 15 kp, with a further 10 mm elongation reached at approximately 100 kp.

Results

The average age of the population was 27 years with a 3:1 ratio of males to females. Sixty-two patients were followed for a minimum of 2 years. Their Lysholm score was 61 points preoperatively and 96 points at approximately 2 years. The pivot shift test was negative in 53%, 1 + in 39%, and 2 + in 8%; the Lachman test was negative in 70%, 1 + in 25%, and 2 + to 3 + in 5%. Laximetry recorded a 2.3-mm gain in stability. Ruptures and severe synovial reactions each had an incidence of about 5%.

Stryker Dacron (44)

This cruciate ligament implant is made of polyethylene terephthalate and has a rupture strength of 300 kp and a maximum strain of 18%. The force-elongation curve of the dacron ligament closely resembles that of human ACL. The ligament is implanted using the MacIntosh technique (MacIntosh 1973, 1974; MacIntosh and Darby 1976; MacIntosh and Tregonning 1977), i.e., a tibial tunnel and an over-the-top femoral placement, both ends attached with staples. Autologous tissue (fascia lata or patellar tendon) was originally used with the prosthesis, but today the dacron band is generally used alone.

Approximately 600 dacron ligaments were implanted from 1979 through 1984 (210 in the shoulder, 233 in the knee). More than half the patients participated in strenuous sports, and 1/3 engaged in light exercise. Only 15% of the patients had had previous knee operations; half of these were medial meniscectomies, and there were 59 extraarticular transfers and 8 lateral meniscectomies. In 1/3 of patients the medial meniscus was removed at the time of the cruciate ligament replacement, and 9% underwent a concomitant medial reconstruction.

Results

Results with the Arpège system were excellent in 71.1% of cases, good in 22.8%, and poor in 6.1%. Two-thirds of the patients were pain-free, and 24% experienced pain, which generally was exertion-dependent. Ten percent experienced frequent pain and were unable to participate in sports. While 85% of the patients rated their stability as good, 15% complained of instability, especially when walking on uneven ground or when running. Ninety percent of the patients had equivalent ranges of motion in both knees, and 10% retained a mild flexion deficit in the operated joint.

Postoperative complications (7%):

– Reflex sympathetic dystrophy: 6
– Hematoma evacuation: 12
– Effusion or synovitis: 19 (3.3%)
– Ligament rupture: 13 (2.2%)
– Venous thrombosis: 10
– Superficial infection: 5
– Deep infection: 2

Discussion

Dacron is biocompatible and causes relatively little intraarticular irritation. Fibrous tissue growth binds the ligament to the bone, especially the tibia, and after several years the tibial tunnel is no longer visible on X-rays. Thirteen ruptures were documented, some occurring in the area of the femoral attachment and some near the intraarticular mouth of the tibial tunnel. No rupture occurred earlier than 6 months postoperatively. Bacteriologically sterile synovitis developed in 10% of cases (not including the 13 ruptures). A fibrous sheath containing multiple giant cells (foreign body reaction) forms around the dacron band. The problems of synovitis and ruptures are the strongest evidence that there is room for further improvement in the dacron prosthesis.

Telos (Trevira High Strength, Type 730)

The ideal material for a prosthetic ligament is a woven polymeric material that is chemically stable in the physiologic milieu, resists fatigue, transmits linear loads efficiently, has a nearly physiologic compliance, can be twisted for anatomic positioning, and can be manufactured in an appropriately small size.

The Telos ligament is a PET band 300 mm long, 10 mm wide, and 1 mm thick woven from 60 longitudinal fibers (chain) and 16 transverse fibers (throw), each fiber composed of 20 individual elements with an average diameter of 23 µm. Previous animal experiments have been *extra*articular (e.g., in the sheep foreleg), so their implications are unclear. A tensile load of 500 N produces 2% strain, and the maximum tensile load is 3600 N.

Clinical Experience (Contzen 1985)

From August, 1980, to April, 1985, the Telos ligament was implanted in 71 patients with chronic ligamentous knee instability, some of whom had had multiple previous operations. ACL replacement was done in

44 patients, PCL replacement in 4, and peripheral reconstructions in the others.

Results

Drawer motion was radiographically absent in 75% of the patients, 3–5 mm in 20%, and 6–8 mm in 5%. Half the patient had a complete range of motion, and the other half showed mild limitation (10°–20°). The overall outcome rating focused on the stability of the ligaments, the condition of the muscles, and the function of the joint. Objectively, 50% of the cases were rated excellent, 30% good, and 20% fair to satisfactory. Subjectively, 64% of the patients stated that they had no problems with the operated knee, although only 36% felt that the operated knee was as good as the opposite knee. Thirty-nine percent reported occasional pain, while 83% said they had no laxness or instablity. Approximately 60% reported a vague "feeling of weakness" in the knee.

Tendon Allografts and Xenografts

One issue relating to the use of homologous and heterologous tendon grafts involves the reaction of the graft bed to donor tissue obtained from a different individual or even a different species. Two theories have been advanced to address this question. Herzog (1963) and Seiffert (1967) state that the allograft or xenograft functions as a stent for endogenous tissue ingrowth, with eventual integration of the foreign tissue, while Jäger claims that the graft becomes enveloped by endogenous tissue and is gradually absorbed ("creeping replacement") (Ansorge and Franke 1978; Kleining 1977; Salamon et al. 1970; Voorhoeve and Hierholzer 1975). The latter theory is favored in the literature owing to the discovery of granulation tissue, plasma cells, and eosinophils at the graft/bed interface consistent with a foreign body response (Kleining 1977; Voorhoeve and Hierholzer 1975). This protracted foreign body reaction in the graft bed is the essential disadvantage of using tendon allografts and xenografts, whose antigenic action cannot always be adequately suppressed despite appropriate chemical and thermal storage methods (Kleining 1977). Voorhoeve and Hierholzer (1975) reported on techniques for the plastic reconstruction of the collateral and cruciate ligaments of the knee. Reports on the use of tendon allografts and xenografts for knee ligament reconstruction have indicated good results in 85% of cases, fair in about 10%,

and poor in 11% (Jäger and Wirth 1978; Voorhoeve and Hierholzer 1975). Particular preference has been given to the use of freeze-dried allografts in recent years (Rosenberg, personal communication).

Animal Experiments

Curtis et al. (1985) transected the ACL in 16 dogs, replacing it with a freeze-dried fascia lata allograft. Eight of the grafts were placed through tibial and femoral bone tunnels, and 8 used a tibial tunnel with an over-the-top femoral placement. In all cases the graft was passed beneath the lateral collateral ligament and fixed to the tibia for extraarticular reinforcement. Histologic studies and biomechanical tests were conducted at 3, 6, 12, and 24 weeks. At reoperation all of the grafts appeared intact, and none showed gross evidence of incompatibility. The knees displayed a mild degree of instability. Histologically, the grafts appeared to provide a collagen scaffold for revascularization and progressive fibrovascular replacement. The rupture force at 24 weeks was approximately 530 N, compared with 800 N in the contralateral knee with an intact ACL.

Bovine Xenograft (Drobny 1986)

Rupture of this graft – composed of glutaraldehyde-stabilized bovine tendon – in uniaxial tensile tests generally occurred at the attachment site. The calculated maximum load is 2000 N, the tensile strength at failure 70 N/mm^2 (both values are slightly higher than those of the human ACL).

Animal Experiments

Experiments in sheep (Drobny 1986) demonstrated the following:

Revascularization

The earliest, very sparse capillary invasion was seen microangiographically at 3 months. In plain sections the graft still presented the appearance of a foreign body in cross section after 1 year.

Rupture Tests

Bone-ligament-bone specimens from 2 ovine knees with the ACL xenograft were removed for rupture testing 1 year after operation. One had a fatigue fracture at the proximal attachment when exposed and was excluded from testing. In the 2nd specimen, a force of approximately 200 N tore the graft completely from the femoral tunnel, implying that there was deficient incorporation of the graft within the tunnel. The graft itself was markedly stiff and showed no intramural substance loss.

Based on these experimental results in sheep, the bovine xenograft was judged to be unsuitable as a cruciate ligament replacement material.

Most animal experiments have involved the extra-articular application of the xenograft, which is not helpful for assessing its use as an intraarticular ACL substitute.

An experimental series in rabbits with a maximum follow-up of 1 year demonstrated patial or complete ensheathment of the graft by synovium. Tissue ingrowth in the bone tunnels was observed along the natural clefts in the xenograft (fibrocartilage). The histology of the intraarticular portion was not described.

Clinical Experience

The xenograft has been used clinically in the U.S. for about 4 years. As of 1985 it had been implanted in 395 patients at 50 centers; 252 were cruciate ligament replacements. The 30 *complications* (7.5%) included 26 cases of postoperative synovitis and/or graft failure. Twenty-nine complications were classified as non-graft-related, 8 due to faulty tightening of the graft or nonisometric tunnel placement, 8 to patient noncompliance. There were 12 cases of infection, 9 by *Staphylococcus aureus*. In 2 series (McMaster et al. 1985, 98 cases; Whipple 1985, 64 cases) the xenograft was implanted under arthroscopic control. Ten patients developed transient synovitis 4–6 months postoperatively, 2 with significant limitation of knee motion. A total of 4 ruptures occurred during the 1st year. Cystic swellings were occasionally noted at the exit sites of the graft on the tibia due to intraarticular fluid leakage through the bone tunnel.

Summary

Cruciate reconstruction with the bovine xenograft, implanted arthroscopically or by open surgery, is a relatively simple procedure that can afford good stability. On the negative side, the complication rate is approximately 25% during just the 1st year. Also, experiments in ovine knees have shown that the bioprosthesis remains essentially as dead material within the joint and at best may show a peripheral ingrowth of nondirectional fibrous tissue.

Discussion

The following problems still have to be overcome in the use of artificial ligaments:

- Material technology in the selection of a ligament
- Practical surgical difficulties during implantation of the ligament (operating technique)
- Long-term performance under high loads
- Ethical problems

Material Technology in Ligament Selection

Autologous reconstructions, discussed extensively in previous chapters, have a reported success rate of 75%–80% in recent publications. While it appears that tendon xenografts are declining in importance as intraarticular cruciate ligament substitutes, allografts (e.g., Achilles tendon) have been used increasingly in recent years with good results (Rosenberg, personal communication). *Three principles* have emerged in the clinical application of alloplastic ligament materials: use of a synthetic band to reinforce an autologous graft (augmentation), use of a synthetic scaffold that induces secondary *fibrous tissue ingrowth* and replacement, and finally use of an inert prosthesis for *definitive replacement*. *Carbon fibers*, formerly uncoated, today are more commonly used in a coated form for better strength and handling. The induction of fibrous tissue formation by carbon fiber implants has been confirmed clinically and experimentally, but the coating on the fibers, intended to prevent fiber destruction, alters the porous surface and hampers tissue ingrowth. The friability of the carbon fibers and the deposition of carbon particles in the joint itself and in parenchymatous organs are known complications. Consequently, carbon fibers can no longer be recommended today for intraarticular cruciate ligament reconstruction. The *polymers* currently preferred as synthetic ligament materials are polyamides, polyester, and polyethylene. *Permanent prosthetic devices* made of these materials include Gore-Tex (polytetrafluoroethylene), Proflex (polyethylene terephthalate), and the Stryker Meadox graft (dacron with a velour surface coating). This type of synthetic ligament, known also as a *total prosthesis*, can function for only a limited time since it does not induce the formation of autologous replacement tissue. The implants will eventually stretch or rupture with passage of time. They have limited biocompatibility, and their implantation incites a classic foreign body response, with histologic studies revealing material damage. Protracted synovitis complicates approximately 20% of cases, even with an unruptured ligament, but generally responds well to single or multiple arthroscopic irrigations. So far, microbiologic evaluation of the synovitis has not revealed the presence of infectious organisms. Synovitis appears to be less common in association with synthetic augmentations (LAD) or ligaments receptive to tissue ingrowth (carbon, Leeds-Keio, Stryker and Telos). In terms of biomechanical properties, carbon fiber implants cannot provide strength in the immediate postoperative period. Some time is needed for fibrous tissue ingrowth to occur. Prosthetic ligaments for permanent substitution all display adequate mechanical strength. They resist all anticipated loads, and cyclic rupture tests in the laboratory yield favorable results. The elasticity of prosthetic ligaments still lags behind that of the human cruciate ligament, which can undergo 10%–15% elastic elongation; this degree of elongation in prosthetic ligaments generally enters the range of plastic deformation, causing the artificial ligament to stretch before it fails. There is disagreement in published data on the forces that develop in the ACL and its maximum rupture strength. While Chen and Black (1980) found a value of 630 N, Noyes and Grood (1976) reported 1700 N for the ACL of younger individuals, also stating that the yield point (limit of elastic deformation) is reached at 1100 N. Since an artificial ligament lacks protection by proprioceptive fibers, it must have greater mechanical strength than the natural ACL. One difficulty in the testing of artificial ligaments (Instron) is the necessary time compression, where ligaments are loaded in rapid sequence with inadequate recovery periods between loads.

Practical Surgical Problems

Practical surgical problems relate to handling of the ligaments and the need to make compromises in the search for optimum isometry. Carbon fibers are particularly sensitive to handling and are easily damaged by instruments or when pulled through a joint. The advantage of a total prosthesis (Gore-Tex, dacron, Telos, Proflex, etc.) is that it obviates the need to sacrifice autologous tissue, resulting in a simpler operative technique. Originally the dacron ligament was used in conjunction with autologous tissue (fascia lata) for augmentation, but today it is employed chiefly as a total prosthesis and thus runs counter to the philosophy of augmentation. In their review, Mansat et al. (1984) noted a slight advantage of dacron as a total prosthesis over dacron with autologous tissue, although the differences were not sta-

tistically significant. With regard to implantation technique, most surgeons have come to favor the over-the-top route, since transcondylar positioning apparently increases the risk of ligament rupture. Most ruptures in over-the-top reconstructions occur distally, near the entry of the ligament into the tibial tunnel. An exception is the Gore-Tex prosthesis, whose proximal, extraarticular portion tends to rupture past the over-the-top segment and before entry into the femoral tunnel.

Fixation by stapling is not ideal, especially on the tibial side, where screw fixation, as recommended by Gore-Tex, appears to be more effective. The Leeds-Keio system offers an interesting solution in which the woven dacron tube is secured in the tunnel with a bone plug. This appears to provide reliable fixation. Retention during postoperative rehabilitation is independent of the mode of fixation. The attachment of the ligament to the bone inside the tunnels varies among different devices. With a dacron graft, a fibrous attachment is formed. Animal experiments with the Gore-Tex and Telos ligaments have demonstrated some ingrowth of osseous tissue into the prosthesis.

Long-Term Performance Under High Loads

The major complications of prosthetic ligament surgery are *synovitis* and *ruptures*. Ruptures generally occur within a relatively short time after surgery (e.g., during the first 2 years with dacron and Gore-Tex). Even "traumatic" ruptures should probably be interpreted essentially as fatigue failures. Prosthetic ligaments placed in the transcondylar position tend to rupture near the femur, while ligaments routed "over the top" tend to rupture intraarticularly near the tibia. If the tibial tunnel is placed too far anteriorly, the rim of the intercondylar notch exerts a guillotine action that can culminate in shearing and rupture. Synovitis is a more frequent complication of prosthetic replacements than of autologous reconstructions. Its incidence ranges between 3% and 10%, and its causes are not yet fully understood. Mansat et al. (1984) attempted to classify postreconstruction synovitis into 3 types: mild, marked, and infection-related. Mild synovitis represents a self-limiting foreign body reaction, with white cell counts in aspirated fluid reaching 3000–7000. Generally this reaction subsides without treatment after the synthetic ligament has acquired a synovial investment. Marked synovitis is associated with leukocyte counts up to 20,000, massive fibrin formation, and an elevated ESR. It may result from a chemical reaction to the antoxidants or an allergic response to the synthetic material (usually polyester). Infectious organisms have not been detected in this type of synovitis. If the inflammation is not controlled by single or multiple arthroscopic irrigations, the ligament must be removed or replaced. Finally, septic synovitis is associated with all the features of a knee infection. In augmentation procedures, necrosis of the autologous material has been suggested as a potential cause of the synovitis (Gacon 1986).

The carcinogenic risks of artificial ligaments are difficult to assess. Dacron has been used in vascular surgery for more than 30 years, so it is reasonable to assume a minimal carcinogenic risk. Carbon particles have been found in most parenchymatous organs following the rupture of carbon fiber ligaments in the knee. We may expect that fluorine-containing particles from a ruptured Gore-Tex ligament, for example, would undergo a similar dissemination. Mechanical tests (Instron, etc.) cannot precisely reproduce intraarticular conditions, due largely to the absence of normal recovery periods for the stressed ligaments. Chen and Black (1980) report that forces up to 630 N develop physiologically in the ACL. Noyes and Grood (1976) state that the a force of 1700 N is needed to rupture the ACL in young, athletically trained individuals, with plastic deformation commencing at 1100 N. Because an artificial ligament lacks natural protection by proprioceptive fibers, the synthetic ligament must be stronger than the natural ligament (at least 1500 N). In Instron tests of the Proflex ligament, a load of 1500 N produced 5% residual elongation after 500 cycles. Loading at 2500 N caused an irreversible change of elasticity, with consequent elongation of the ligament. The ACL of a marathon runner is subjected to approximately 20,000 tensile load cycles, with forces equivalent to about one-half the body weight. Chen and Black (1980) estimate that the ACL of an athlete will undergo an average of 1.5 million cyclic tensile loads per year. Since few authors can report on more than 5 years' clinical experience with synthetic ligaments, we still can only speculate as to the long-term performance of these devices.

Ethical Problems

Significant ethical questions arise in connection with the use of synthetic knee ligaments. Should artificial ligaments, like joint replacement arthroplasty, be essentially reserved for older patients? Should synthetic ligaments be used in young patients despite the risk that a good early result may encourage a premature return to overvigorous activities? Is total replacement of the cruciate ligament feasible, or should we use augmentation techniques or materials receptive to long-term endogenous tissue ingrowth? Should autologous tissue be spared when a synthetic is used so that, in the event of failure, a classic ligament reconstruction can still be carried out? Even with autologous tissue transfers, there is still much diversity in the assessment of long-term results. Finally, some authors claim that synthetic ligaments should be reserved for salvage cases, i.e., severely unstable knees in which multiple previous operations have been performed and there is virtually no prospect for a successful autologous reconstruction. While this may be a valid indication for prosthetic replacement, there would be a correspondingly higher risk of complications.

The application of prosthetics to ligamentous knee surgery still poses a great many problems. Yet we are still in the initial stages of this discipline, much as we were 30 years ago with respect to joint replacement arthroplasty. Thus, we may anticipate further progress in prosthetic ligament surgery, leading to more consistent and permanent successes. It is reasonable to expect that this technique will become an established and important subspecialty of ligamentous surgery. In all cases the potential complications of the procedure should be thoroughly discussed with the patient beforehand in a preoperative consultation.

References

Alm A (1973) Survival of part of patellar tendon transposed for reconstruction of anterior cruciate ligament. Acta Chir Scand 139: 443–447

Ansorge D, Franke A (1978) Anwendungsmöglichkeiten homologer citalitkonservierter Sehnen und Bänder. Zentralbl Chir 2: 98–107

Arnoczky SP, Tarvin GB, Marshall JL (1982) Anterior cruciate ligament replacement using patellar tendon. An evaluation of graft revascularization. J Bone Joint Surg [Am] 64: 217–224

Arvidsson I, Eriksson E, Häggmark T, Johnson RJ (1981) Isokinetic thigh muscle strength after ligament reconstruction in the knee joint: Results from a 5–10 year follow-up after reconstructions. Int J Sports Med 2: 7–11

Burri C, Claes L (1983) Alloplastischer Bandersatz. In: Aktuelle Probleme in Chirurgie und Orthopädie, Bd 25. Huber, Bern Stuttgart Wien

Burri C (1980) Grundlagen des Kniebandersatzes durch Kohlenstoff. Unfallheilkunde 83: 208–213

Burri C, Neugebauer R (1981) Technik des alloplastischen Bandersatzes mit Kohlefasern. Unfallchirurgie 7: 289–297

Cabaud HE, Feagin JA, Rodkey WG (1982) Acute anterior cruciate ligament injury and repair reinforced with a biodegradable intraarticular ligament. Am J Sports Med 10/5: 259–265

Chen EH, Black J (1980) Materials design analysis of the prosthetic anterior cruciate ligament. J Biomed Mater Res 14: 567

Claes L, Burri C, Neugebauer R, Wolter D (1981) Biomechanische Untersuchungen zum alloplastischen Ersatz von Bändern mit elastischen Kohlenstoffaserbandprothesen. Rheumamedizin 3: 63-64

Clancy WG, Nelson DA, Reider B, Narechania RG (1982) Anterior cruciate ligament reconstruction using one-third of the patellar ligament, augmented by extra-articular tendon transfers. J Bone Joint Surg [Am] 64: 352-359

Contzen H (1963) Grundlagen der Alloplastik. Habilitationsschrift, Johann Wolfgang Goethe Universität Frankfurt/Main

Contzen H (1969) Biologische Grundlagen der Alloplastik. In: Handbuch der plastischen Chirurgie, Bd 1. de Gruyter, Berlin S 1-36

Contzen H (1981) Die Korrektur veralteter Kniebandverletzungen mit textilem Kunststoffband. 17. Tagung der Österreichischen Gesellschaft für Unfallchirurgie

Contzen H (1981) Mechanical properties of polyester ligament replacement alloplastic ligament replacement. Symposium on alloplastic ligament, Reisenburger Workshop 4.-5. 12. 1981

Contzen H (1985) Materialtechnische Voraussetzungen und biologische Grundlagen für den alloplastischen Kniebandersatz. Unfallchirurgie 2/5: 242-246

Contzen H, Straumann F, Paschke G (1967) Grundlagen der Alloplastik mit Metallen und Kunststoffen. Thieme, Stuttgart, S 77-163

Contzen M (1983) Experimentelle Untersuchungen zur Rekonstruktion isolierter Bandstrukturen durch alloplastisches Bandmaterial. Med. Dissertation, Johann-Wolfgang-Goethe-Universität, Frankfurt/Main

Curtis RJ, Delee JC, Drez DJ (1985) Reconstruction of the anterior cruciate ligament with freeze dried fascia lata allografts in dogs. Am J Sports Med 13: 408-414

Drobny T (1986) Kreuzbandersatz im Tierexperiment. Vortrag ACL Study Group, Zermatt

Eriksson E (1976) Reconstruction of the anterior cruciate ligament. Orthop Clin North America 7: 167-179

Forster JW (1976) A study of the mechanism by which carbon fibre acts as a tendon prosthesis. J Bone Joint Surg [Br] 58: 376

Forster JW (1978) Biological reactions to carbon fibre implants. Clin Orthop 131: 300-307

Fox JM (1985) Prosthetic ligament reconstruction. In: UCLA Extension (ed) 2nd annual symposium prosthetic ligament reconstruction of the knee. Palm Springs/CA, pp 137-147

Fujikawa K (1985) Clinical study of cruciate ligament reconstruction with Leeds-Keio artificial ligament. In: UCLA Extension (ed) 2nd annual symposium prosthetic ligament reconstruction of the knee. Palm Springs/CA, pp 126-128

Fujikawa K (1986) Clinical study of the Leeds-Keio artificial ligament. In: UCLA Extension (ed) 3rd annual symposium prosthetic ligament reconstruction of the knee, 10.-12. 4.

Gacon G (1986) Problèmes généraux posés par l'utilisation des ligaments artificiels en chirurgie du genoux. J Traumatol Sport 3/1: 3-5

Götz H (1974) Kunststoffkompatibilitätsstudien. Langenbecks Arch Chir 335: 95-126

Gore-Tex (1988) SL Gore & Associates (UK) Ltd. Kirkton Campus Livingston West Lothian Scotland EH54 7BH. Gore Tex Ligament, United States Clinical Investigation

Henning CE (1979) Anterior cruciate ligament reconstruction with fat pad coverage: Six years experience. First Congress of the International Society of the Knee, Lyon

Herzog KH (1963) Experimentelle Grundlagen der Transplantation von konserviertem Sehnengewebe. Langenbecks Arch Chir 303: 303-324

Homsy A (1981) Proplast knee ligament implants. Symposium on alloplastic ligament, Reisensburger Workshop 4.-5. 12. 1981

Hughston JC, Barrett GR (1983) Acute anteromedial rotatory instability. Long-term results of surgical repair. J Bone Joint Surg [Am] 65: 145-153

Jäger M, Wirth CJ (1978) Kapselbandläsionen. In: Biomechanik, Diagnostik und Therapie. Thieme, Stuttgart, S 124-170

James SK, Kellam JF, Slocum DB, Larsen RL (1983) Der Proplast-Ligament-Ersatz für die Kreuzbänder des Kniegelenkes. In: Burri C (Hrsg) Aktuelle Probleme in Chirurgie und Orthopädie. Huber, Bern Stuttgart Wien (Alloplastischer Bandersatz, Bd 25, S 124-129)

Jenkins D, Jenkins HR (1977) Induction of tendon and ligament formation by carbon implants. J Bone Joint Surg [Br] 59: 53-57

Jenkins DHR (1980) The role of flexible carbon-fibre implants as tendon and ligament substitutes in clinical practice. J Bone Joint Surg [Br] 62: 497-499

Johnson RJ, Eriksson E, Haggmark T, Pope MH (1984) A five to ten year follow-up after reconstruction of the anterior cruciate ligament. Clin Orthop 183: 122

Jones KG (1980) Results of use of the central one-third of the patellar ligament to compensate for anterior cruciate ligament deficiency. Clin Orthop 147: 39

Kennedy JC (1978) Late reconstruction of injured ligaments of the knee. In: Schultz HP, Krahl H, Stein WH (eds) Late reconstructions of injured ligaments of the knee. Springer, Berlin Heidelberg New York, p 30

Kennedy JC (1983) The use of a ligament augmentation device (L. A. D.) in the anterior cruciate deficient knee. Vortrag, American Academc of Orthopaedic Surgeons, Anaheim

Kennedy JC, Fowler PJ (1971) Medial and anterior instability of the knee. An anatomical and clinical study using stress machines. J Bone Joint Surg [Am] 53: 1257-1270

Kennedy JC, Willis RB (1976) Synthetic cruciate ligaments — preliminary report. J Bone Joint Surg [Br] 58: 142

Kennedy JC, Weinberg MW, Wilson AS (1974) The anatomy and function of the anterior cruciate ligament. As determined by clinical and morphological studies. J Bone Joint Surg [Am] 56: 223-235

Kennedy JC, Hawkins RJ, Willis RB, Danylchuk KG (1976) Tension studies of human knee ligaments. Yield point, ultimate failure, and disruption of the cruciate and tibial collateral ligaments. J Bone Joint Surg [Am] 58: 350-355

Kennedy JC, Stewart R, Walker DM (1978) Anterolateral rotary instability of the knee point. An early analysis of the Ellison procedure. J Bone Joint Surg [Am] 60: 1031-1039

Kinzl L et al. (1976) Gewebeverträglichkeit der Polymere Polyäthylen, Polyester und Polyacetatharz. Z Orthop 114: 777-784

Kleining R (1977) Behandlung älterer Bandverletzungen am Kniegelenk mit freien homologen und heterologen Transplantaten. Hefte Unfallheilkd 129: 179-181

Konikoff J (1974) Development of a single stage active tendon prosthesis. J Bone Joint Surg [Am] 56: 848

Larson RL (1988) Prosthetic Replacement of Knee Liga-

530   U. Munzinger

ments: Overview. In: Feagin JA (ed) The crucial ligaments. Churchill-Livingstone, New York, pp 495–506

Lysholm J, Gillquist J, Liljedahl SO (1981) Long term results after early treatment of knee injuries. Acta Orthop Scand 53: 109

Mansat C, Gacon G, Lalain JJ (1984) Plastie antéro-externe du genou - interêt du Dacron à propos de 500 cas revus. 5èmes Journées Lyonnaises de Chirurgie du Genou, Lyon, pp 263–269

McIntosh DL (1973) The lateral pivot shift: Symposium on knee injuries. ACS Clinitape, C73–OR3

McIntosh DL (1974) Acute tears of the anterior cruciate ligament. Over the top repair. Vortrag, AAOS Meeting in Dallas, Texas

McIntosh DL, Darby TA (1976) Lateral substitution reconstruction. J Bone Joint Surg [Br] 58: 142

McIntosh DL, Tregonning RJA (1977) A follow-up study and evaluation of „over the top" repair of acute tears of the anterior cruciate ligament. J Bone Joint Surg [Br] 59: 511

McMaster WC, Greenwald AS, Springer SI (1985) Properties and clinical applications of bioprosthetic tendons and ligaments. In: UCLA Extension (ed) 2nd annual symposium prosthetic ligament reconstruction of the knee. Palm Springs/CA, pp 105–111

Mironova S (1978) Spätresultate der Rekonstruktion des Bandapparates des Kniegelenkes mit Lawsan. Zentralbl Chir 103: 432–434

Mockwitz J (1985) Der alloplastische Ersatz der veralteten isolierten Kreuzbandruptur. Unfallchirurgie 11/6: 295–301

Mockwitz J et al. (1980) Erweiterte Diagnostik der Kapselbandverletzung am Kniegelenk. Unfallchirurgie 6/2: 94–100

Neugebauer R (1980) Der Kreuzbandersatz durch Kohlenstoffaser. Hefte Unfallheilkd 148: 259–262

Neugebauer R, Burri C (1981) Ergebnisse nach alloplastischem Bandersatz mit Kohlenstoffasern. Unfallchirurgie 7: 298–304

Neugebauer R (1981) In Vitro- und in Vivo-Untersuchungen zur Fixation von Kohlenstoffasersträngen als Bandersatz am Kniegelenk. Rheumamedizin 3: 21–24

Nicholas JA (1973) The five-one reconstruction for anteromedial instability of the knee. Indications, technique and the results in fifty-two patients. J Bone Joint Surg [Am] 55: 899–922

Noyes FR (1977) Functional properties of knee ligaments and alterations induced by immobilization: A correlative biomechanical and histological study in primates. Clin Orthop 123: 210–239

Noyes FR, Grood ES (1976) The strength of the anterior cruciate ligament in humans and rhesus monkeys. Age-related and species-related changes. J Bone Joint Surg [Am] 58: 1074

Noyes FR, Grood ES (1977) Knee ligament function and failure. Clinical application of biomechanics, biomechanical test and concepts. Vortrag, American Orthopaedic Society of Sport Medicine, Las Vegas

Noyes FR, Sonstegard DA, Arbor A (1973) Biomechanical function of the pes anserinus of the knee and the effect of its transplantation. J Bone Joint Surg [Am] 55: 1225–1241

Noyes FR, De Lucas J, Torvik PJ (1974 a) Biomechanics of anterior cruciate ligament failure: An analysis of strain-rate sensitivity and mechanism of failure in primates. J Bone Joint Surg [Am] 56: 236–253

Noyes FR, Torvik PJ, Hyde WB (1974 b) Biomechanics of ligament failure. An analysis of immobilization, exercise and reconditioning effects in primates. J Bone Joint Surg [Am] 56: 1406

Noyes FR, Butler DL, Grood ES, Basset RW, Hosea T (1978) Clinical paradoxes of anterior cruciate instability and a new test to detect its instability. Orthop Trans 2: 36

Noyes FR, Bassett RW, Grood ES, Butler DL (1980 a) Arthroscopy in acute traumatic hemarthrosis of the knee. Incidence of anterior cruciate tears and other injuries. J Bone Joint Surg [Am] 62: 687

Noyes FR et al. (1980 b) Arthroscopy in acute traumatic hemarthrosis of the knee. J Bone Joint Surg [Am] 62: 687–695

Noyes FR, Mooar PA, Matthews DS, Butler DL (1983 a) The symptomatic anterior cruciate-deficient knee. Part I. The long-term functional disability in athletically active individuals. J Bone Joint Surg [Am] 65: 154

Noyes FR, Butler DL, Paulos LE, Grood ES (1983 b) Intraarticular cruciate reconstruction. 1. Perspectives on graft strength, vascularization, and immediate motion after replacement. Clin Orthop 172: 71

Olson EJ (1988) The biocompatibility of anterior cruciate ligament replacements: Current clinical, histological and biochemical knowledge, with a protocol for failed ligament retrieval. 55th Annual Meeting, Atlanta/GA, Feb-ruary 4–9

Oretorp N, Gillquist J, Liljedahl SO (1979) Long term results of surgery for non acute anteromedial rotatory instability of the knee. Acta Orthop Scand 50: 329–336

Poppon P, Prudhon JL (1977) Techniques et résultats de l'intervention de Kenneth Jones. Chirurgie du Genou, 3èmes Journées, Lyon, pp 92–93

Rehm KE, Schultheis KH (1985) Bandersatz mit Polydioxanon (PDS) Unfallchirurg 11, 5: 264–273

Roth JH et al. (1985) PP braid augmented and non-augmented intraarticular ACL reconstruction. Am J Sports Med 13/5: 321

Roth JH (1985) Simultaneous clinical follow-up of polypropylene augmented and non-augmented anterior cruciate ligament reconstructions. In: UCLA Extension (ed) 2nd annual symposium prosthetic ligament reconstruction of the knee. Palm Springs/CA, pp 65–98

Salamon A (1970) Der experimentelle Ersatz des vorderen Kreuzbandes im Kniegelenk durch Transplantate verschiedenen Typs. Bruns Beitr Klin Chir 218: 182–191

Seedhom B (1985) The Leeds-Keio ligament. In: UCLA Extension (ed) 2nd annual symposium prosthetic ligament reconstruction of the knee. Palm Springs/CA, pp 115–125

Seiffert KE (1967) Biologische Grundlagen der homologen Transplantation konservierter Bindegewebe. Hefte Unfallheilkd

Semlitsch M u. Wittert HG (1980) Implantat-Werkstoffe für Gelenkendoprothesen an der oberen Extremität. Orthopade 9: 108–118

Volkov MV (1982) Behandlung von Knieschäden bei Sportlern. 10. Internationales Symposium über spezielle Probleme der orthopädischen Chirurgie, Luzern

Voorhoeve A, Hierholzer D (1975) Ergebnisse bei Transplantation homologer und heterologer Sehnen als Bandersatz bei instabilem Knie. Hefte Unfallheilkd 125: 117–123

Weiss AB (1985) Ligament and tendon replacement about the knee with absorbable polymer-carbon fiber scaffolds - clinical experience. In: UCLA Extension (ed) 2nd annual symposium prosthetic ligament reconstruction of the knee. Palm Springs/CA, p 100

Whipple TL (1985) Reconstruction of the anterior cruciate ligament using bovine xenograft prosthesis under arthroscopic control. In: UCLA Extension (ed) 2nd annual symposium prosthetic ligament reconstruction of the knee. Palm Springs/CA, pp 112-114

Williams DF (1973) Implants in Surgery. Sunders, London Philadelphia Toronto

Wirth CJ (1984) Die komplexe vordere Knie-Instabilität. Thieme, Stuttgart, New York

Wolter D (1978) Der alloplastische Ersatz des medialen Knie-seitenbandes durch beschichtete Kohlenstoffasern. Unfallheilkunde 18: 390-397

Wolter D (1979) Untersuchungen zur intraossären Verankerung des alloplastischen Bandersatzes mit Kohlenstofffasern beim Schaf. Langebecks Arch Chir [Suppl]: 221-224

Woods W (1979) Proplast leader for use in cruciate ligament reconstruction. Am J Sports Med 7: 314-320

Synthetic Augmentation of Anterior Cruciate Ligament Repairs and Reconstructions

M. Wagner and R. Schabus

New discoveries in the functional anatomy of the knee joint and the pathophysiology of ligament healing have influenced and significantly altered the surgical management of acute ligamentous injuries and chronic knee instabilities. For example, we now know the critical importance of cruciate ligament isometry and the major significance of early functional rehabilitation after surgery. Early functional therapy contributes to the rapid restoration of joint motion while preventing or reducing cartilaginous and muscular morbidity. This type of therapy can be instituted at low risk if the cruciate ligament reconstruction has been reinforced by a concomitant synthetic augmentation to create an "internal splint." Through augmentation, we have achieved marked improvement in our late results of cruciate ligament reconstructions.

Synthetic augmentation is based on the temporary use of an alloplastic device to reinforce and protect a cruciate ligament repair or autologous reconstruction. It may involve:

- The synthetic augmentation of a repaired anterior cruciate ligament (ACL) that has been freshly torn from its proximal attachment
- The synthetic augmentation of an autologous ACL reconstruction (free patellar tendon graft, central one-third, bone-tendon-bone graft) for chronic anterior knee instability or a fresh midsubstance tear of the ACL (composite reconstruction)

We have used the Kennedy LAD for our synthetic augmentations.

The *decision for surgical treatment* in patients with a cruciate ligament injury depends on whether the lesion is chronic or acute. With an acute injury, the decision is difficult because the physician must "foresee" the resulting laxity and the possible associated need for operative treatment. The decision is easier with chronic instabilities, since the patient is already handicapped by functional instability.

The following factors influence patient selection for a cruciate ligament operation:

- Patient profile (compliance, work, recreation)
- Activity level (work or leisure activies with a high risk of pivot-shift episodes)
- Willingness or ability to modify activities
- Age of the patient: these procedures are contraindicated before skeletal maturity (open growth plates)
- Degree of instability (AP translation, pivot shift, rotation);
- Type of cruciate ligament tear (complete or incomplete, proximal or midsubstance)
- Interval from injury to diagnosis or surgery
- Associated peripheral capsuloligamentous injuries
- Associated cartilage damage
- Associated meniscal injuries
- Subluxation of the patella
- Knee type: ACL-dominated (hyperextension and genu recurvatum) or quadriceps-dominated)
- Limb axis (varus morphotype)
- Generalized ligamentous laxity

Besides the usual local and general contraindications to knee ligament surgery, skeletal immaturity is a contraindication to this operative method.

The operation should be scheduled as soon after the injury as possible, but under optimum conditions (competent, experienced knee surgeon), so a prompt diagnosis is essential. A capsuloligamentous injury requiring operative treatment is a *traumatologic emergency with delayed urgency*.

Further postponement of surgery would mean loss of time and emotional distress for the patient. Hemarthrosis and pain have deleterious effects on ligament strength, the cartilage, and the muscle. Also, the damaged ligament will undergo degeneration and retraction with passage of time.

Before surgery the patient should be *informed* about the possible risks and complications of the cruciate ligament operation. The patient should understand that synthetic material and fixation screws will be implanted about the joint, and that a second, minor operation will be needed to remove the implants. In particular, the patient should be made aware that postoperative rehabilitation will be demanding and will require much cooperation.

A single dose of systemic antibiotics is given immediately before the operation. The operative area is shaved and covered with a sterile dressing.

The procedure is performed under general or epidural anesthesia, commencing with stability testing (Lachman, pivot shift, drawer, KT-1000, varus/valgus stress) after anesthesia has been induced. With the patient supine, the thigh is secured in a leg holder with tourniquet, the knee is flexed, and the lower leg and foot are covered with a sterile stocking.

Operating Technique

Augmented Repair of the Acutely Torn ACL

Following repeat stability testing, the interior of the knee joint is inspected by fluid arthroscopy to locate the site of the ACL tear, identify the type of tear, and disclose associated injuries. Arthroscopy evaluates whether the tear is partial or complete, the integrity of the synovial sleeve, and the level of the tear.

This method of repair is recommended only for femoral avulsions or proximal-third tears of the ACL with a good ligamentous structure.

Diagnostic arthroscopy is followed by the arthroscopic treatment of associated meniscal injuries (repair or resection). A miniarthrotomy incision 3–4 cm long is made just medial to the patellar tendon, and a 2nd small, oblique skin incision is made over the medial tibial condyle, 3 cm distal to the joint line, for preparing the tibial bone tunnel.

The slitlike tibial bone tunnel is created using a 2.5-mm drill wire and 8-mm chisel. The intraarticular tunnel opening should be at the posteromedial border of the tibial attachment of the ACL.

Next a supracondylar skin incision 3.5 cm long is made on the lateral side of the knee. The vastus lateralis muscle is released from the lateral intermuscular septum and retracted anteriorly to expose the lateral surface of the lateral femoral condyle.

A transcondylar bone tunnel 3 mm in diameter is drilled through the lateral femoral condyle, and a pullout suture is passed through it for subsequent attachment to the "posterolateral bundle" of the repair sutures. The over-the-top route is prepared by subperiosteal dissection with a curved clamp, perforating the posterior joint capsule near the cap of the lateral condyle; another pullout suture is passed through this route. The stump of the ACL is pierced from anteromedial to posterolateral with at least 4 atraumatic No. 2 Vicryl sutures to establish uniform tension over the full length and cross section of the ligament. The

first, posterolateral bundle of the repair sutures is pulled through the transcondylar drill hole.

The LAD is implanted by first pulling the device up into the joint through the tibial tunnel, positioning the LAD so that it is posteromedial and parallel to the ACL. The braid is passed over the top of the lateral femoral condyle together with the second, anteromedial bundle of the repair sutures (Fig. 1).

For fixation of the LAD, the knee is extended or slightly flexed (0°–10°, depending on the length increase associated with the over-the-top placement). First the proximal end is fixed with a 6.5-mm cancellous bone screw and metal washer. Then the LAD is tightened to a tension of 8–10 kg, and the distal end is secured in the same way (Fig. 2). Then the ACL is reattached proximally by tying the sutures over the osseous bridge with the knee flexed 30° (Figs. 3, 4).

The operation is concluded by closing the wounds in layers over suction drains. The knee is immobilized in 20° flexion with a bivalve plaster cast or locked motion splint.

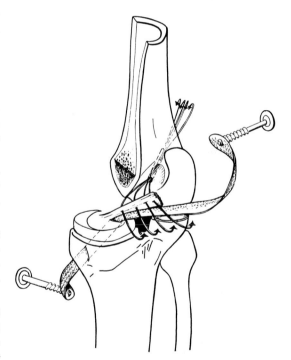

Fig. 1. Technique for repairing a fresh proximal rupture of the ACL by suture reattachment and synthetic augmentation (right knee, posteromedial aspect; medial femoral condyle has been removed for clarity). The repair sutures form 2 bundles: One is passed through the lateral femoral condyle, the other is routed over the top along with the LAD. The LAD is attached with a 6.5-mm AO/ASIF cancellous bone screw driven through the eyelet at each end. The intraarticular mouth of the tibial tunnel for the LAD opens posteromedial to the tibial attachment area of the ACL

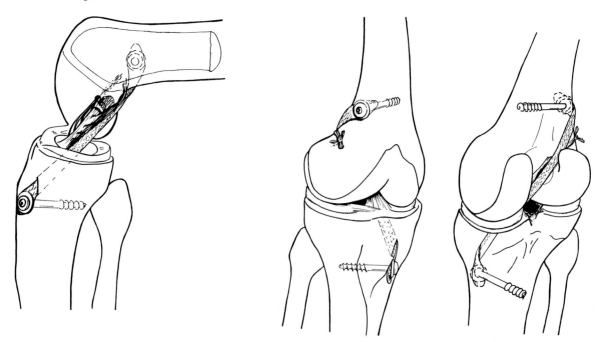

Fig. 2. Technique for repairing a fresh proximal rupture of the ACL by suture reattachment and synthetic augmentation (right knee, medial aspect following removal of the medial femoral condyle). The repair sutures have been tightened, and the LAD has been attached to the bone at both ends

Fig. 3 *(left).* (Technique for repairing a fresh proximal rupture of the ACL (right knee, anterolateral aspect). The repair sutures have been tied, and the LAD has been fixed to the femur and tibia with screws and metal washers

Fig. 4 *(right).* Technique for repairing a fresh proximal rupture of the ACL by suture reattachment and synthetic augmentation (right knee, posteromedial aspect). The LAD runs posteromedial to the reattached ACL and passes upward by the over-the-top route

Composite Reconstruction of the ACL (Autograft and Augmentation)

Arthroscopy is performed to evaluate meniscal or cartilage injuries, check for osteophytic narrowing of the intercondylar notch, scars, and to identify the type of ACL lesion (acute midsubstance rupture or chronic insufficiency, i. e., ACL absent or represented by scar tissue).

Following arthroscopy, an anterior incision is made over the patellar tendon. The central third of the patellar tendon is harvested along with proximal and distal bone blocks from the patella and tibial tuberosity. The bone-tendon-bone graft is augmented with a Kennedy LAD 15 cm long and 8 mm wide; this is done by enveloping the device inside the tubed autologous graft, without suturing the LAD directly to the graft (composite graft). After the composite graft has been detached, the joint is entered by a transligamentous arthrotomy with incision of the fat pad (Fig. 5). The intercondylar notch is widened as required, and any meniscal or cartilage lesions are treated.

A lateral incision is made at the supracondylar level, and the lateral femoral condyle is exposed over the intermuscular septum.

The bone tunnels are prepared by first drilling guidewires through the tibia from the outside in and through the femur from the inside out with the knee flexed 120°.

After testing of isometry, the guidewires are overdrilled with a cannulated reamer (8–12 mm) from the outside in. The edges of the tunnel openings are chamfered. The over-the-top route for the proximal end of the LAD is prepared by perforation of the posterior capsule.

The composite graft is pulled upward into the joint through the tibial tunnel, making sure that the distal bone block is anterior to the LAD inside the tunnel. The proximal bone block is pulled into the femoral bone tunnel until it is flush with the intraarticular tunnel opening. The proximal end of the LAD is placed in the over-the-top position.

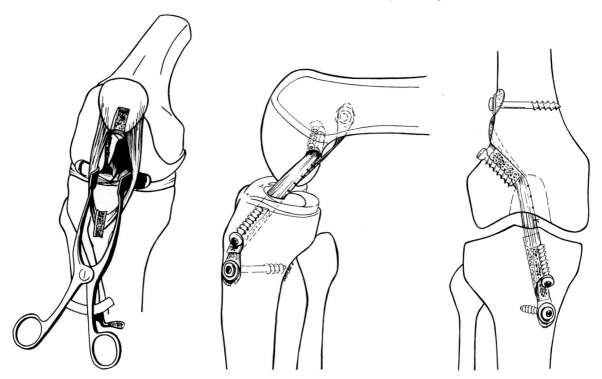

Fig. 5 *(left).* Transligamentous approach for osteotomizing the central third of the patella for a bone-tendon-bone graft. The infrapatellar fat pad is split, and the interior of the knee joint is exposed through the donor defect

Fig. 6 *(middle).* Autologous ACL reconstruction with synthetic augmentation (right knee, medial aspect after removal of the medial femoral condyle). The bone-tendon-bone graft from the central third of the patellar tendon has been fixed with inter-

ference-fit screws, and the LAD has been fixed with 6.5-mm cancellous bone screws inserted through the eyelets over washers. Implanted over the top, the LAD becomes markedly lax with knee flexion

Fig. 7 *(right).* Autologous reconstruction of the ACL with synthetic augmentation (right knee, anterior aspect). The bone block in the femoral tunnel should fit flush with the surface of the intercondylar notch

For definitive fixation of the composite graft:

- The proximal end of the LAD is attached to the femur with a 6.5-mm AO/ASIF cancellous bone screw with metal washer (eyelet technique).
- The femoral bone block is secured by interference-fit fixation with a screw (6.5-mm AO/ASIF cancellous bone screw, 30 mm long).
- The LAD is pulled taut to a tension of 8–10 kg, and with the knee extended, the distal end of the LAD is attached to the tibia with a 6.5-mm AO/ASIF cancellous bone screw over a metal washer.
- With the knee flexed 30°, the tibial bone block is fixed inside the tunnel with an interference-fit screw (Figs. 6–9).

The wounds are closed in layers over suction drains, and the knee is immobilized in 20° flexion with a bivalve cast or locked motion splint.

Postoperative Treatment

A bivalve plaster cast or locked motion splint holds the knee in approximately 20° of flexion during the period of wound healing (2 weeks). In the hospital the cast or splint is taken off daily to allow passive range-of-motion exercises from 10° to 70° flexion, as permitted by effusion and pain. Following suture removal, the patient wears a limited motion splint for a total of 8 weeks postoperatively. The splint is gradually adjusted to extend the arc of motion (Fig. 10); a range of 10°–85° is reached by the end of 8 weeks.

In patients with associated collateral ligament injuries that have been surgically repaired, the knee is immobilized in a cast for 3–4 weeks before treatment with the motion splint is initiated.

Partial weight-bearing ambulation is permitted using 2 forearm crutches, and weight bearing is progressively increased according to pain tolerance. A longer period of non-weight-bearing is required in patients

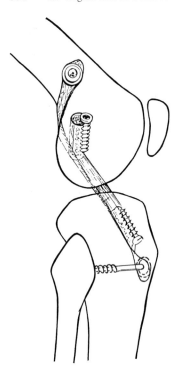

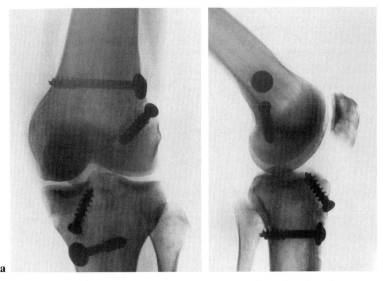

Fig. 8. Autologous reconstruction of the ACL with synthetic augmentation (right knee, lateral aspect)

Fig. 9 a, b. Postoperative AP and lateral radiographs taken after a composite reconstruction of the ACL. The bone blocks are secured by interference fit fixation using bone screws. Each end of the LAD is fixed with a 6.5-mm AO/ASIF cancellous bone screw driven through the eyelet over a metal washer

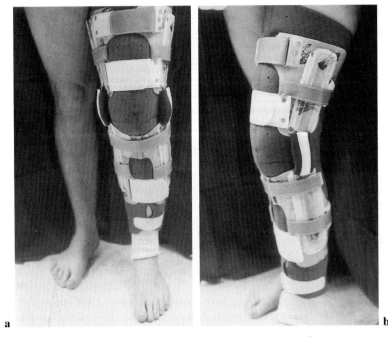

Fig. 10 a, b. Postoperative limited motion splint (Salzburg model). A neoprene stocking is worn to control swelling and prevent window edema. The splint has an adjustable arc of flexion-extension and is fixed to the thigh and lower leg with velcro fasteners. The patient initially ambulates with 2 forearm crutches and partial weight bearing

with articular cartilage damage or a meniscus repair.

Cryotherapy is administered in the immediate postoperative period to reduce swelling and relieve pain. Isometric exercises and electrotherapy are prescribed starting on the 2nd postoperative day.

Hardware Removal and Repeat Arthroscopy

The metal fixation devices are removed 6–12 months after the operation (by 1986 the period had been reduced to 6 months), permitting dynamic stabilization of the LAD system. By this time the LAD is securely fixed by fibrous tissue growth and should not loosen. Repeat arthroscopy was routinely performed in almost all patients.

Clinical Population and Late Results

Primary Repair of the ACL with Synthetic Augmentation

This procedure was performed in 74 patients from 1983 to 1985. All had an acute, complete rupture of the ACL in its proximal third (near the femoral attachment). The Lachman and pivot shift tests were positive in all cases.

Sixty-four of the 74 patients were followed an average of 3.5 years (13.5% were lost to follow-up). The patients were followed continuously, with an average interval of 40.8 months from the operation to the last follow-up examination. This clinical series comprised 39 men and 25 women with an average age of 29 years.

Seventy percent of the patients had their operation within 1 week of the injury. Coexisting injuries of the collateral ligaments, menisci, or cartilage were surgically treated in 52 cases. Tenodesis of the iliotibial tract was performed in the 80% of patients who had a 2+ or 3+ pivot shift when tested preoperatively under anesthesia.

The results of the follow-up study are represented by the findings of the last follow-up examination, conducted an average of 40.8 months after the operation. Anteroposterior stability testing (measured by the KT-1000 arthrometer) showed that the translation in 19% of cases was less than on the uninjured side. There was no difference in 16%, a difference of only 1 mm in 34%, 2 mm in 23%, and 3–4 mm in 8%. The Lachman test was negative in 67% of cases, 1+ in 30%, and 2+ in 3%. A 1+ pivot shift was elicited in only 2%.

In 84% of cases, extension was unrestricted relative to 0° extension in the healthy leg; in 8% there was 6°–10° limitation of extension on the operated side. There was unrestricted flexion in 77% of cases, a flexion deficit of 1°–5° relative to the uninjured side in 16%, and a 6°–10° deficit in 3%. Four percent exhibited a flexion deficit greater than 10°. The "one-leg hop test for distance" index was greater than 91 in 68%, and 81–90 in 19%. Eleven percent of the patients were unable or refused to perform the test.

Some 97% of the patients returned to sports activities, with 83% returning at their preinjury level and 14% experiencing some degree of disability. With regard to overall subjective impression, 70% of the patients said that the injured, operated knee gave them "no problems," 28% reported "slight problems," and 2% reported "serious problems."

None of the 64 patients in our series developed an infection, and there was no evidence of effusion at last follow-up. One patient complained of severe femoropatellar problems, another had complaints relating to a previous bout of reflex sympathetic dystrophy, and another had problems relating to a herniation of the vastus lateralis muscle.

Follow-up arthroscopy at the time of metal removal disclosed a rupture of the Kennedy LAD in 7 patients (11%). All ruptured LADs were removed. Arthroscopic scrutiny of the ACL showed a good, solid, intact structure in 4 of these 7 cases, and 5 showed good results in the stability and function tests.

Autologous Graft with Synthetic Augmentation (Composite Reconstruction)

From 1983 to 1986, 87 patients underwent a composite reconstruction for chronic anterior instability or a midsubstance tear of the ACL.

Additionally, a tractopexy was performed in 88.5% of these patients, and a notch plasty was performed in 23.1%. Articular cartilage damage was noted intraoperatively in 25.6%.

Eighty of the 87 patients were available for follow-up more than 3 years postoperatively.

Stability

KT-1000 measurements: Seven knees (9%) were found to be unstable (>3 mm translation). In 4 of these cases arthroscopy confirmed a ruptured LAD.

Pivot shift test: A positive pivot shift was elicited in 5 kness (6.4%). In 2 of these cases arthroscopy disclosed a ruptured LAD.

Lachman test: Lachman mobility was 2 + in 3 joints (5.1%) and 3 + in 1 joint (1.3%).
Seventy of the knees (89.7%) were judged to be stable.

Range of Motion

Extension: There was no limitation of extension in 49 joints (62.8%). One joint (1.3%) had an extension deficit greater than 10°.

Flexion: Fifty-five patients (70.5%) had no limitation of flexion, and 1 (1.3%) had a flexion deficit greater than 10°.
Limitation of motion was judged to be present in 10 knees (12.8%).

Clinical Symptoms

Six patients (7.8%) complained of significant disability relating to the operated knee. One of the patients could recall an antecedent history of adequate reinjury.

Athletic Activity (n = 77)

When questioned about their current ability to engage in sports, 52 patients (67.5%) stated that they could participate at the same level as before their ligament injury. Four patients (5.2%) stated that they were unable to participate in any sports activities.

Return to Sports Participation (n = 67)

Twenty-five patients (37.3%) stated that they were able to resume sports activities within 5 months. By 1 year, 53 patients (79.1%) were again participating in sports.

Function Test (n = 74)

In 41 patients (55.4%) the operated limb achieved at least 91% of the function of the opposite limb. Overall, the difference relative to the uninjured side was less than 20% in 61 of the patients (78.2%).

Complications

Twelve LAD ruptures (15.4%) were detected arthroscopically. One patient sustained a massive reinjury. At the present time, 8 of these knees are stable and 4 are unstable.

Discussion

The follow-up of acute, complete proximal-third ruptures of the ACL managed by primary surgical repair and concomitant synthetic augmentation indicates good results.

The anticipated disadvantages of the bony fixation of the LAD at both ends – stress shielding, foreign body reaction, higher infection rate, risk of material fatigue or rupture – were not clinically apparent at the time of follow-up.

The advantage of this technique of synthetic augmentation is that it protects the original, repaired cruciate ligament. The augmentation device serves as an internal splint and prevents excessive stretching of the autologous tissue in the initial postoperative months. It also permits early postoperative rehabilitation.

Implanting the LAD by the over-the-top route protects the repaired ACL during extension while still permitting functional stimulation of the autologous tissue in flexion. This stimulus is needed to ensure functional remodeling ("ligamentization") of the transplanted tissue.

Every synthetic augmentation leads to a slight alteration of natural joint motion. The augmentation moves the proximal tibia to a position of posterior subluxation and slight external rotation. This emphasizes the need to avoid excessive tension in the composite graft that would increase the pressure between the articular surfaces. We have shown experimentally that the over-the-top positioning of a synthetic augmentation band is necessary to provide "stress protection" of the autologous tissue in extension while permitting "stress formation" in flexion. The augmentation device should be tightened to a primary tension of 8–10 kp with the knee in extension (Fig. 11).

At the start of our clinical series, we found that full range-of-motion recovery was delayed in patients with an excessively tight LAD, though we did not find excessive cartilage wear at follow-up. The primary tension of the LAD protects the autologous reconstruction from excessive loads during the early postoperative period, but it also weakens the formative stimulus on the graft (stress shielding). Implanting the LAD by the through-the-top route leads to increased material fatigue, and rotation up to 90° on the prestressed LAD can cause the device to rupture at the intraarticular rim of the femoral bone tunnel.

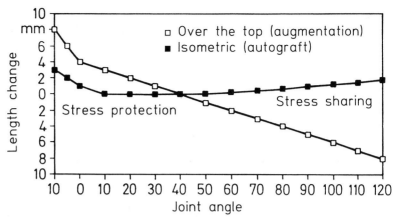

Fig. 11. Graphic representation of the biomechanics of a synthetically augmented autologous reconstruction. The augmentation should protect the autograft from excessive loads during active extension but permit appropriate loading of the graft during flexion

Stability

The instability rate was 3.6% in the ACL repair cases and 10.3% in the augmented reconstructions. Rupture of the LAD was detected arthroscopically in a large percentage of the unstable joints. Only 2 of the 21 LAD ruptures occurred in knees where an over-the-top implantation had been performed.

Range of Motion

While the failure rate in terms of mobility was 6% in the repaired knee joints, limitation of motion was twice as frequent (12.8%) in joints reconstructed with a bone-tendon-bone graft. This may have resulted from nonisometric placement of the graft or from scarring of the capsule.

Sports

Two years after the operation, 87% of the patients with an augmented ACL repair returned to their pre-injury level of sports activity, as opposed to 67.5% of the patients with a bone-tendon-bone graft. The overall ratio of athletically fit patients to patients no longer able to participate in sports was 4:1. There was less difference between the 2 patient groups with regard to the interval between the operation and the return to sports. By 1 year, 88% of the patients with an augmented ACL repair and 79% of the patients with an augmented reconstruction had resumed sports. Although postoperative sports participation is largely dependent on individual factors, it should be emphas-

ized that the majority of patients with an augmented reconstruction suffered from chronic instability and had already curtailed their athletic involvement for some time prior to surgery.

Function Test

A less than 20% functional discrepancy relative to the uninjured side was present in more than 85% of the patients with an augmented repair and in 78.2% of patients with an augmented reconstruction. Of course this test also depends on other circumstances such as the condition of the ankle and the patient's coordination and level of conditioning.

Posterior Cruciate Ligament

We still have not found an entirely satisfactory solution to the problem of the surgical treatment of posterior cruciate ligament (PCL) injuries, or of posterior instabilities of the knee. For a "favorable" rupture located near the attachment of the PCL, we combine reattachment of the ligament with a synthetic augmentation. If substitution is indicated, we reconstruct the PCL with a composite graft (one-third of the patellar tendon plus LAD). The patient is repositioned intraoperatively to permit a technically and anatomically correct attachment of the graft to the posterior surface of the upper tibia.

At present, however, we still do not have enough clinical experience to offer a general recommendation with regard to the synthetic augmentation of the PCL.

Summary

Reconstruction of the ACL with synthetic augmentation permits early rehabilitation with a rapid return to sports participation.

LAD-augmented repair of the ACL can correct post-traumatic instability in more than 95% of cases. Eighty-eight percent of the patients in our series were able to resume sports participation by 1 year after operation.

Reconstruction of the ACL with an LAD-augmented patellar tendon graft can correct the original instability in 90% of cases, and 79% of our patients were able to resume sports participation by 1 year after surgery.

The authors are grateful to Mrs. H. Doppler for providing the illustrations of the operative technique and to our colleagues at the First University Trauma Surgery Clinic who participated in the follow-up study.

Instability and Osteoarthritis

Instability-Related Osteoarthritis: Special Indications for Osteotomies in the Treatment of the Unstable Knee

R. P. Jakob

Development of Osteoarthritis in the Cruciate-Deficient Knee

An untreated rupture of the anterior cruciate ligament (ACL) leads to osteoarthritic changes in a large percentage of cases (Dejour et al. 1987; Jacobsen 1977; McDaniel and Dameron 1983). In 10- and 14-year follow-ups of untreated ACL ruptures, McDaniel and Dameron (1983) found an 84% incidence of meniscal lesions and an 86% incidence of osteoarthritic changes of varying degree, such as squaring of the medial femoral condyle, marginal osteophyte formation, joint-space narrowing, subchondral sclerosis, and peaking of the intercondylar eminence. An obvious relationship was noted between medial meniscectomy, joint-space narrowing with osteoarthritic changes, and varus deformity. Other associated factors were heavy body weight, lateral meniscectomy, age, and restricted activity level. This unique compilation provides a representative cross section of untreated ACL ruptures and demonstrates the relevant aspects of its natural history. The pathogenesis of the predominantly medial joint deterioration is based on various factors. The repeated giving-way episodes, whose clinical correlate is the pivot shift, reflect an episodic subluxation of the lateral and medial compartments. While the lateral compartment is inherently less constrained and can better distribute the forces of compression and shear, the forces in the medial compartment are greater per square centimeter of cartilage surface area due to the concavity of the medial tibial plateau. In an analysis of the division of load between the lateral and medial compartments of the knee during gait, Johnson et al. (1980) found that the medial compartment shares a greater portion of the load than a static analysis would imply, except in knees that have more than 5° of valgus deformity. Because the mechanical axis of the leg in monopodal stance crosses the medial compartment due largely to the action of extrinsic varus forces (body weight), the medial compartment is more susceptible to cartilage lesions, cartilage wear, and meniscal pathology. These factors are accentuated by the varus morphotype

common in athletic individuals. The varus may be increased by loss of lateral coaptation ("décoaptation externe" of Bousquet), laxness of peripheral structures in the arcuate complex, and perhaps following extensive extraarticular transfers that have compromised the ability of the iliotibial tract to support lateral coaptation (Hey Groves 1920; Jakob 1987). Another significant factor is body weight, which amplifies the extrinsic varus component (Fig. 1).

Single-compartment osteoarthritis, whether occurring as an isolated sequel to cruciate deficiency or, more commonly, in conjunction with meniscal pathology, may be associated with instability of the medial or lateral collateral ligament.

Osteoarthritis associated with clinically symptomatic instability must be regarded differently from osteoarthritis in an adequately stabilized joint. Finally, attention must be given to cartilage pathology and accompanying osteoarthritis in the femoropatellar compartment.

The study by Dejour et al. (1987) in 2 different patient groups is valuable in the analysis of instability-related osteoarthritis. In an initial series of 150 patients followed for 3 years or more after ACL reconstruction with the patellar tendon and an extraarticular transfer, osteoarthritic changes were found in 13.3%. In a second series of 64 patients who had undergone a valgus osteotomy of the proximal tibia, the histories suggested a ACL rupture sustained 10–50 years earlier with an average "tolerance time" of 35 years. Dejour stated that the most important features of osteoarthritis were osteophytosis in the intercondylar notch and on the posterior margin of the medial tibial plateau, medial joint-space narrowing, and posterior subluxation of the medial femoral condyle, which was clearly appreciated on the lateral weight-bearing radiograph. The osteoarthritis developed rapidly in joints that remained unstable despite surgical treatment, especially when preosteoarthritic changes had already been noted at operation. Other unfavorable prognostic signs were the persistence of an "active" Lachman sign, medial meniscectomy, the development of varus deformity due to posterior erosion of the medial tibial plateau,

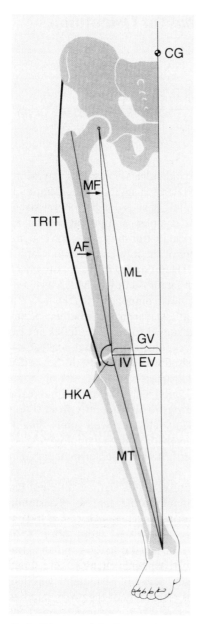

Fig. 1. Diagram of the forces acting on the knee joint in genu varum. The intrinsic varus component is compensated by the iliotibial tract, which functions as a dynamic lateral tension band. The extrinsic varus component increases with body weight. Even with genu varum, the lateral side remains active as a tension band. *AF*, Anatomic femoral axis; *MF*, mechanical femoral axis; *MT*, mechanical tibial axis; *ML*, mechanical limb axis; *TRIT*, iliotibial tract; *IV*, intrinsic varus component; *EV*, extrinsic varus component (body weight); *GV*, global varus component; *HKA*, hip-knee-ankle angle; *CG*, center of gravity

coexisting lateral laxity, constitutional genu varum, and hamstring weakness.

The evolution of osteoarthritis is profoundly influenced by the success of the ACL reconstruction and the elimination of a positive Lachman sign (anterior drawer near extension). The spontaneous destruction or surgical removal of the medial meniscus initiates a vicious cycle of deterioration that promotes posterior subluxation of the medial condyle and lateral coaptation loss with increased varus tibiofemoral angulation in the one-legged stance. Thus, the preservation of stability and of the medial meniscus are the most important guarantees of good long-term results.

Another factor that can promote osteoarthritis is deficiency of the posterolateral corner of the knee, which can occur in association with ACL deficiency, especially in patients with constitutional genu varum. Muscular balance is also a significant factor, because individuals who have hyperlax ligaments with recurvatum tend to have weak hamstrings that cannot compensate for the increasing laxness of the posteromedial corner. Hamstring rehabilitation, therefore, is important in the prevention of osteoarthritis.

Finally, the "surgical insult" can significantly accelerate the onset of osteoarthritis in cases where the surgeon has ignored certain basic principles of technique.

Ligament transfers and reconstructions should be done sparingly in joints that already display significant intraarticular cartilage pathology and meniscal lesions or defects involving the medial compartment. The presence of even minimal joint-space narrowing, squaring of the femoral condyles, and osteophytosis of the intercondylar notch and posterior medial tibial plateau are warning signs that an intraarticular reconstruction might greatly accelerate the degenerative process, especially in patients over 30 years of age. We feel that the articular forces must be reduced by combining the ligament reconstruction with a proximal tibial valgus osteotomy in patients who have loss of lateral coaptation accompanied by significant constitutional varus deviation.

A Lemaire-type anterolateral transfer and similar procedures used to relieve instability can promote osteoarthritis if the posteromedial corner is lax and the medial meniscus is absent, because they rotate the knee externally to a position in which the medial femoral condyle is posteriorly subluxed. Failed extraarticular transfers cause loss of lateral coaptation by weakening the important lateral tension band.

The decision whether to operate in an unstable knee should be based chiefly on the functional disability that is present, i.e., the patient's subjective instability.

But the decision should be made while the athletically and vocationally active patient is still young, because there is a better chance of preventing osteoarthritis if appropriate surgery is performed reasonably soon after the ACL lesion is sustained, and thus before the development of significant meniscal and cartilage pathology and posteromedial laxity that could jeopardize the ligament reconstruction. The major goal is to relieve functional disability, although it is unclear whether osteoarthritic deterioration of the joint will continue to progress despite adequate stabilization. For example, Fried et al. (1985) found that up to 85% of patients whose knees had been successfully stabilized by a combined intraarticular and extraarticular ACL reconstruction experienced an increase in the severity of preoperative osteoarthritis with pain, stiffness, and swelling. Their study supports the value of early stabilization prior to the development of meniscal and cartilage pathology.

Lynch et al. (1983) noted a progression of osteoarthritis in adequately stabilized knees in which a partial or complete meniscectomy had been performed. These authors emphasize the need to preserve the meniscus by repairing the tear or by leaving a stable, asymptomatic tear alone.

Another potential cause of osteoarthritic degeneration may be faulty surgical technique used to restore stability while preserving unrestricted joint motion. Observations in our own series (Jakob et al. 1988) confirm the high incidence of (mild) postoperative flexion and extension deficits (see chapter by Kipfer et al., p. 389 ff.). An extraarticular transfer and especially an imprecise intraarticular cruciate reconstruction can alter joint kinematics in a way that causes abnormal rolling and gliding of the condyles, limited motion, and contracture. The efforts of the physiotherapist to overcome these contractures – e.g., a 20° extension loss due to overtightening of an over-the-top graft or a flexion loss caused by attaching the femoral end of the graft too far anteriorly – will impose unphysiologic compressive loads on the articular cartilage and may initiate osteoarthritic change. In general it may be said that any restriction of joint motion that necessitates manipulation under anesthesia and arthrolysis can promote cartilage deterioration. This can be avoided by withholding cast immobilization postoperatively and mobilizing the operated limb immediately after surgery.

An unknown percentage of patients, then, will seek orthopedic treatment for osteoarthritic knee problems 10–20 years after an untreated rupture of the ACL or after undergoing a cruciate and collateral ligament reconstruction with meniscectomy.

There are limits to what can be done therapeutically for osteoarthritis initiated by instability and meniscectomy. Besides joint-stabilizing procedures, which must be considered carefully according to the severity of osteoarthritis, measures directed at the cause of the arthritis should be considered only when osteoarthritis is confined to one compartment of the knee. Severe global osteoarthritis of the knee in middle-aged patients falls within the therapeutic domain of nonoperative orthopedics and rheumatology. In patients over 60 years of age, prosthetic arthroplasty is added to the therapeutic options. Patients with moderately severe, unicompartmental osteoarthritis of the knee are the best candidates for an osteotomy.

Below we shall consider options that are available for the treatment of instability-related osteoarthritis of the knee. Selected examples will illustrate how the operator can seek solutions to this problem through a combination of hard- and soft-tissue surgical techniques.

Patient Selection

Patient selection and preoperative planning require a complete evaluation of the status of the knee. This includes (in the sequence indicated):

- Assessment of constitutional laxity
- Identification of weight-bearing morphotype while the limb is inspected from the front and side (varus, valgus or normal angulation, recurvatum or antecurvatum)
- Accurate assessment of range of motion, especially with regard to a flexion or extension deficit. If the affected knee has an extension loss of 5° but can hyperextend to 15°, the patient can extend the knee while walking despite an effective extension loss of 20°. The same 20° extension loss in a "tight-jointed" individual who can extend the healthy knee to 0° will have far greater functional significance and will cause a limping gait. The significance of a flexion loss also varies according to whether the healthy knee can flex to 135° or 155°.
- Detection of instability by moving the knee in all 6 degrees of freedom (3 translation, 3 rotations). The subjective tests are objectified by obtaining standard comparative bilateral radiographic views in a positioning device. With concomitant deficiency of the anterior and posterior cruciate ligaments, the amount of anterior and posterior translation is ascertained. A distinction is drawn be-

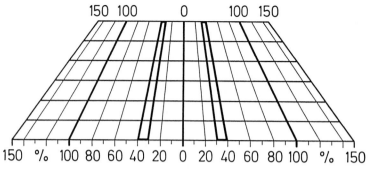

Fig. 2. Template dividing the medial and lateral tibial plateus each into a 100% grid for identifying the point where the mechanical limb axis crosses the plateau on the frontal plane

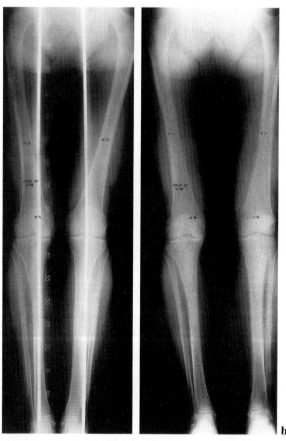

Fig. 3 a,b. Weight-bearing radiographs showing the points where the mechanical limb axes cross the plane of the knee joint. **a** With the weight distributed evenly on both legs, the mechanical axis passes through a point 30% medial to the midpoint of the tibial eminence. **b** With the right leg bearing 90% of the weight, the mechanical axis passes through a point 40% medial to the midpoint. (After Fujisawa et al. 1979)

tween varus-valgus opening due to collateral ligament laxity and joint-space narrowing due to absence of the meniscus, cartilage damage, or depression of the articular surface.

– Testing the cartilage status by flexion-extension with varus stress for the lateral side and valgus stress for the medial side; meniscal tests (MacMurray test, hyperextension pain); test for femoropatellar crepitus by extending the knee against a resistance

– Detection of synovitis with capsular thickening and joint effusion

– Roentgen examination, which includes the following views prior to osteotomy: long-leg AP weight bearing in 10°–20° flexion, 45° tunnel view, lateral weight bearing in 30° flexion (to detect anterior tibial subluxation), patellar sunrise view

– Varus-valgus stress of 20 kg in a special positioning device to detect ligament instability or joint-space narrowing due to thinning of the cartilage (normal cartilage width 4 mm). Full-length AP standing film of both legs (orthoradiograph) with 90% weight bearing on the affected limb, checked on a household scale with the patient standing on a board to equalize the limb lengths. The 10% load on the opposite limb ensures a straight, upright body posture; the 90% load on the affected side provides for compression of the articular cartilage by the body weight.

– Assessment of axial geometry by determining the point where the mechanical limb axis crosses plane of the tibial plateau on a percentage grid whose zero point is midway between the tibial spines (bibliography in Fujisawa et al. 1979) (Figs. 2, 3)

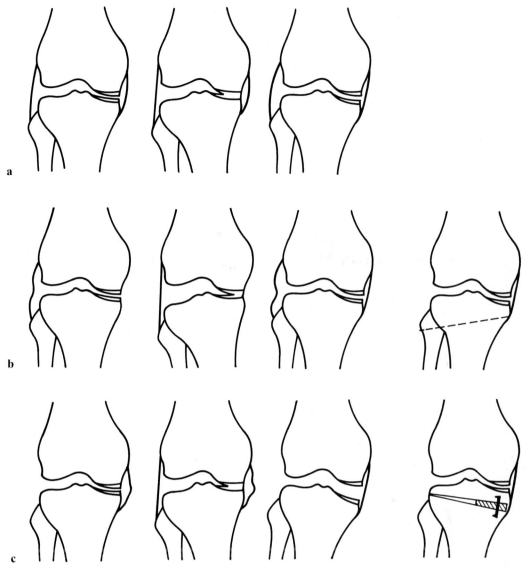

Fig. 4a–c. Combined deformities due to osteoarticular and ligamentous causes compound the difficulty of preoperative planning. **a** The supine examination shows medial joint space narrowing with normal tightness of both collateral ligaments. **b** Supine examination shows medial narrowing and lateral opening of the joint space, appreciated best on the varus stress film. Valgus stress opens the medial compartment by the thickness of the lost cartilage. A closed-wedge osteotomy is indicated. **c** The valgus stress film demonstrates marked opening of the medial joint space. An open-wedge osteotomy is indicated

This detailed clinical and radiographic workup can effectively evaluate bony, cartilaginous, and ligamentous deformities about the knee joint (Figs. 4–6). We consider performing a proximal tibial valgus osteotomy when:

- There are early but definite osteoarthritic changes in the medial compartment.
- The limb shows a varus morphotype.
- The varus morphotype is compounded by lateral instability.

- The lateral compartment shows no degenerative changes on the valgus stressradiograph.

We use a closed-wedge osteotomy combined with a fibular osteotomy when 10° or more of angular correction is required (Fig. 4b). We perform a medial open-wedge osteotomy at the supraligamentous level if it is also necessary to tighten the medial collateral ligament and the goal does not go beyond restoring a normal limb axis by 5°–6° of correction, or if the osteotomy is to be combined with an ACL reconstruction (Fig. 4c).

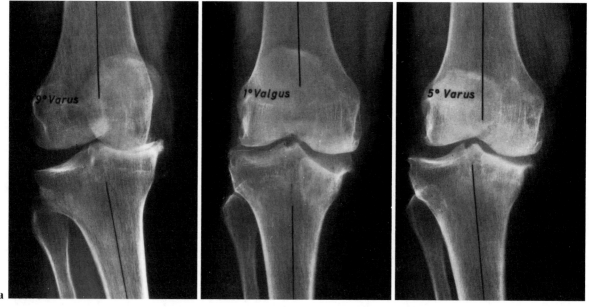

Fig. 5. Knee as in Fig. 4b, with excessive lateral joint-space opening due to laxness of the lateral collateral ligament (monopodal radiograph) (**a**) and medial narowing due to bone loss from the tibial plateau ("pagoda sign"), best appreciated on the valgus stress film (**b**). The best planning document is an axial stress film with pressure applied to the sole of the foot (**c**) or an orthoradiograph with the body weight evenly distributed

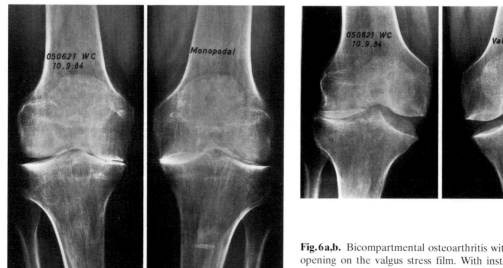

Fig. 6a,b. Bicompartmental osteoarthritis with marked medial opening on the valgus stress film. With instability of this severity, an orthoradiograph with the affected leg bearing 90% of the body weight should be used to plan the osteotomy

The osteotomy is combined with an ACL reconstruction when osteoarthritis is mild, motion is not restricted, and symptoms relating to anterior instability are subjectively and objectively disabling.

Another indication for proximal tibial osteotomy is severe posterolateral instability, which may be associated with anterior instability. The procedure may be done with or without a ligament reconstruction.

Varus osteotomies are less commonly performed for genu valgum with lateral osteoarthritis secondary to ligamentous deficiency.

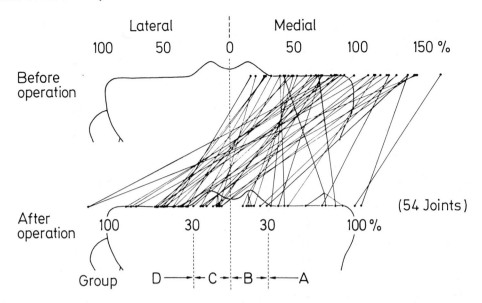

Fig. 7. Diagram from Fujisawa et al. (1979). Before surgery the crossing points of the mechanical axis are scattered over a broad range in the medial compartment. After surgery the best cartilage regeneration is seen arthroscopically in joints where the mechanical axis crosses the lateral compartment 30%–40% from the midpoint

Closed-Wedge Proximal Tibial Valgus Osteotomy

Determining the Correction Angle

The size of the osteotomy wedge depends on the severity of the unicompartmental osteoarthritis. With moderately severe to severe medial osteoarthritis in which the joint space is narrowed from 4 to 0–2 mm, we follow the recommendations of Fujisawa et al. (1979) and Hernigou et al. (1987) (Fig. 7). In long-term follow-ups of 54 knees that had undergone proximal tibial osteotomy, the Japanese authors observed arthroscopic cartilage regeneration in cases where the mechanical limb axis crossed the knee 30%–40% lateral to the midpoint of the tibial eminence. This observation is consistent with that of Hernigou et al., who found that results were best when the hip-knee-ankle angle was 183°–186° but were unfavorable when there was under- or overcorrection outside that range. In both methods preoperative planning is based on an orthoradiograph, which demonstrates axial alignment in relation to limb length. It is known that the angle between the femoral and tibial anatomic axes is greater in individuals of small stature than in tall individuals. Thus the ana-

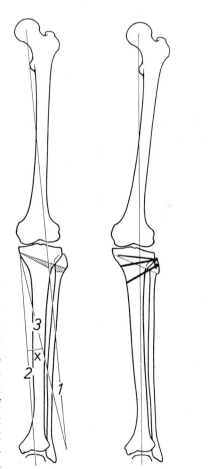

Fig. 8. Calculation of the wedge angle needed to move the mechanical axis to an ideal position (30%–40%) in the lateral compartment. *1*, New mechanical axis; *2*, line from the osteotomy hinge point to the existing center of the ankle joint; *3*, line from the hinge point to the new center of the ankle joint; *x*, required correction angle. (After Miniaci et al. 1989)

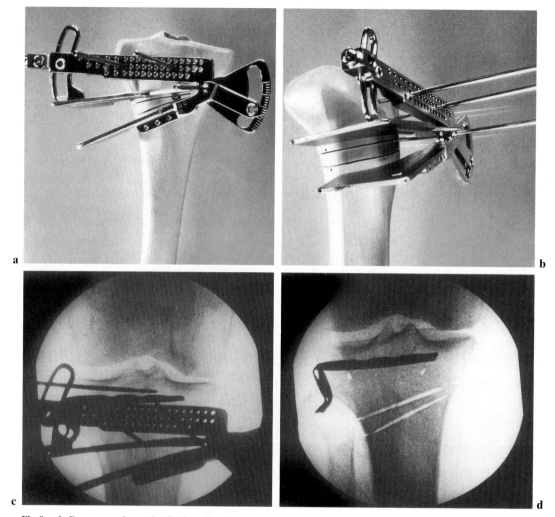

Fig. 9 a–d. Prototype of a cutting jig that allows precise definition and resection of the osteotomy wedge. The osteotomy cuts meet at the hinge point

tomic axis is a somewhat imprecise index for preoperative planning, and we no longer use it.

How, then, can the osteotomy be performed with such precision that the mechanical axis crosses the lateral compartment at 30%–40% and the postoperative hip-knee-ankle angle is 183°–186°? Figure 8 illustrates our geometric technique for calculating the resection angle for a proximal tibial closed-wedge valgus osteotomy. The new mechanical axis is drawn on an orthoradiograph with 90% weight bearing on the affected limb. (If lateral joint opening is markedly pathologic, we use only 50% weight bearing to plan the osteotomy; otherwise the resection angle could be too large.) The hinge point for the closed-wedge osteotomy is placed 1.5–2 cm distal to the medial joint space, and a line is drawn connecting it to the center of the ankle joint. A second line is drawn from the hinge point to the new center of the ankle joint.

The angle × between the lines equals the angle of the resected wedge, which is now drawn in. The orientation of the wedge will be more transverse or more oblique depending on the desired direction. The 90% weight-bearing orthoradiograph taken 4 months postoperatively must confirm the desired course of the mechanical axis. When making the preoperative drawing, we use a tibial plateau template, shown to scale in Fig. 2, which can be adjusted to the width of the tibial plateau on the X-ray film. The ideal placement of the mechanical axis at 30%–40% of the plateau width is marked on the template.

A precision cutting jig is used to transfer the planned angle of resection to the tibia (Fig. 9). Pure visual estimation is unsatisfactory as it may produce an imprecise wedge resection and compromise stability by disrupting the cortical hinge.

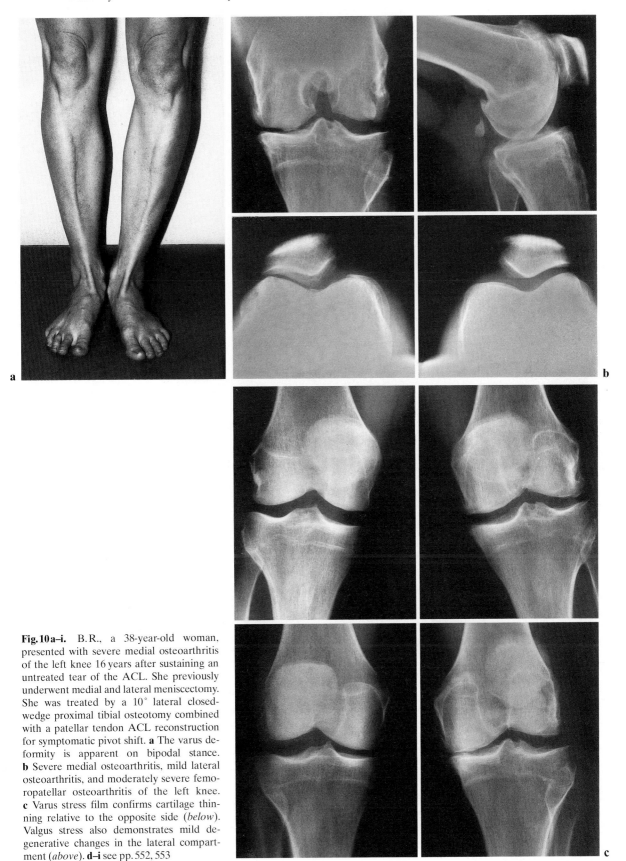

Fig. 10a–i. B.R., a 38-year-old woman, presented with severe medial osteoarthritis of the left knee 16 years after sustaining an untreated tear of the ACL. She previously underwent medial and lateral meniscectomy. She was treated by a 10° lateral closed-wedge proximal tibial osteotomy combined with a patellar tendon ACL reconstruction for symptomatic pivot shift. **a** The varus deformity is apparent on bipodal stance. **b** Severe medial osteoarthritis, mild lateral osteoarthritis, and moderately severe femoropatellar osteoarthritis of the left knee. **c** Varus stress film confirms cartilage thinning relative to the opposite side (*below*). Valgus stress also demonstrates mild degenerative changes in the lateral compartment (*above*). **d–i** see pp. 552, 553

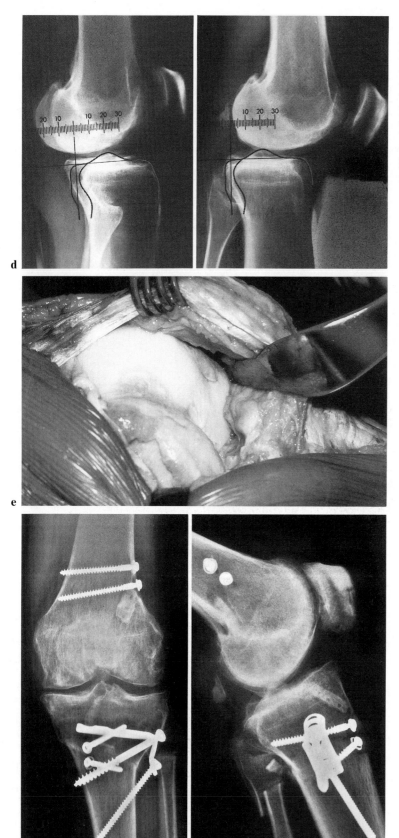

Fig. 10. d Anterior and posterior drawer films show massive anterior instability despite the osteoarthritis. **e** Operation confirms osteoarthritic involvement of the medial condyle and of the lateral condyle to a lesser degree. **f** A patellar tendon ACL reconstruction augmented with a Kennedy LAD was performed concurrently with the valgus osteotomy, which was kept minimal due to the imperfect lateral compartment. The osteotomy was fixed with a bent 5-hole semitubular plate using the modified Weber-Brunner technique (1982)

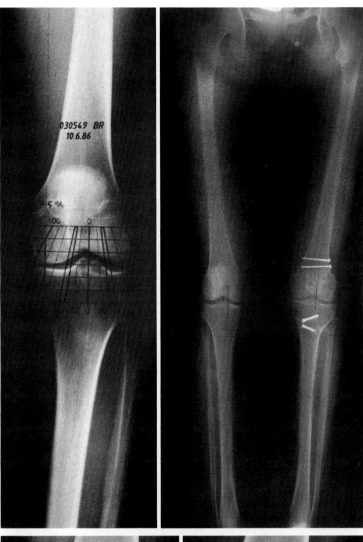

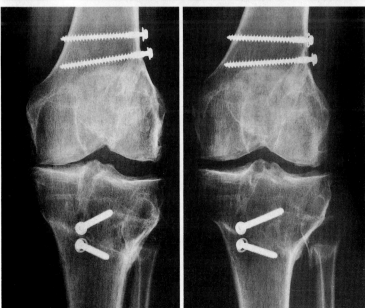

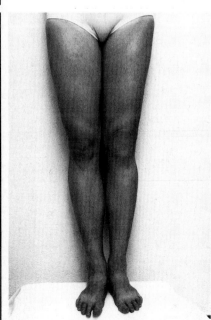

Fig. 10. g The 90% weight-bearing ortho-radiograph at 2 years shows a shift of the mechanical limb axis from 75% varus pre-operatively to a point 13% lateral to the tibial eminence. **h** Varus-valgus stress films at 2 years confirm no change in medial os-teoarthritis, with a markedly wider lateral joint space. **i** Clinical photo shows mild genu valgum on the left side. Stability is good, and residual complaints mainly affect the femo-ropatellar joint

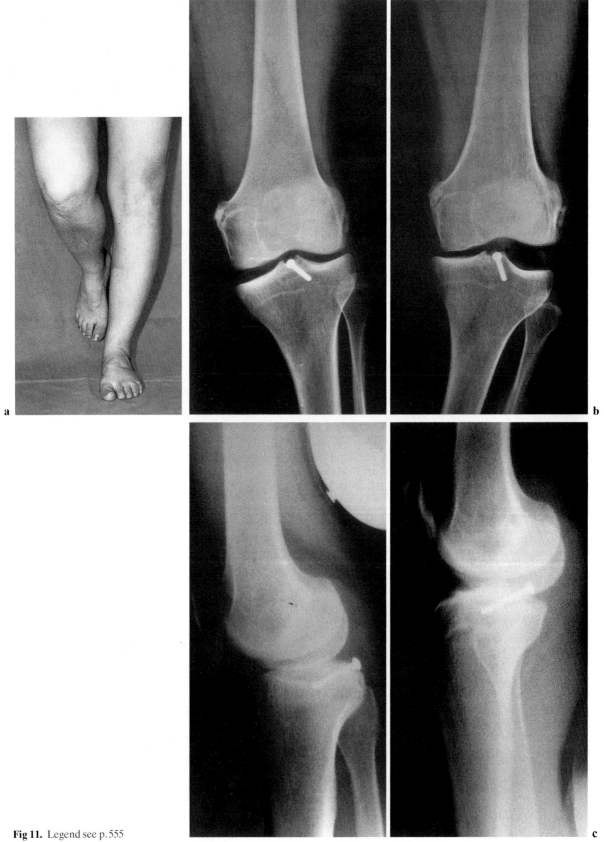

Fig 11. Legend see p. 555

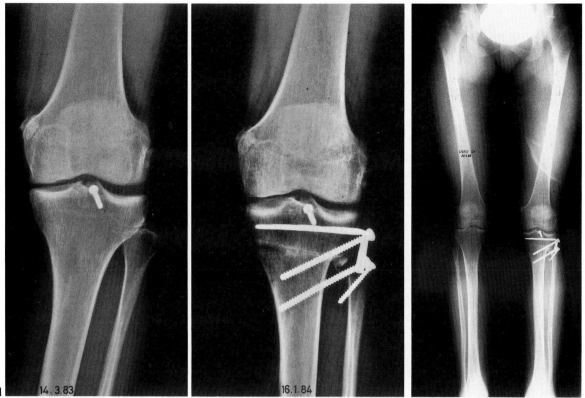

◁ **Fig. 11 a–f.** S.H., a 26-year-old woman, was seen 8 years after her knee injury and 6 years after a posterolateral repair with osseous reattachment of the PCL. She had pronounced varus instability with a marked antero-posterolateral component. It was decided in 1985 to correct the varus deformity by a 10° valgus osteotomy before proceeding with the ligament reconstruction originally planned. The patient was very pleased with the result of the osteotomy and largely free of complaints, so ligament reconstruction was withheld despite the persistence of significant objective instability. **a** Monopodal stance confirms the left varus component, accentuated by the coexisting ligamentous instability. **b** Valgus stress film shows slight medial opening with good cartilage in the lateral compartment. Varus stress evokes massive lateral opening with medial translation of the tibia beneath the femur. **c** Drawer stress films show mild posterior and marked anterior translation of the tibia. **d, e** Monopodal weight-bearing radiographs show the preoperative varus (*d*) and absence of varus after the tibial osteotomy (*e*). Screws were driven through the fibula in an attempt to reduce lateral instability by pressing the fibular head distally. **f** The 90% weight-bearing orthoradiograph at 4 years confirms absence of varus instability following displacement of the mechanical axis into the lateral compartment

Further loss of correction in this situation can be avoided only by performing a technically complex internal or external fixation. Figures 10–12 illustrate our standard osteotomy and fixation technique, modified from Weber and Brunner (1982); in Fig. 12 an adolescent hip plate is used in place of the less stable 1/2-tubular plate. While a lateral closing-wedge osteotomy is appropriate for severe osteoarthritis of the medial compartment, it is not justified if degenerative changes are mild (varus morphotype) and the goal is simply to achieve a normal axial alignment, following the principle of Bousquet. In this case only 5° of correction may be desired, shifting the mechanical limb axis, say, 20% into the lateral compartment. If there is coexisting laxity of the medial collateral ligament, we correct the deformity with a medial open-wedge tibial osteotomy proximal to the superficial attachment of the ligament (Figs. 13, 14). If the surgeon prefers a medial open-wedge osteotomy in every case, the medial collateral ligament must be detached subperiosteally on a piece of bone to avoid excessive loading of the medial compartment. This type of valgus osteotomy is advantageous in that it provides good stability, heals rapidly through the use of tricortical iliac bone grafts, can be fixed with staples or a medial T- or L-plate, and avoids fibular osteotomy. Because this osteotomy is less invasive and is associated with less morbidity, it is easier to combine it with a cruciate ligament reconstruction in the same sitting.

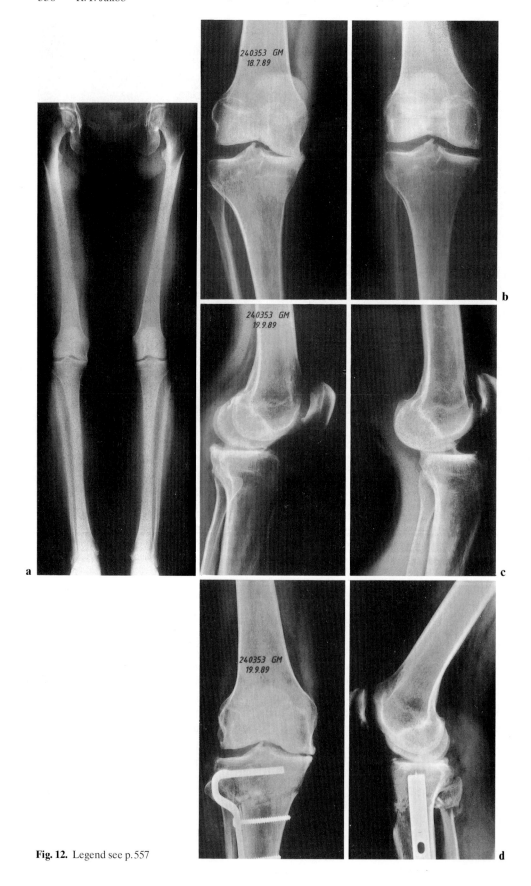

Fig. 12. Legend see p. 557

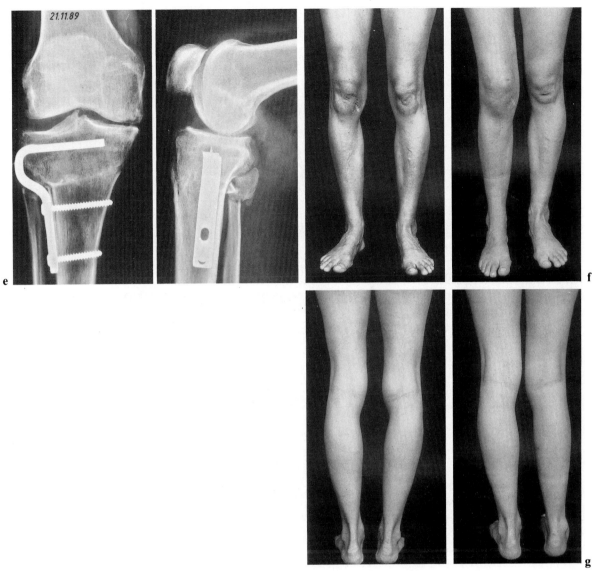

◁ **Fig. 12 a–g.** G. M., a 36-year-old woman, was seen 15 years after sustaining an untreated tear of the ACL and after undergoing medial meniscectomy. She presented with severe medial osteoarthritis and subjectively disabling, objectively pronounced anterior instability. Two-stage operative treatment began with a proximal tibial valgus osteotomy fixed with an ASIF adolescent hip plate (50-mm blade length, 15-mm arch) (we now use this plate routinely as it provides better stability than the 1/2-tubular plate). Arthroscopic abrasion chondroplasty was performed in the same sitting (before the osteotomy), followed by 2 months of intensive physiotherapy with cane ambulation to relieve stress in the medial compartment while stimulating fibrocartilage regeneration. **a** Orthoradiograph shows medial compression with a straight tibia. **b** Varus stress shows deficient medial cartilage, valgus stress shows good lateral cartilage. **c** Drawer stress films show pronounced anterior instability despite osteoarthritis (translation > 20 mm). **d** Postoperative radiographs show fixation of the osteotomy with an adolescent hip plate. **e** Radiographs at 2 months show union of the osteotomy. **f** Pre- and postoperative clinical appearance from the front and **g** from behind

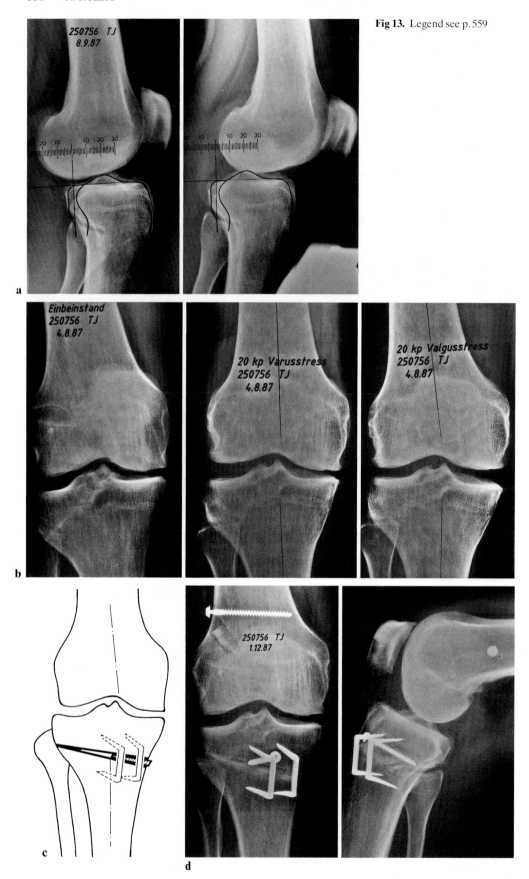

Fig 13. Legend see p. 559

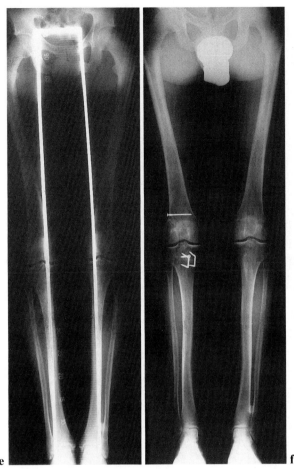

e   f

◁ **Fig. 13a–f.** T.J., a 31-year-old man with a 5-year history of ACL deficiency, was seen 6 years after medial meniscectomy on the affected side. He presented with marked subjective and objective anterior instability, medial osteoarthritis, and a radiographically healthy-appearing lateral compartment (**a**). A patellar tendon reconstruction was performed concomitantly with a proximal tibial 6° open-wedge valgus osteotomy secured with 3 tricortical iliac crest bone grafts and 2 staples. Exercises were commenced right away from a posterior splint, and the osteotomy united at 7 weeks with progressive loading. With a normoaxial correction, we attempt to move the mechanical axis into the 10%–20% region of the lateral compartment. **a** Drawer stress films demonstrate 20 mm of anterior translation. **b** Radiographs with monopodal weight bearing, varus stress, and valgus stress confirm medial osteoarthritis with absence of lateral compartment disease. **c** Proximal tibial open-wedge osteotomy. **d** Postoperative radiographs. **e** The mechanical axis on the preoperative orthoradiograph crossed the knee at 10% varus; **f** postoperatively it crosses the knee at 20% valgus

As a general rule, all valgus osteotomies for osteoarthritis of the knee with varus deformity are performed on the proximal tibia, regardless of the associated instability or meniscus problems.

By contrast, we perform virtually all varus osteotomies for lateral compartmental osteoarthritis on the distal femur (Fig. 15). We expose the supracondylar portion of the femur through a lateral approach, direct the wedge osteotomy medially upward on a lateral hinge, remove a medial 2/3-shaft wedge, and fix the osteotomy with a lateral 7-hole condylar plate that incorporates an interfragmental lag screw. We have found that healing is less satisfactory when the osteotomy is fixed medially with a hip plate. In a series of 35 supracondylar varus osteotomies, we noted 4 cases of delayed union, nonunion, and correction loss in 14 osteotomies that were plated medially, but we saw no complications in any of the 21 osteotomies fixed by lateral plating (Grossmann et al. 1990). We avoid a closed-wedge varus tibial osteotomy for genu valgum due to the danger of jointline obliquity with respect to the mechanical axis. As for the lateral open-wedge proximal tibial osteotomy, we have used it 3 times for various indications in recent years, and each case was complicated by some degree of peroneal nerve palsy due to stretching or neurapraxia. As a result, we cannot recommend this procedure. Nerve recovery was complete in 2 cases and partial in 1. Even exposure of the peroneal nerve, done in 2 cases during preparation for the osteotomy, could not prevent nerve damage. One way to avoid this is to define the "safe" degree of varus correction on a preoperative varus stressradiograph, confine the osteotomy to the tibia, and perform a sagittal fibular head osteotomy parallel to the proximal tibiofibular articulation so that the lateral tibial plateau can glide past the intact fibula (Fig. 16). This osteotomy can produce a maximum correction of about 8° while restoring tension to the lateral collateral ligament, iliotibial tract, and arcuate complex. Another option would be an osteotomy using the Ilizarov technique, which involves a gradual application of distraction and angular correction.

An open-wedge osteotomy that establishes a normal or overcorrected axial alignment while indirectly restoring ligamentous tension permits immediate postoperative mobilization of the operated limb. This is even more desirable when the osteotomy is combined with arthroscopic debridement and an abrasion chondroplasty in which eburnated cartilage sites are abraded to bleeding subchondral bone. This has a resonable chance of inducing fibrocartilage regeneration only if the knee is kept non-weight-bearing for approximately 3 months, continuous mobilizaton of the knee is started immediately after surgery, and excessive compartmental loading has been eliminated.

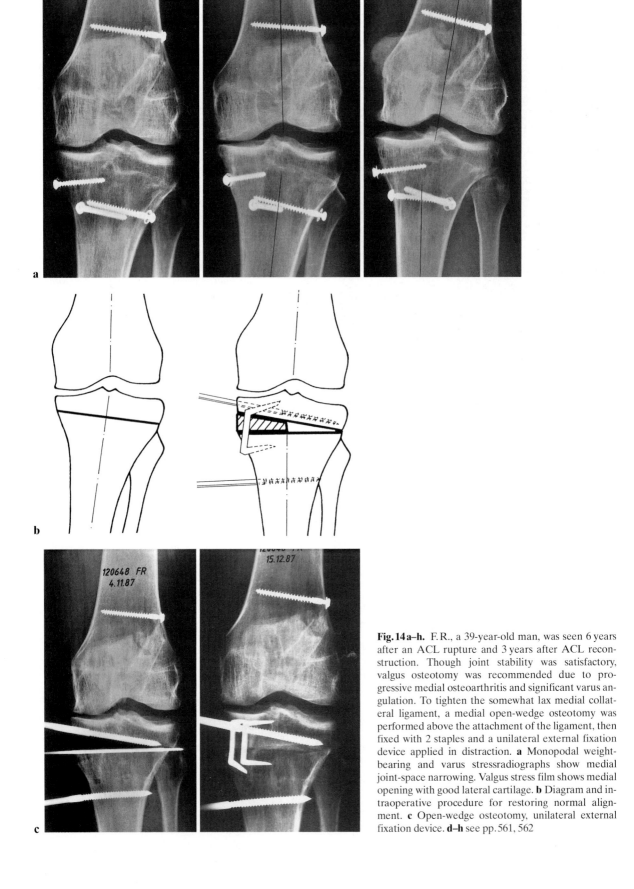

Fig. 14a–h. F.R., a 39-year-old man, was seen 6 years after an ACL rupture and 3 years after ACL reconstruction. Though joint stability was satisfactory, valgus osteotomy was recommended due to progressive medial osteoarthritis and significant varus angulation. To tighten the somewhat lax medial collateral ligament, a medial open-wedge osteotomy was performed above the attachment of the ligament, then fixed with 2 staples and a unilateral external fixation device applied in distraction. **a** Monopodal weight-bearing and varus stressradiographs show medial joint-space narrowing. Valgus stress film shows medial opening with good lateral cartilage. **b** Diagram and intraoperative procedure for restoring normal alignment. **c** Open-wedge osteotomy, unilateral external fixation device. **d–h** see pp. 561, 562

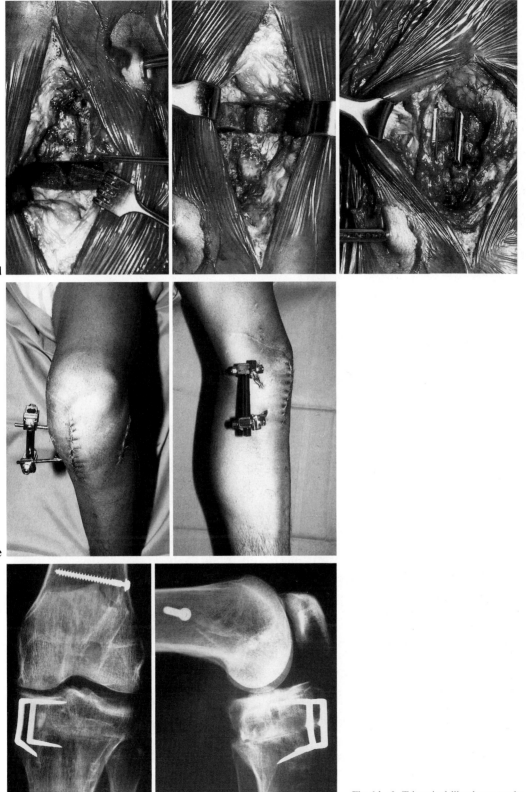

Fig. 14. d Tricortical iliac bone grafts are inserted into the osteotomy and protected by 2 staples. **e** External fixation is maintained for 9 weeks. **f** Osteotomy is consolidated at 11 months

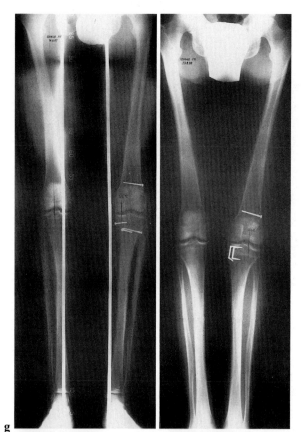

Fig. 14. g Orthoradiographs: mechanical limb axis crosses medial compartment preoperatively (45%) and lateral compartment (20% valgus) postoperatively, representing a normal axial alignment. **h** Clinical comparison: monopodal stance preoperatively (genu varum); bipodal stance with external fixation device; monopodal stance postoperatively, showing correction of genu varum

g

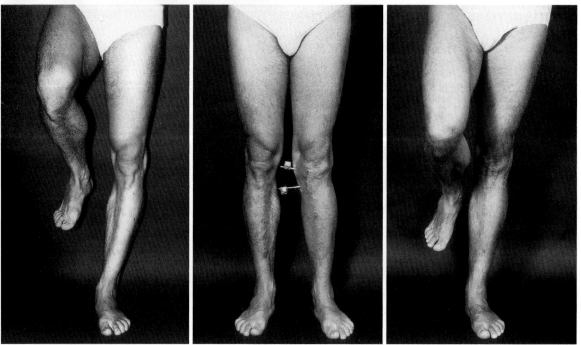

h

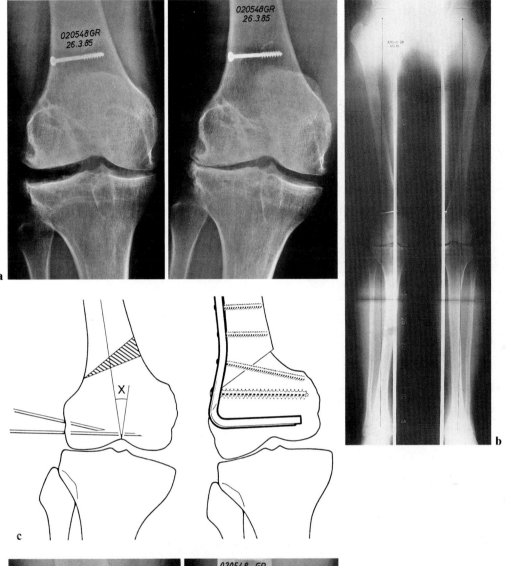

Fig. 15 a–d. G. R., a 38-year-old man, sustained tears of the ACL and lateral meniscus at 18 years of age, managed by lateral meniscectomy. A Jones reconstruction of the ACL was performed at age 29, and a partial medial meniscectomy at age 36. At age 38 the patient underwent a distal femoral osteotomy with 12° correction in varus and 10° in extension for significant lateral osteoarthritic complaints. Two years later the clinical result was good, with slight varus overcorrection. **a** Varus-valgus stress films show a well-preserved medial compartment with complete loss of lateral cartilage. **b** Orthogradiograph shows constitutional genu valgum with the mechanical axis crossing the lateral compartment at 60%. **c** Diagram of the supracondylar varus osteotomy, fixed with a lateral 7-hole condylar plate. **d** Preoperative and postoperative weight-bearing films show slight overcorrection in varus. Technique of supracondylar varus osteotomy for osteoarthritis with valgus deformity, fixation with a 7-hole condylar plate

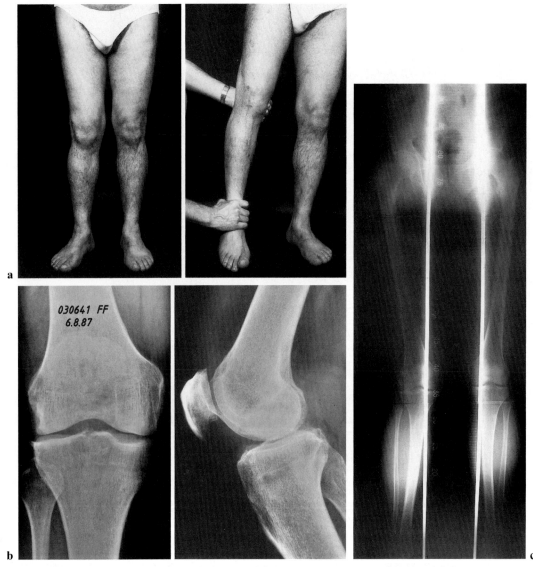

Fig. 16 a–h. F.F., a 46-year-old man, was seen 2 years after a posterolateral ligament injury and lateral meniscectomy with osteoarthritis of the lateral compartment, cartilage loss and valgus deformity. Marked varus instability prohibited a simple supracondylar varus osteotomy. Posterolateral ligament repairs are difficult, of dubious benefit, and would interfere with the goal of immediate mobilization. An osteotomy was planned that would simultaneously correct the valgus deformity and restore lateral ligamentous tension. A transverse osteotomy was performed through the upper tibia, and the fibular head was os- teotomized parallel to the proximal tibiofibular articulation. The open-wedge osteotomy tightened the lateral collateral liga- ment, established a normal axis without overcorrection, and re- stored good lateral stability. The site was fixed with tricortical iliac bone grafts and staples. **a** Clinical appearance in bipodal stance with right venu valgum, demonstration of varus insta- bility. **b** AP and lateral radiographs do not demonstrate the se- verity of lateral compartmental osteoarthritis. **c** Orthoradio- graph shows the mechanical axis crossing the knee at 90% valgus. **d–h** see pp. 565, 566

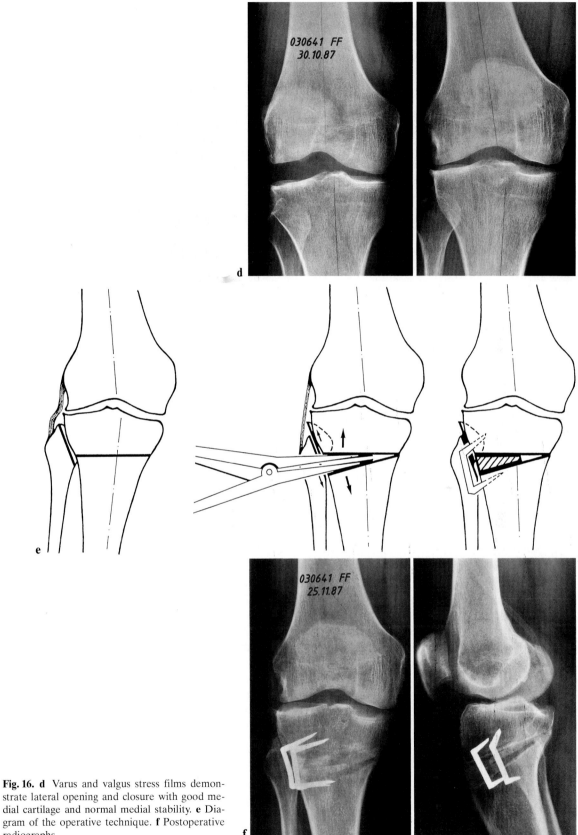

Fig. 16. d Varus and valgus stress films demonstrate lateral opening and closure with good medial cartilage and normal medial stability. **e** Diagram of the operative technique. **f** Postoperative radiographs

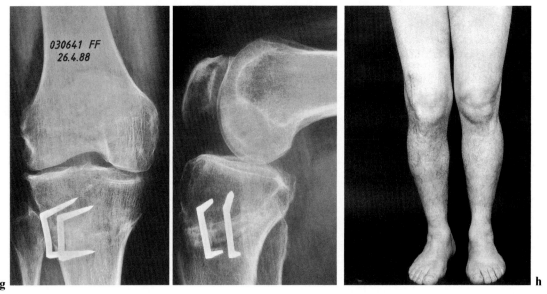

Fig. 16. g Radiographs at 11 months show physiologic valgus. **h** Clinical appearance: normal limb axis

Osteotomy and Ligament Reconstruction

If the osteoarthritis is associated with episodes of subjective instability, it may be appropriate to combine the osteotomy with an arthroscopic or transligamentous ACL reconstruction, which in turn will facilitate early rehabilitation with minimal pain. The surgeon who has not mastered arthroscopic cruciate reconstruction is advised to perform the 2 procedures separately, approximately 3–6 months apart, to reduce the surgical insult. It would be counterproductive to stop half way by addressing the ligament problem alone.

With regard to synthetic cruciate ligament reconstructions, it should be noted that a cruciate reconstruction, whether autologous, homologous, or synthetic, is generally subject to increased loads in the osteoarthritic knee. Presumably this is due largely to the alteration of joint kinematics by the osteoarthritic changes but may also relate to the synovitis and bathing of the graft by enzyme-enriched synovial fluid, which can attack the autologous graft and disrupt the remodeling of its fibers. In any case the stability achieved with an autologous graft in these cases is markedly inferior to that achieved in nonosteoarthritic joints. This led us several years ago to attempt to "salvage" several unstable osteoarthritic knees by performing a prosthetic cruciate ligament reconstruction. Unfortunately, unaccountable failure of the prosthesis occurred in several patients within just a few months – a problem that is specifically mentioned by some manufacturers of prosthetic ligaments. We must conclude that prosthetic cruciate reconstruction is not a valid alternative for osteoarthritic knees. On the other hand, we have had encouraging results with augmentation of the autologous patellar tendon graft by a thin artificial band, a technique that has become routine for the challenging indications described here.

Finally, the natural history of a knee with progressive osteoarthritis is marked by the formation of grooves and buttressing osteophytes that tend to stabilize the joint on the sagittal plane. Operative stabilization may be omitted in these cases. Self-stabilization at this stage, however, is evidenced by a significant, demonstrable loss of articular motion.

Effective treatment is difficult in patients with bicompartmental osteoarthritis, which will not benefit from ligament stabilization and corrective osteotomy. Arthroscopic joint debridement and irrigation may afford temporary relief in such cases. Total knee arthroplasty should be considered for severe osteoarthritis, whether uni-, bi- or tricompartmental, in patients over 60 years of age.

References

Bousquet G, Rhenter J-L, Bascoulergue G, Millon J (1982) Illustré du genou. Mure, Le Coteau

Dejour H, Walch G, Deschamps G, Chambat P (1987) Arthrose du genou sur laxité chronique antérieure. Rev Chir Orthop 73: 157-170

Fried JA, Bergfeld JA, Weiker G, Andrish JT (1985) Anterior cruciate reconstruction using the Jones-Ellison procedure. [Am] J Bone Joint Surg 67: 1029-1033

Fujisawa Y, Masuhara K, Shiomi S (1979) The effect of high tibial osteotomy on osteoarthritis of the knee. Orthop Clin North Am 10: 585-608

Grossmann SP, Miniaci A, Jakob RP (1988) Supracondylar femoral varus osteotomy in the treatment of valgus deformity about the knee. Am J Knee Surg

Hernigou P, Medevielle D, Debeyre J, Goutallier D (1987) Proximal tibial osteotomy for osteoarthritis with varus deformity. [Am] J Bone Joint Surg 69: 332-354

Hey Groves EW (1920) The crucial ligaments of the knee joint: Their function, rupture and the operative treatment of the same. Br J Surg 7: 505-515

Jacobsen K (1977) Osteoarthrosis following insufficiency of the cruciate ligaments in man: A clinical study. Acta Orthop Scand 48: 520-526

Jakob RP (1987) Pathomechanical and clinical concepts of the pivot shift sign. Semin Orthop 1: 9-17

Jakob RP, Kipfer W, Klaue K, Stäubli HU, Gerber C (1988) Etude critique de la reconstruction du ligament croisé antérieur du genou par la plastie pédiculée sur le Hoffa à partir du tiers médian du tendon rotulien, 50 genoux opérés avec recul de 2 à 4 ans. Rev Chir Orthop 74: 44-51

Johnson F, Leitl S, Waugh W (1980) The distribution of load across the knee: A comparison of static and dynamic measurements. J Bone Joint Surg [Br] 62: 346-349

Lynch MA, Henning CE, Glick KR (1983) Knee Joint surface changes: Long-term follow-up meniscus tear treatment in stable anterior cruciate ligament reconstructions. Clin Orthop 172: 148-153

McDaniel WJ, Dameron TB (1983) The untreated anterior cruciate ligament rupture. Clin Orthop 172: 158-163

Weber BG, Brunner CF (1982) Special techniques in internal fixation. Springer, Berlin Heidelberg New York

Miniaci A, Ballmer FT, Ballmer PM, Jakob RP (1989) Proximal tibial osteotomy - a new fixation technique. Clin Orthop 246: 250-259

Monopodal Weight-Bearing Radiography of the Chronically Unstable Knee

H. Dejour, P. Neyret, and M. Bonnin

Radiographs taken of the chronically unstable knee while the patient bears full body weight on the affected limb (monopodal weight-bearing films) are of interest in that they provide diagnostic and prognostic information on the joint as a function of several factors: the limb morphotype on the frontal and sagittal planes, muscular equilibrium, body weight, and body size. It is well known that a rupture of the anterior cruciate ligament (ACL) can have different functional and radiographic consequences in different individuals. Monopodal weight-bearing radiographs often provide the key to understanding these differences.

Monopodal films can be obtained only in patients with a unilateral ACL deficiency, since comparison with the healthy knee is necessary in order to evaluate the role of laxity. We obtain 3 monopodal standing views of the knee joint: (1) an AP projection with the knee extended but not hyperextended and the quadriceps tense, (2) a lateral projection with the knee flexed 20°–30° and the quadriceps contracted, and (3) a lateral projection in maximum hyperextension (only in patients with recurvatum).

Frontal Equilibrium

Joint symmetry is evaluated by comparing the heights of the medial and lateral joint spaces on the AP radiograph. We say that "decoaptation" is present when one of the joint spaces is wider, signifying loss of contact between the femoral condyle and tibial plateau. Lateral decoaptation is much more common than medial decoaptation in accordance with the varus-producing forces that are active during weight bearing. Lateral decoaptation is measurable as the angle between the femoral and tibial joint planes. It may be a "pure" decoaptation, with the medial joint space retaining a normal width, or there may be associated narrowing of the medial joint space in relation to the opposite knee. There may also be a rotatory femorotibial component, but this is difficult to assess and so we disregarded it. Lateral decoaptation is not pathologic in itself, as it occurred in 40% of the healthy controls that we examined radiographically. It definitely relates to anatomic varus but must depend on other factors as well.

A rupture of the ACL is frequently accompanied by lateral decoaptation. Lateral decoaptation with medial joint-space narrowing is very common and signifies damage to the medial meniscus and articular cartilage, which is more important than the lateral ligamentous lesions. In such cases it is important to identify those patients who additionally have congenital genu varum. We shall see that lateral decoaptation can also coexist with anterior subluxation of the medial tibial plateau; this is visible on the lateral film. Such knees tend to progress to medial femorotibial osteoarthritis. Lateral decoaptation without medial narrowing is very unusual (less than 10% of cases). It implies a lesion of the posterolateral corner. In a patient with a normal morphotype and mild valgus angulation in the supine position, a knee with this form of decoaptation can slip into varus during ambulation; this can be documented on the monopodal weight-bearing film.

As common as lateral decoaptation is, it is not observed in all cases. Chronic ACL instability may process to medial femorotibial narrowing with no lateral decoaptation or to global osteoarthritis. Global degeneration that is "equilibrated" shows narrowing of both the medial and lateral joint spaces; it is more common in patients with constitutional genu valgum.

We have never seen "medial decoaptation" as an accompanying feature of a ruptured ACL.

An isolated rupture of the posterior cruciate ligament (PCL) appears to have no effect on lateral decoaptation provided there are no associated peripheral lesions of posterolateral structures.

Sagittal Equilibrium

Rupture of the ACL leads to a disruption of joint kinematics that is manifested only in certain weight-bearing situations. Supine, non-weight-bearing radiographs in various positions of flexion will show that the knee maintains an essentially constant center of rotation. But if the film is taken while the patient is standing on the affected limb with the knee flexed 30°, anterior translation of both tibial plateaus will be apparent. The amount of subluxation decreases as the knee is flexed further, and it increases if the forces across the knee joint are increased (jumping or landing from a jump). Thus, the anterior tibial translation measured on the lateral radiograph does not correspond to the maximum anterior translation. The degree of anterior translation is dependent on secondary intraarticular traumatic lesions and the osteoarthritis resulting from ACL deficiency.

We believe that the monopodal weight-bearing film is very important for the assessment of sagittal laxity. This is done by measuring the subluxation actively produced by quadriceps contraction while the knee is bearing weight; this corresponds to natural, everyday situations when the knee is not subjected to maximum loading.

Generally we measure the distance between two lines parallel to the posterior tibial cortex, one passing through the posterior border of the medial tibial plateau and the other tangential to the most posterior point on the medial femoral condyle (see Fig. 4c). Constitutional laxity in the healthy knee joint typically permits an anterior displacement of about 3 mm.

It is essential, then, to compare the affected knee with the opposite healthy knee. Rupture of the ACL leads to progressive anterior translation of the medial tibial plateau. With an isolated ACL lesion of recent occurrence, healthy menisci, and competent secondary posteromedial restraints, the anterior translation (affected knee minus healthy knee) will equal no more than 1–2 mm or may be absent. But if medial meniscectomy has been performed and there is a lateral rotatory drawer with a pivot shift in external rotation, these lesions will result in distention of the posteromedial corner, causing a significantly greater net anterior displacement – perhaps more than 1 cm – relative to the opposite side.

The following factors can additionally influence the degree of anterior translation:

– The slope of the tibial plateau: We define this as the angle between the slope of the medial plateau and the long axis of the tibia (minus 90°). The average value is 6°. We first became aware of this morphologic aspect of the tibial plateau in a patient with bilateral congenital aplasia of the ACL (Dejour et al. 1987b). The proximal tibial epiphysis was abnormally developed and showed a flexion deformity of 20°. There was 20 mm of anterior translation, the condyles appearing to slip backward on both tibial plateaus. Ligament reconstruction in this case had to be supplemented by a corrective osteotomy. Another patient with a chronic ACL rupture had undergone a flexion osteotomy and ACL reconstruction 8 years before. Although the subjective result was good initially, anterior tibial translation gradually increased with the condyles slipping down the slope of the tibial plateau. This impression has been confirmed for tibial slopes of about 15°, which lead to significant anterior translation.

The relationship between the tibial slope and anterior tibial translation on monopodal weight bearing has been demonstrated in an analysis of 281 cases of unilateral rupture of the ACL (Bonnin 1990). There was a linear relationship between the tibial slope and the anterior tibial translation that is highly significant for both affected knees and the contralateral normal knees ($p < 0.0001$). This means that as the slope of the tibial plateau increases, so does the anterior tibial translation. The regression line showed that for every 10° increase in the backward inclination of the tibial plateau, anterior tibial translation is increased by 6 mm (Fig. 1).

It remains unclear whether ligamentous stability tends to deteriorate when the tibial plateau slope is greater than 12°, or whether these factors are causally interrelated.

Muscular tone or rigidity can alter the degree of anterior translation. Although this is easy to demonstrate clinically, it is difficult to quantify, and it could account for certain clinical-radiographic inconsistencies. There is no way of confirming, however, that good proprioceptive control or muscular rigidity is manifested by an absence or reduction of translation in monopodal stance.

Rupture of the PCL leads to a posterior translation of the tibia that appears to depend on the degree of the posterior slope. Significantly, this translation loosens the peripheral structures, especially on the medial side. This may account for the infrequency of medial femorotibial osteoarthritic changes after an isolated rupture of the PCL, since the osteoarthritis is more likely to be in the lateral compartment or tricompartmental.

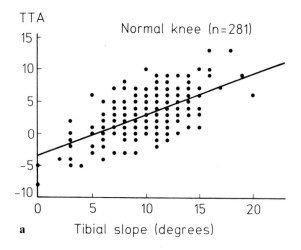

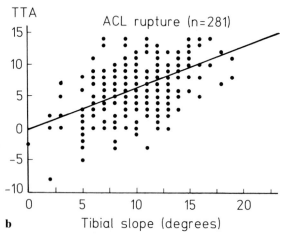

Fig. 1a,b. Relationship between tibial slope and anterior tibial translation (ATT) on monopodal weight bearing. **a** Normal knees. **b** Knees with ruptured ACL

Relationship between Frontal and Sagittal Equilibrium

With "straight" anterior subluxation of the proximal tibia, both plateaus subluxate to the same degree with a minimal rotatory component. In "equilibrated" osteoarthritis, the anterior translation of the medial tibial plateau can increase so that the knee moves into a position of external rotation. This reflects the progressive distention of the posteromedial corner and leads to a scalloped erosion of the posterior tibial plateau. The medial femorotibial narrowing and the anterior translation of the tibia develop on the plane of the instant center of rotation of the knee. Thus, the femorotibial narrowing is accompanied by loss of lateral coaptation. Medial narrowing, lateral decoaptation, and anterior subluxation are closely interre-

lated, therefore. A concept that reduces the process to a purely seesaw-like action on the frontal plane, with one side rising while the other descends to produce medial narrowing and lateral decoaptation, disregards the processes on the sagittal plane and so is incomplete.

A lesion of the posterolateral corner combined with a rupture of the ACL is likewise reflected in lateral decoaptation on the AP monopodal weight-bearing film. This is associated with a loosening of the lateral structures that affects the lateral collateral ligament less than the posterolateral restraints. These lesions would permit an increased anterior translation of the lateral tibial plateau by reducing the distance between the attachment sites of the lateral collateral ligament, leading to increased lateral decoaptation in the monopodal stance.

Role of Tibial Osteotomy in Chronic Laxity

Proximal Tibial Valgus Osteotomy

The monopodal weight-bearing radiograph is useful in assessing the need for proximal tibial valgus osteotomy. An isolated rupture of the ACL in itself does not alter the axial alignment as shown on the AP monopodal film. As discussed earlier, the greater the extent of secondary peripheral lesions accompanying the ACL rupture, the greater their impact on the width of the lateral and medial femorotibial joint spaces on the frontal plane.

It is a therapeutic axiom that every anomaly that appears on the monopodal weight-bearing radiograph cannot be corrected by a simple ligament reconstruction. The forces responsible for lateral decoaptation are so large that they will loosen or disrupt any ligament reconstruction aimed at relieving lateral instability. To correct lateral decoaptation, then, it is necessary to supplement the ligament reconstruction with an osteotomy that will neutralize the lateral distending forces.

By the same token, the proximal tibial valgus osteotomy can reduce the scope of indications for ACL reconstruction. A recent study (Dejour et al. 1987b) has shown that ACL reconstruction can initiate the development of osteoarthritis. This especially occurred in knees that displayed preoperative radiographic changes such as more than 50% joint-space narrowing or had a previous medial meniscectomy, in patients over 50 years of age, and in patients with more than 8° of varus deformity. All of these patients would be candidates for an operation combining

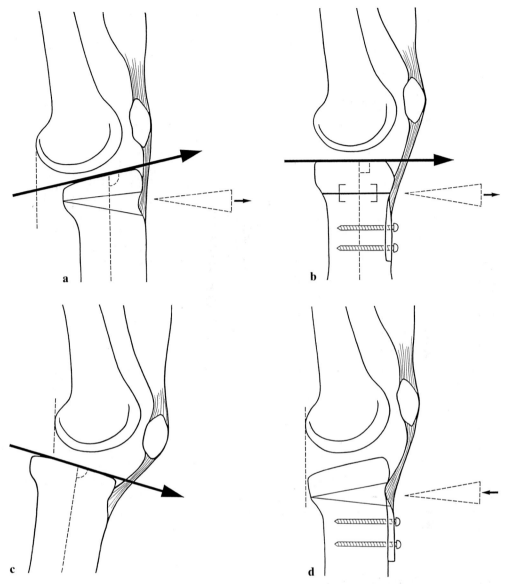

Fig. 2a,b. The slope of the tibial plateau is defined as the angle formed by the tibial shaft axis and the tangent to the medial tibial plateau, minus 90°. The epiphysis in a recurvatum knee would yield a negative slope angle (as in **c**: 85°-90° = -5°). When there is a strongly positive slope of the tibial plateau as in **a** (105°-90°), an anterior closed-wedge osteotomy of the proxi- mal tibia will reduce anterior tibial subluxation by leveling the plateau. **c, d** A negative slope promotes anterior gliding of the femoral condyles. This has an unfavorable effect in a knee with chronic PCL deficiency. An anterior open-wedge osteotomy of the proximal tibia is helpful in controlling this subluxation

proximal tibial valgus osteotomy with ACL recon- struction.

Proximal tibial valgus osteotomy is mandatory for ad- vanced femorotibial osteoarthritis secondary to chronic instability of the ACL (Dejour et al. 1987a). In these cases where disabling subjective and objec- tive instability coexist, we prefer to combine the osteotomy with an extraarticular rather than intraar- ticular reconstruction.

As we have seen, this osteotomy can be done concur- rently with a ligament reconstruction or as an isolated procedure, and either an open-wedge or closed- wedge technique may be used. The medial open- wedge osteotomy is more precise and is appropriate for the correction of an excessive varus morphotype. If the surgeon wants to achieve overcorrection for severe medial osteoarthritis, or if radiographs dem- onstrate pre-osteoarthritic changes or lateral decoap- tation, a lateral closed-wedge osteotomy is preferred.

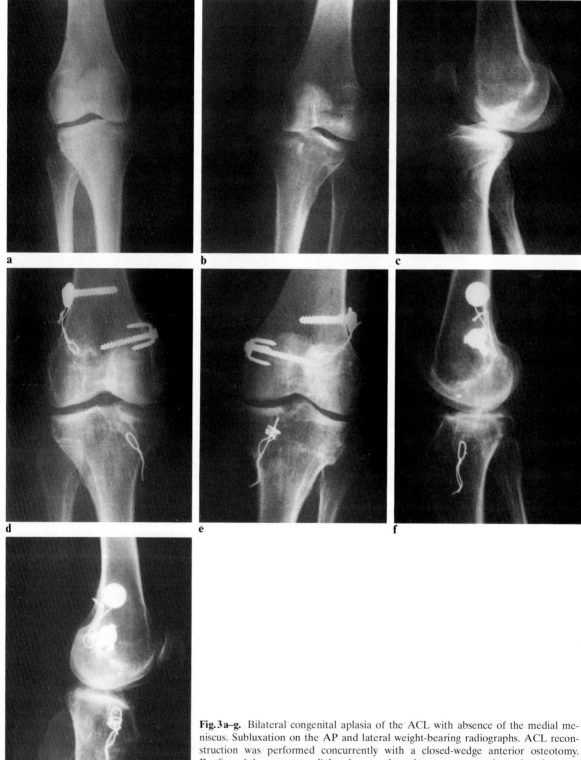

Fig. 3 a–g. Bilateral congenital aplasia of the ACL with absence of the medial meniscus. Subluxation on the AP and lateral weight-bearing radiographs. ACL reconstruction was performed concurrently with a closed-wedge anterior osteotomy. Reefing of the posteromedial and posterolateral corners was performed at the same time. The result at 3 years is good, with good correction of the subluxation in monopodal stance

Fig. 4. Athlete who underwent a medial meniscectomy and lateral extraarticular reconstruction at 24 years of age presented to us in 1982 with pre-osteoarthritic changes. An ACL reconstruction alone in this situation can greatly accelerate osteoarthritic progression. A proximal tibial valgus osteotomy combined with a patellar tendon reconstruction of the ACL permits early resumption of sports activities. The result at 2 years is shown ▷

Fig. 5 a–c *(below).* A 24-year-old man presented 2 years after ACL rupture and repair (Lemaire reconstruction, partial meniscectomy in the left knee) with severe, rapidly progressive medial osteoarthritis and lateral decoaptation. No signs of instability were seen (**a**). An open-wedge valgus osteotomy was performed in 1984. Five years later the slope of the tibial plateau measures 8° in the healthy knee and 14° in the affected knee. This increased tibial slope is unfavorable for it cannot restrain anterior tibial subluxation and promotes posterior gliding of the condyles. The patient also exhibits a flexion contracture of 10°. A metaphyseal valgus-recurvatum osteotomy is planned to relieve stress on the eroded medial compartment (**c**)

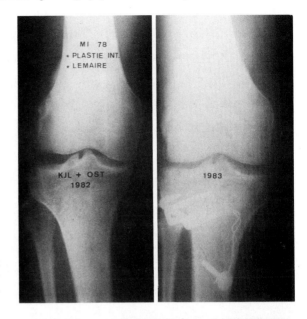

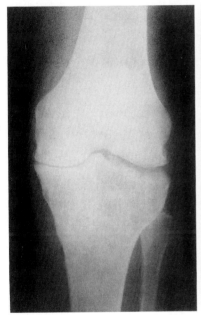
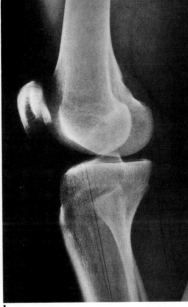
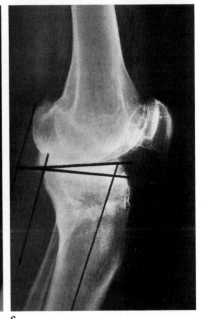

a   b   c

Tibial Extension Osteotomy

The lateral monopodal weight-bearing film enables us to study the relationship between the slope of the tibial plateau and anterior subluxation. Based on the disappointing results of ligament reconstructions alone for the correction of significant anterior subluxation accompanied by a tibial plateau slope greater than 15°, whether congenital, constitutional or iatrogenic in origin, we recommend adding an anterior open-wedge osteotomy of the proximal tibia (Figs. 2–7). Unlike the proximal tibial valgus osteotomy, this procedure has rarely been practiced in humans (Slocum and Devigne 1983). When the tibial slope is in the range of 10°–15°, we lack the statistical data to justify a recommendation for anterior open-wedge proximal tibial osteotomy. In any case this degree of slope would require very little correction.

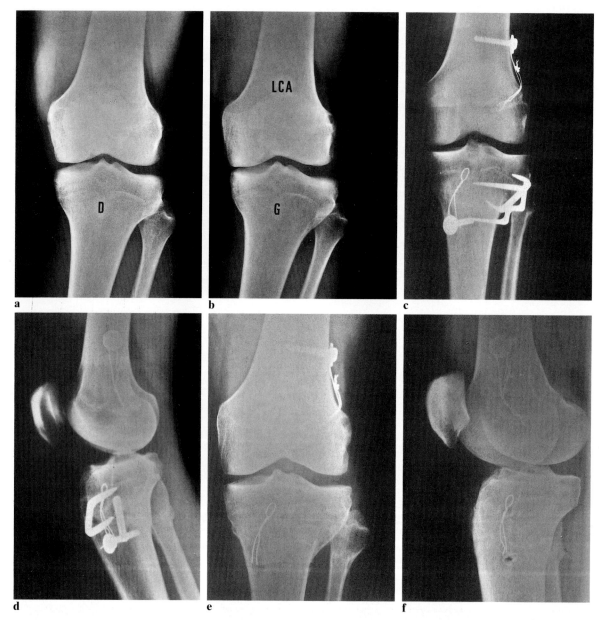

Fig. 6 a–f. Male 25 years of age with lateral decoaptation in both knees, more pronounced on the left side, apparent on the AP monopodal weight-bearing film. Anterolateral instability (deficiency of ACL and posterolateral corner). Proximal tibial valgus osteotomy is combined with intraarticular reconstruction of the ACL

Interaction between Valgus and Extension Osteotomy of the Proximal Tibia

Since 1970 we have performed 180 proximal tibial valgus osteotomies for chronic laxities, 10 of them for posterior instability. The correction on the frontal plane was consistently combined with a modification of the plateau slope.

With a lateral closed-wedge osteotomy, an extension effect is achieved on the tibial plateau by directing the osteotomy obliquely. This appears to be beneficial in knees with anterior instability. Proof of this effect is offered by an analysis of lateral closed-wedge proximal tibial osteotomies in knees with chronic posterior laxity. In these cases we have observed an anterior gliding of the tibial plateau with forward displacement of the area of femorotibial contact. By contrast, a medial open-wedge osteotomy not only preserves the posterior slope of the tibial plateau but even increases it; this restrains posterior subluxation

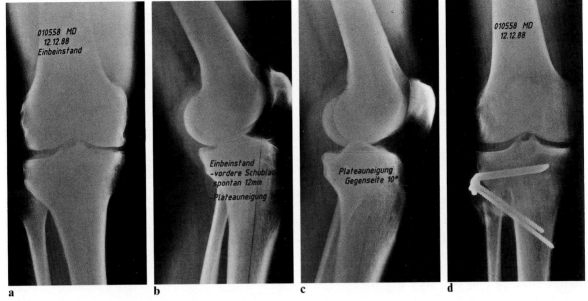

a   b   c   d

Fig. 7a–d. Male 30 years of age with chronic ACL instability. The AP monopodal weight-bearing film (**a**) shows narrowing of the medial joint space. The lateral weight-bearing film shows 12 mm of spontaneous anterior subluxation with a 14° tibial slope (**b**). A lateral film of the opposite knee shows a plateau slope of only 10°. Proximal tibial valgus osteotomy also redirected the tibial plateau to a more favorable slope. The course to date has been satisfactory, so cruciate ligament reconstruction has been withheld

of the tibia by promoting posterior gliding of the femoral condyles on the tibial plateau (Fig. 8).

In summary, the technique of a proximal tibial valgus osteotomy (open- or closed-wedge, obliquity) is of major interest because it can have a positive or negative effect on stability in the sagittal plane. An open-wedge osteotomy produces a flexion effect on the tibial plateau that is unfavorable in anterior instability but favorable in posterior instability, where it opposes tibial subluxation while preserving tension in the peripheral structures. Thus, a proximal tibial valgus osteotomy must not exacerbate bony recurvatum in a knee with posterior instability.

Monopodal Stance, Osteotomy, and Rehabilitation

The lateral monopodal weight-bearing radiograph also has important implications for rehabilitation. If the difference in subluxation between the healthy and affected knees is pronounced (more than 4 mm), we do not permit weight bearing for 6 weeks postoperatively; premature weight bearing would place an excessive strain on the graft before the bony fragments have become incorporated. If the difference is less than 4 mm, we permit earlier weight bearing protected by an elevated heel that prevents hyperextension.

Correction of the abnormalities visible on the monopodal weight-bearing film serves to protect ligament reconstructions. Again, the knee should be rehabilitated in flexion, especially if an extension osteotomy has been performed on the upper tibia. We have observed no static or functional problems associated with a weight-bearing knee pivot in athletes who have had an anterior closed-wedge osteotomy of the proximal tibia (without overcorrection).

Conclusion

Radiographs in monopodal stance convey an accurate impression of functional reality. They permit us to interpret the pathophysiology of chronic instabilities. They help us to understand the mechanism of secondary traumatic intraarticular lesions and their role in the pathogenesis of osteoarthritis. Also, they aid in the selection of patients for osteotomies and support the rehabilitation of chronic anterior knee laxity.

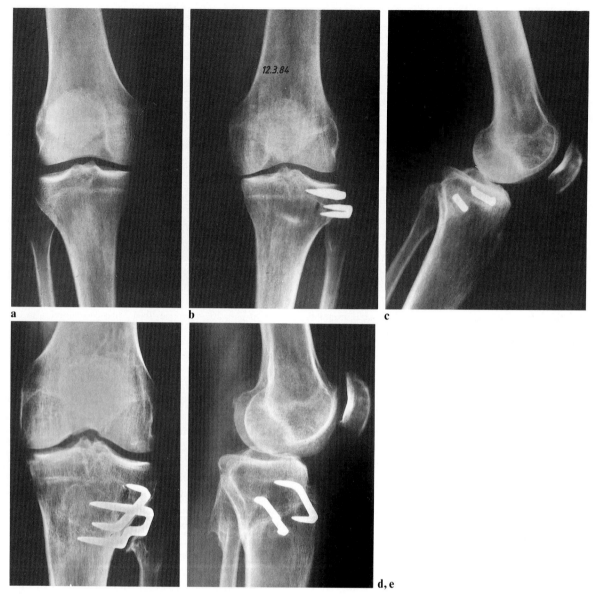

Fig. 8a–e. Acute repair of posterior and posterolateral lesions sustained in a skiing injury was followed by residual instability, varus overload in monopodal stance compared with the opposite side, and slight narrowing of the medial joint space. One year later a lateral closed-wedge proximal tibial valgus osteotomy was performed; the original staples were removed and new staples inserted to fix the osteotomy. This yielded a negative plateau slope angle (– 3°) which, unfortunately, cannot restrain posterior subluxation and anterior gliding of the femoral condyles. It would have been better to achieve a flexion effect with the osteotomy, reorienting the plateau to a 10° slope

References

Bonnin M (1990) La subluxation tibiale antérieure en appui monopodal dans les ruptures du ligament croisé antérieure; étude clinique et biomechanique. Thèse Medecin no .180, Lyon

Dejour H, Walch G, Deschamps G, Chambat P (1987 a) Arthrose du genou sur laxité chronique antérieure. Rev Chir Orthop 73: 157–170

Dejour H, Walch G, Neyret P, Adeleine P (1987 b) Résultats des laxités chroniques antérieures. À propos de 251 cas opérés et revus avec un recul minimum de 3 ans. Rev Chir Orthop 7: 622–636

Dejour H, Neyret P, Eberhard P, Walch G (1990) Absence congénitale bilatérale du ligament croisé antérieur et du ménisque interne. A propos d'un cas. Rev Chir Orthop (in press)

Slocum B, Devigne T (1983) Crucial tibial thrust: a primary force in the canine stifle. J Am Vet Med Assoc 183/4: 456–459

Role of Unicompartmental Arthroplasty in Femorotibial Osteoarthritis with a Deficient Central Pivot

P. Cartier

The coexistence of stage IV unicompartmental osteoarthritis with anterior cruciate ligament (ACL) insufficiency poses a difficult problem, especially when anatomic factors (lack of bone loss) and low patient age mandate the selection of a minimal arthroplastic procedure. When osteoarthritis is mild, we favor a proximal tibial osteotomy combined with a Lemaire-type extraarticular reconstruction, which has yielded good results.

For a number of authors, absence of the ACL means repeated failures and reoperations with osteoarthritic deterioration that may eventually prompt a recommendation for total knee arthroplasty. In this article we shall examine the conditions that would contraindicate a proximal tibial osteotomy while favoring a unicompartmental arthroplasty, with or without a functioning cruciate ligament. We shall also discuss various anatomic situations involving a deficient central pivot and their frequency. Finally we shall address some technical points that merit special consideration.

Indications for Unicompartmental Arthroplasty in which Tibial Osteotomy is Contraindicated

The ideal candidate for a proximal tibial osteotomy is a patient under 65 years of age with genu varum, less than 15° of flexion deformity, little or no ligamentous laxity, and no true anteroposterior femorotibial subluxaton. These conditions are not always satisfied, however, and contraindications to proximal tibial osteotomy are common, especially in the ACL-deficient knee.

Age

In patients over 70 years old with genu varum, we favor a unicompartmental arthroplasty except in patients who have less than 10° of varus deformity, who are biologically younger than their chronological age,

and in whom the scope of indications for osteotomy can be extended.

In patients over 65 years of age with genu valgum, we consistently favor unicompartmental arthroplasty using a 7-mm-thick femoral component.

Valgus or Varus > 8° with Predominant Femoral Deformity

In these cases proximal tibial osteotomy would create an oblique joint line with femorotibial subluxation and a progression of osteoarthritic deterioration on both the medial and lateral sides.

The decision between femoral osteotomy and unicompartmental arthroplasty depends chiefly on patient age but also on the presence of varus bowing of the tibial diaphysis with dysplasia of the lateral condyle.

Pronounced Instability

In patients with varus and pronounced ligamentous instability, other authors have recommended a proximal tibial valgus osteotomy with an overcorrection of 7°–10° past the mechanical axis. In many cases, however, this laxity is not a ligament problem but relates directly to the loss of bony substance. This situation can be clarified by the evaluation of varus-valgus stress films.

Overcorrection signifies a true ligamentous instability (varus-valgus laxity), while undercorrection confirms that the problem is one of bone loss (joint-space narrowing). In such cases we believe that, for esthetic (overcorrected limb axis) and functional reasons, unicompartmental arthroplasty is superior to osteotomy. The patient is unlikely to appreciate the pronounced "iatrogenic deformity" of the postosteotomy valgus, especially if the opposite knee is in varus. From a functional standpoint, varus on one side and valgus on the other creates an unstable situation that can quickly lead to an exacerbation of the non-operated genu varum. In such cases the pros-

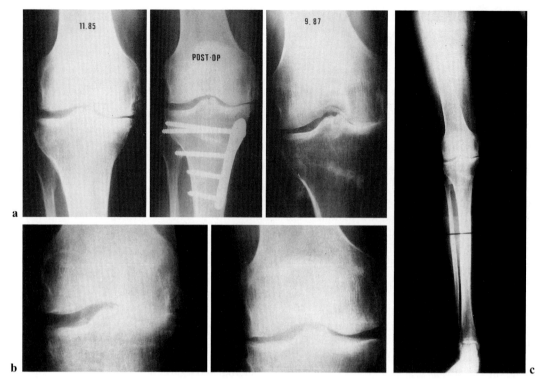

Fig. 1 a–c. Failed proximal tibial osteotomy with joint obliquity in a patient with medial femorotibial arthrosis secondary to an old rupture of the ACL, straight tibia. (The ideal indication for osteotomy is medial osteoarthritis with varus bowing of the tibia)

thetic revision of a failed proximal tibial osteotomy would necessitate a total knee replacement with far greater bone loss than a primary unicompartmental arthroplasty. Moreover, pronounced genu valgum in these older patients will have adverse effects on the ankle joints and the lumbar spine.

Valgus or Varus Deviation without Bowing of the Tibial Shaft

Tibial osteotomy may be appropriate in cases where there is varus or valgus angulation of a straight tibia, as long as the deviation is less than 5°. With greater deviation, osteotomy would produce an oblique joint line, leading in turn to excessive loading of the compartment that requires decompression (Figs. 1, 2). Especially in genu varum, the more valgus correction is applied, the greater the tendency for persistence of pain on the medial side. The best way to avoid these problems is to use a goniometer preoperatively to determine the 3 components of the deviation (femoral, tibial, articular) when the tibia is clinically and radiographically straight.

This aspect merits special consideration. A significant number of patients develop a purely articular medial femorotibial osteoarthritis that leads secondarily to varus deviation, since the cartilage loss and subsequent bone loss on the medial side are not the result of an accompanying abnormal curvature of the tibial shaft. Varus cases in which the tibia is perfectly straight with no anterior bowing invariably do poorly after valgus osteotomy. Their etiology is based entirely on articular pathology, and a valgus osteotomy that "breaks a straight bone" will produce joint obliquity, as will any joint deformity that is corrected at the diaphyseal-metaphyseal level in a patient without varus or anterior bowing of the tibia.

Accordingly, osteotomy is contraindicated in patients who show varus deviation of a straight tibia due to local joint pathology with secondary chondritis following giving-way episodes and old meniscus lesions. The treatment of choice is unicompartmental arthroplasty, except in cases with largely bicompartmental involvement that will necessitate a total prosthesis.

In patients with a failed proximal tibial osteotomy, unicompartmental arthroplasty can be used to correct mild obliquities. If the deformity exceeds 10°, total arthroplasty is indicated. Thus, unicompartmental arthroplasty is the best therapeutic option for

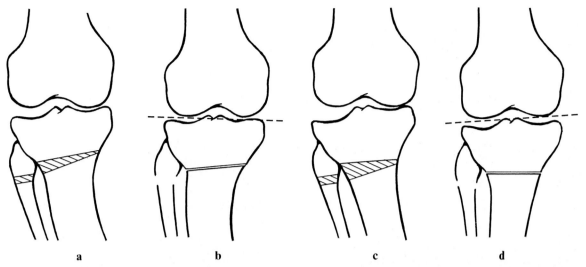

Fig. 2a–d. With varus bowing of the tibia, a valgus osteotomy will produce a horizontal joint line (**a, b**). With a straight tibia and medial osteoarthritis, valgus osteotomy will produce an oblique joint line that is lower on the lateral side (**c, d**)

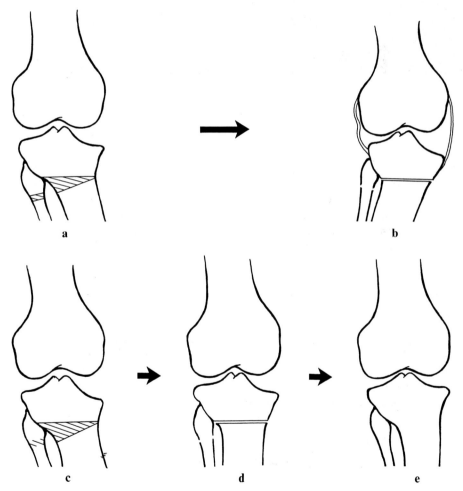

Fig. 3a–e. With a pagoda-like slope of the medial plateau caused by osteoarthritic erosion, it is very difficult to calculate the necessary wedge size. If the wedge is too small, the tibia will drift back into varus; if too large, there will be overcorrection accentuated by the concomitant medial instability

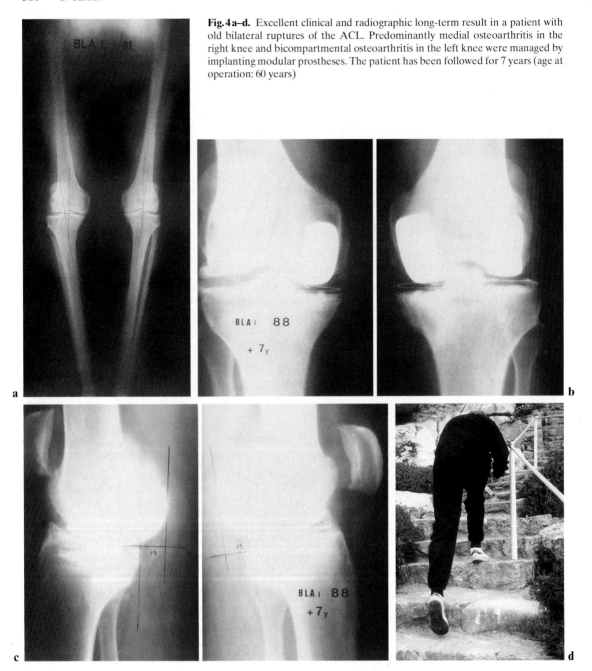

Fig. 4 a–d. Excellent clinical and radiographic long-term result in a patient with old bilateral ruptures of the ACL. Predominantly medial osteoarthritis in the right knee and bicompartmental osteoarthritis in the left knee were managed by implanting modular prostheses. The patient has been followed for 7 years (age at operation: 60 years)

femorotibial, medial, or lateral degenerative arthritis associated with a straight tibia.

Pagoda-Like Deformity of the Tibial Plateau (Fig. 3)

This heavy erosion of substance from the tibial plateau invariably leads to failure of an over- or undercorrected osteotomy. Unicompartmental arthroplasty is the only appropriate treatment.

Anteroposterior Subluxation (Figs. 4–6)

This instability is demonstrated by weight-bearing radiographs of the fully extended knee. Standard lateral projections of the slightly flexed knee with the patient in a supine position are unsatisfactory for demonstrating this femorotibial anteroposterior subluxation. A proximal tibial osteotomy in these cases cannot halt the progresson of femorotibial subluxation and leads to:

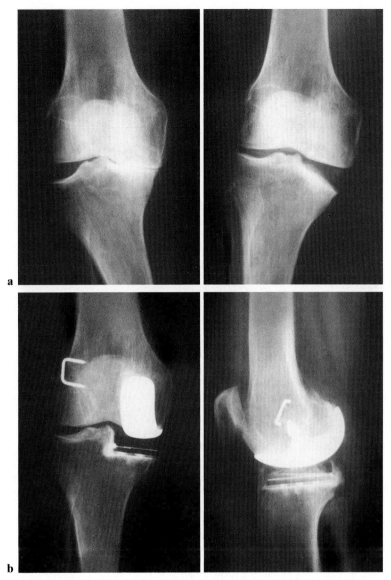

Fig. 5 a,b. Long-term results of a unicompartmental arthroplasty combined with a Lemaire lateral extraarticular reconstruction for severe medial osteoarthritis in an ACL-deficient knee with a persistent pivot shift that necessitated the lateral repair. A proximal tibial osteotomy would not have produced adequate equilibration of ligamentous and bony stability due to the pronounced medial bone loss. Intentionally, the knee was not overcorrected to 3°–4° of valgus. *Under*correction is the guiding principle of unicompartmental arthroplasty

– An exacerbation of femorotibial osteoarthritis
– Femoropatellar pain and instability

There are 2 types of anteroposterior subluxation (Fig. 7): that associated with anterior osteophytes that displace the tibia posteriorly, and that associated with an oblique, usually medial erosion of the tibial plateau that displaces the tibia forward.

The only way to control the subluxation is by hemiarthroplasty. An intraoperative radiograph in full extension is taken to check the reduction of the subluxation following insertion of the unicompartmental prosthesis.

Flexion Contracture > 15° (Figs. 7, 8)

If the sagittal deformity is corrected by resecting a proximal tibial wedge that is larger anteriorly than posteriorly, this will produce an anterior downslope of the joint line followed by a unicompartmental progression of osteoarthritis.

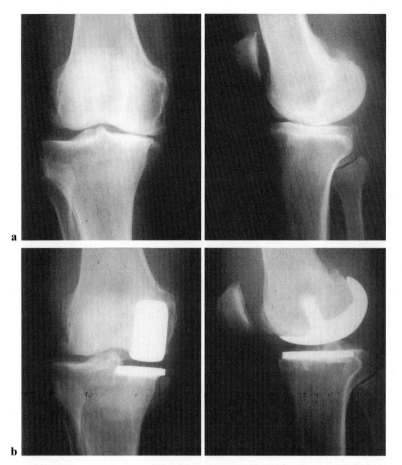

Fig. 6 a,b. Good clinical and radiographic result 2 years after a medial unicompartmental arthroplasty in a woman with varus gonarthrosis secondary to an old ACL rupture. The undercorrection avoids overloading of the lateral compartment, which also shows partial osteoarthritic involvement

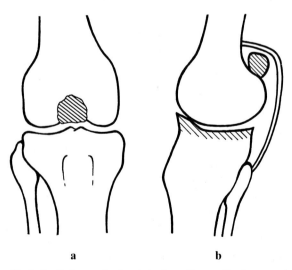

Fig. 7 a,b. Patterns of osteophyte formation on the femur and tibia associated with chronic instability of the ACL

Unlike some authors, we believe that flexion deformity of the osteoarthritic knee is not the result of a posterior capsular contracture, but of bony obstructions on the anterior part of the tibial plateau and within the intercondylar notch, and that this abnormality is frequently pronounced in one compartment. Resection of the obstructing osteophytes and leveling of the joint line by a unicompartmental arthroplasty make it possible to achieve complete or subtotal extension in a large percentage of cases.

Femoropatellar Osteoarthritis

Femoropatellar osteoarthritis does not automatically contraindicate unicompartmental arthroplasty. It is important to distinguish 3 different situations:

– The most common situation is an unfavorable femoropatellar alignment resulting from valgus or

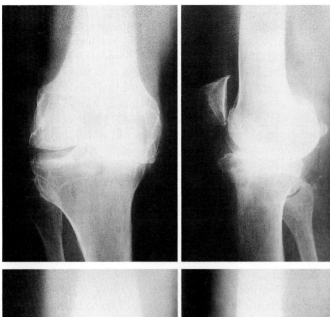

Fig. 8 a–c. Excellent 4-year clinical and radiographic result in a patient with predominantly medial osteoarthritis and flexion contracture following an old ACL rupture, managed by unicompartmental arthroplasty with a Marmor prosthesis

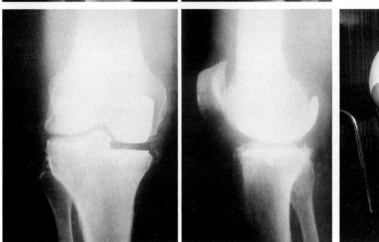

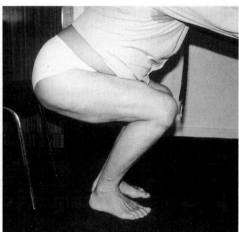

varus deviation of the tibia. Generally the pain is dramatically improved by correcting the alignment of the knee joint.

- Faulty femoropatellar alignment necessitates soft-tissue surgical measures and occasionally transposition of the tibial tuberosity. A concomitant proximal tibial osteotomy can yield good results in these cases.
- Finally, severe femoropatellar osteoarthritis may necessitate a patellar prosthesis with an artificial trochlear surface combined with unicompartmental arthroplasty in order to restore normal knee anatomy.

Forms of ACL Insufficiency

Three etiologies are of importance. The first is a slow progressive rupture in the setting of an evolving degenerative process. In these cases the slow rate of progression permits a stabilizing adaptation of the knee joint with retraction of peripheral soft-tissue structures (capsule, ligaments) and no clinical signs of instability. The anterior drawer sign, Lachman sign, and pivot-shift test are negative or trace positive. At operation the ACL is found to be absent, and the intercondylar notch is filled with bone. The cartilage of the contralateral compartment is usually still intact except for a narrow strip of cartilage erosion (on the medial aspect of the lateral condyle in genu varum, on the lateral aspect of the medial condyle in genu valgum), which should be debrided during unicompartmental arthroplasty.

The second form is true post-traumatic ACL insufficiency, usually preceded years earlier by a severe knee sprain followed by recurrent bouts of instability. The patients are typically young, and many have had one or more meniscectomies and have undergone intra- or extraarticular cruciate reconstructions. Absence of the ACL is noted at operation, but the intercondylar notch is not obliterated by bone. The opposite compartment frequently exhibits chondropathic changes; fortunately these are relatively mild in most cases, making it possible to perform a unicompartmental arthroplasty with axial undercorrection, provided the tibial curvature is physiologic. The anterior drawer, Lachman, and pivot-shift tests are positive.

The third form is ACL laxity relating to the erosion of bone. This etiology merits greater attention, because surgeons who have not mastered unicompartmental arthroplasty may otherwise perform an unnecessary total joint replacement. Arthrotomy reveals a slender, lax cruciate ligament that is constricted by intercondylar osteophytes, but whose laxness is also caused by bone loss in one compartment. This may be overlooked by a cursory intraoperative inspection. Indeed, such a ligament may retain good quality and tension following anatomic reorientation (notch plasty), transverse resection of the eroded area, and resurfacing of the tibial plateau by a unicompartmental arthroplasty. Thus, rather than make a superficial assessment of ACL instability in the face of severe osteoarthritis, the surgeon should exhaust the possibilities of a conservative resection and arthroplasty that could preserve or restore cruciate ligament function. It should be remembered that, in contrast to rheumatoid arthritis, the histologic and biomechanical quality of the ACL in osteoarthritis is generally satisfactory.

Case Material and Results

Our latest series of arthroplasties with the Marmor prosthesis, in use since 1974, for which follow-up data are available included several patients with severe osteoarthritis coexisting with ACL insufficiency who underwent a unicompartmental arthroplasty. When the patients were reexamined in 1986, we used radiographs and surgical notes to identify the cases with absence of the ACL and were able to confirm that favorable long-term results could be achieved (see Fig. 4). Unfortunately, there is no reliable randomized study that takes into account the factor of cruciate ligament instability.

One technical point should be noted: the need to place the tibial component of the arthroplasty back from the anterior cortex to avoid upward tilting of the artificial plateau. Initially this problem was not related to absence of the ACL. Since 1984 we have used the new MOD III prosthesis and have also made more detailed notes on the status of the joint as seen at operation, recording all changes including the condition of the cruciate ligaments. In a series of 100 unicompartmental arthroplasties in which the MOD II prosthesis was inserted medially (91 cases) or laterally (9 cases) for grade IV osteoarthritis, the ACL was found to be normal in 82 cases, lax in 6 cases, and absent in 12. Of the 18 patients with a lax or absent ACL, 16 had an excellent or very good result at 2–4 years' follow-up, and 2 had a satisfactory result (1 patella baja, 1 case with prior hemiplegia and quadriceps insufficiency) unrelated to the ACL deficiency. Radiographic follow-up confirmed this favorable impression, showing no cases of deterioration relative to the intraoperative or immediate postoperative instability. The study confirms that, when certain technical aspects are taken into account, absence of the central pivot does not compromise the success of a unicompartmental arthroplasty.

Technical Problems in Unicompartmental Arthroplasty When the ACL is Absent

Except in cases where the ACL is merely lax and its function (tension) can be restored by removing obstructing osteophytes and restoring the joint line to a normal level, absence of the ACL necessitates technical precautionary measures that are essential to a successful clinical and radiographic outcome.

A perfectly horizontal tibial resection is of prime importance. Any joint-line obliquity on the sagittal plane will promote the progressive subluxation of an unconstrained unicompartmental prosthesis. A precise resection is ensured by using a cutting guide placed against the front of the tibia (Fig. 9).

Next, it is important to establish perfect congruity between the anterior edges of the condylar and tibial components in full extension so that the condylar component is flush with the tibial component or projects slightly past it anteriorly. In the ACL-deficient knee, this requires placing the tibial component in a somewhat more posterior position. If the trial prosthesis is placed anteriorly, its front edge will have a tendency to tilt upward like a ducks' beak. As soon as the component is moved posteriorly by several millimeters, or perhaps as much as 1 cm, this phenome-

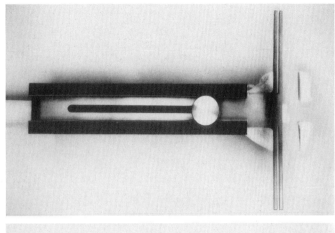

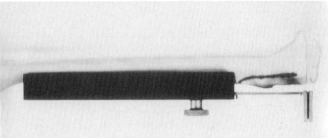

Fig. 9 a,b. Pretibial cutting guide allows for a precise horizontal resection in the frontal and sagittal planes

non disappears, and the components will be properly congruent when the knee is extended.

We attribute this to the fact that the new position corresponds to the "corrected Lachman position" within the arthroplasty. It is easily understood that the problem of nonrecognition leads relatively often to unfavorable results which actually are due to absence of the ACL, compounded by an excessive posterior downslope of the tibial osteotomy or by placing the condylar component farther posteriorly than usual to avoid patellar problems. Once the trial tibial component has been ideally positioned, a reference mark is placed at the level of the intercondylar eminence, and the definitive prosthesis is inserted. If the tibial component projects past the posterior cortex due to the small anteroposterior diameter of the tibial plateau, the patient must be cautioned later to avoid a full squatting position if at all possible. After

the components have been inserted, the pivot-shift maneuver is attempted. If a pivot shift is elicited in an older patient, he or she should be followed at regular intervals. In younger patients, we routinely perform a Lemaire reconstruction 6–8 weeks later (Fig. 5).

Conclusions

Insufficiency of the central pivot is not a contraindication to proximal tibial osteotomy or unicompartmental arthroplasty, although special attention must be paid to the implantation technique and the condition of the cartilage in the opposite compartment. The stability noted at the end of the operation may warrant a secondary procedure in younger, active patients, depending on their age and activity level.

Complications
of Anterior Cruciate Ligament
Reconstruction

Intra- and Postoperative Complications

H.-U. Stäubli and R. P. Jakob

Typical complications may arise during and after reconstruction of the anterior cruciate ligament (ACL). We distinguish errors of operating technique from complications that arise during the course of healing. In this article we shall discuss several technical pitfalls, identify their causes, and recommend steps and measures for avoiding these complications.

Complications during ACL Reconstruction

Problems of Bone Tunnel Placement

Tibial Bone Tunnel

Frontal plane: If the tibial bone tunnel is placed *too far medially*, there may be encroachment of the cruciate ligament graft into the articular cartilage of the medial tibial plateau (Fig. 1 a). This can damage the articular surface of the medial tibial plateau or cause the graft to impinge against the medial femoral condyle or posterior cruciate ligament (PCL), with risk of secondary insufficiency. If the tunnel is placed *too far laterally* in relation to the tibial geometric area of attachment, the graft will impinge against the intercondylar surface of the lateral femoral condyle. The restraining action of the graft to anterior subluxation can be compromised by repetitive microtrauma during rotation. Unremoved osteophytes along the osteochondral junction of the intercondylar wall of the lateral condyle can damage the graft through a shearing effect.

Sagittal plane: If the transtibial tunnel is placed *too far anteriorly*, the following complications may arise:

– Damage to the transverse ligament that interconnects the anterior horns of the menisci, or damage to the anterior horn of the medial meniscus
– Anterior graft impingement with secondary loss of extension, graft hypertrophy, and difficult rehabilitation
– Chronic microtraumatization of the cruciate graft at the anterior rim of the intercondylar roof with secondary graft insufficiency

Placing the tibial tunnel *too far posteriorly* results in inadequate graft length, which can lead to limitation of motion, depending on the femoral tunnel placement, or to inadequate restraint with secondary insufficiency (Fig. 2).

Femoral Bone Tunnel

If the transfemoral tunnel is placed *too far medially*, as it generally is in the one-tunnel technique (Good et al. 1987), the resultant graft function will be anisometric or anisotonic, and the graft will give inadequate restraint to anterolateral subluxation. If the femoral tunnel is in continuity with the superomedial third of the intercondylar notch, reaming by the outside-in technique can cause iatrogenic damage to the PCL or portions of it including its synovial investment. Besides an iatrogenic PCL lesion, this can lead to fraying of the graft as it is pulled through the joint. Occasionally the anterior meniscofemoral ligament (of Humphry) is damaged by placing the graft too far medially.

If the femoral tunnel is *too far lateral*, it generally will be anisotopic on the sagittal plane as well. Placing the tunnel *too far anteriorly* leads to an alteration of graft length and tension that may exceed the maximum physiologic elongation of 13%–15% depending on the isometric zone (Fig. 3 a). The result is restricted motion or graft loosening. The monopodal weight-bearing radiograph documents residual anterior laxity, while stress films allow for quantitation of residual compartmental displacements following reconstruction of the ACL (Fig. 3 b). Placing the femoral tunnel *too far posteriorly* can lead to posterior tunnel fracture if the knee is inadequately flexed during reaming. With part of the posterior tunnel wall missing, it is difficult to fix the bone block in the femoral tunnel so that it will be stable on motion and partial weight bearing. Primary fixation is inadequate, and isometry is not ensured (Sidles et al. 1988; Hefzy et al. 1989; Graf 1987). If the femoral tunnel is too large, too anterior, and too lateral (Fig. 4 a), the residual sagittal laxity (Fig. 4 b) may be accompanied

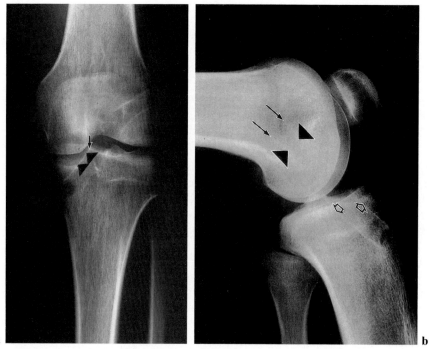

a   b

Fig. 1. a The tibial bone tunnel was placed too far medially. The patient experienced recurrent giving-way episodes 1 year after the intraarticular reconstruction. Radiographs show that the tibial tunnel is too far medial (*arrowheads*), causing partial destruction of the tibial articular cartilage (*arrow*). **b** Here the outlet of the femoral bone tunnel (*arrowheads*) is too high and too anterior. The tibial bone tunnel (*open arrows*) is slightly too posterior on the sagittal plane

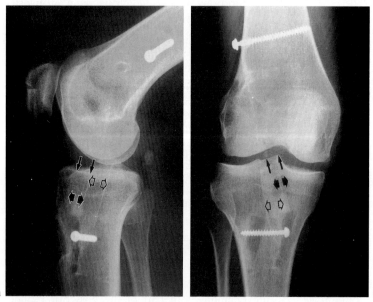

a   b

Fig. 2. a The tibial bone tunnel was placed too far posteriorly (*open arrows*) for an open ACL reconstruction using the central third of the patellar tendon. Five years later the patient had significant secondary instability with an incarcerated peripheral bucket-handle tear of the medial meniscus. The meniscal tear was repaired arthroscopically, followed by transarthroscopic reconstruction of the ACL with correct placement of the tibial tunnel (*solid arrows*) on the sagittal plane. **b** Initial (*open arrows*) and transarthroscopic (*solid arrows*) tibial bone tunnel, which opens in the anteromedial portion of the tibial attachment area

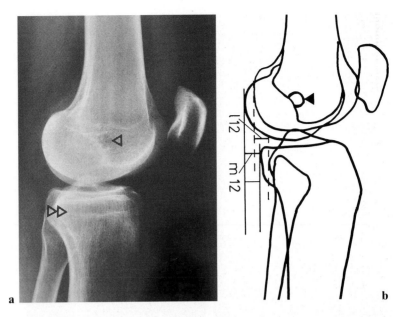

Fig. 3. a Lateral view of the knee shows that the femoral attachment (*arrowhead*) is too far anterior, leading to residual anterior laxity (*double arrowhead*). **b** Anterior drawer stressradiograph after anisotopic reconstruction documents residual anterior translations of 12 mm with an anisotopic femoral attachment (*solid arrowhead*)

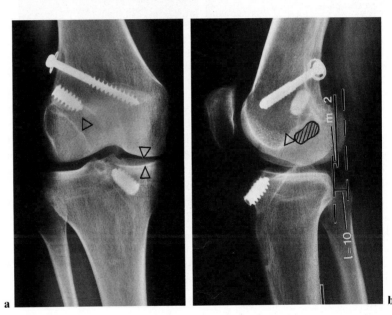

Fig. 4a,b. The femoral attachment is too lateral (*open arrowhead*) and too anterior. The monopodal weight-bearing film shows a combined anterior residual laxity of 10 mm for the lateral compartment and 2 mm for the medial compartment

by varus laxity (Fig. 5a) with unphysiologic compression of the medial compartment. The articular cartilage of the lateral compartment generally remains intact (Fig. 5b).

Faulty bone tunnel placement can be avoided by carefully planning the location and orientation of the tunnel openings prior to operation. Standard radiographic views are excellent for determining the positions of the tunnel inlets and outlets and thus defining the course of the graft. They enable the surgeon to adapt the femoral and tibial attachment sites to the 3-dimensional relationships of the individual knee joint

(Graf 1987). The ideal site for the intraarticular opening of the tibial tunnel is in the anteromedial portion of the tibial attachment area; the corresponding most isometric femoral attachment site is in the area where the anteromedial bundle attaches to the intercondylar aspect of the lateral femoral condyle (Hefzy et al. 1989).

In arthroscopic reconstructions of the ACL, correct placement of the tibial attachment generally presents no difficulties when the extensor apparatus is centered. In an open reconstruction through a medial approach, the patella generally is subluxated laterally to

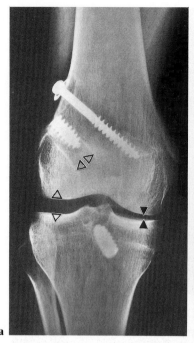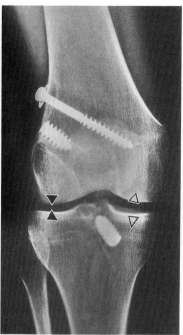

a   b

Fig. 5. a Residual varus laxity in the right knee with medial compression (*solid arrowheads*) and lateral distraction (*open arrowheads*) due to excessive lateral and anterior placement of the intercondylar outlet of the femoral tunnel (*small double arrowheads*). **b** Valgus stress film

obtain a better view of the intercondylar notch. This maneuver in the ACL-deficient knee leads to anteromedial subluxation and lateral translation of the tibia through traction on the patellar tendon, making correct placement of the tibial outlet difficult. Thus, the graft placement should be checked arthroscopically or visually in full extension with a reduced extensor apparatus and with maximum internal and external rotation of the tibia.

Before definitive reaming, the geometry of the femoral attachment can be checked by observing the position of the Kirschner guidewires using an image intensifier with a cross-table projection.

Complications of an Anisometric or Anisotopic Primary Repair of the ACL

An ACL repair using transcondylar pullout wire and primary fascia lata augmentation that is anisotopic on the frontal and sagittal planes (Fig. 6 a,b) can lead to varus decoaptation (Fig. 6 c) with an intact lateral compartment (Fig. 6 d), combined anterolateral (Fig. 6 e) and posterior residual laxity (Fig. 6 f), or to breakage of the reattachment wire (Fig. 6 g).

In the case illustrated, the medial submeniscal metallic foreign body had to be removed transarthroscopically. Nine years after the primary repair there was persistent, symptomatic knee instability with marked narrowing of the intercondylar notch by ectopic ossification about the anisotopic reattachment site. The anisotopic repair necessitated early manipulation under anesthesia to mobilize the knee. As a result, patella infera (Fig. 6 i) was apparent 20 months after the primary repair in comparison with the normal opposite side (Fig. 6 h).

Complications Involving the Graft Donor Site

Patella Baja and Ectopic Ossifications

Varying degrees of patellar descent (patella baja, patella infera) may develop following removal of the central one-third of the patellar tendon (Figs. 6 g, 7). It is still uncertain whether this relates to the technique of defect closure, scar contracture of the residual tendon, scarring of the infrapatellar fat pad, or a dystrophic factor in association with constitutional factors. A beak-like excrescence at the distal pole of the patella and foci of heterotopic ossification along the graft donor bed are commonly observed after reconstructions using the central third of the patellar tendon. Due to metaplasia, ectopic ossification in the cruciate ligament graft may be observed after reconstructions of the ACL and PCL.

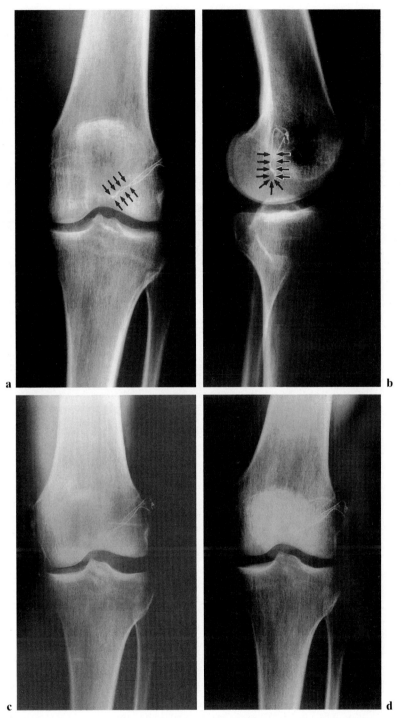

Fig. 6a–d. Nine years after an anisotopic transfemoral ACL repair and augmentation with a fascia lata strip. **a, b** The transcondylar reattachment site is too low and anterior (*arrows*). Monopodal weight-bearing films in the AP and lateral projections.

c, d Varus decoaptation (varus stress test) with an intact articular cartilage surface in the lateral compartment (valgus stress test). **e–i** see p. 594

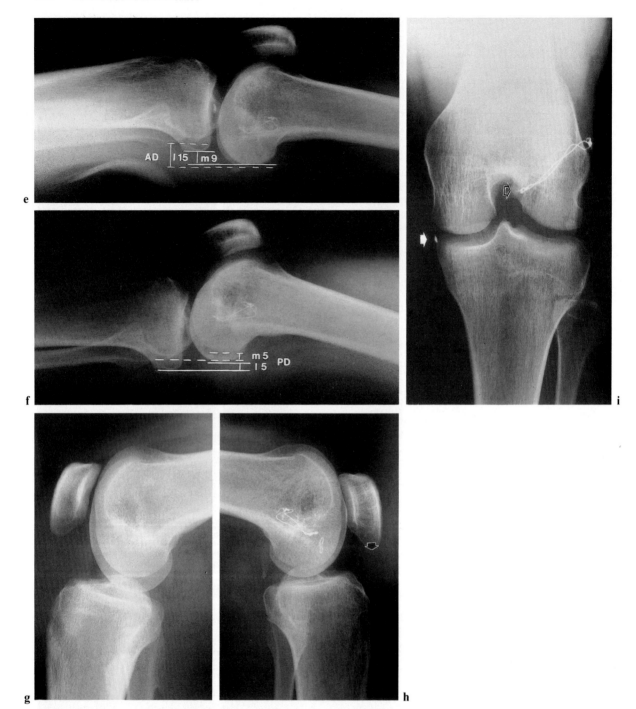

Fig. 6 e–i. Stressradiographs under anesthesia. **e** Residual anterolateral subluxation with anterior displacement (*AD*) of 9 mm medially and 15 mm laterally. **f** Residual posterior displacement (*PD*) of 5 mm on each side. *Broken line*, lateral compartment; *solid line*, medial compartment. **g** Narrowing of the intercondylar notch with sites of heterotopic ossification (*open arrow*), medial submeniscal fragment of the broken ligament repair wire (*white arrow*). **h** Normal patellar position. **i** Patella infera (*arrow*) 2 years after an anisotopic transfemoral repair

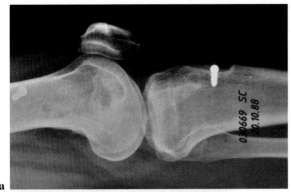

a

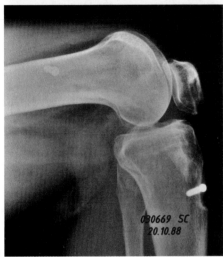

b

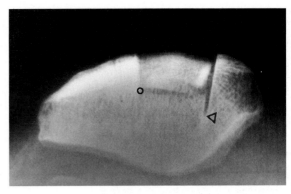

Fig. 8. If the surgeon cuts too deeply into the patella when harvesting the bone block (*arrowhead*), a longitudinal fissure fracture can occur. Rounding the ends of the bone block (*circle*) reduces stress concentration at those sites

◁

Fig. 7. a Patella baja in extension. Arthrofibrosis and low-riding patella after harvesting of the central third of the patellar tendon and correction of tunnel placement. **b** Patella baja in flexion. A low-riding patella is occasionally observed in both flexion and extension following transfer of the central portion of the patellar tendon

Fracture of the Patella in the Donor Region

If the oscillating saw cuts too deeply during removal of the patellar bone block, it can cause longitudinal fissuring of the patella (Fig. 8). To avoid this complication, we recommend rounding the ends of the bone block with a 2.0-mm drill bit to avoid stress concentration at those sites. Chisels with a conical point that might split the patella should be replaced by flat-tipped chisels. Applying transverse compression across the patella with a bone forceps can help avoid this complication during excision of the bone block. If a fissure fracture of the patella occurs during the procedure, it can be fixed and stabilized with bone sutures, using the anterior galea aponeurotica as an anterior tension band. Care is taken to preserve this structure during the surgical approach and when harvesting the graft. Complete longitudinal fractures are anatomically reduced and stabilized by internal fixation with lag screws (Fig. 9). Bone-graft donor defects can be repaired with cancellous bone plugs obtained during the primary reconstruction. This eliminates areas of bone loss while preventing secondary complications of bone block removal despite early mobilization.

Transverse Patellar Fractures

Three months after undergoing a proximal tibia valgus osteotomy combined with an ACL reconstruction using the quadriceps tendon and a bone block from the base of the patella, one patient fell onto the knee while hiking and sustained a transverse fracture of the patella in the former bone-graft donor bed (Fig. 10) with a complete rupture of the passive auxiliary extensor apparatus. The patellar fracture was stabilized with a wire-loop tension band and transverse lag screw, and the residual anterior defect was repaired by cancellous grafting. The tears in the retinacula and the anterior portion of the iliotibial tract were repaired with sutures.

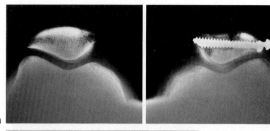

a

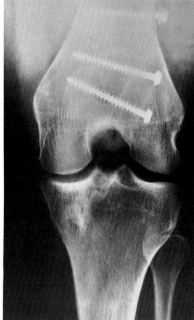

b

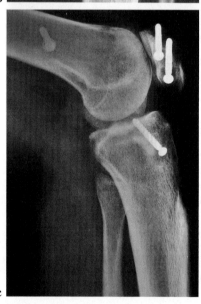

c

Fig. 9 a–c. Cutting the patella too deeply or using conical chisels to harvest the bone block can cause an iatrogenic longitudinal patellar fracture. This can be treated by internal fixation with lag screws and by filling the anterior defect with autologous cancellous bone taken from the tibial or femoral bone tunnel. Additionally, the anterior galea aponeurotica is oversewn to produce an anterior tension-band effect

Rupture of the Patellar Tendon in the Donor Region

Patients with general ligamentous laxity tend to have a narrow patellar tendon, so the removal of a 10-mm-wide graft can significantly weaken the patellar tendon and predispose to secondary rupture. Primary augmentation can be performed by swinging a flap from the prepatellar galea aponeurotica into the donor defect.

Residual Complaints Involving the Donor Site on the Tibial Tuberosity

Sharp edges formed by removal of the bone block from the tibial tuberosity should not be left in an area that is a weight-bearing zone for the patient (test pre-operatively by having the patient kneel and marking the contact area). Fine rasps can be used to smooth the bone edges.

Complications Relating to a Narrow Intercondylar Notch

An adequate notch plasty is recommended to prevent graft impingement against the intercondylar aspect of the lateral femoral condyle and the anterior roof of the intercondylar notch. If the notch is too narrow laterally and superiorly (Fig. 11), round burs, rounded chisels, or arthroplastic shavers are used to enlarge it adequately, i.e., to the original intercondylar notch configuration (see Fig. 11). An excessive reduction osteotomy of the intercondylar portion of the lateral femoral condyle should be avoided as it might further compromise the joint guidance and stability that the bony geometry provides.

Varus Gonarthrosis and Chronic ACL Insufficiency

In patients with unstable postmeniscectomy varus osteoarthritis with narrowing of the medial joint compartment and loss of lateral varus coaptation

▷

Fig. 10. a ACL reconstruction using the quadriceps tendon on a patellar bone block combined with proximal tibial osteotomy. **b** Three months after transarthroscopic ACL replacement and high tibial valgus osteotomy, the patient sustained a transverse fracture and longitudinal fissure of the patella (direct fall onto the knee while walking downhill). **c** Fractures were stabilized by internal fixation with an anterior tension band and sagittal lag screw; postoperative rehabilitation

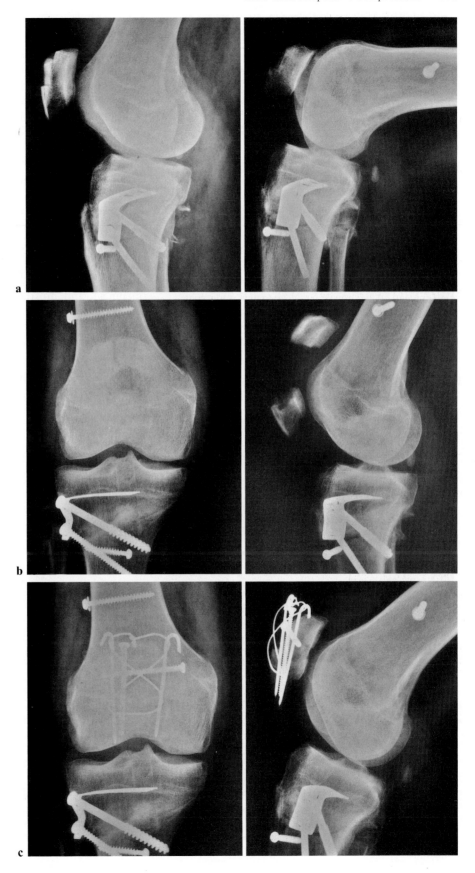

Fig. 10. Legend see p. 596   c

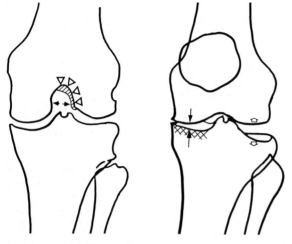

Fig. 11. A narrow intercondylar fossa (*arrows*) should be widened to its original intercondylar configuration (*arrowheads*)

Fig. 12 *(right).* With unstable postmeniscectomy varus gonarthrosis and lateral joint-space widening, a proximal tibial valgus osteotomy should be performed in addition to intraarticular ACL reconstruction and tightening of the arcuate complex to avoid secondary graft distention. A possible alternative is a medial open-wedge upper tibial osteotomy with bone graft insertion

(Fig. 12), the recommended procedure is a proximal tibial valgus osteotomy combined with an adequate notch plasty, transarthroscopic reconstruction of the ACL, and tightening of the arcuate complex. This avoids the gradual secondary graft elongation that commonly occurs in these joints while reducing the pressure and shear loads on the medial compartment.

Complications of Prosthetic Cruciate Reconstruction

The following complications have been described following prosthetic reconstruction of the ACL:

– *Biomechanical damage.* This type of damage includes loss of graft tension due to creep, the generation of wear debris at bony edges (e.g., tunnel openings), and prosthesis rupture with residual subluxation (Fig. 13).
– *Biochemical damage.* The activation of synovial cells by particulate wear debris leads to an increased production of cartilage-damaging proteinases. This "synthetic arthritis" is characterized by

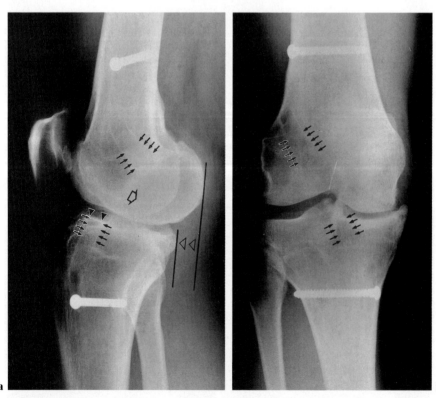

Fig. 13. a Rupture of a prosthetic cruciate ligament. The tibial tunnel is anisotopic and placed too far anteriorly (*small solid arrowheads*); the femoral tunnel is likewise placed too far anteriorly (*small arrows*). Anterior roof osteophyte (*open arrow*), significant anterior subluxation (*open arrowheads*). **b** Postmeniscectomy varus gonarthrosis with a ruptured cruciate ligament prosthesis

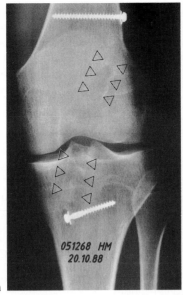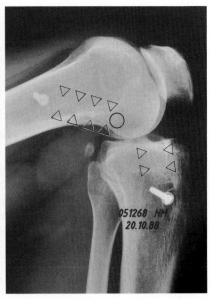

a   b

Fig. 14 a, b. Anatomically sound, isometric ACL reconstruction in the AP (**a**) and lateral (**b**) projections. Placement of the tibial tunnel in the anteromedial portion of the tibial attachment site, of the femoral tunnel in the anteromedial portion of the femo- ral attachment site high on the intercondylar aspect of the lateral femoral condyle, and adequate primary graft fixation are the conditions necessary for an early start of functional rehabilitation

recurrent effusions and local heat due to reactive synovitis. Hypertrophic synovial villi and foreign-body giant cell granulomas are noted in biopsy material. Kang et al. (1989) have shown that microparticles from various synthetic ligaments significantly increase the activity of collagenases, gelatinase, and stromalysin under in vitro and in vivo conditions. These neutral proteinases can break down the structural components of articular cartilage. The same proteinases have been detected in patients with chronic destructive arthritis. Wear debris from synthetic ligaments thus provides a human model for iatrogenically induced arthritis.

– *Chemical damage.* Cases of chemical arthritis with secondary arthrofibrosis have been incited by the fixatives (glutaraldehyde) present in bovine allograft materials.

– *Structural damage to cartilage and bone.* In time, biomechanical and biochemical damage to the three compartments of the knee joint leads to cartilage damage and eventual bone damage at the subchondral level. The Gigli-saw effect of too-rigid implants can cause local cartilage destruction. The removal of a prosthesis inserted through bone tunnels generally results in bony channel defects that involve portions of the physiologic cruciate ligament attachment sites on the tibia or femur.

Reconstruction Options with a Ruptured ACL Prosthesis

Treatment begins with transarthroscopic synovectomy and copious joint lavage. After removal of the failed prosthesis, the anisotopic bone tunnels are curetted and widened with cutting bits of appropriate diameter and then filled in with size-matched autologous bone plugs or bone replacement material (tricalcium phosphate). After the synthetic tricompartmental synovitis has subsided and the bone plugs have consolidated at the isometric sites, an arthroscopic or open autologous reconstruction is performed.

Septic Arthritis with a Prosthetic Ligament in Place

After copious arthroscopic joint lavage and synovectomy, the prosthesis is removed, and the tunnels are curetted and drained. Infected bone tunnels are drilled out to healthy bone with a cannulated reamer, followed by the insertion of a suction-irrigation drain or repetitive arthroscopic joint lavage. After inflammatory signs have subsided, the defects are repaired with autologous bone plugs.

When an early infection develops, the chondronocive effect can occasionally be controlled by repeated arthroscopic irrigations and synovectomy following removal of the prosthesis and all wear debris.

A late infection with arthrofibrosis and septation of the joint space by adhesions is generally managed by an open synovectomy with joint debridement and curettage of the bone tunnels after the foreign material has been removed.

Factors That Lower the Complication Rate

A knowledge of anatomy, three-dimensional preoperative planning based on an individual analysis of standard radiographic views, intraoperative check of Kirschner wire placement before definitive reaming of the bone tunnels, appropriate graft selection and preparation, atraumatic intraarticular positioning of the graft, isometric graft placement, stable primary fixation, and early rehabilitation can reduce the incidence of intra- and postoperative complications. An awareness of the possible complications permits an early recognition of risk factors. Reconstructive procedures that are too technically complex and poorly reproducible should be rejected in favor of simple reconstructive techniques with predictable donor pathology. Intraoperative or postoperative arthroscopic scrutiny, supplemented by radiography, can be helpful in reducing immediate and longer-term complications. Dystrophies and infections should be diagnosed as early as possible and appropriately treated. A reconstruction that closely approximates the anatomy and isometry of the natural ACL (Fig. 14) permits early, goal-oriented functional rehabilitation of the operated knee. Frequent follow-up visits and personal guidance of the patient will help to avoid the complications described above. Perioperative arthroscopy has a major diagnostic and interventional role in the early detection and treatment of primary or secondary complications.

References

Good L, Odensten M, Gillquist J (1987) Precision in reconstruction of the anterior cruciate ligament. Acta Orthop Scand 58: 658–661

Graf B (1987) Isometric placement of substituts for the anterior cruciate ligament. In: Jackson DW, Drez D (eds) The anterior cruciate deficient knee. St. Louis Washington/DC Toronto, pp 102–113

Hefzy MS, Grood ES, Noyes FR (1989) Factors affecting the region of most isometric femoral attachments Part II: The anterior cruciate ligament. Am J Sports Med 17: 208–216

Kang J, Fu FH, Oeson E, Evans C (1989) The biochemical response to artificial wear particles in-vitro and their histological response in-vivo. 6th Congress of the International society of the knee, Rome, 8–12th May 1989

Marshall DM (1989) Patella baja. An uncommon but important cause of anterior knee pain. 6th Congres of the International society of the knee, Rome, 8–12th May 1989

Sidles JA, Larson RV, Garbin JL, Matsen FA (1988): Ligament length relationships in the knee. University of Washington

Stäubli H-U (1988) Preoperative planning to determine anatomic attachment areas in anterior cruciate ligament reconstruction. ACL study group conference, Snowmass, Aspen/CO, March 19–26th, pp 37–38

Role of Arthroscopy in the Diagnosis and Treatment of Complications of ACL Reconstruction

A. Gächter

Arthroscopy is very helpful for evaluating the postoperative course following reconstruction of the anterior cruciate ligament (ACL). It is particularly useful for establishing the cause of a chronic synovitis and for evaluating graft insufficiency, traumatic or "pseudotraumatic" graft rupture, secondary cartilage lesions, meniscal pathology, and secondary ligament deficiencies. The rare cases of infection following ACL reconstruction are another good indication for arthroscopic evaluation as well as therapeutic arthroscopic irrigation.

Chronic Synovitis

Chronic synovitis following an operative procedure in the knee can have various causes. The extraarticular causes include muscular insufficiency. Poor muscular guidance (especially of patellar tracking) can induce secondary chondromalacia, and laxness of the capsule can create a vacuum effect inside the joint leading to recurrent effusions. Other causes that merit investigation are cartilage lesions that incite a "chondrodetritic synovitis" and meniscal lesions, which can provoke effusion through mechanical irritation. Incarcerated portions of the graft are another potential cause of effusion. At arthroscopy, the effusion can be removed by arthroscopic irrigation, and concomitant procedures can be done to remove lesions that perpetuate the synovitis (e.g., meniscectomy, resection of frayed graft sites, etc.).

Graft Insufficiency

There can be many reasons for postoperative ligament insufficiency. Some increase in laxity is to be expected during the first 6–8 months after an autologous ACL reconstruction. Swelling of the graft and the remodeling processes associated with graft revascularization can lead to elongation of the central pivot. With passage of time, the graft will usually regain some of its lost tension.

Another potential cause of graft insufficiency is stretching of the substitute ligament by increased knee flexion. This can occur only in grafts that have been placed in a nonisometric position, however. An additional cause is inadequate fixation of the graft ends.

Graft Rupture

Graft ruptures can have exactly the same presentation as an acutely torn cruciate ligament, including the same mechanism of injury, posttraumatic hemarthrosis, and the arthroscopic picture of torn, tangled fiber bundles. Thus, graft ruptures can occur in response to adequate trauma to the knee. In other cases a very minor trauma can cause graft rupture if the central pivot has been excessively loaded due to insufficiency of the secondary restraints.

Over a period of years the graft may undergo degenerative changes in the form of chondrification, ossification, or mucoid-cystic change. Arthroscopy is useful for assessing the quality and position of the graft. It can also assess possible varus-valgus instability by demonstrating increased joint-space opening on the medial or lateral side. Recurrent hemarthrosis should direct suspicion toward graft insufficiency, as tearing of the synovial sheath can be a source of recurrent bleeding.

Cartilage Lesions

The traumatic mechanism causing rupture of the ACL generally damages the articular cartilage as well. The proximal femoropatellar cartilage is the most common site of involvement. An external rotation-valgus injury, for example, can additionally cause lateral subluxation of the patella (or in some cases complete dislocation). Arthroscopy can demonstrate cartilage impaction at that site shortly after the injury. Often this type of lesion can significantly complicate the postoperative course and prolong rehabilitation. If there is concomitant destruction in the medial compartment and corresponding angular deformity, a proximal tibial valgus osteotomy is indicated. Radiographic findings alone do not always supply adequate information. The shifting produces transverse chondral fractures on the lateral femoral condyle that can spread to produce complete cartilage defects.

The intercondylar notch may become progressively narrowed as a result of osteoarthritis. Typically an osteophyte forms at the border of the intercondylar notch, usually on the femoral side, which constricts the notch and may have a sharp edge that can wear through the graft. Motorized instruments can be used to trim the edge back until it no longer interferes with graft motion.

Meniscal Lesions

Acute locking of the knee joint is not uncommon following cruciate ligament reconstructions. The most frequent cause is a bucket-handle tear of the medial or lateral meniscus. Continued shifting usually causes damage to the lateral meniscus (with associated transverse chondral fractures on the lateral femoral condyle). An initially small posterior horn tear of the medial or lateral meniscus can in time spread anteriorly, resulting in a complete, incarcerated bucket handle tear. It needs to be determined in these cases whether a meniscus repair is feasible. Smaller flap tears are best managed by arthroscopic resection of the tag.

Ligament Insufficiency

A functional evaluation of the knee joint under arthroscopic control is excellent for the assessment of ligament deficiencies on both the medial and lateral sides. Usually it can be determined whether the insufficiency is more meniscotibial or meniscofemoral. Particular attention must be given to the (rare) complete proximal detachment of the long and superficial structures of the medial collateral ligament: Because the proximal ligament attachment blends with the adductor tendon, stability is good in the extended knee but decreases markedly with flexion as the whole ligament-tendon complex slips posteriorly over the condyle.

Infection

Although infections are rare in the wake of ACL reconstructions, arthroscopic irrigation should be performed whenever an infection is suspected. This irrigation, repeated as necessary and combined with systemic antibiotics, will cure the infection without synovectomy in the majority of cases. Also, the clearing of hemarthrosis by postoperative irrigation can eliminate a good culture medium for infectious organisms. Arthroscopic irrigation is also very beneficial for chondrodetritic synovitis and synovitis incited by synthetic wear debris (cruciate ligament prosthesis).

Graft Hypertrophy

It is a fairly recent discovery that a great many extension deficits following ACL reconstructions do not develop because they are "necessary for stability" but result from massive scarring and thickening of the graft. An increasingly painful extension loss occurring between 4 and 8 months postoperatively is characteristic of graft hypertrophy. It is usually found to be due to incorrect positioning of the implant. If the graft is attached too far anteriorly on the tibia, it will impinge against the roof of the intercondylar notch, inciting the formation of a small hematoma. As the hematoma becomes organized, the graft thickens further and sustains even greater trauma from notch impingement. This can give rise to a grotesque, tense, spherical intraarticular mass that occasionally may fill the intercondylar notch, causing severe limitation of motion. For this reason extension should never be forced during the initial postoperative months, since experience has shown that forced extension exercise or dynamic splintage exacerbates the degree of hypertrophy. Histologic examination reveals hyperplastic scar tissue, so it would be more accurate to speak of graft *hyperplasia* than hypertrophy. The pain elicited by forced extension is localized mainly to the infrapatellar fat pad or popliteal fossa. We can explain the popliteal pain by noting that, during forced extension, the hyperplastic mass in the intercondylar fossa lifts the femoral condyle from the tibial plateau, thereby stretching pain receptors in the posterior capsule. This is especially common when the ACL has been replaced by a vascularized graft based on the infrapatellar fat pad.

The recommended treatment is debulking of the hyperplastic graft by arthroscopic shaving. This may be combined with an arthroscopic notch plasty as re-

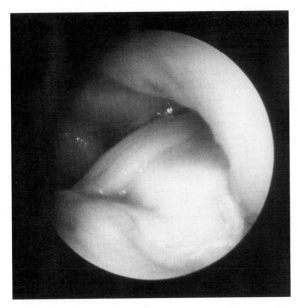

Fig. 1. Arthroscopic view of an insufficient graft 2 years after operation. The fiber bundles are elongated and indurated. The insufficiency is not very pronounced

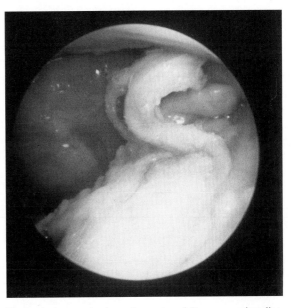

Fig. 2. Arthroscopic view of a ruptured Dacron cruciate ligament graft. The individual bundles tend to tear at different levels. The small light reflections are from synthetic particles that have become embedded in the synovium

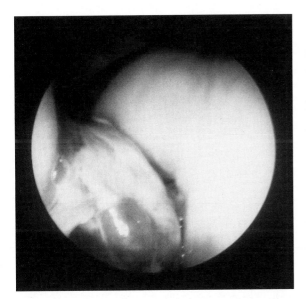

Fig. 3. Graft hyperplasia following a patellar tendon reconstruction of the ACL. The femur and intercondylar notch are visible at the top of the image, the graft below; in between is the hyperplastic mass with sites of fresh internal hemorrhage. Symptoms are pain and limitation of extension

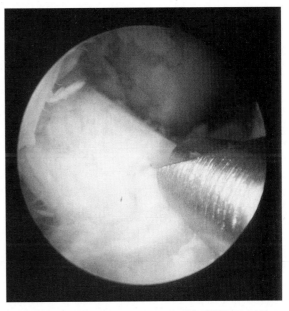

Fig. 4. The hyperplastic tissue can be removed with a shaver. The line of demarcation between the mass and the actual graft is easily identified. This arthroscopic procedure should restore a full range of knee extension

quired. In rare cases the graft must be moved to a different attachment site on the tibial plateau.

In summary, while arthroscopic follow-up of ACL reconstructions is technically demanding (visualization, adhesions, evaluation, etc.), it contributes greatly to the early detection of complications and, when properly interpreted, can improve the operative techniques that are applied. Arthroscopy is particularly rewarding in the assessment and treatment of postreconstruction infection and graft hypertrophy.

References

Gächter A (1988) Die Bedeutung der Arthroskopie beim Pyarthros Hefte Unfallheilkd 200: 132–136

Gächter A (1989) Arthroskopische Spülung zur Behandlung infizierter Gelenke. Operat Orthop Traumatol 1: 196–199

Gächter A, Kohler D (1988) Transplantathypertrophie – eine wichtige Indikation für arthroskopische Kontrollen nach vorderer Kreuzbandplastik. In: Beck E (Hrsg) Arthroskopie bei Instabilität des Kniegelenkes. Fortschritte in der Arthroskopie, Bd 4. Enke, Stuttgart, S 104–109

Rehabilitation and Evaluation

Aspects of Rehabilitation
in the Anterior Cruciate Ligament-Deficient Knee

C. Gerber

Rehabilitative measures and equipment are subjects of intense debate as they apply to the prophylaxis and treatment of anterior cruciate ligament (ACL) lesions. In this article we shall explore the role of rehabilitative methods in the prevention, treatment, and postoperative reconditioning of these injuries.

Prophylaxis

Perfect rehabilitation and optimum coordination training are believed to have a prophylactic effect with regard to ligamentous knee injuries. While this preventive effect is likely to occur in uninjured patients, it has been only sparsely documented.

Prophylaxis

Knee injuries, especially when sports-related, are based on trauma mechanisms that are common in the given sport and explain why the same types of injury tend to recur. In a 1969 study of knee injuries at the West Point Military Academy, it was found that 80% of the knee injuries sustained by cadets were second or third injuries. This led to the institution of a screening program for newly enrolled cadets. If asymmetry of the thigh muscles was noted, the cadet was placed on a rehabilitation program, and participation in the contact sport was not allowed until symmetrical muscular development had been achieved. This measure significantly reduced both the incidence and severity of knee injuries among cadets (Abbott 1969). In 1971 Callahan conducted a study in 61,000 New York high school students. The likelihood of a 2nd or 3rd football knee injury in this population was 15 to 17 times higher than that of an initial knee injury. In these students as well, the incidence of injuries was significantly reduced by rehabilitation.

Although no conclusive studies have been done on the optimum mode of rehabilitation, there is no question that a perfect muscular status in a previously injured patient has prophylactic value in the prevention of further knee injuries.

Prophylactic Braces

A variety of prophylactic knee braces are currently used for the prevention of knee injuries, especially in the United States. Contrary to expectations, however, there is no good evidence that prophylactic bracing has been able to lower the incidence of these injuries. Indeed, the foremost studies indicate an increased rate of injuries associated with prophylactic knee bracing among collegiate football players. In summary, we must conclude from available studies (Garrick and Regna 1987; Hewson et al. 1986; Rovere et al. 1987; Teitz et al. 1987) that knee bracing has no value as a prophylactic measure.

Therapeutic Rehabilitation of the ACL-Deficient Knee

The functional disability associated with an anatomically confirmed ACL insufficiency varies greatly among different patients. Some patients have practically no disability and can participate in sports, while others may experience multiple painful subluxation episodes daily, with rapidly ensuing meniscal lesions and degenerative joint changes.

The first conservative therapeutic measure to be considered is activity modification. Often the patient can no longer participate in contact sports at a competitive level. If the patient is satisfied with a reduced activity level, or if he or she changes to a sport that puts little stress on the ACL (alpine skiing, cycling), it is often unnecessary to treat the condition further. If the patient is unwilling to accept activity modification, more specific treatment must be instituted.

Braces

We have shown (Gerber et al. 1983) that the manually tested AP translation in a knee with a ruptured ACL can be reduced by approximately one-half with a Lenox-Hill brace (Fig. 1). Clinical studies (Colville et al. 1986; Coughlin et al. 1987) have shown that the pivot-shift phenomenon is not completely suppressed. Neither can bracing normalize the kinematics of an unstable knee joint. Nevertheless, many patients report improvement in subjective stability, thus accounting for the subjective clinical success of this treatment method in patients who are willing to wear a brace.

Muscular Training

ACL insufficiency leads to selective quadriceps muscle atrophy and, within the quadriceps apparatus, to selective atrophy of the vastus medialis (Gerber et al. 1985). This correlates with a relative weakness of the knee extensors in patients with persistent ACL insufficiency (Arvidson et al. 1981). Solomonow et al. (1987) showed that loading of the ACL stimulates a direct reflex activation of the hamstrings with a concomitant inactivation of the quadriceps. Thus, even at the reflex level, the hamstrings appear to perform a protective function for the ACL. In at least one clinical experiment (Walla et al. 1985), optimum hamstring utilization was apparently able to compensate for subjective instability, at least to a degree.

An unstable knee displays an abnormal motion pattern (Gerber et al. 1983) in which the joint is subjected to stresses it is not designed to withstand. Although it may be possible to improve subjective instability by muscular training, we reject rehabilitation with the aim of returning the patient to vigorous sport without operative treatment. If a rehabilitation program were coupled with activity modification, however, we would favor such an approach. Hamstring training is paramount in cases of ACL instability, where there is no rationale for systematic quadriceps conditioning.

Postoperative Rehabilitation

Postoperative rehabilitation after ACL reconstruction is intended to restore the condition not just of the lower extremity but also of the injured patient as rapidly and completely as possible. Postoperative immobilization, practiced routinely in former years,

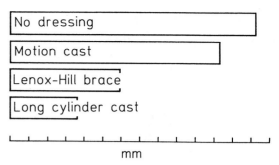

Fig. 1. Manually tested AP displacement of the knee in various protective dressings (n = 8)

leads to changes in the articular cartilage, capsuloligamentous structures, and the periarticular muscles. These changes are clearly deleterious and have been described fully in other publications (Gerber et al. 1980). The AO group (Association for the Study of Internal Fixation) has always advocated the early postoperative mobilization of joints, and the work of Salter et al. (1980) in particular has lent scientific support to this concept as it applies to lesions of the articular cartilage. If some degree of immobilization must be accepted, then attention must be given to the biomechanical principles that influence the rehabilitation of ACL lesions.

Biomechanical Principles

A variety of theoretical (Morrison 1969) and experimental studies have shown in essence that the quadriceps is a powerful antagonist of the ACL, especially near extension. The calculated forces that develop in the ACL, posterior cruciate ligament (PCL), medial and lateral collateral ligaments, quadriceps, hamstrings, and gastrocnemius muscles are summarized in Table 1. These findings are consistent with the experimental data of Henning et al. (1985) (Fig. 2), who found that downhill walking and quadriceps contraction near extension imposed large tensile stresses on the ACL, whereas crutch walking, cycling, and jumping rope placed virtually no stress on the ACL. Arms et al. (1984) confirmed the antagonistic role of the quadriceps mechanism and showed that quadriceps contraction up to 45° of flexion caused significant loading of the ACL. This antagonistic effect is accentuated by a varus or internal rotation stress on the lower leg. Building on these experiments, Renström et al. (1986) showed that the potentially harmful effect of the quadriceps is not abolished by simultaneous contraction of the hamstrings. During muscular training, the farther distally

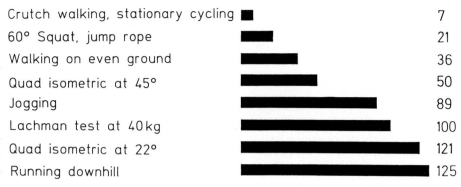

Crutch walking, stationary cycling	7
60° Squat, jump rope	21
Walking on even ground	36
Quad isometric at 45°	50
Jogging	89
Lachman test at 40 kg	100
Quad isometric at 22°	121
Running downhill	125

Fig. 2. Relative tensile loading of the ACL in vivo (40-kg Lachman test equals 100%). (After Henning et al. 1982)

Table 1. Calculated maximum stresses (after Morrison 1969)

Mean calculated maximum force (kg)

Activity	Anterior cruciate ligament	Posterior cruciate ligament	Medial collateral ligament	Lateral collateral ligament	Quadriceps	Hamstrings	Gastrocnemius
Walking on even ground	17	36	8	22	87	140	119
Walking up a ramp	7	65	7	71	80	109	152
Walking down a ramp	45	27	8	28	195	86	–
Climbing stairs	3	123	4	70	196	80	36
Descending stairs	10	46	8	36	172	40	70

a resistance is exerted on the tibia, the greater the degree of displacement of the tibia on the femur during quadriceps contraction (Jurist and Otis 1985).

The key biomechanical discoveries relating to the rehabilitation of ACL lesions can be summarized as follows: The ACL becomes increasingly tense with progressive extension, whether passive or active. The quadriceps is an antagonist of the ACL, and extreme quadriceps tension not only can rupture a healthy ACL but can also stretch or tear a reconstructed ACL during quadriceps training in the slightly flexed knee. Hamstring contraction can protect the ACL, but not with concomitant innervation of the extensor group.

Biological Considerations

Healing processes in ACL grafts are discussed elsewhere in this volume. Here we shall note only that the most commonly used patellar tendon grafts do not achieve the strength of the normal ACL even by 1 year after operation (Fig. 3) (Paulos et al. 1981). The healing of various ACL substitutes calls for different levels of aggressiveness in rehabilitation. Prosthetic substitutes may be regarded as primarily stable.

Certain extraarticular stabilizations are not significantly jeopardized by rehabilitation, but intraarticular biologic grafts are distensible during the revascularization period and cannot tolerate large mechanical loads.

Until a few years ago, ACL reconstructions were routinely immobilized in a plaster cast for 6–8 weeks. Under the influence of Burri et al. (1971), mobile casts and braces were introduced that restricted joint motion, especially near terminal extension, while still permitting an arc of motion that would not endanger

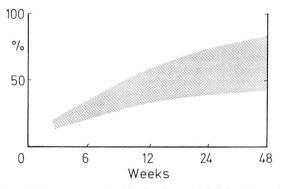

Fig. 3. Rupture strength of healing ligaments in laboratory animals. (After Paulos et al. 1981)

the ACL. Skyhar et al. (1985) startled the orthopedic community by reporting that continuous passive motion tended to compromise rather than promote the nutrition of the ACL, while Burks et al. (1984) showed that continuous motion in the early postoperative period could lead to the loosening or failure of certain types of ACL reconstruction. These experimental concerns have been qualified, however, by clinical experience in prospective studies (Noyes et al. 1987; Sandberg et al. 1987) showing unquestionably that early postoperative mobilization does not compromise postoperative stability. In our own randomized prospective study of 42 patients who underwent ACL reconstructions, we found no difference in stability between knees that had been immobilized and those that had been functionally mobilized. On the other hand, a complete range of motion was recovered earlier in patients who received functional therapy, and muscular atrophy was less pronounced (Fig. 4). While immobilization in a long cylinder cast affects the degree of atrophy, the form of immobilization does not alter the distribution of fiber types: the slow Type 1 fibers in the vastus lateralis muscle become less numerous postoperatively and then normalize again by approximately 6 months. The relative decrease in Type 1 fibers during the first 9 postoperative weeks is offset mainly by an increase in 2b fibers (Fig. 5). Contrary to expectations, our studies showed no decrease in femoropatellar complaints or incidence of osteoarthritis when a functional rehabilitation program was followed.

In summary, the deleterious effect of joint immobilization is well documented in experimental studies, but it is less well established clinically. Available clinical evidence indicates that rigid immobilization does not significantly improve the final stability achieved after a reconstruction. Also, given the low patient acceptance of casting, we do not believe that a rationale exists today for the routine use of rigid cast immobilization after surgery.

Postoperative Electrotherapy

Some studies appear to show that transcutaneous electrical stimulation can reduce postoperative pain and muscular atrophy (Eriksson et al. 1981; Morrissey et al. 1985), while other studies have been unable to demonstrate such an effect (Sisk et al. 1987). More recent investigations show that the therapeutic effect is dependent on the voltage (Wong 1986) and current frequency (Kramer 1987) that are employed. But even the latter study was unable to show a significant advantage over maximum active contractions based

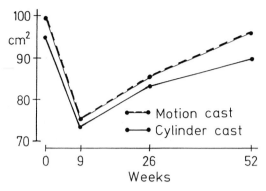

Fig. 4. Effect of immobilization on the cross-sectional area of the distal thigh muscle (n = 42)

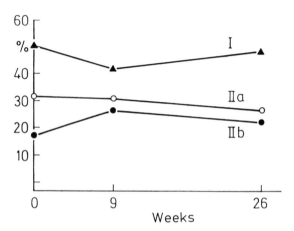

Fig. 5. Postoperative course of fiber-type distribution in the vastus lateralis muscle (n = 28)

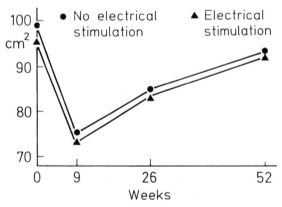

Fig. 6. Effect of electrical stimulation (8-s contraction; 11,000 Hz, 3×30 min/day) on cross-sectional area of distal thigh muscle (n = 28)

on isokinetic measurements. We are currently completing a study in 28 patients that has shown no significant beneficial effect of electrical stimulation in reducing muscle atrophy or altering the distribution of muscle fiber types (Fig. 6).

In summary, there is still no definitive evidence to support or refute the value of electrical stimulation. Available data are inadequate, however, to justify the routine use of this modality. Our own results have caused us to view electrical stimulation with skepticism.

The major questions about rehabilitation today relate to the form of postoperative immobilization and the value of electrostimulation. The importance of mobilization for the rapid restoration of mobility is undisputed; other benefits of early mobilization have been documented experimentally but not clinically, at least in the long term. It does not appear that muscular training is significantly enhanced by electrical stimulation. Rehabilitation and rehabilitation research have helped to prove the unsoundness of earlier concepts such as forced quadriceps training. On the other hand, an optimized rehabilitation program apparently is unable to compensate for a mediocre operating technique. In this sense rehabilitation should again be viewed essentially as a supplement to optimum surgical treatment. The concept of replacing appropriate surgery by an ambitious rehabilitation is no longer tenable.

References

Abbott HG (1969) Reconditioning in the prevention of knee injuries. Arch Phys Med Rehabil 50: 326–333

Arms SW, Pope MH, Johnson RJ, Fischer RA, Arvidsson I, Eriksson E (1964) The biomechanics of anterior cruciate ligament rehabilitation and reconstruction. Am J Sports Med 12: 8–18

Arvidsson I, Eriksson E, Häggmark T, Johnson RJ (1981) Isokinetic thigh muscle strength after ligament reconstruction of the knee joint: Results from a 5–10 year follow-up after reconstructions of the anterior cruciate ligament in the knee joint. Int J Sports Med 2: 7–11

Burks R, Daniel D, Losse G (1984) The effect of continuous passive motion on anterior cruciate ligament reconstruction stability. Am J Sports Med 12: 323–327

Burri C (1971) Funktionelle Behandlung nach Bandnaht und Plastik am Kniegelenk. Langenbecks Arch Klin Chir [Suppl 112]

Callahan WT (1971) A statewide study designed to determine methods of reducing injury in interscholastic football competition by equipment modification. New York State, Public High School Athletic Association, Albany

Colville MR, Lee CL, Ciullo JV (1986) The Lenox Hill brace. An evaluation of effectiveness in treating knee instability. Am J Sports Med 14: 257–261

Coughlin L, Oliver J, Berretta G (1987) Knee bracing and an-

terolateral rotatory instability. Am J Sports Med 15: 161–163

Eriksson E, Häggmark T, Kiessling KH, Karlsson J (1981) Effect of electrical stimulation on human skeletal muscle. Int J Sports Med 2: 18–22

Garrick JG, Requa RK (1987) Prophylactic knee bracing. Am J Sports Med 15: 471–476

Gerber C, Matter P (1983) Biomechanical analysis of the knee after rupture and repair of the anterior cruciate ligament. J Bone Joint Surg [Br] 65: 391–399

Gerber C, Matter P, Chrisman OD, Langhans M (1980) Funktionelle Rehabilitation nach komplexen Knieverletzungen. Wissenschaftliche Grundlagen und Praxis. Schweiz Sportmed 28: 37–56

Gerber C, Jakob RP, Ganz R (1983) Observations concerning the limited mobilisation cast after anterior cruciate ligament surgery. Arch Orthop Trauma Surg 101: 291–296

Gerber C, Hoppeler H, Claassen H, Robotti G, Zehnder R, Jakob RP (1985) The lower-extremity musculature in chronic symptomatic instability of the anterior cruciate ligament. J Bone Joint Surg [Am] 67: 1034–1043

Henning CA, Lynch MA, Glick KA (1985) An in vivo strain gauge study of elongation of the anterior cruciate ligament. Am J Sports Med 13: 22–26

Hewson GF, Mendini RA, Wang JB (1986) Prophylactic knee bracing in college football. Am J Sports Med 14: 262–266

Jurist KA, Otis JC (1985) Anteroposterior tibiofemoral displacements during isometric extension efforts. The roles of external load and knee flexion angle. Am J Sports Med 13: 254–258

Kramer JF (1987) Effect of electrical stimulation current frequencies on isometric knee extension torque. Phys Ther 67: 31–38

Morrison JB (1969) Function of the knee joint in various activities. Biomed Eng: 573–580

Morrissey MC, Brewster CE, Shields CL, Brown M (1985) The effects of electrical stimulation on the quadriceps during postoperative knee immobilization. Am J Sports Med 13: 40–45

Noyes FR, Mangine RE, Barber S (1987) Early knee motion after open and arthroscopic anterior cruciate ligament reconstruction. Am J Sports Med 15: 149–160

Paulos L, Noyes FR, Grood E, Butler DL (1981) Knee rehabilitation after anterior cruciate ligament reconstruction and repair. Am J Sports Med 9: 140–149

Renström P, Arms SW, Stanwyck TS, Johnson RJ, Pope MH (1986) Strain within the anterior cruciate ligament during hamstring and quadriceps activity. Am J Sports Med 14: 83–87

Rovere GD, Haupt HA, Yates CS (1987) Prophylactic knee bracing in college football. Am J Sports Med 15: 111–116

Salter RB, Simmons DF, Malcolm EB, Rumble EZ, McMichael D, Clements ND (1980) The biological effects of continuous passive motion on the healing of full thickness defects in articular cartilage. J Bone Joint Surg [Am] 62: 1232–1251

Sandberg R, Nilsson B, Westlin N (1987) Hinged cast after knee ligament surgery. Am J Sports Med 15: 270–274

Sisk TD, Stralka SW, Deering MB, Griffin JW (1987) Effect of electrical stimulation on quadriceps strength after reconstructive surgery of the anterior cruciate ligament. Am J Sports Med 15: 215–220

Skyhar MJ, Danzig LA, Hargens AR, Akeson WH (1985)

612   C. Gerber

Nutrition of the anterior cruciate ligament. Effects of continuous passive motion. Am J Sports Med 13: 415–418

Solomonow M, Baratta R, Zhou BH, Shoji H, Bose W, Beck C, D'Ambrosia R (1987) The synergistic action of the anterior cruciate ligament and thigh muscles in maintaining joint stability. Am J Sports Med 15: 207–213

Teitz CC, Hermanson BK, Kronmal RA, Diehr PH (1987) Evaluation of the use of brances to prevent injury to the knee in collegiate football players. J Bone Joint Surg [Am] 69: 2

Walla DJ, Albright JP, McAuley E, Martin RK, Eldridge V, El-Khoury G (1985) Hamstring control and the unstable anterior cruciate ligament-deficient knee. Am J Sports Med 13: 34–39

Wong RA (1986) High voltage versus low voltage electrical stimulation. Phys Ther 66: 1209–1214

Functional Rehabilitation
after Anterior Cruciate Ligament Reconstruction

B. Fandrey, B. Grünig, and R. P. Jakob

This article on the rehabilitation of patellar-tendon reconstruction of the anterior cruciate ligament (ACL) is intended to guide patients, physical therapists, and physicians in establishing a time frame for regaining motion and returning the patient to activity. The individual constitutional (hyper- or hypomobility) and conditioning status of the patient will determine the pace at which rehabilitation should proceed.

We begin by reviewing some basic principles of biomechanical force transmission in the knee joint and some physiotherapeutic concepts relevant to the postoperative treatment regimen (Arms et al. 1984; Baratta et al. 1984; Biedert and Stauffer 1989; Daniel et al. 1985; Draganich et al. 1987; Egger and Bur 1985; Einsingbach et al. 1988; Frisch 1989; Henning et al. 1985; Paulos et al. 1981, 1987; Solomonov et al. 1987; Steadman and Higgins 1988; see also chapter by Kipfer et al., p. 619 ff.).

Force Transmission in the Knee

Since the quadriceps muscle is an antagonist of the ACL, the biomechanical factor of quadriceps tension has a crucial bearing on all phases of rehabilitation:

0°–40° Flexion

In this range the patella is anterior to the tibia tuberosity in relation to the anterior tibial border, and quadriceps traction across the patella generates an anteriorly directed force (Fig. 1 a).

50°–70° Flexion

The patella and tibial tuberosity are even with the anterior tibial border (Fig. 1 b).

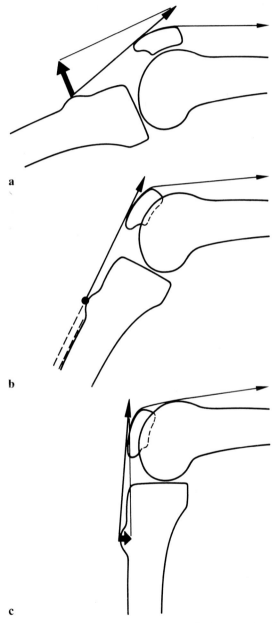

Fig. 1. a The tibia glides anteriorly, the ACL is taut. **b** Quadriceps tension no longer exerts an anteriorly directed force. The ACL is unstressed in this position. **c** The quadriceps cannot exert an anterior pull. Its force vector is directed posteriorly

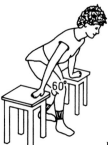

Fig. 2. "Duck standing"

90° Flexion

The patella is behind the tibial tuberosity in relation to the anterior tibial border (Fig. 1 c).

Terminology

Co-Contraction

Co-contraction denotes the simultaneous contraction of the knee flexors (hamstrings) and extensors (quadriceps) for the controlled muscular guidance of the joint at the biomechanically favorable angle of 60°.

"Duck Standing" (Fig. 2)

In the starting position for this exercise the knee is flexed 60° with quadriceps-hamstring co-contraction, the hip is flexed 90°, the back is straight, the center of body gravity is over the knee, and the entire foot is bearing weight. First the patient assumes the position on the right or left foot while bracing himself on side supports, then he stands freely, bearing full weight with the knee flexed 60°.

The load produced by this exercise is favorable for:

– Proprioception in the joint (pressure or tension)
– Innervation of the muscles
– Metabolic processes that counteract osteoporosis (decalcification) of the patella
– Cartilage nutrition
– Strengthening of tendons and ligaments

Duck Walking

The starting position for duck walking is the same as that for duck standing. The object is to covert the static position of the duck stance into locomotion. This places an increased demand on the muscular sta-

bilization of the joint during shifting and braking of the body weight.

Neuromuscular Coordination Training

Here the goal is to train the interaction of the nervous system (reception, transmission, and processing of motor impulses) and muscles (reactive contraction) within a specific, planned motor sequence so that the action can be performed economically, with the lowest possible energy expenditure. By delaying muscular fatigue, coordination is essential for training strength, quickness, and endurance.

Removal of the graft from the patellar tendon, which is exceptionally rich in free nerve endings (pain receptors), creates a structural and neurogenic deficit that significantly impairs proprioception and thus coordination.

Static and Dynamic Muscular Training

Static Training

Static muscular effort relies on isometric muscle contraction and serves to maintain a given body or limb position. Static training mainly improves intramuscular coordination, in which high demands are placed on a precisely adapted innervation and recruitment of individual muscle fibers.

When the patient can perform maximum static contractions without pain, he may progress to the 2nd phase of muscular rehabilitation involving dynamic concentric contractions.

Dynamic Training

The muscular effort in dynamic training may be concentric or eccentric.

– Dynamic concentric (positive dynamic) training: Positive dynamic muscular effort relies on isotonic muscle tension, in which the muscle shortens as its tension increases. The force expended in this type of exercise is greater than the resistance to be overcome. Positive dynamic muscle training mainly improves intermuscular coordination.
– Dynamic eccentric (negative dynamic) training: In this type of exercise the muscle lengths as it slowly yields to a resistance (e.g., lowering a weight). Negative dynamic training allows peak stresses higher than those in static and concentric training. Thus, eccentric contractions should always be painless,

since pain signifies overloading of the muscle tissue.

In the early phase of muscular rehabilitation, the emphasis is on the training of innervation and coordination (reversal of motion). The resistance in these exercises should always be matched to the patient's neuromuscular capabilities. Both the static and dynamic (positive/negative) training aspects of duck standing and duck walking utilize the patient's own body weight as the resistance. Depending on the level of muscular control, the resistance can be decreased

by permitting hand and arm support, or it can be increased by imposing greater weight bearing. As rehabilitation progresses, dynamic concentric and eccentric training with an elastic strap (e.g., Medflex, available in 3 resistances; Fig.3) allows for a graded increase of resistance matched to individual neuromuscular capacities. The tensile force exerted by the strap places rigorous demands on the coordination, power, and endurance of a specific muscle group that continue to provide an effective training stimulus even in the late phase of rehabilitation (Fig.4).

Isokinetic Training

For isokinetic contractions, equipment is used to maintain a constant, preset speed of movement during a particular exercise. The mechanical resistance accommodates fully to whatever force is exerted. For each joint position, the concentrically contracting muscle (agonist and antagonist) can develop the corresponding maximum tension at a uniform contraction velocity.

The 4 phases of our rehabilitation program are outlined in Table 1, and Fig.5 shows the postoperative progress sheet that is given to the patient so that he can chart his own progress.

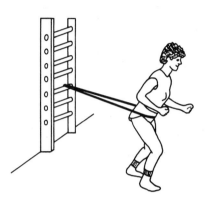

Fig.3. Jogging against the resistance of an elastic strap

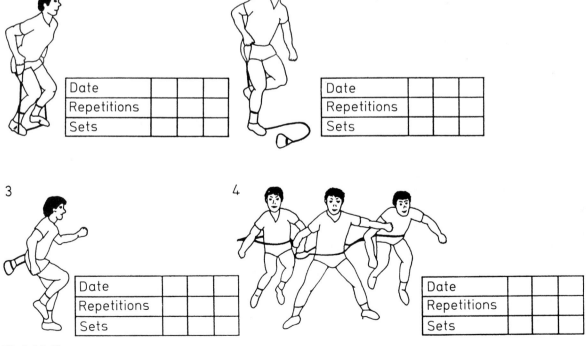

Fig.4. Medflex program

Name of hospital

Date of operation: _____

Operative technique: _____
_____
_____
_____

Name:

Postoperative Progress Sheet

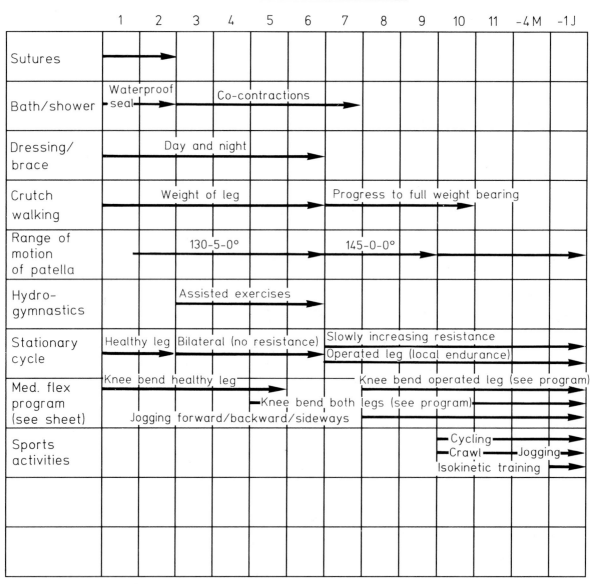

	1	2	3	4	5	6	7	8	9	10	11	-4M	-1J
Sutures	→→→												
Bath/shower	Waterproof seal →		Co-contractions →→										
Dressing/ brace	Day and night →→→												
Crutch walking	Weight of leg →→						Progress to full weight bearing →						
Range of motion of patella	130-5-0° →→						145-0-0° →→			→→→→			
Hydro-gymnastics	Assisted exercises →												
Stationary cycle	Healthy leg →	Bilateral (no resistance) →					Slowly increasing resistance →→						
							Operated leg (local endurance)						
Med. flex program (see sheet)	Knee bend healthy leg →				Knee bend both legs (see program) →		Knee bend operated leg (see program) →→						
							Jogging forward/backward/sideways →						
Sports activities										Cycling →→			
										Crawl → Jogging →			
										Isokinetic training →			

Next visit: _____

Modified for Dr. R. Steadman

Fig. 5. Postoperative progress sheet

Table 1. Rehabilitation program

Phase I	First 6 weeks (1st follow-up visit)		**Phase II**	Weeks 7–10

Phase I — First 6 weeks (1st follow-up visit)

Goals:
Range of motion 120–5–0°
Full patellar mobility
Mastery of co-contractions at 40°–60° flexion
  (with high-riding patella: more flexion):
1. while leg raising against gravity
2. while duck standing (see Fig. 2)
3. while duck walking
Neuromuscular coordination of knee flexors
  and knee extensors, closed kinetic chain

Physical therapy:
Static and dynamic muscular training between
  100°–45° against a low resistance
Hydrogymnastic pool: as soon as the patient can
  raise the leg against gravity while co-contracting
  quadriceps and hamstrings
Goal: coordinated motor guidance
Stationary cycle: if controlled guidance of the limb
  is present
Load: low resistance, pedal with hamstring innervation (no foot straps)
Goals: promote blood flow, improve cartilage
  nutrition, prevent patellar decalcification

Patient:
Partial weight bearing (weight of leg)
Firm elastic bandage day and night
Home program (exercises with elastic strap)

Phase II — Weeks 7–10

Goals:
Range of motion 130–5–0°
Free patellar mobility
Full weight bearing
Neuromuscular coordination of knee flexors
  and extensors with weight bearing

Physical therapy:
Duck walking with increasing extension (-5°)
Strength, endurance, reactive training of quadriceps (especially vastus medialis) from 120° to
  45° with *no* distal resistance
Medflex training at 40°–60° (jogging against
  elastic strap)
Ambulatory training: transition to full weight
  bearing

Patient:
Full weight bearing between weeks 8 and 10
  (depending on individual)
Straight leg raising (-5°) with co-contraction
No muscular effort against resistance from
  45° to 0°
Hydrogymnastic pool and stationary cycle as in
  Phase I
Driving a car: after full weight bearing has been
  achieved
Home program (increase strap program)

Phase III — From week 11 to 4 months

Goals:
Full range of motion to end of Phase III
Free patellar mobility
Well-stretched muscles
Jogging without a limp against elastic strap re-
  sistance (end of Phase III)

Physical therapy:
Note:
During the first 4 months the ACL is undergoing
  revascularization and is relatively weak during
  that period.
Static and dynamic training in extension
End of 4 months:
Light jogging on even ground under supervision
  of physical therapist
Criterion: can jog without a limp against elastic
  strap resistance (forwards/backwards/sideways)
  (see Fig. 3)

Patient:
Cycling on even ground (in lower gears)
Individualized home program

Phase IV — 5 to 12 months

Goal:
Restoration of symmetrical strength to within
  10% (gradual increase)

Physical therapy:
Individualized training for:
– Coordination
– Endurance
– Power
– Muscle length
Supervision by physical therapist

Patient:
Muscular effort against resistance from 45° to 0°
  (increase 5° per week toward full extension)
Patient may engage in sports that do not involve:
– exposure to uncontrolled forces (contact
  sports);
– abrupt stopping or changing of direction;
– rotary maneuvers (cutting, pivoting).
Caution: The rupture strength of the ACL at
  1 year is no more than 50%–80% that of the
  normal ACL.

The physician and physical therapist can modify the sheet according to how the patient is progressing.

Posterior Cruciate Ligament

The treatment regimen must be modified somewhat when posterior instability is present. When the posterior cruciate ligament (PCL) is unstable, rehabilitation is frequently complicated by pain in the overstressed femoropatellar joint. Gravity causes posterior drawing of the tibia, which stresses the reconstructed ligament when the patient sits upright with his feet resting on the floor or lies in the supine position.

Quadriceps strengthening to protect the femoropatellar joint is effectively accomplished by performing concentric and eccentric exercises between 0° and 45° of knee flexion with the patient in the prone or lateral position.

It is difficult to train the vastus lateralis and tensor fasciae latae muscles in their function as knee extensors in the last 30° of extension, and terminal rotation should be avoided if at all possible. The quadriceps and gastrocnemius are stimulated and trained, especially at the start of rehabilitation, to function more effectively as PCL agonists. Based on the tension diagram of the PCL, the hamstrings can be trained between 0° and 45° of flexion. Special emphasis is placed on the medial hamstrings when posterolateral instability is present, because they restrain posterior gliding of the lateral tibial condyle.

When there is damage to the medial collateral ligament, certain functional exercises, such as the valgus-producing breast stroke in swimming, are contraindicated.

References

Arms SW, Pope MH, Johnson RJ, Fischer RA, Arvidsson I, Eriksson E (1984) The biomechanics of anterior cruciate ligament rehabilitation and reconstruction. Am J Sports Med 12 (1): 8-18

Baratta R, Solomonow M, Zhou BH, Letson D, Chuinard R, D'Ambrosia R (1988) Muscular coactivation. The role of the antagonist musculature in maintaining knee stability. Am J Sports Med 16 (2): 113-122

Biedert R, Stauffer E (1989) Proprioceptivity of the knee joint. J Orthop Res (in preparation)

Daniel DM, Malcolm LL, Losse G et al. (1985) Instrumented measurements of anterior laxity of the knee. J Bone Joint Surg [Am] 67: 720-726

Draganich PD, Jaeger RJ, Kralj AR (1987) Coactivation of the hamstrings and quadriceps during extension of the knee. Bone Joint Surg [Am] 71: 1075-1081

Egger JP, Bur M (1985) Krafttraining. Trainer-Bulletin, Schweizer Skiverband

Einsingbach T, Klümper A, Biederman L (1988) Sportphysiotherapie und Rehabilitation. Thieme, Stuttgart New York

Frisch H (1989) Programmierte Untersuchung des Bewegungsapparates, 3. Aufl. Springer, Berlin Heidelberg New York Tokyo

Henning CE, Lynch MA, Glick K (1985) An in vivo strain gage study of elongation of the anterior cruciate ligament. Am J Sports Med 13: 22-26

Paulos LE, Corry Payne III F, Rosenberg TD (1987) Rehabilitation after anterior cruciate ligament surgery. In: Jackson DW, Drez D (eds) The anterior cruciate deficient knee. Mosby, St. Louis Washington/DC Toronto, pp 291-314

Paulos LE, Noyes FR, Grood E, Butler DL (1981) Knee rehabilitation after anterior cruciate ligament reconstruction and repair. Am J Sports Med 9: 140-149

Solomonow M, Baratta R, Zhou BH, Shoji H, Bose W, Beck C, D'Ambrosia R (1987) The synergistic action of the anterior cruciate ligament and thigh muscles in maintaining joint stability. Am J Sports Med 15 (3): 207-213

Steadman JR, Higgins RW (1988) ACL injuries in the elite skiers. In: Feagin JA (ed) The crucial ligaments. Churchill Livingstone, New York Edinburgh London Melbourne, pp 471-482

Isokinetic Testing to Evaluate Quadriceps and Hamstring Strength after a Primary Anterior Cruciate Ligament Repair or Reconstruction

W. C. Kipfer, B. Grünig, P. M. Ballmer, R. Zehnder, and R. P. Jakob

Muscular strength can be quantitatively assessed either by manual testing or by an objective, examiner-independent measuring system (Davies 1984; Scharf and Noack 1987) (Table 1).

The physical force parameters that are measurable in humans occur as a result of the ability of muscles to generate a force. Two basic types of muscular contraction must be differentiated (Table 2).

The advantage of isokinetic force testing is that it can measure the torques that are developed at a constant, preset level of exertion in any angular direction (Davies 1984; Eggli 1987). The speed of the exercise can even be 0°/s (isometric exercise). The resistance provided accommodates completely to the force that is exerted, providing a maximum load with no peak loads throughout the arc of motion. The feeling of an "accommodating resistance" is most closely approximated by moving the limbs under water (Weineck 1986). The data obtained by isometric testing under standardized conditions of positioning and fixation are objective, reproducible, and permit comparisons

with everyday functional movements and with loads specific to a given type of sport.

Cybex II Testing

The Cybex II system consists of a dynamometer, a parallel goniometer, a device for preselecting and maintaining a constant speed of exercise (0–300°/s), and a desktop computer with a two-channel chart recorder.

Cybex measurements furnish information on the current state of training of the tested muscle groups, such as the extensor and flexor muscles of the knee. The data can be displayed as a force-velocity curve, permitting a quantitative and qualitative assessment of the muscular forces that develop in each phase of the movement (Schart and Noack 1987). The results are evaluated on the basis of the force-velocity curves (Fig. 1) and the values determined with the Cybex Data Reduction Computer (CDRC).

The Cybex system permits the following quantities to be determined:

– The *maximum torque* in newton meters (Nm), as a measure of the force that is developed. Normally the static torque (static maximum force) is greater than the dynamic torque (dynamic maximum force) (Weineck 1986). The maximum force that can be developed decreases with increasing angular velocity (Fig. 2) (Thorstensson et al. 1976). The shape of the curve also indicates the angular position of maximum torque and the angular range of the torque deficit (see Fig. 1).

Table 1. Quantitative assessment of muscular strength

Manual methods (subjective)	Mechanical methods (objective)
Girth measurement	Torque measurement by
Visual and palpable findings during muscular contraction	isokinetic testing
Muscle testing (0–5[a])	
Force measurement with spring scale	

[a] Activity levels according to British Medical Research Council

Table 2. Types of muscular contraction

Type of contraction	Muscle length	Resistance	Speed	Measurable force
Isometric	*Constant*	Variable	*Constant* (0°/s)	Static
Eccentric	Lengthened	*Constant*	Variable	
Concentric	Shortened	*Constant*	Variable	} Dynamic
Isokinetic	Shortened	Variable	Constant	

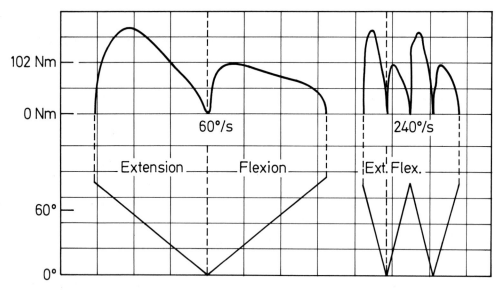

Fig. 1. Development of force (torque) (patient DT 060551, healthy knee)

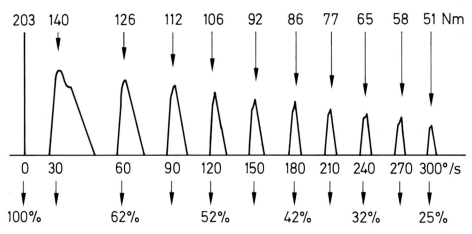

Fig. 2. Torque versus speed of movement

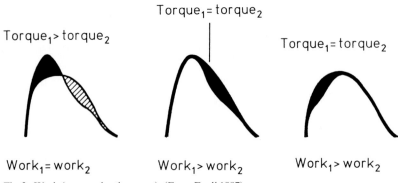

Fig. 3. Work (area under the curve). (From Eggli 1987)

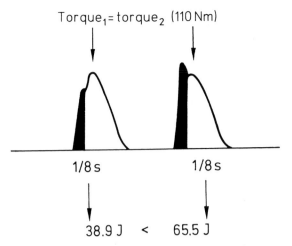

Fig. 4. Torque acceleration energy. (From Eggli 1987)

- *Work* in joules. This represents the area under the curve (integral). As Fig. 3 shows, work is independent of torque and motion amplitude.
- The *torque acceleration energy*, defined as the work (J) performed during the first 0.125 s, furnishes information on the explosiveness of a muscular contraction (Bührle and Schmidt-Steicher 1981). This reflects the ability to increase the expended force at the fastest possible rate (Fig. 4). Acceleration energy is independent of angular velocity.
- The *average power* (W) represents the average muscle work per unit time that is performed during the testing of several repetitions. Muscle power initially increases with angular velocity up to about 180°/s, then slowly declines (Davies 1984). Power analysis gives useful information on the state of training of a subject, especially when the operated and nonoperated sides are compared.

Additional parameters can also be computed:

- The *H/Q ratio*, or the ratio of the maximum force developed by the hamstrings (H) and quadriceps (Q) (agonist and antagonist). In calculating this ratio, the normally stronger extensor force is taken as 100%. Both muscle groups are in a physiologic balance that depends on the individual state of training (Grace et al. 1984; Scharf and Noack 1987; Spring, personal communication). The slightly lower flexor strength is attributable to prestretching of the flexors in the usual test position and to their predominantly postural function (Janda 1979).
- Determination of the *percentage difference between the right and left extremities*, regardless of the subject's state of training, has both clinical and therapeutic significance. A right-left disparity of 10% or less is within normal limits according to Grace et al. (1984) and Wyatt and Edwards (1981).

An accurate analysis of the force curves as a function of test speed is essential (Davies 1984). The curves indicate, for example, the portion of the exercise in which a "depression phenomenon" is observed (Fig. 5). A feeling of instability and pain can significantly reduce force generation at low angular velocities ($\leqslant 60°/s$), for low speeds are associated with relatively long contraction times that enable a high tension to be developed. A "force deficit" can also result from reflex pain inhibition, which usually is confined to a certain angular range (see Fig. 5). Our clinical experience indicates that pain inhibition lessens with increasing angular velocity.

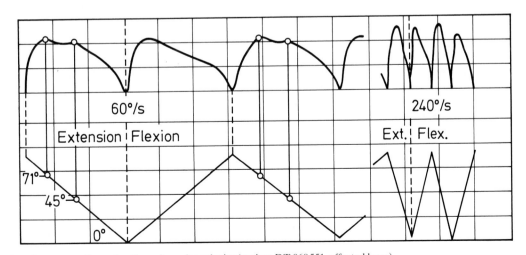

Fig. 5. "Depression phenomenon" as a function of angular velocity (patient DT 060551, affected knee)

Materials and Methods

We performed isokinetic testing as part of the follow-up of 114 patients (38% female) who underwent a primary repair of the anterior cruciate ligament (ACL) (see chapter by Ballmer et al., p. 293 ff.). The patients consisted of both athletically active and inactive individuals; their average age was 33 years. The average interval from operation to follow-up was 5 1/2 years.

The isokinetic tests were performed with a Cybex II dynamometer under standardized conditions: sitting position with the upper body, pelvis, and thigh immobilized. Each test began with a 5-min warmup phase on a stationary cycle. All tests were conducted by the same examiner (B. E. G.). The test protocol consisted of 5 cycles of exercise at an angular velocity of 60°/s and 50 cycles at a velocity of 240°/s. The maximum torque at 60 and 240°/s was investigated for the extensor and flexor muscles in addition to torque acceleration energy, work, and average power measured at 240°/s.

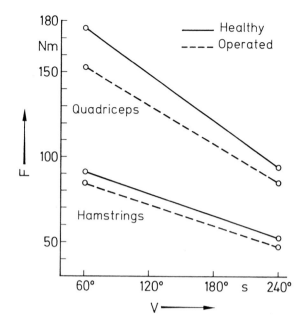

Fig. 6. Force-velocity diagram for the extensors and flexors of the healthy and operated limbs

Results

The *maximum torque* of the extension exercise at the lower test speed occurred at an average angle of 55° for both extremities. Comparing the maximum torque of the quadriceps and hamstrings in the operated leg with the nonoperated leg, we see that the maximum torque deficit of the quadriceps was greater than that of the hamstrings at both test velocities (Table 3).

The *force-velocity diagrams* showed different behaviors in the two muscle groups. They were consistent with the findings of Scharf and Noack (1987). Starting from a higher initial value, the quadriceps curve fell more sharply with increasing velocity than the hamstring curve, and both curves showed a converging trend (Fig. 6).

The *H/Q ratio* at 60°/s was 57% on the operated side and 52% on the nonoperated side. At 240°/s, the value was 56% for both legs.

On *comparing the sides*, we found that 40% of all the patients showed less than a 10% difference between the operated and healthy sides in all the Cybex parameters tested.

There was no direct relationship between the *patients' evaluations* and the Cybex data. Thus, 75% of the patients who rated their knee as "good" showed more than a 10% right-left discrepancy in all the Cybex values.

We also found no direct connection between *athletic activity* and Cybex data. Some 62% of the patients who injured their knee during sports returned to the same type of sport, yet half of them showed more than a 10% right-left discrepancy in each of the Cybex parameters recorded.

In the patients who had *difficulty stair climbing* (14% of our series), we noted a marked force deficit for both the quadriceps and hamstrings at the lower test speed (Table 4).

In patients with *retropatellar pain* and symptomatic crepitation, right-left comparison at a test speed of 60°/s showed a decrease of up to 17% in quadriceps strength on the affected side. The right-left difference in patients with no femoropatellar symptoms averaged less than 10% for both muscle groups.

We also compared the maximum torque at 60°/s with the findings of *clinical stability testing* (Lachman test).

Table 3. Percentage difference between the quadriceps (Q) and hamstrings (H) on the operated and nonoperated sides

Parameters	Velocity			
	60°/s		240°/s	
	Q	H	Q	H
Maximum torque	13%	8%	10%	9%
Average acceleration energy			6%	10%
Work			10%	9%
Average power			7%	7%

Table 4. Difficult stair climbing and maximum torque at a test speed of 60°/s. Percentage difference between the right and left sides

Subjective assessment		Q deficit	H deficit
No problems	98	10%	6%
Going up stairs	4	21%	16%
Going down stairs	6	24%	20%
Going up and down	6	37%	18%
Total	114		

Table 5. Lachman test and maximum torque at a test speed of 60°/s. Percentage difference between the right and left sides

Anterior drawer in 15° flexion	Q deficit	H deficit
0– 3 mm	13%	10%
3– 5 mm	13%	8%
5–10 mm	12%	1%

We found no relationship between the right-left quadriceps differences and clinically detectable instability. In the evaluation of the hamstrings, however, we found that the difference between the healthy and operated sides decreased with increasing instability (Table 5), signifying an increase of flexion strength in the affected extremity.

Discussion

The quantitative measurement of muscle strength is gaining increasing importance in the evaluation of muscular rehabilitation following operative procedures on the musculoskeletal system. Isokinetic testing is advantageous because it can measure effective muscle strength at a functional speed (0°–300°/s) in various joint positions. The reproducible measurements describe the current state of training of the tested muscle groups, and analysis of the data permits the recognition of functional disturbances.

In the knee that has undergone a repair or reconstruction of the ACL, active muscular stabilization is weakened, often for months, as a result of immobilization and disuse. Consequently, muscular protection of the repair or graft is not ensured. This weakness chiefly affects the extensor muscles of the knee. For example, Schart and Noack (1987) found a decrease in maximum quadriceps strength for up to 1 year after capsuloligamentous reconstructions in the knee. In cases with persistent instability, Arvids-

son et al. (1981) and Gerber et al. (1985) were able to demonstrate quadriceps weakness and atrophy even after a period of years. Grace et al. (1984) note, however, that a right-left percentage difference of up to 10% is still within physiologic limits. Goslin and Charteris (1979) additionally found a significant discrepancy between the dominant and nondominant legs. Wyatt and Edwards (1981) supplemented this finding by noting that it was true only for males. In our population, the difference in strength between the quadriceps muscles on the operated and non-operated sides was greater than 10% mainly at a lower angular velocity (60°/s). Contrary to the observations of Arvidsson et al. (1981), we found no increase in the right-left quadriceps difference as a function of clinically demonstrable residual instability. However, we did note an appreciable decrease in the strength difference between the right and left hamstrings with increasing instability, implying a relative increase in flexion strength on the operated side.

This observation can be explained by noting that the hamstrings are agonists of the ACL and thus are subject to increased loading when the ACL is deficient (Giove et al. 1983; Renström et al. 1986). Also, since they function chiefly as postural muscles, they are less prone to atrophy than the medial and lateral portions of the quadriceps (Janda 1979).

We likewise attribute the relatively gradual slope of the force-velocity curve for the hamstrings to the postural maintenance function of this muscle group (Spring 1981).

Maximum torque of the extensors is attained at 60°/s between 50° and 60° of flexion (Thorstensson et al. 1976; Arvidsson et al. 1981; Wyatt and Edwards 1981; Scharf and Noack 1987). With this amount of flexion, quadriceps activity does not yet impose excessive stresses on the ACL (Arms et al. 1984). In this position the ACL is relatively well protected, as tension measurements in the ACL by Renström et al. (1986) confirm. We feel that greater attention should be given to this fact during rehabilitation.

The H/Q ratio of clinically healthy subjects is 55%–60% at angular velocities of 60°/s, an observation also made by Spring (personal communication) in alpine ski racers and by Scharf and Noack (1987) in an athletic population. Wyatt and Edwards (1981) measured H/Q ratios of 72% in the males and 71% in the females of their study population, which numbered 100 subjects. As Spring (personal communication) points out, we should strive to achieve a physiologic balance between the extensors and flexors so that the ACL will have optimum muscular protection from potentially disruptive forces.

Conclusions

Isokinetic testing can be widely utilized for the evaluation of muscular forces, especially since it permits an objective assessment of specific properties of muscle groups. We agree with Arvidsson et al. (1981) that the initial Cybex study after cruciate ligament surgery should be performed shortly before the end of the rehabilitation program, or at least before the resumption of competitive athletics that are stressful to the knee. If the study is performed too early, the healing ACL may be damaged by the forces that develop during the test. The dynamometer can only measure forces, it cannot control them, so the force vectors that act on the ligament cannot be calculated (Paulos et al. 1987).

References

Arms SW, Pope MH, Johnson RJ, Fischer RA, Arvidsson I, Eriksson E (1984) The biomechanics of anterior cruciate ligament rehabilitation and reconstruction. Am J Sports Med 12: 8-18

Arvidsson I, Eriksson E, Häggmark T, Johnson RJ (1981) Isokinetic thigh muscle strength after ligament reconstruction in the knee joint: Results from a 5-10 year follow-up after reconstructions of the anterior cruciate ligament in the knee joint. Int J Sports Med 2: 7-11

Bührle M, Schmidt-Steicher D (1981) Komponenten der Maximal- und Schnellkraft. Sportwissenschaft 11: 11-27

Davies GJ (1984) A compendium of isokinetics in clinical usage. S and S., La Crosse/WI

Eggli D (1987) Maßvolles Training: Einsatz isokinetischer Systeme. In: Ow D, Hüni G (Hrsg) Muskuläre Rehabilitation. Interdisziplinäre Physiotherapie und Rehabilitation 3. Perimed, Erlangen, S 117-124

Eggli D (1987) Maßstab für Kräfte. In: Ow D, Hüni G (Hrsg) Muskuläre Rehabilitation. Interdisziplinäre Physiotherapie und Rehabilitation 3. Perimed, Erlangen, S 86-98

Gerber C, Hoppeler H, Claassen H, Robotti G, Zehnder R, Jakob RP (1985) The lower-extremity musculature in chronic symptomatic instability of the anterior cruciate ligament. J Bone Joint Surg [Am] 67: 1034-1043

Giove TP, Miller SJ, Kent BE, Sanford TL, Garrick JG (1983) Non-operative treatment of the torn anterior cruciate ligament. J Bone Joint Surg [Am] 65: 184-191

Goslin BR, Charteris J (1979) Isokinetic dynamonetry: Normative data for clinical use in lower extremity (knee) cases. Scand J Rehab Med 11: 105-109

Grace TG, Sweetser ER, Nelson MA, Ydens LR, Skipper BJ (1984) Isokinetic muscle imbalance and knee joint injuries. J Bone Joint Surg [Am] 66: 734-740

Janda V (1979) Muskelfunktionsdiagnostik; Muskeltest, Untersuchung verkürzter Muskeln, Untersuchung der Hypermobilität. E. Fischer, Heidelberg

Paulos IE, Payne FC, Rosenberg TD (1987) Rehabilitation after anterior cruciate ligament surgery. In: Jackson DW, Drez D (eds) The anterior cruciate deficient knee. Mosby, St. Louis, pp 241-314

Renström P, Arms SW, Stanwyck TS, Johnson RJ, Pope M-H (1986) Strain within the anterior cruciate ligament during hamstring and quadriceps activity. Am J Sports Med 14: 83-87

Scharf HP, Noack W (1987) Die Bedeutung isokinetischer Kraftmessung in Sport und Rehabilitation. Sportverletzung Sportschaden 3: 142-149

Spring H (1981) Muskelfunktionsdiagnostik nach Janda: Ergebnisse einer Untersuchung an Skifahrern der Nationalmannschaften Schweiz und Lichtenstein. Schweiz Z Sport Med 29: 143-146

Thorstensson A, Grimby G, Karlsson J (1976) Force-velocity relations and fiber composition in human knee extensor muscles. J Appl Physiol 40: 12-16

Weineck J (1986) Sportbiologie. Beiträge zur Sportmedizin 27. Perimed, Erlangen

Wyatt MP, Edwards AM (1981) Comparison of quadriceps and hamstrings torque values during isokinetic exercise. J Orthop Sports Phys Ther 3: 48-56

Concluding Remarks

Rationale and Benefit of Treating Cruciate Ligament Lesions: The Payer's Perspective

E. W. Ramseier

The study by Rubin (1983) focuses on the late outcomes of traumatic knee injuries involving the cruciate ligaments. It is interesting to compare these results from the era of conventional knee surgery with the results of present-day knee traumatology, which were discussed in a recent paper (Ramseier 1987).

Rubin (1983) reports on 467 cases from the period 1972–1974. The great majority of these cases were combined injuries; there were only 45 isolated injuries of the anterior cruciate ligament (ACL) and 10 isolated tears of the posterior cruciate ligament (PCL). Twenty-five percent of all knee injuries involving the cruciate ligaments ended with the awarding of a disability pension from the Swiss Accident Insurance Agency (SUVA). In 2/3 of cases the level of the disability assessment was between 10% and 20%.

The best therapeutic results were achieved in patients with an isolated ACL lesion managed by primary operative treatment; results were significantly poorer in the cases managed nonoperatively. It was found, moreover, that the results of secondary cruciate ligament operations (cruciate reconstructions) were markedly poorer than those of primary operations.

On the whole, an analysis of the knee injuries treated in the early 1970s shows that primary operative treatment and secondary interventions yielded results that were just as unsatisfactory as those of primary conservative treatment with a cast brace.

The only exception to this general rule was isolated tears of the ACL managed by primary surgical repair. In these cases the results were markedly better than with primary nonoperative treatment or a secondary reconstructive procedure. This finding is not statistically significant, however, due to the insufficient case numbers.

These relatively unfavorable results are probably due to an inadequate clinical evaluation and unsatisfactory arthroscopic workup compared with present-day methods. Exploratory arthrotomy was still a frequent practice, and arthroscopy was very rarely performed.

How do these results compare with those achieved in modern knee traumatology? Following preliminary studies by Zollinger and Dietschi (1982), we published a study in 1984 on the late outcomes of cruciate ligament injuries (Ramseier and Zollinger 1984). This additional body of data reveals some interesting trends:

First, we noted a marked rise in the overall incidence of cruciate ligament injuries during the past 14 years (Tables 1, 2).

The percentage of knee injuries sustained in industrial accidents has declined during that period (Table 3). This is probably due in large measure to the tireless efforts of the SUVA to improve occupational safety.

Meanwhile, the percentage of knee injuries sustained in nonindustrial accidents, especially cruciate liga-

Table 1. Cruciate ligament involvement in knee injuries according to SUVA statistics for the period 1970–1983

Year	Knee injuries	Cruciate ligament injuries
1970	12,640	280
1972	13,490	120
1974	15,500	210
1976	13,520	420
1978	13,710	590
1980	15,500	1170
1982	16,020	1620
1983	17,210	1690

Table 2. Cost analysis of cruciate ligament injuries for 1970–1983 (treatment cost index not including daily costs and pensions, total cost based on wage sum index; index 1/1/1970 = 1)

Year	Number	Disability time/case (days)	Treatment cost index/case (SFr.)	Total cost index/case (SFr.)
1970	280	88	1466	12,037
1972	120	125	4074	24,072
1974	210	66	2032	21,637
1976	420	87	3313	17,646
1978	590	86	2649	14,382
1980	1170	89	2583	10,565
1982	1620	99	2826	11,459
1983	1690	102	2727	9,012

Table 3. Proportion of industrial injuries relative to all cruciate ligament injuries in 1970, 1974, and 1982

Year	Total	Industrial
1970	100	20
1974	60	10
1982	280	30

Table 4. Proportion of nonindustrial injuries relative to all cruciate ligament injuries in 1970, 1974, 1979, and 1982

Year	Total	Vehicular	Skiing	Soccer
1970	180	10	30	40
1974	150	50	40	30
1979	630	120	140	170
1982	1340	220	270	510

Table 5. Late results of cruciate ligament injuries for the period 1970–1983

Year	Number	SUVA pensions	Percentage
1970	280	64	23
1972	120	53	44
1974	210	90	43
1976	420	104	25
1978	590	113	19
1980	1170	141	12
1982	1620	186	11
1983	1690	138	8

ment injuries (Table 4), has risen dramatically, with the greatest increases occurring in motor vehicle accidents and especially in sports-related injuries. This has focused much attention on ways to prevent these nonindustrial injuries, a task that in Switzerland has been spearheaded by the Advisory Center for Accident Prevention (BFU). Much has been published in recent years on skiing-related injuries of the lower extremity, where the marked decline in malleolar and tibial fractures owing to improved safety bindings and modern boot designs have been paralleled by a dramatic rise in knee injuries. As our statistics show, however, there have also been marked increases in the incidence of knee injuries sustained in soccer and other types of sport.

There are various reasons behind the tremendous *increase in the diagnosis of cruciate ligament injuries*: One factor is undoubtedly a true rise in the incidence of cruciate ligament injuries based on an increased risk posed by certain types of sport. Another factor is improved diagnostic techniques, which enable physicians to detect many more cruciate ligament injuries than before. Particular progress has been made in clinical evaluation and arthroscopy, while computed tomography has contributed to the diagnosis of acute knee injuries only in highly selected cases. Initial experience with magnetic resonance imaging suggests that MRI will one day provide a safe, noninvasive, highly accurate diagnostic modality, although its costs are still high.

Another noteworthy trend accompanying the marked rise in cruciate ligament injuries has been an equally pronounced *decline in disability rates* following cruciate ligament lesions. This decline has been well above 50% during recent years (Table 5). We can easily attribute this to the significantly better outcomes of modern reconstructive surgery. Also, improved diagnostic techniques provide a more comprehensive view of the injured structures, enabling the surgeon to formulate a more specific and selective plan of treatment. This led us in 1984 to speculate about the future impact of transarthroscopic surgery and the "miniarthrotomy" (Ramseier and Zollinger 1984).

The substantial improvement of therapeutic results, reflected in the marked, steady decline of pension cases, has financial implications as well (see Table 2). In considering financial costs, we must not overlook the fact that we are dealing with the mixed results of various conservative and operative treatment methods. The average disability time ranges from 3 to 4 months and has not increased significantly since 1970.

By contrast, the (inflation-adjusted) medical treatment costs have approximately doubled during the same period to reflect the increased sophistication of procedures in diagnosis, treatment, and rehabilitation. Fortunately, however, the total cost index per case (treatment cost + daily cost + pension) has fallen slightly as a result of improved treatment outcomes.

In summary, improved clinical methods and diagnostic aids for evaluating the injured knee have resulted in the diagnosis of many more cruciate ligament injuries than before, permitting their prompt referral for primary repair or secondary reconstruction with a significant improvement in late outcomes. The higher costs of diagnostic and therapeutic procedures, including costly posttraumatic rehabilitation, are balanced by a marked reduction in disability rates.

References

Ramseier EW (1987) Häufigkeit und Spätresultate von Kreuzbandverletzungen am Kniegelenk. Hefte zur Unfallheilkunde 189: 993–995

Ramseier EW, Zollinger H (1984) Problematik der Knieverletzungen aus der Sicht der SUVA. Helv Chir Acta 51: 499–504

Rubin J (1983) Kreuzbandläsionen. Dissertation, SUVA

Zollinger H, Dietschi C (1982) Kreuzbandläsionen, eine medizinisch-statistische Analyse. Sozial- und Präventivmedizin 27: 33–37

Future Outlook

A. Gächter

Insurers will no doubt provide the impetus for a fundamental change in the operative techniques for replacement of the anterior cruciate ligament (ACL). Accident insurers will no longer be willing to reimburse the costs of protracted rehabilitation and job disability.

As a result, surgeons will be forced to perform a minimally invasive procedure that will require a minimal length of rehabilitation. The benefit of the operation should be maximal not just for the patient but also in terms of reducing the cost to the insurer.

Present-day operative methods can satisfy these requirements only in rare cases, so we must look in new directions. Two approaches are of particular interest in this regard:

The first is the *arthroscopically assisted cruciate ligament reconstruction*. Although this technique is very demanding, it can shorten the rehabilitation time. The drill guides used for the reconstruction must be perfected further so that the procedure will permit an optimum graft placement despite the use of minimal incisions.

An important goal is to determine what implant is best suited for the arthroscopic method. When an autologous patellar tendon strip is used, the procedure is comparable to an open operation, so there are no basic advantages to the arthroscopic technique. American and Japanese surgeons also use patellar tendon allografts, which of course are compatible with minimal incisions. Another option is the pes anserinus, whose tendons can be harvested with a stripper through very small incisions and transplanted under arthroscopic control. This can be done to best advantage, however, only if synthetic materials are used to reinforce the graft. A number of arthroscopically guided procedures are already in use, and little additional progress is anticipated in this area.

The second major approach is the use of *synthetic materials* for cruciate ligament reconstruction. Previously used synthetics have various disadvantages, however. Their resistance to fatigue failure is still so poor that they succomb to wear at an early stage. With most implants, however, the exact time to fatigue failure is not predictable or controllable in

any given case and may range from a few months to several years. There is still hope that a synthetic material can be developed that will satisfy the requirements of biocompatibility while also meeting the most stringent requirements in terms of rupture strength. Much developmental work remains to be done not just on the material itself (e.g., Kevlar) but also on techniques of attachment.

Besides biocompatibility and strength, a synthetic ligament material also must have favorable elastic properties to prevent the occurrence of peak loads during motion that could cause premature wear in certain portions of the joint. A basic rationale for replacement of the ACL is not just to restore stability but also to prevent instability-associated osteoarthritic changes.

Today it is widely agreed that autologous grafts undergo a "crisis period" between about the 3rd and 8th months after implantation. During this time the graft undergoes edematous swelling and seeks to establish an adequate blood supply, which temporarily compromises the viability of the graft. It is known that the stability of the joint deteriorates during this period. This poses a significant mechanical threat to the graft, which may become overloaded, stretched, and deficient. For many years there has been interest in bridging this critical period. One attempt in this direction has been the use of synthetic augmentation devices (e.g., the Kennedy LAD), whose purpose is to protect and support the graft until the latter can acquire a functionally competent structure. Synthetic augmentation devices are still controversial: While it is true that the device absorbs some of the stress that would otherwise act on the reconstructed ligament, there is concern that the device will absorb too much stress and cause excessive "stress shielding" of the biologic graft. Thus, devices of this kind need to be dynamized at the appropriate time, i.e., a greater share of the stress should be transmitted to the graft after a certain interval has passed. This interval varies among different individuals, however, and is not easily identified.

Today there is growing interest in developing *absorbable synthetics* that would gradually dissolve over a period of 6–12 months after implantation. This would provide an effective bridge between the periods of graft protection and graft self-sufficiency while eliminating the need for a second operation to increase load sharing by the graft. Current research is focusing heavily on absorbable synthetic materials. Such an augmentation would permit more vigorous functional rehabilitation, accelerate recovery, and presumably would improve long-term stability.

Attention must continue to be focused on instrumentation. Refinements in this area allow for a more precise conduct of the operating technique while reducing tissue trauma and nerve disruption. Refined instrumentation can bring advantages to open methods that are similar to those in arthroscopically controlled procedures. Special devices are already available for identifying isometric attachment sites, and further improvements are anticipated. Graft tension measurements prior to definitive fixation should help to ensure an optimum placement of the cruciate ligament substitute. Simple spring scales are too inaccurate for this task.

But the major challenge in ACL reconstruction, now and in the future, is not a problem of technique selection but one of patient selection. The question of when to reconstruct is particularly critical in the case of an acute ACL injury. We still lack the crieria needed to furnish an answer. In many cases operative treatment is withheld only to prove necessary later on. But if it were possible to apply specific criteria in the acutely injured patient that would establish whether an ACL reconstruction would eventually become necessary, at least the patient selection problem would be solved. It is already known that certain condylar shapes and certain relationships between the condylar circumference and tibial articular surface either necessitate a cruciate ligament reconstruction or imply that such a procedure is unnecessary. A rupture of the ACL in a patient with general ligamentous laxity is usually a much more urgent indication than in a very muscular patient with tight ligaments.

In the future, we hope that 3-dimensional computer models can be used to identify the patients and patterns of injury for which a cruciate ligament reconstruction is indicated. We would no longer have to wait for patients to develop an incapacitating pivot shift, and adequate operative treatment could be selectively provided while the tear is still fresh. It is also hoped that the apparatus used for instability measurements will one day furnish reproducible results.

One implication of these technical advances is that cruciate ligament reconstruction will become increasingly more technical and complex, so increasingly it will become the province of highly specialized surgeons.

The future holds other possibilities as well, such as the potential use of pharmacologic agents or magnetic fields to control graft remodeling. One day we might even be able to produce a "laboratory" cruciate ligament or introduce a cruciate ligament cell culture into the knee that would grow in vivo into a stable ligament.

Subject Index